ENDOSCOPIC ONCOLOGY

ENDOSCOPIC ONCOLOGY

Gastrointestinal Endoscopy and Cancer Management

Edited by

DOUGLAS O. FAIGEL, MD, FACG, FASGE

Associate Professor of Medicine, Director of Endoscopy
Oregon Health and Science University, Portland, OR

MICHAEL L. KOCHMAN, MD, FACP, FASGE

Professor of Medicine and Surgery, Co-Director Gastrointestinal Oncology,
Hospital of the University of Pennsylvania, Philadelphia, PA

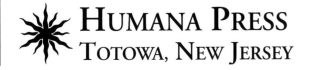

HUMANA PRESS
TOTOWA, NEW JERSEY

© 2006 Humana Press Inc.
999 Riverview Drive, Suite 208
Totowa, New Jersey 07512

humanapress.com

For additional copies, pricing for bulk purchases, and/or information about other Humana titles, contact Humana at the above address or at any of the following numbers: Tel: 973-256-1699; Fax: 973-256-8341; E-mail: orders@humanapr.com or visit our website at www.humanapress.com

This publication is printed on acid-free paper. ∞
ANSI Z39.48-1984 (American National Standards Institute)
Permanence of Paper for Printed Library Materials.

Production Editor: Melissa Caravella

Cover design by Patricia F. Cleary

Cover illustration: From Fig. 5B in Chapter 3, "Image Enhancement Endoscopy," by Stephan M. Wildi and Michael B. Wallace; Fig. 2 in Chapter 13, "Diagnosis and Management of Gastrointestinal Lymphoma," by John G. Kuldau, Peter R. Holman, and Thomas J. Savides; and Fig. 1A in Chapter 15, "Carcinoid Tumors," by Willscott E. Naugler and Gordon C. Hunt.

Printed in the United States of America. 10 9 8 7 6 5 4 3 2 1

eISBN 1-59745-172-X

Library of Congress Cataloging-in-Publication Data

Endoscopic oncology : gastrointestinal endoscopy and cancer management / edited by Douglas O. Faigel, Michael L. Kochman.
        p. ; cm.
   Includes bibliographical references and index.
   ISBN 1-58829-532-X (alk. paper)
   1. Endoscopy. 2. Gastrointestinal system--Cancer--Endoscopic surgery. 3. Gastrointestinal system--Diseases--Diagnosis.
   [DNLM: 1. Neoplasms--therapy. 2. Endoscopy, Gastrointestinal--methods. QZ 268 E556 2006] I. Faigel, Douglas O. II. Kochman, Michael L.
   RC804.E6E53 2006
   616.99'407545--dc22
                                2005036564

Preface

Cancer is the second most common cause of death in Americans (*see* www.cdc.gov). Colorectal cancer kills more Americans than any other malignancy except for lung cancer. The incidences and mortalities of the major gastrointestinal (GI) malignancies are shown in Table 1. Taken as a group, the five most common GI malignancies account for more cancers and more cancer deaths than for any other site.

Flexible endoscopy has given physicians unprecedented access to the GI tract. The ability to endoscopically visualize, biopsy, and apply therapy has had implications for the management of all the major GI malignancies. Accepted applications of endoscopy range from detection of malignant and premalignant lesions (e.g., colonoscopy for colon cancer screening), prevention of cancers through removal of precursor lesions (e.g., polypectomy), surveillance of premalignant conditions (e.g., Barrett's esophagus), palliation of symptoms (e.g., placement of stents for biliary or esophageal obstruction) or staging of cancers to allow stage directed therapy (e.g., endoscopic ultrasound), and, in selected circumstances, definitive therapy for early stage neoplasms (e.g., endoscopic mucosal resection). This partial list of applications demonstrates the central role that endoscopy plays in management for those at risk for or with a GI malignancy. The wide variety of endoscopic techniques applied suggests a new subspecialty of endoscopy: "endoscopic oncology." This is similar to "surgical oncology," as it concerns itself with the subset of endoscopic procedures directly applied for the management of neoplastic and precancerous conditions.

It becomes apparent that a substantial proportion of endoscopies are performed for a cancer-related indication. To determine what proportion of endoscopic procedures are done out of a concern for cancer or a premalignant condition, a large national database of endoscopic reports (Clinical Outcomes Research Initiative [CORI]) was queried. Indications related to cancer were defined by convening an expert panel (Table 2).* We then queried the CORI database to determine the proportion of endoscopies done for these indications. The CORI database encompassed 105 practice sites in 28 states and had data on 245,971 patients.

The results demonstrated that the majority of endoscopic procedures (63.5%) in these practices were performed owing to a primary concern for cancer (Fig. 1). In fact, only for EGD were the majority not done for a cancer-related indication (32.7%). The great majority of colonoscopy (84.4%), ERCP (59.9%), and EUS (98.7%) procedures are

Table 1
Incidence and Mortality of the Five Most Common Gastrointestinal Malignancies

Site	Incidence[a]	Mortality[a]
Colorectum	53.9	21.6
Pancreas	11.1	10.6
Stomach	9.1	4.9
Liver/intrahepatic bile ducts	6.2	4.4
Esophagus	4.5	4.3

Data from SEER database 1992–2002 (www.seer.cancer.gov).
[a]Per 100,000.

Table 2
Cancer-Related Indications for Endoscopic Procedures

EGD	Dysphagia, Barrett's, anemia, f/u gastric ulcer, familial polyposis, abnormal X-ray
Colonoscopy	Heme+, CRC screen/surveillance, ulcerative colitis screening, polyp on flex sig, family history, hematochezia, f/u polyp abnormal X-ray
ERCP	Jaundice, biliary obstruction, stricture, pancreatic duct obstruction, stent placement, abnormal X-ray
EUS	Cancer staging, fine needle aspiration, submucosal tumor, stricture, pancreatic mass/cyst, lymphadenopathy, abnormal X-ray

done for cancer-related indications. For colonoscopy, the major cancer-related indications are surveillance of patients with prior polyps (21.3% of cancer-related indications), evaluation of hematochezia (26.2%), follow-up of a positive hemoccult test (15.6%), or surveillance in a patient with a family history of colorectal cancer (17.8%). For EGD, dysphagia was the most common cancer-related indication (62.4%) followed by anemia (23%) and Barrett's screening/surveillance (12.2%). For ERCP, 98% of the cancer-related indications are related to bile duct obstruction. For EUS, the primary indications related to cancer are FNA of a mass (26%), stage a known cancer (23%), or evaluate a pancreas lesion (23%).

*Faigel DO, Lieberman DA, Falk GW, et al. Endoscopic oncology: cancr as an indication for gastrointestinal endoscopy in the United States. Gastrointest Endosc 2002; 55(5):AB164.

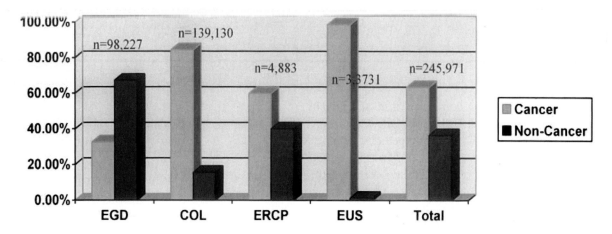

Fig. 1. Proportion of endoscopic procedures done for cancer-related indications. (Data from the CORI database.)

With nearly two-thirds of all endoscopic procedures being done out of a primary concern for cancer, it is apparent that all of us who do endoscopy are endoscopic oncologists!

This textbook examines the interface between endoscopy and oncology. It is organized anatomically: esophagus, stomach, colorectum, and pancreaticobiliary. For each site, the relevant cancers and premalignant conditions are addressed and the use of endoscopy in their diagnosis, management, and treatment discussed in detail. Additionally, the reader will find chapters summarizing the state-of-the-art for nonendoscopic medical and surgical cancer treatment.

This book was written with the practicing endoscopist in mind. However, given the multidisciplinary approach of modern cancer care, this book will be of interest to all health care professionals who take care of cancer patients, including medical oncologists, radiation oncologists, and surgeons.

Douglas O. Faigel, MD, FACG
Michael L. Kochman, MD, FACP

Contents

Contributors

NUZHAT A. AHMAD, MD, *Division of Gastroenterology, Hospital of the University of Pennsylvania, Philadelphia, PA*

KEVIN G. BILLINGSLEY, MD, *Department of Surgery, Oregon Health and Science University, Portland, OR*

CHARLES D. BLANKE, MD, *Division of Hematology and Oncology, Oregon Health and Science University, Portland, OR*

WILLIAM R. BRUGGE, MD, *Department of Medicine, Massachusetts General Hospital, Boston, MA*

CHRISTOPHER A. CANNING, MD, *Department of Radiation Oncology, Oregon Health and Science University, Portland, OR*

MARCIA I. CANTO, MD, MHS, *Division of Gastroenterology and Hepatology, Johns Hopkins University School of Medicine, Baltimore, MD*

AMITABH CHAK, MD, *Division of Gastroenterology, University Hospitals of Cleveland, Case Western Reserve University, Cleveland, OH*

YANG K. CHEN, MD, *Professor of Medicine, Gastrointestinal Practice Director/Director of Endoscopy, University of Colorado Hospital, Anschutz Outpatient Pavilion Aurora, CO*

RAQUEL E. DAVILA, MD, *Division of Gastroenterology, Oregon Health and Science University, Portland, OR*

JASON A. DOMINITZ, MD, MHS, *Associate Professor of Medicine, Division of Gastroenterology, VA Puget Sound Health Care System and University of Washington School of Medicine, Seattle, WA*

JEFFREY DREBIN, MD, PhD, FACS, *Department of Surgery and Abramson Cancer Center, University of Pennsylvania School of Medicine, Philadelphia, PA*

GLENN M. EISEN, MD, MPH, *Division of Gastroenterology, Oregon Health and Science University, Portland, OR*

DOUGLAS O. FAIGEL, MD, FACG, *Associate Professor of Medicine, Director of Endoscopy, Oregon Health and Science University, Portland, OR*

GREGORY G. GINSBERG, MD, *Professor of Medicine, Division of Gastroenterology, Director of Endoscopic Services, University of Pennsylvania Health Systems, Philadelphia, PA*

DEEPAK V. GOPAL, MD, FRCP(C), FACP, *Assistant Professor of Medicine, Section of Gastroenterology and Hepatology, University of Wisconsin School of Medicine, Madison, WI*

TAKUJI GOTODA, MD, *Endoscopy Division, National Cancer Center Hospital, Tokyo, Japan*

WILLIAM M. GRADY, MD, *Assistant Member, Clinical Research Division, Fred Hutchinson Cancer Research Center; Assistant Professor of Medicine, Division of Gastroenterology, University of Washington School of Medicine; Staff Physician, VA Puget Sound Health Care System, Seattle, WA*

DIANE HERSHOCK, MD, PhD, *Department of Hematology/Oncology, Abramson Cancer Center, Hospital of the University of Pennsylvania, Philadelphia, PA*

JOHN M. HOLLAND, MD, *Department of Radiation Oncology, Oregon Health and Science University, Portland, OR*

PETER R. HOLMAN, MD, *Division of Hematology/Oncology, University of California, San Diego, CA*

WENDY C. HSU, MD, *Department of Radiology, Hospital of the University of Pennsylvania, Philadelphia, PA*

ARTHUR Y. HUNG, MD, *Department of Radiation Oncology, Oregon Health and Science University, Portland, OR*

GORDON C. HUNT, MD, *Division of Gastroenterology, University of California, San Diego, CA*

ANDREW IPPOLITI, MD, *Division of Gastroenterology, Department of Medicine, Cedars-Sinai Medical Center, Los Angeles, CA*

BRIAN C. JACOBSON, MD, MPH, *Boston University School of Medicine, Boston Medical Center, Boston, MA*

SANJAY JAGANNATH, MD, *Division of Gastroenterology and Hepatology, Johns Hopkins University School of Medicine, Baltimore, MD*

VAMAN JAKRIBETTUU, MD, *Division of Gastroenterology, University of Colorado Health Sciences Center, Denver, CO*

MICHAEL L. KOCHMAN, MD, FACP, *Professor of Medicine and Surgery, Co-Director Gastrointestinal Oncology, Hospital of the University of Pennsylvania, Philadelphia, PA*

JOHN G. KULDAU, MD, *Division of Gastroenterology, University of California, San Diego, CA*

MARC S. LEVINE, MD, *Department of Radiology, Hospital of the University of Pennsylvania, Philadelphia, PA*

GEORGE A. MAKAR, MD, *Division of Gastroenterology, Hospital of the University of Pennsylvania, Philadelphia, PA*

KEVIN MCGRATH, MD, *Division of Gastroenterology, Hepatology, and Nutrition, University of Pittsburgh Medical Center, Pittsburgh, PA*

JON MORRIS, MD, *Department of Surgery and Abramson Cancer Center, University of Pennsylvania School of Medicine, Philadelphia, PA*

WILLSCOTT E. NAUGLER, MD, *Division of Gastroenterology, University of California, San Diego, CA*

DOUGLAS B. NELSON, MD, *Division of Gastroenterology, Minneapolis VA Medical Center, Professor of Medicine, University of Minnesota, Minneapolis, MN*

IAN D. NORTON, MBBS, PhD, FRACP, *Department of Gastroenterology and Hepatology, Concord Hospital, Sydney, Australia*

GREGORY OLDS, MD, *Division of Gastroenterology, University Hospitals of Cleveland, Case Western Reserve University, Cleveland, OH*

GEORGIOS I. PAPACHRISTOU, MD, *Division of Gastroenterology, Hepatology, and Nutrition, University of Pittsburgh Medical Center, Pittsburgh, PA*

GANAPATHY A. PRASAD, MD, *Division of Gastroenterology and Hepatology, Mayo Clinic, Jacksonville, FL*

MASSIMO RAIMONDO, MD, *Division of Gastroenterology and Hepatology, Mayo Clinic, Jacksonville, FL*

STEPHEN E. RUBESIN, MD, *Professor of Radiology, University of Pennsylvania School of Medicine and Department of Radiology, Hospital of the University of Pennsylvania, Philadelphia, PA*

THOMAS J. SAVIDES, MD, *Department of Gastroenterology, University of California, San Diego, CA*

MANDEEP S. SAWHNEY, MD, *Division of Gastroenterology, Minneapolis VA Medical Center, Assistant Professor of Medicine, University of Minnesota, Minneapolis, MN*

JAMES M. SCHEIMAN, MD, *Division of Gastroenterology, University of Michigan Medical Center, Ann Arbor, MI*

VANESSA M. SHAMI, MD, *Division of Gastroenterology, University of Virginia, Charlottesville, VA*

OMID A. SHAYE, MD, *Division of Gastroenterology, Department of Medicine, Cedars-Sinai Medical Center, Los Angeles, CA*

EVAN S. SIEGELMAN, MD, *Department of Diagnostic Radiology, Hospital of the University of Pennsylvania, Philadelphia, PA*

ADAM SLIVKA, MD, PhD, *Division of Gastroenterology, Hepatology and Nutrition, University of Pittsburgh Medical Center, Pittsburgh, PA*

ROY M. SOETIKNO, MD, *Division of Gastroenterology, Palo Alto VA Medical Center, Palo Alto, CA*

JOHN STROTHER, MD, *Division of Hematology and Oncology, Oregon Health and Science University, Portland, OR*

WEIJING SUN, MD, *Department of Surgery and Abramson Cancer Center, University of Pennsylvania School of Medicine, Philadelphia, PA*

JONATHAN P. TERDIMAN, MD, *Division of Gastroenterology, University of California, San Francisco, CA*

MADHULIKA G. VARMA, MD, *Division of Gastroenterology, University of California, San Francisco, CA*

FERNANDO S. VELAYOS, MD, *Division of Gastroenterology, University of California, San Francisco, CA*

JASON VOLLWEILER, MD, *Department of Gastroenterology and Hepatology, Cleveland Clinic Foundation, Cleveland, OH*

MICHAEL B. WALLACE, MD, MPH, *Division of Gastroenterology and Hepatology, Mayo Clinic, Jacksonville, FL*

ERIK-JAN WAMSTEKER, MD, *Division of Gastroenterology, University of Michigan Medical Center, Ann Arbor, MI*

KENNETH K. WANG, MD, *Division of Gastroenterology and Hepatology, Mayo Clinic, Jacksonville, FL*

IRVING WAXMAN, MD, *Section of Gastroenterology, The University of Chicago, Chicago, IL*

STEPHAN M. WILDI, MD, *Division of Gastroenterology, University of Zurich, Switzerland*

TIMOTHY WOODWARD, MD, *Division of Gastroenterology and Hepatology, Mayo Clinic, Jacksonville, FL*

KENNETH H. YU, MD, *Division of Hematology/Oncology, University of Pennsylvania, Philadelphia, PA*

GREGORY ZUCCARO, JR., MD, *Department of Gastroenterology and Hepatology, Cleveland Clinic Foundation, Cleveland, OH*

List of Color Plates

Color Plates follow p. 84

ESOPHAGUS 1

1   Barrett's Esophagus
Screening, Diagnosis, and Management

Glenn M. Eisen, MD, MPH

CONTENTS

1. INTRODUCTION

Barrett's esophagus (BE) or columnar lined esophagus, is an acquired condition associated with chronic gastroesophageal reflux disease (GERD). BE is strongly associated with GERD. Numerous endoscopic studies have demonstrated high rates of BE in patients with chronic GERD *(1–3)*. It is a condition in which the normal stratified squamous epithelium of the tubular esophagus is replaced by a metaplastic columnar epithelium. The overriding concern for patients with BE is its malignant potential. BE is accepted as the precursor in most cases of esophageal adenocarcinoma. This malignancy has been linked to chronic GERD and obesity as has BE *(4,5)*. Three case–control studies have demonstrated a strong association between adenocarcinoma of the esophagus and GERD *(4–7)*. The incidence of this malignancy has been rising at a rate of 5–10% for the past three decades in western Europe and the United States, faster than any nondermatological malignancy *(8)*. The Surveillance, Epidemiology, and End Results registry noted more than a 100% increase in the incidence of this tumor between 1976 and 1987 *(9)*. The increasing incidence of esophageal adenocarcinoma appears to be continuing *(10)*. Before the 1970s, esophageal adenocarcinoma accounted for less than 5% of esophageal malignancies. The increased incidence of this lesion is unlikely to be explained by alterations in the use of diagnostic testing (i.e., endoscopy) because this tumor has been found to have a significant male predilection. Also, misclassifying distal esophageal adenocarcinomas as gastric cardiac adenocarcinomas is unlikely to account for this trend because cardia malignancies are increasing in incidence as well. Epidemiological studies have consistently shown esophageal adenocarcinoma to be most common in males (7:1 ratio to females) and whites *(11,12)*.

From: *Endoscopic Oncology: Gastrointestinal Endoscopy and Cancer Management.* Edited by: D. O. Faigel and M. L. Kochman © Humana Press, Totowa, NJ

The prognosis is poor once symptomatic cancer develops, the 5-yr relative survival rate being less than 7%. This dismal prognosis has prompted efforts at endoscopic screening and surveillance, in order to identify earlier staged cancers and dysplastic lesions. There is some preliminary data that suggests that esophageal adenocarcinoma detected by endoscopic surveillance is detected at an earlier stage than when individuals present with dysphagia *(13)*. However, there are currently no randomized clinical trials formally assessing the utility of screening for or surveillance of BE.

2. PATHOGENESIS

2.1. GERD AND BE

It is currently accepted that BE develops as a complication of chronic GERD. The evidence that mucosal injury to the esophagus as a result of GERD can cause BE and lead to adenocarcinoma of the esophagus is compelling *(14,15)*. The estimated prevalence of reflux in the general population is between 25 and 35% (at least one episode per week). Approximately 10–15% of the population experience reflux daily. Overall, it has been estimated that more than 60 million American adults experience reflux symptoms on a regular basis. BE has been identified in 10–20% of individuals undergoing upper endoscopy for reflux symptoms and in 0.4% at autopsy *(16)*. Recent studies have demonstrated a direct correlation between the rates of endoscopy and the discovery of BE *(17)*. The incidence of clinically diagnosed BE (>3 cm) increased 28-fold between 1965–1969 and 1995–1997 in the Olmstead County catchment area, suggesting that the more we look for BE, the more we find. Utilizing these estimates of prevalence, BE may be present in almost 700,000 adults in the United States. It thus appears that GERD is quite common, as it is the development of BE. The concern is that those individuals with BE are at greater risk of developing esophageal adenocarcinoma than the general population.

A recent prospective assessment of asymptomatic male veterans older than 50 yr determined that 25% had BE *(18)*. This finding suggests that many individuals without GERD, or at least subclinical GERD may still develop BE. Lagergren et al. *(4)* also found that in their case–control study of GERD and esophageal adenocarcinoma, 40% of those with this malignancy did not note antecedent GERD. These study results are disconcerting, because screening is currently focused on symptomatic individuals only, and to screen entire populations would be untenable. There appears to be limited familial clustering of BE, accounting for perhaps 10% of all cases *(19,20)*. Nongenetic factors appear to predominate, although satisfactory answers regarding why white males remain the highest risk group remain unknown. Neither tobacco use nor alcohol ingestion are strong risk factors, unlike in the case of squamous cell carcinoma of the esophagus.

2.2. RISK OF ESOPHAGEAL ADENOCARCINOMA

The presence of BE is associated with a risk of developing esophageal adenocarcinoma that is 30–125 times that of the general population *(21)*. However, this relative risk does not correspond with a high absolute risk. The incidence of colorectal cancer remains approx 20-fold higher than the incidence of esophageal adenocarcinoma in the United States *(22)*.

Individuals with BE develop adenocarcinoma at a rate of 0.8–1.3% per year, based on small retrospective and prospective cohorts *(23)*. The natural history of BE progression to cancer is limited to a handful of prospective endoscopic studies comprising 285 patients followed from 1 to 5 yr. Of the 150 patients without dysplasia at study onset, 5 developed cancer over an interval of 3.4–10 yr. There has been significant variation in the reported incidence of BE as well as its progression to esophageal adenocarcinoma. However, the absolute risk may be somewhat overstated owing to publication bias inherent for small cohorts *(24)*. The overall risk appears to be approx 1 per 100 patient-years. It appears that the overall cancer risk is somewhat small, and the majority of patients will not develop esophageal adenocarcinoma. Nevertheless, current guidelines suggest both screening for those at risk and surveillance once BE is detected.

3. DIAGNOSIS AND SURVEILLANCE

3.1. DIAGNOSING BE

BE can be detected on upper endoscopy but must be verified by histological assessment. On endoscopic examination the distal esophageal mucosa appears velvety reddish and extends cephalad from the gastroesophageal junction (GEJ). This mucosa can extend circumferentially or in the form of "tongues" of mucosa. Segments of BE have been somewhat arbitrarily separated into short and long segments, with a long segment considered 3 cm in length or greater *(25)*. Incomplete intestinal metaplasia (IM) of the tubular esophagus is the histological hallmark of BE. Special stains (e.g., Alcian blue) are frequently employed to identify goblet cells indicating IM, which is termed "incomplete" because the clomnuar cells lack a brush border. The endoscopist and pathologist must ascertain that the biopsies do not originate from the proximal stomach *(26)*. Prior studies have found frequent IM at the GEJ, but its significance

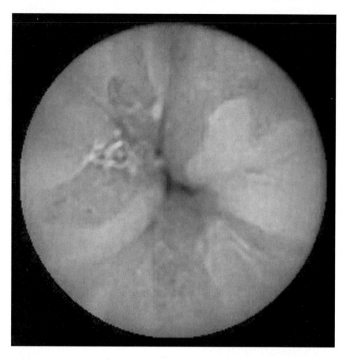

Fig. 1. Capsule endoscopy image of the distal esophagus demonstrating tongues of salmon-colored columnar epithelium consistent with BE.

remains unclear and practice guidelines do not recommend routine biopsies of this area *(27)*. Other types of mucosa have been considered Barrett's epithelium in the past include cardiac and fundic type epithelia. However, these cell types do not appear to have the same malignant potential as intestinal metaplastic tissue and should no longer be considered Barrett's *(28)*.

Other diagnostic modalities such as thin caliber endoscopy and capsule endoscopy have been recently utilized to diagnose BE, but biopsy is not always possible, potentially limiting their utility *(29,30)* (Fig. 1). Barium upper gastrointestinal series should not be utilized for Barrett's screening because of its lack of sensitivity to detect columnar-lined epithelium. Nonendoscopic balloon cytology to retrieve dysplastic or nondysplastic Barrett's epithelium has proved disappointing in research trials and should not be employed in clinical practice *(31)*.

Although not generally validated, standard endoscopic biopsy technique usually involves four quadrant biopsy of the visible Barrett segment at 2-cm intervals, with focused biopsying of any ulceration or raised lesion within the segment. Utilization of jumbo biopsy forceps has been suggested to improve diagnostic yield, but a recent study suggested this technique was just as fallible as standard biopsy forceps in detecting unsuspected malignancy in patients harboring high-grade dysplasia (HGD) *(32)*. A Seattle group has advocated using jumbo biopsy forceps for Q1 cm biopsies as a research technique, but this has not been generally utilized in clinical practice *(33)*.

Other novel endoscopic techniques have been utilized in research settings in the hope of identifying abnormalities within a Barrett's segment rather than relying on the "needle in the haystack" method of random biopsies. Chromoendoscopy using methylene blue has been shown to detect 95% of IM *(34)*.

Magnification endoscopy in addition to methylene blue installation maybe useful in identifying HGD and early cancer in the absence of visible lesions within a Barrett's segment *(35)*. Sharma et al. *(36)* performed chromoendoscopy with indigo carmine staining combined with magnification endoscopy in patients with BE and found the ridge/villous pattern had a 92% positive predictive value for IM. Other techniques have been attempted for detecting either IM and/or dysplasia including fluorescence spectroscopy and optical coherence tomography *(see* Chapter 3). The elusive goal remains to develop a sensitive, noninvasive modality to identify those at high risk for malignancy. Thus far clinical practice has not adopted any of these investigational techniques—continuing to rely on random four-quadrant biopsies of visualized columnar-lined epithelium.

There has been intense interest in developing markers of progression to malignancy in patients with BE. Risk stratification by histology, immunohistochemistry, and molecular pathology has been evaluated. Despite all this research effort, the only currently clinically accepted and utilized marker is dysplasia. This remains a purely morphological term. Riddell et al. *(37)* defined dysplasia as "an unequivocal neoplastic epithelium confined within the glandular basement membrane." The degree of dysplasia is determined based on the degrees of morphological abnormality. Unfortunately, there remains significant interpathologist interpretation variability with κ-scores ranging from 0.43 to 0.66 *(38,39)*. Therefore, a second opinion is warranted, especially in cases in which clinical decision making will be affected.

3.2. SCREENING/SURVEILLANCE OF BE

It appears that most cases of esophageal adenocarcinoma develop through a sequence of cellular changes leading to progressive dysplasia and ultimately carcinoma. This process affords endoscopists the opportunity to detect dysplasia and intervene before the development of malignancy. Current recommendations suggest biannual endoscopic surveillance examinations for individuals with BE. A healthy 30 yr old might be expected to undergo 25 endoscopies over the course of his/her lifetime. Multiply these frequent endoscopies by the estimated 1–2% in the United States with BE and this leads to a significant health expenditure, not to mention the complication risks and loss of work time. Furthermore, this practice, although widely endorsed and utilized, has not been clearly linked to improved patient outcomes.

Updated guidelines for the diagnosis and surveillance of BE were published by the American College of Gastroenterology (ACG) in 2002 *(40)*. Recommendations from two other gastroenterology societies were given during preparation of this document and "incorporated into the final document whenever possible." The recommendation for endoscopic screening states: "patients with chronic GERD symptoms are those most likely to have BE and should undergo upper endoscopy." This guideline remains quite vague, but in general individuals 50 and over with GERD symptoms for 5 or more years should be considered for screening. However, the published clinical guideline permits wide variation in screening practices. A recent AGA consensus conference concluded that

Table 1
Surveillance for Barrett's Esophagus *(40)*

Dysplasia	Documentation	Follow-up endoscopy
None	Two EGDs with biopsy	3 yr
Low grade	Highest grade on repeat	1 yr until no dysplasia
High grade	Repeat EGD with biopsy	Focal every 3 mo
	Expert pathologist confirmation	Multifocal intervention Mucosal irregularity EMR

EGD, esophagogastrodudonoscopy; EMR, endoscopic mucosal resection.

there was insufficient evidence to support screening for BE in adults over the age of 50, regardless of the duration of reflux symptoms *(41)*.

Endoscopic surveillance is recommended in patients with documented BE. These patients are recommended to have two examinations with biopsy. If there is no dysplasia on two consecutive endoscopies with biopsy, then a 3-yr interval from thereon is considered appropriate *(23)* *(see* Table 1). There have been several decision models developed concerning Barrett's screening and surveillance practices. One of the first models only evaluated endoscopic surveillance and determined that endoscopic surveillance every 2–3 yr appears most cost-effective *(42)*. The ACG practice parameters committee has concurred with this determination, but has cited the significant limitations of present data.

Despite the increasing incidence of esophageal adenocarcinoma in the United States and western Europe, the overall cancer rates are still small as demonstrated earlier. Inadomi et al., employing a Markov model and literature-based estimates, found that screening followed by surveillance in BE patients with dysplasia appears economically acceptable with an incremental cost-effectiveness ratio (ICER) of $10,440 compared with no screening. However, surveillance in patients without dysplasia appears prohibitively expensive with ICERs between $381,543 and $596,184, depending on an interval of between q2 and 5 yr *(43)*. These authors questioned the utility of surveillance in patients not demonstrated to have dysplasia.

There are currently no large-scale, multicenter studies evaluating the natural history of BE, severely limiting our ability to make evidence-based decisions on diagnosis, surveillance, and risk stratification. Further, all available research has come from tertiary endoscopy centers potentially biasing the findings.

Once patients with BE develop dysplasia, the risk of cancer increases dramatically. Patients with HGD (who do not have cancer at baseline) have a high risk of progression to cancer of 14–59% during follow-up of 3–7 yr *(44–46)*. The natural history of low-grade or indeterminate dysplasia is less certain, with reported rates of progression of neoplasia from 7 to 28% *(47)*. Sampliner analyzed data from five centers that have performed prospective studies from 2.7 to 7.3 yr, finding that 7% of patients with low-grade dysplasia and 2% of patients with no dysplasia developed cancer during follow-up *(23)*.

4. MANAGEMENT OF BE

Theoretically, eliminating the Barrett's epithelium could decrease or eliminate the cancer risk. In addition, the burden for endoscopic surveillance might also diminish. Unfortunately, despite several trials, neither medical (profound acid inhibition) or surgical (fundoplication) therapies appear to achieve complete regression of BE and elimination of its cancer risk *(48–50)*.

Patients diagnosed with advanced dysplasia in a BE segment are advised to undergo more frequent surveillance or esophagectomy, owing to the significant cancer risk. Between 5 and 60% of patients with HGD enrolled in surveillance will develop cancer over 1–7 yr *(51,52)*. Prophylactic esophagectomy has been recommended by many experts for patients with known HGD, because 30 and 40% may already harbor malignancy *(53,54)*. However, esophagectomy is associated with significant morbidity (20–47%) and mortality (average 4%) even at experienced centers *(55,56)*. The results may be more disappointing at other sites, although data is lacking.

Also, some patients with HGD may not be surgical candidates owing to significant comorbidity. It has been estimated that the mean age at diagnosis of Barrett's associated adenocarcinoma is 64 yr old *(57)*. An ideal therapy would be able to eliminate the premalignant epithelium and remove the need for further endoscopic evaluation. Furthermore, this intervention could be targeted for individuals with BE at high risk for developing cancer.

Recently, it has been shown that if the metaplastic epithelium is endoscopically ablated and subsequently healed in an anacid environment, the neoepithelium may become normal squamous mucosa *(58)*. Following this seminal report, there have been numerous small, uncontrolled trials evaluating various ablative methods to eliminate early esophageal adenocarcinoma, dysplastic tissue, and even nondysplastic BE. There has been considerable enthusiasm for these techniques despite the lack of prospective randomized controlled trials to establish their efficacy.

5. CONCLUSIONS

BE is an accepted malignant precursor for esophageal adenocarcinoma. This tumor's incidence has continued to rise at a rapid rate over the past 30 yr. Current practice guidelines recommend screening individuals with chronic GERD symptoms for the presence of BE. These guidelines are somewhat vague and millions of patients fit these criteria for screening. Despite minimal evidence that screening or surveillance is effective, these are the current practice standards.

The number of new cases of cancer of the esophagus in 2003 was 14,250 *(59)*. If we assume that approximately one-half of these cases are adenocarcinoma, there are about 7000 new cases of adenocarcinoma per year. Three recent studies (two population-based studies and a systematic review of the literature) found that less than 7% of patients with adenocarcinoma had known BE prior to the cancer diagnosis *(60,61)*. Surveillance cannot work if the vast majority of patients who ultimately develop cancer are not enrolled in surveillance programs. Despite this, it continues to be endorsed.

Currently, conventional upper endoscopy is recommended as a screening tool, but potentially other modalities, such as small caliber endoscopes and capsule endoscopy, may provide a more cost-effective mechanism for screening. Once BE is diagnosed, by the presence of IM, then surveillance intervals are based on whether dysplasia is present. Medical management includes antisecretory therapy primarily for GERD symptom relief. There are no studies demonstrating that PPI or H2RA therapy eliminates Barrett's metaplasia or cancer risk. This holds true for surgical fundoplication as well. Endoscopic ablation of BE should be reserved for patients with dysplastic epithelium (*see* Chapter 5).

There remain significant information gaps that could aid in our management of patients with BE. Discerning truly high-risk groups for esophageal adenocarcinoma could lead to targeted screening and surveillance. Further work on validating molecular markers for BE progression is necessary as well, given the interobserver variability of dysplasia assessment and its moderate concordance with subsequent neoplasia.

REFERENCES

1. Winters C, Spurling TJ, Chobanian SJ, et al. Barrett's esophagus: A prevalent occult complication of gastroesophageal reflux disease. Gastroenterology 1987; 92:118–124.
2. Lieberman DA, Oehlke M, Helfand M, GORGE Consortium. Risk factors for Barrett's esophagus in community-based practice. Am J Gastroenterol 1997; 92:1293–1297.
3. Eisen GM, Sandler RS, Murray S, Gottfried M. The relationship between gastroesophageal reflux disease and its complications with Barrett's esophagus. Am J Gastroenterol 1997; 92:27–31.
4. Lagergren J, Bergstrom R, Lindgren A, Nyren O. Symptomatic gastroesophageal reflux as a risk factor for esophageal adenocarcinoma. N Engl J Med 1999; 340(11):825–831.
5. Lagergren J, Bergstrom R, Nyren O. Association between body mass and adenocarcinoma of the esophagus and gastric cardia. Ann Int Med 1999; 130(11):883–890.
6. Chow WH, Finkle WD, McLaughlin JK, Frankl H, Ziel HK, Fraument JF Jr, The relation of gastroesophageal reflux disease and its treatment to adenocarcinomas of the esophagus and gastric cardia. JAMA 1995; 274:474–477.
7. Farrow DC, Vaughan TL, Sweeney C, et al. Gastroesophageal reflux disease, use of H2 receptor antagonists and risk of esophageal and gastric cancer. Cancer Causes Control 2000; 11:231–238.
8. Blot WJ, McLaughlin JK. The changing epidemiology of esophageal cancer. Semin Oncol 1999; 26(5 Suppl 15):2–8.
9. Blot WJ, Devesa SS, Kneller RW, et al. Rising incidence of adenocarcinoma of the esophagus and gastric cardia. JAMA 1991; 265:1287–1289.
10. Bollschweiler E, Wolfgraten E, Gutschow C, et al. Demographic variations in the rising incidence of esophageal adenocarcinoma in white males. Cancer 2001; 92:549–555.
11. Powell J, McConkey CC. The rising trend in oesophageal adenocarcinoma and gastric cardia. Eur J cancer Prev 1992; 1:265–269.
12. Hansson LE, Sparen P, Nyren O. Increasing incidence in both histological types of esophageal carcinoms among men in Sweden. Int J Cancer 1993; 54:402–407.
13. Sampliner RE. Adenocarcinoma of the esophagus and gastric cardia: is there progress in the face of increasing cancer incidence? Ann Int Med 1999; 130(1):67–69.
14. Shaheen N, Ransohoff DF. Gastroesophageal reflux, Barrett esophagus and esophageal cancer. Scientific Review. JAMA 2002; 287:1972–1981.
15. Falk GW. Barrett's esophagus. Gastroenterology 2002; 122:1569–1591.

16. Cameron AJ, Zinsmeister AR, Ballard DJ, et al. Prevalence of columnar-lined (Barrett's) esophagus. Comparison of population-based clinical and autopsy findings. Gastroenterology 1990; 99:918–922.

17. Conio, M, Cameron AJ, Romero Y, et al. Secular tends in the epidemiology and outcome of Barrett's oesophagus in Olmsted County, Minnesota. Gut 2001; 48:304–309.

18. Gerson LB, Shetler K, Triadafilopoulos G. Prevalence of Barrett's esophagus in asymptomatic individuals. Gastroenterology 2002; 123(2):461–467.

19. Chak A, Lee T, Kinnard MF, et al. Familial aggregation of Barrett's oesophagus, oesophageal adenocarcinoma and oesophagogastric junctional adenocarcinoma in Caucasian adults. Gut 2002; 51:323–328.

20. Romero Y, Cameron AJ, Locke GR 3rd, et al. Familial aggregation of gastroesophageal reflux in patients with Barrett's esophagus and esophageal adenocarcinoma. Gastroenterology 1997; 113:1449–1456.

21. Spechler SJ, Goyal RK. Barrett's esophagus. N Engl J Med 1986; 315:362–371.

22. Eisen G, Lieberman D, Fennerty MB, Sonnenberg A. Screening and surveillance in Barrett's esophagus: a call to action. Clin Gastroenterol Hepatol. 2004; 2(10):861–864.

23. Drewitz DJ, Sampliner RE, Garewal HS. The incidence of adenocarcinoma in Barrett's esophagus: a prospective study of 170 patients followed 4.8 years. Am J Gastroenterol 1997; 92(2):212–215.

24. Shaheen NJ, Crosby MA, Bozymski EM, Sandler RS. Is there publication bias in the reporting of cancer risk in Barrett's esophagus? Gastroenterology 2000; 119(2):333–338.

25. Sharma P, Morales TG, sampliner RE. Short segment Barrett's esophagus—the need for standardization of the definition and endoscopic criteria. Am J Gastroenterol 1998; 93:1033–1036.

26. Paull A, Trier JS, Dalton MD, et al. The histologic spectrum of Barrett's esophagus. N Engl J Med 1976; 295:476–480.

27. Spechler SJ. Intestinal metaplasia at the gastroesophageal junction. Gastroenterology 2004; 126(2):567–575.

28. Haggitt RC. Adenocarcinoma in Barrett's esophagus: a new epidemic? Hum Pathol 1992; 23:475–476.

29. Eliakim R, Yassin K, Shlomi I, et al. A novel diagnostic tool for detecting oesophageal pathology: the PillCam oesophageal video capsule. Aliment Pharmacol Ther 2004; 20(10):1083–1089.

30. Sorbi D, Gostout CJ, Henry J, Lindor KD. Unsedated small-caliber esophagogastroduodenoscopy (EGD) versus conventional EGD: a comparative study.Gastroenterology 1999; 117(6):1301–1307.

31. Falk GW, Chittajallu R, Goldblum R, et al. Surveillance of patients with Barrett's esophagus for dysplasia and cancer with balloon cytology. Gastroenterology 1997; 112(6):1787–1797.

32. Falk GW, Rice TW, Goldblum JR, Richter JE. Jumbo biopsy forceps protocol still misses unsuspected cancer in Barrett's esophagus with high-grade dysplasia. Gastrointest Endosc 1999; 49(2):170–176.

33. Reid BJ, Blount PL, Rubin CE, et al. Flow cytometric and histological progression to malignancy in Barrett's esophagus: prospective endoscopic surveillance of a cohort. Gastroenterology 1992; 102:1212–1219.

34. Canto MI, Setrakian S, Petras R, et al. Methylene blue selectively stains intestinal metaplasia in Barrett's esophagus. Gastrointest Endosc 1996; 44:1–6.

35. Yagi K, Nagamura A, Sekine A. Accuracy of magnifying endoscpy with methylene blue in the diagnosis of specialized intestinal metaplasia and short-segment Barrett's esophagus in Japanese patients without Helicobacter pylori infection. Gastrointest Endosc 2003; 58–65.

36. Sharma P, Weston AP, Topalovski M, et al. Magnification chromoendoscopy for the detection of intestinal metaplssia and dysplasia in Barrett's oesophagus. Gut 2003; 52:24–27.

37. Riddell RH, Goldman H, Ransohoff DF, et al. Dysplasia in inflammatory bowel disease: standardized classification with provisional clinical applications, Hum Pathol 1983; 14:931–968.

38. Montgomery E, Bronner MP, Goldblum JR, et al. Reproducibility of the diagnosis of dysplasia in Barrett esophagus: a reaffirmation. Hum Pathol 2001; 32:368–378.

39. Alikhan M, Rex D, Khan A, et al. Variable pathologic interpretation of columnar lined esophagus by general pathologists in community practice. Gastrointest Endosc 1999; 50:23–26.

40. Sampliner RE. Updated guidelines for the diagnosis, surveillance and therapy of Barrett's esophagus. Am J Gastroenterol 2002; 97: 1888–1895.

41. Sharma P, McQuaid K, Dent J, et al. A critical review of the diagnosis and management of Barrett's esophagus: the AGA Chicago workshop. Gastroenterology 2004; 127:310–330.

42. Provenzale D, Kemp JA, Arora S, et al. A guide for surveillance of patients with Barrett's esophagus. Am J Gastroenterol 1994; 89:670–680.

43. Inadomi JM, Sampliner R, Lagergren J, Lieberman D, Fendrick AM, Vakil N. Screening and surveillance for Barrett's esophagus in high-risk populations: A cost-utility analysis. Ann Intern Med 2003; 138:176–186.

44. Reid BJ, Levine DS, Longton G, et al. Predictors of progression to cancer in Barrett's esophagus: baseline histology and flow cytometry identify low and high-risk patient subsets. Am J Gastroenterol 2000; 95:1669–1676.

45. Buttar NS, Wang KK, Sebo TJ, et al. Extent of high grade dyaplasia in Barrett's esophagus correlates with risk of adenocarcinoma. Gastroenterology 2001; 120:1630–1639.

46. Schnell TG, Sontag SJ, Chejfec G, et al. Long-term management of Barrett's esophagus with high grade dysplasia. Gastroenterology 2001; 120:1607–1619.

47. Falk GW. Barrett's esophagus. Gastroenterology 2002; 122:1569–1591.

48. Gore S, Healey CJ, Sutton R, et al. Regression of columnar lined (Barrett's) oesophagus with continuous omeprazole therapy. Aliment Pharmacol Ther 1993; 7:623–628.

49. Sampliner RE, Garewal HS, Fennerty MB, Aickin M. Lack of impact of therapy on extent of Barrett's esophagus in 67 patients. Dig Dis Sci 1990; 35:93–96.

50. Sharma P, Sampliner RE, Camargo E. Normalization of esophageal pH with high dose proton pump inhibitor therapy does not result in regression of Barrett's esophagus. Am J Gastroenterol 1997; 92(4):582–585.

51. Reid BJ, Levine DS, Longton G, Blount PL, Rabinovitch PS. Predictors of progression to cancer in Barrett's esophagus: baseline histology and flow cytometry identify low-high risk patients subsets. Am J Gastroenterol 2000; 95:1669–1676.

52. Schnell TG, Sontag SJ, Chejfec G, et al. Long-term nonsurgical management of Barrett's esophagus with high grade dysplasia. Gastroenterology 2001; 120:1607–1619.

53. Pera M, Trastek VF, Carpenter HA, Allen MS, Deschamps C, Pairolero PC. Barrett's esophagus with high grade dysplasia: an indication for esophagectomy? Ann Thorac Surg 1992; 54:199–204.

54. Rice TW, Falk GW, Achar E, Petras RE. Surgical management of high grade dysplasia in Barrett's esophagus. Am J Gastroenterol 1993; 88:1832–1836.

55. Daly JM, Fry WA, Little AG, et al. Esophageal cancer: results of an American College of Surgeons patient care evaluation study. J Am Coll Surg 2000; 190:548–559.

56. Heitmiller RF, Redmond M. Hamilton SR. Barrett's esophagus with high grade dysplasia. Ann Surg 1996; 224:66–71.

57. Cameron AJ, Lomboy CT. Barrett's esophagus: age, prevalence, and extent of columnar epithelium. Gastroenterology 1992; 103:1241–1245.

58. Sampliner RE, Hixson LJ, Fennerty MB, Garewal HS. Regression of Barrett's esophagus by laser ablation in an anacid environment. Dig Dis Sci 1993; 38(2):365–368.

59. Jemal A, Murray T, Samuels A, Ghafoor A, Ward E, Thun MJ. Cancer Statistics 2003. CA Cancer J Clin 2003; 53:5–26.

60. Corley DA, Levin TR, Habel LA, Weiss NS, Buffler PA. Surveillance and survival in Barrett's adenocarcinomas: A population-based study. Gastroenterology 2002; 122:633–640.

61. Dulai GS, Guha S, Kahn KL, Gornbein J, Weinstein WM. Preoperative prelvalence of Barrett's esophagus in esophageal adenocarcinoma: A systematic review. Gastroenterology 2002; 122:26–33.

2 Endoscopic Screening for Squamous Cell Carcinoma of the Esophagus

BRIAN C. JACOBSON, MD, MPH

CONTENTS

1. INTRODUCTION

Although the relative incidence of esophageal squamous cell carcinoma (SCC) has been declining steadily in the United States and Europe compared to that of adenocarcinoma (1,2); esophageal SCC continues to be the more common form of esophageal malignancy worldwide (3). There are approx 6000 new cases of esophageal SCC diagnosed in the United States annually (4). The global incidence and gender ratio vary widely according to geographic region, likely reflecting environmental and dietary factors more than genetic predisposition. Several risk factors for esophageal SCC have been identified, making screening a potential option for specific populations. This chapter outlines conditions or behaviors that are strongly associated with this malignancy, describes methods for improving the endoscopic detection of early squamous cell dysplasia, and suggests specific instances in which screening for esophageal SCC may be appropriate.

2. RATIONALE FOR SCREENING

In general, screening for a disease should be undertaken when early detection will result in improved patient survival or quality of life. Typically, the number of people deriving benefit from screening for a malignancy is small, whereas the majority of those screened face potential morbidity, both physical and psychological, from screening procedures (5). It is for this reason that screening is often reserved for specific high-risk populations. For instance, current guidelines recommend screening endoscopy for Barrett's esophagus among patients with chronic gastroesophageal reflux disease, and for

surveillance endoscopy for dysplasia among those with known Barrett's esophagus (6,7), even though the annual incidence of esophageal adenocarcinoma among those with Barrett's esophagus is approx 0.4–0.5% (8–12). Screening for esophageal SCC, however, has not been widely advocated despite the high mortality associated with this malignancy (13). Long-term survival correlates directly with stage at diagnosis (14), suggesting that detection of very early cases should improve outcomes. The infrequency of esophageal SCC makes population-based screening inappropriate. Nonetheless, certain individuals with an increased risk for SCC of the esophagus exist (Table 1), and an understanding of their risk may help guide clinicians and patients in making decisions about screening and surveillance.

3. HIGH-RISK ASSOCIATIONS

3.1. RACE, GENDER, AND GEOGRAPHIC ASSOCIATIONS

Based on data in the National Cancer Institute's Surveillance, Epidemiology, and End Results (SEER) cancer registry, black men in the United States have a nearly fivefold greater annual risk for developing esophageal SCC than non-Hispanic white men (15). Black women have a twofold greater risk compared with non-Hispanic white men, and a nearly fourfold greater risk compared with women of all other races and ethnicities (15). Asian men are also at increased risk, having twice the incidence as non-Hispanic white men. Particular regions of the world have also been identified in which the incidence of esophageal SCC is extremely high, approaching 1 case per 1000 adults (16). These locations include eastern Turkey, northern Iran and Afghanistan, southern regions of the former Soviet Union including Turkmenistan and Uzbekistan, northern China and India, regions of Brazil, Argentina, and Uruguay, and the Transkei region of Cape Province and Kenya (3,16). These demographic

From: *Endoscopic Oncology: Gastrointestinal Endoscopy and Cancer Management.* Edited by: D. O. Faigel and M. L. Kochman © Humana Press, Totowa, NJ

Table 1
Conditions or Exposures Strongly Associated
With Esophageal SCC

Condition or exposure	Relative risk for esophageal SCC
Chronic alcohol use	+ + +
Chronic tobacco use	+ +
Poverty	+
Current or prior cancer of the upper aerodigestive tract	+ + + +
Caustic esophageal stricture	+ + +
Tylosis (type A)	+ + + + +
Achalasia	+

and geographic associations are most likely explained by environmental exposures, such as tobacco, alcohol, and particular dietary factors (discussed later), although differences in susceptibility to exposures may still account for some of these observations (17).

3.2. CHRONIC TOBACCO AND ALCOHOL USE

As many as 80–90% of cases of esophageal SCC can be attributed to tobacco and alcohol use (14,16). The risk associated with cigarette smoking increases directly with increasing pack-years of exposure, with those smoking more than 54 pack-years having a relative risk that is sixfold higher than nonsmokers (18). Former smokers continue to have an increased risk, although this begins to improve in the second decade after cessation. It is postulated that several components of tobacco products, such as nitrosamines, aromatic amines, aldehydes, and phenols have direct carcinogenic effects (3). These may be ingested as tobacco condensates, and thereby come into direct contact with esophageal mucosa (19). Alcohol consumption also demonstrates a dose-dependent increase in risk, with those consuming more than 30 drinks per week having a greater than sevenfold increased risk over nondrinkers (18). Liquor and beer are likely associated with a greater risk than wine, although overall quantity of alcohol consumed may be more important than the specific form (20). The combined, chronic use of large amounts of alcohol and tobacco appears to confer the greatest risk for esophageal SCC, and likely identifies one of the largest at-risk populations in the United States.

3.3. PREVIOUS SCC OF THE UPPER AERODIGESTIVE TRACT

Esophageal SCC is often associated with synchronous or metachronous SCC of the head and neck. The reported incidence of an esophageal SCC associated with a current or prior cancer of the upper aerodigestive tract ranges from 3.7 to 30% (16,21). This variation in rates is likely explained by differences in populations studied and their differing duration of follow-up. A synchronous esophageal SCC has also been found in up to 31% of resected esophageal specimens, many of which were confined to the mucosa or submucosa (22,23). In one prospective study, 14% of patients undergoing endoscopic mucosal resection for early stage (mucosal or submucosal involvement) esophageal SCC were found to develop metachronous esophageal SCC between 14 and 58 mo post-treatment (24). In addition, among patients with esophageal SCC,

surveillance pharyngolaryngoscopy can frequently detect metachronous head and neck cancers (25). These findings have lent support to the "field effect" theory, suggesting that the entire squamous epithelium of the upper aerodigestive tract in susceptible individuals is at high risk of malignancy after prolonged exposure to some damaging agent. However, in another prospective study investigators systematically screened 331 men with *any* current or prior nonesophageal cancer, not necessarily upper aerodigestive tract SCC, and found 2.7% harbored esophageal SCC (26). Even after excluding 51 patients with head and neck cancer, the prevalence of esophageal SCC in that study was still 2.1%, a number higher than expected. This suggests that individuals who have experienced any form of cancer may be at increased risk for esophageal SCC.

3.4. DIETARY FACTORS AND POOR SOCIOECONOMIC STATUS

The consumption of salt-pickled or cured foods, sun-dried foods, moldy foods, and smoked fish have all been associated with esophageal SCC (16). It is postulated that these foods expose the esophageal mucosa to high levels of carcinogenic *N*-nitroso compounds or fungal toxins. In addition, diets deficient in fruits, vegetables, zinc, vitamins A, C, E, niacin, and riboflavin, and other micronutrients have also been associated with an increased risk of esophageal SCC (16). Iron deficiency may be associated with esophageal SCC in connection with the Plummer-Vinson syndrome, a combination of iron deficiency anemia and a cervical esophageal web (16,27). Unfortunately, the relative risks associated with specific nutrient exposures or deficiencies have not been well established and dietary questionnaires would likely be impractical for identifying individuals for screening endoscopy. A more useful distinction arises from a condition closely associated with poor nutritional status, namely low socioeconomic status. Poverty has been strongly linked with esophageal SCC (18,28), and may represent a more meaningful way to risk-stratify individuals when considering specific populations for screening.

Another interesting dietary factor that has been associated with esophageal SCC is the frequent consumption of extremely hot beverages, a practice common in regions of Central and South America, China, Iran, and India (16). One such beverage, mate, is an infusion of the herb *Ilex paraguayensis* that is often consumed at extremely hot temperatures. This drink, popular in parts of Argentina, Uruguay, Paraguay, and Brazil, results in thermal esophagitis (29), and it is only those who drink hot mate (as opposed to warm mate), that appear to have increased cancer risk (30). It is therefore the thermal injury from this practice that has been postulated to result in dysplastic changes of the esophagus. In fact, consumption of extremely hot tea and coffee have also been linked to esophageal SCC (31).

3.5. CAUSTIC INGESTION

The risk for developing esophageal cancer in the setting of an esophageal stricture following caustic ingestion is increased 1000-fold compared with the general population (7). The reported interval between ingestion of a caustic substance (e.g., lye) and the subsequent development of cancer ranges from 14 to 47 yr, and the tumor typically develops within the stricture itself. The mechanism of increased risk is unknown, but may relate to chronic inflammation within the stricture.

3.6. ACHALASIA

Achalasia is a condition of unknown etiology in which there is loss of neurons within the esophageal wall and lower esophageal sphincter. It is clinically manifested by dysphagia to both solid food and liquids, with eventual dilation of the esophagus and chronic stasis of ingested foods. It is this stasis and subsequent inflammation that is postulated to impart an increased risk of esophageal cancer to those with achalasia. This risk has been estimated to be 7- to 33-fold greater than normal, and includes risks for adenocarcinoma and, more commonly, SCC *(16)*. One prospective, *hospital-based* study followed 195 patients with achalasia with periodic endoscopy for a total follow-up of 874 person-years *(32)*. During that time three patients developed esophageal SCC a mean of 5.4 yr after their diagnosis of achalasia. This cancer incidence of 3.4 per 1000 patients per year was significantly higher than that expected in the general population. Two of the three patients demonstrated long-term survival after treatment for their cancer. The only prospective, *population-based* study to address this issue included 1062 patients with a combined total of 9864 yr of follow-up *(33)*. These patients, however, were not necessarily enrolled in a cancer surveillance program. Excluding cases likely present at study entry, the incidence of cancer was 20-fold greater among men and eightfold greater among women with achalasia compared with the general population. Of the 24 cases of cancer reported in that study, 14 were SCC, 6 were adenocarcinoma, and 4 were undifferentiated. Previous reports had suggested that cancer risk rises 15–20 yr after symptoms of achalasia first develop *(16)*. However, in the prospective, population-based study the risks were similar for each time frame after initial diagnosis examined (1–4, 5–9, and 10–24 yr) *(33)*. This suggests that surveillance, if advocated, should begin immediately after diagnosis. The frequency and cost-effectiveness of endoscopic surveillance in achalasia has not been determined. Whether definitive therapy for achalasia (e.g., surgical myotomy) changes cancer risk has also not been determined.

3.7. TYLOSIS (DIFFUSE PALMOPLANTAR KERATODERMA)

This rare, autosomal-dominant, fully penetrant condition is marked by hyperkeratosis of the palms and soles, in addition to a thickening of the oral and esophageal mucosa. Two phenotypes, A and B, have been identified and appear to be linked to mutations in keratin genes clustered on chromosomes 17q23 and 12q11–q13, respectively *(34,35)*. Type B presents in infancy, is associated with gingival hyperplasia, and regions of hyperkeratosis have sharply demarcated edges that can extend onto wrist flexures *(36)*. This form has not been associated with an increased risk of esophageal cancer. In contrast, type A presents in childhood to young adulthood and is associated with buccal leukoplakia and regions of hyperkeratosis that have blurred edges that can affect weight-bearing regions *(36)*. Patients with type A tylosis have an extremely high risk of developing SCC of the esophagus, with a 50% incidence by age 45 and a more than 90% incidence by age 65 *(37)*. Early dysplasia may be endoscopically invisible, suggesting surveillance biopsies should be taken from multiple sites at various levels of the esophagus.

3.8. RADIATION THERAPY TO THE CHEST

There is a fivefold increased risk of esophageal SCC 10 or more years after radiation therapy for breast cancer compared with women who did not receive radiation therapy for their breast cancer *(38)*. However, the overall risk in this setting is still low, with one study documenting only 72 primary esophageal SCCs among 220,000 women with more than 1 million person-years of follow-up *(38)*.

3.9. LICHEN PLANUS

Lichen planus is a disease of unknown etiology in which there is T-lymphocyte-mediated inflammation directed against the squamous epithelium of the skin, mouth, esophagus, genitals, and anus *(39)*. In mucocutaneous regions, including the esophagus, lichen planus may manifest as lacelike striae or papular, atrophic, plaque-like, or erosive lesions. Patients with liver disease, including hepatitis C, are at increased risk for this condition, although a pathophysiological mechanism explaining the association remains undefined *(40)*. External skin lesions often resolve within 1–2 yr, but lesions of mucus membranes can persist for decades. Patients with oropharyngeal lichen planus are at increased risk for developing SCC, although the risk appears to be less than 1% *(41)*. There is a single report of a person with chronic esophageal lichen planus developing advanced esophageal SCC despite undergoing annual upper endoscopy *(42)*. That patient was neither a smoker nor a regular user of alcohol, increasing the likelihood that the etiology of her SCC was chronic inflammation associated with lichen planus. The authors of that report suggest regular surveillance for dysplasia for anyone with esophageal lichen planus, although there is no evidence proving the effectiveness of this strategy.

4. METHODS FOR IMPROVING THE ENDOSCOPIC DETECTION OF DYSPLASIA

When performing endoscopy for the early detection of malignancy, any suspicious lesion should be biopsied, with consideration given to taking multiple pieces using large-size (jumbo) biopsy forceps for maximum sensitivity *(43)*. The addition of brush cytology may also improve the diagnostic yield *(44,45)*. However, esophageal SCC most likely develops through a dysplasia–neoplasia sequence similar to other forms of cancer *(3)*. This implies that there are microscopic changes, such as nuclear enlargement and clumping of chromatin, that are present before the development of endoscopically visible lesions. The development of improved endoscopic optics along with the use of special mucosal stains (termed "chromoendoscopy") has proven useful for making these lesions visible during endoscopy. These enhancements may allow an endoscopist to target biopsies, thereby making screening or surveillance procedures more efficient.

4.1. MAGNIFICATION ENDOSCOPY

Magnifying endoscopes use various lenses to enlarge an already high-resolution video image. By using special dials on the endoscope handle, the endoscopist can "zoom in" on an image, magnifying it 1.5–105 times the original size *(46)*. This feature has been used with chromoendoscopy (*see* Section 4.2.) to characterize Barrett's epithelium *(47,48)*, small bowel atrophy in patients with suspected malabsorption *(49)*, colonic polyps, and aberrant crypt foci *(50,51)*.

4.2. CHROMOENDOSCOPY

Chromoendoscopy is the term describing the use of special dyes during endoscopy to highlight histological changes within the gastrointestinal mucosa. A specific dye is applied to the mucosa, typically with the use of a spray catheter passed through the accessory channel of an endoscope. After the application of the dye, careful endoscopic inspection is performed looking for areas that either fails to stain or stain differently than their surroundings. The dye used is chosen based on the particular pathology sought and the choice reflects the different cell types and cell components stained by each dye. In the case of squamous cell dysplasia, iodine is used as the stain based on a chemical reaction between iodine and glycogen *(52)*. The glycogen rich prickle-cell layer of the stratified squamous esophageal epithelium stains greenish brown after the application of a potassium iodide solution or Lugol's iodine. Dysplastic epithelium lacks the glycogen-rich granules in the prickle-cell layer and therefore fails to stain. The brown staining of the normal squamous cells may not be complete but the endoscopist can take biopsies targeted from the least stained regions. Iodine chromoendoscopy can detect early SCC in the esophagus that might otherwise go undetected by conventional endoscopy *(52,53)*. Iodine chromoendoscopy can also be helpful in defining the extent of an esophageal SCC or in better defining the gastroesophageal junction. To perform iodine chromoendoscopy, the esophageal mucosa is typically washed with 40–50 cc of water to remove mucus followed by the application of 10–20 cc of 1.5–3% Lugol's solution. The endoscopist should then wait 1–5 min to ensure sufficient staining before careful inspection. Biopsies are generally taken from unstained or understained regions 5 mm or greater in diameter. Patients may experience heartburn, chest discomfort, dysphagia, fever, tingling, or nausea and the technique should be avoided in those with an allergy to iodine *(52,53)*.

4.3. SPECTROSCOPY AND OPTICAL COHERENCE TOMOGRAPHY

Currently the identification of dysplastic or neoplastic epithelium depends on the histological interpretation of a biopsy specimen by a pathologist. Unfortunately, because normal-appearing epithelium may still harbor dysplasia, "blind" biopsy protocols are still the most commonly used method of tissue sampling during surveillance endoscopy. Yet even the most widely advocated systematic approach using jumbo biopsy forceps can miss adenocarcinoma in the setting of Barrett's esophagus *(54)*. Furthermore, there is significant interobserver variation among pathologists classifying degrees of dysplasia within histological specimens of Barrett's esophagus *(55,56)*. This has led investigators to search for alternative methods for identifying dysplasia that do not rely on tissue processing and histological interpretation. Spectroscopy and optical coherence tomography are two such techniques. They provide information about a tissue using optical technology without the need for taking a biopsy.

Spectroscopy relies on the fluorescent properties of inherent tissue components (fluorescence spectroscopy), the photon-scattering and color-absorption properties of living tissue (light-scattering spectroscopy), and the vibration patterns of specific biological agents (Raman spectroscopy) to aid in the diagnosis of dysplastic foci *(57)*. Optical coherence tomography uses the reflection of infrared light off of living tissue to generate an image similar to that obtained by standard histological processing of a biopsy specimen with 10 µ resolution *(58)*. Although early in clinical applications, these methods are demonstrating great promise for the early detection of esophageal dysplasia *(59,60)*.

5. EFFECTIVENESS OF SCREENING

In some institutions, iodine chromoendoscopy is performed routinely at the end of upper endoscopy for all male patients over the age of 50 *(52)*. This may be appropriate in regions of the world where esophageal SCC is extremely prevalent, but there is no data to support this type of routine use in most locations. However, several investigators have prospectively studied the selective use of upper endoscopy to evaluate specific patients considered to have increased risk for esophageal SCC *(24,26,61–71)*. These patient populations have included those with a history of upper aerodigestive tract malignancy, those with *any* prior malignancy, and those with chronic alcohol/tobacco exposure (Table 2). Some authors regularly performed iodine chromoendoscopy for screening/surveillance, whereas others either used iodine staining selectively, or not at all. When chromoendoscopy was regularly used, there were frequently lesions detected only after the application of Lugol's iodine, supporting its utility in screening. Among a combined total of 3036 patients with a history of current or prior head and neck cancer undergoing screening/surveillance endoscopy, 153 (5%) were found to have either high-grade dysplasia or a synchronous or metachronous esophageal SCC, many of which were confined to the mucosa or submucosa. Among 1504 patients with a history of excessive alcohol use, either alone or in combination with tobacco and hot mate consumption, 60 (4%) were found to have high-grade dysplasia or SCC, many of which were likewise early stage. Given the association between alcohol, smoking, and cancers of the head and neck, it is impossible to determine the exact contribution of each component to the development of esophageal SCC. In addition, the vast majority of patients screened have been male, leaving the utility of screening among women impossible to determine. Nonetheless, a 4–5% yield of dysplasia for a screening endoscopic procedure is quite high and suggests these specific patient populations may benefit from the implementation of a formal screening protocol.

There are, however, different yields between screening (an initial endoscopy) and surveillance (repeat endoscopies over some time interval) endoscopies, with most studies showing that the largest benefit comes an initial screening examination. Different patterns of iodine staining have been noted that may help further risk-stratify patients into those who are more likely to progress to cancer, and therefore more likely to benefit from repeated endoscopy *(24)*. Patients whose esophagus contains numerous tiny (<5 mm) foci of mucosa that fails to stain with iodine appear to be more likely to develop cancer during follow-up *(24,26)*. The yield of iodine chromoendoscopy surveillance in the setting of achalasia has not been reported.

Table 2
Prospective Studies of Screening for Esophageal SCC Among High-Risk Populations

Author	High-risk association	No. of patients	Male (%)	No. of subjects with high-grade dysplasia or cancer (%)	No. of subjects with early-stage[a] lesions (%)
Shiozaki (67)	H&N Ca	178	77	9 (5.1)	7 (78)
Ina (64)	H&N Ca	127	100	8 (6.3)	NR
Muto (65)	H&N Ca	389	83	54 (13.9)	50 (93)
Petit (66)	H&N Ca	1560	NR	50 (3.2)	NR
Scherubl (68)	H&N Ca	148	72	15 (10.1)	10 (67)
Atabek (62)	H&N Ca	574	NR	12 (2.1)	NR
Tincani (70)	H&N Ca and excessive alcohol/tobacco	60	92	5 (8.3)	5 (100)
Shimizu (26)	Prior nonesophageal cancer[b]	331	100	9 (2.7)	9 (100)
Shimizu (24)	Prior esophageal SCC	82	93	12 (14.6)	12 (100)
Yokoyama (71)	Excessive alcohol	901	100	33 (3.7)	31 (94)
Ban (61)	Excessive alcohol	255	100	10 (3.9)	10 (100)
Meyer (69)	Excessive alcohol and/or smoking[b]	158	96	13 (8.2)	NR
Fagundes (63)	Excessive alcohol, smoking, and hot mate drinking	190	100	4 (2.1)	NR

H&N Ca, head and neck cancer; NR, not reported.
[a]Early-stage, high-grade dysplasia or stage I cancer (confined to the mucosa or submucosa without lymph node metastases) (73).
[b]An unreported percentage of subjects also had head and neck cancer.
Note: All studies except Petit, Scherubl, and Atabek reported the routine use of Lugol's iodine chromoendoscopy.

It is extremely important to clarify the definition of effective screening. If one's aim is to simply identify cancer, the data in Table 2 suggest a reasonably high yield for screening endoscopy among patients with head and neck cancer or excessive alcohol and tobacco use. However, when determining the utility of a screening test for malignancy, one should also consider the impact of identifying early cancer on the patient's survival and quality of life. In the case of esophageal SCC, definitive treatment of early-stage lesions can certainly improve survival, but among the patients for whom screening may detect these lesions, overall survival may still be limited. For example, among patients with cancer of the head and neck, a sizeable portion will die from recurrence of this tumor, regardless of therapy for an incidentally identified esophageal cancer. In some cases, surgery for head and neck cancer may limit a surgeon's ability to resect an esophageal cancer, leaving only nonoperative therapeutic options. Finally, patients with chronic alcohol and tobacco exposure are likely to have comorbidities such as cirrhosis or heart disease that predispose to early mortality or limit treatment options for cancer. Therefore, the effectiveness in identifying early esophageal SCC may be limited by an unchanged life expectancy. Two studies of more than 3500 patients with head and neck cancer failed to find much survival benefit from endoscopic screening for esophageal carcinoma (62,66). However, several of the deaths in those series were from esophageal cancer and iodine chromoendoscopy was not routinely used in screening. Therefore very early, otherwise curable lesions may have been underdiagnosed. The question of whether long-term survival can be improved among high-risk populations undergoing optimized screening remains unanswered.

6. CONCLUSIONS AND RECOMMENDATIONS

Although certain exposures significantly increase the risk of developing esophageal SCC, the overall prevalence of this disease should be considered when deciding who might benefit from endoscopic screening. It is probably a combination of factors that conveys the highest risks, and physicians must determine on an individual basis whether screening endoscopy might have a potential impact on a given patient's course. For instance, an impoverished 60-yr-old black man with a long history of alcohol and tobacco use may benefit from a screening endoscopy with iodine chromoendoscopy, whereas a wealthy 60-yr-old nonsmoking white woman who drinks alcohol only occasionally is unlikely to dervie any benefit from screening. Others who may benefit include patients with an early-stage head and neck cancer or patients from a region of the world where the incidence of esophageal SCC is very high. Only patients who can be effectively treated for esophageal cancer should be screened, although early cancers may be amenable to endoscopic mucosal resection in otherwise inoperable patients (72).

According to the American Society for Gastrointestinal Endoscopy (ASGE), patients with tylosis should begin surveillance endoscopy at age 30 and have repeat endoscopy not more than every 1–3 yr (7). This should be limited to patients with type A tylosis. The ASGE also recommends that patients with a history of caustic ingestion with stricture formation undergo endoscopic screening beginning 15–20 yr after the ingestion with surveillance endoscopy not more than every 1–3 yr (7). A role for endoscopic screening among patients with achalasia is less clear, although patients with a prolonged history of dysphagia before diagnosis and treatment may derive benefit. Patients with longstanding esophageal lichen planus may benefit from screening and surveillance, but this remains speculative. There is insufficient evidence to support a role for screening among patients with a history of radiation therapy to the chest. Finally, the cost-effectiveness of endoscopic screening for esophageal SCC among any high-risk population has not been established.

REFERENCES

1. Devesa S, Blot WJ, Fraumeni JF. Changing patterns in the incidence of esophageal and gastric carcinoma in the United States. Cancer 1998; 83:2049–2053.

2. Botterweck AA, Schouten LJ, Volovics A, Dorant E, van den Brandt PA. Trends in incidence of adenocarcinoma of the oesophagus and gastric cardia in ten European countries. Int J Epidemiol 2000; 29:645–654.

3. Stoner GD, Gupta A. Etiology and chemoprevention of esophageal squamous cell carcinoma. Carcinogenesis 2001; 22:1737–1746.

4. Jemal A, Tiwari RC, Murray T, et al. Cancer Statistics, 2004. CA Cancer J Clin 2004; 54:8–29.

5. Cullen J, Schwartz MD, Lawrence WF, Selby JV, Mandelblatt JS. Short-Term Impact of Cancer Prevention and Screening Activities on Quality of Life. J Clin Oncol 2004; 22:943–952.

6. Sampliner RE. Practice Parameters Committee of the American College of Gastroenterology. Practice guidelines on the diagnosis, surveillance, and therapy of Barrett's esophagus. Am J Gastroenterol 1998; 93:1028–1032.

7. American Society for Gastrointestinal Endoscopy. The role of endoscopy in the surveillance of premalignant conditions of the upper gastrointestinal tract. Gastrointest Endosc 1998; 48:663–668.

8. Cameron A, Ott B, Payne W. The incidence of adenocarcinoma in columnar-lined (Barrett's) esophagus. N Engl J Med 1985; 313:857–859.

9. Murray L, Watson P, Johnston B, SLoan J, Mainie I, Gavin A. Risk of adenocarcinoma in Barrett's esophagus: population based study. BMJ 2003; 327:534–535.

10. Shaheen N, Crosby M, Bozymski E, Sandler R. Is there publication bias in the reporting of cancer risk in Barrett's esophagus? Gastroenterology 2000; 119:333–338.

11. Spechler S, Lee E, Ahnen D, et al. Long-term outcome of medical and surgical therapies for gastroesophageal reflux disease: follow-up of a randomized controlled trial. JAMA 2001; 285:2331–2338.

12. Spechler SJ, Robbins AH, Rubins HB, et al. Adenocarcinoma and Barrett's esophagus: an overrated risk? Gastroenterology 1984; 87:927–933.

13. Pisani P, Parkin DM, Bray F, Ferlay J. Estimates of the worldwide mortality from 25 cancers in 1990. Int J Cancer 1999; 83:18–29.

14. Enzinger P, Mayer R. Esophageal cancer. N Engl J Med 2003; 349:2241–2252.

15. Kubo A, Corley DA. Marked multi-ethnic variation of esophageal and gastric cardia carcinomas within the United States. Am J Gastroenterol 2004; 99:582–588.

16. Ribeiro U, Posner MC, Safatle-Ribeiro AV, Reynolds JC. Risk factors for squamous cell carcinoma of the esophagus. Br J Surg 1996; 83:1174–1185.

17. Brown LM, Hoover RN, Greenberg RS, et al. Are racial differences in squamous cell esophageal cancer explained by alcohol and tobacco use? J Natl Cancer Inst 1994; 86:1340–1345.

18. Gammon MD, Schoenberg JB, Ahsan H, et al. Tobacco, alcohol, and socioeconomic status and adenocarcinomas of the esophagus and gastric cardia. J Natl Can Inst 1997; 89:1277–1284.

19. De Stefani E, Barrios E, Fierro L. Black (air-cured) and blond (flue-cured) tobacco and cancer risk. III: Oesophageal cancer. Eur J Cancer 1993; 29A:763–766.

20. Brown LM, Hoover RN, Gridely G, et al. Drinking practices and risk of squamous-cell esophageal cancer among black and white men in the United States. Cancer Cause Control 1997; 8:605–609.

21. Erkal HS, Mendenhall WM, Amdur RJ, Villaret DB, Stringer SP. Synchronous and Metachronous Squamous Cell Carcinomas of the Head and Neck Mucosal Sites. J Clin Oncol 2001; 19:1358–1362.

22. Kuwano H, Ohno S, Matsuda H, Mori M, Sugimachi K. Serial histologic evaluation of multiple primary squamous cell carcinomas of the esophagus. Cancer 1988; 61:1635–1638.

23. Pesko P, Rakic S, Milicevic M, Bulajic P, Gerzic Z. Prevalence and clinicopathologic features of multiple squamous cell carcinoma of the esophagus. Cancer 1994; 73:2687–2690.

24. Shimizu Y, Tukagoshi H, Fujita M, Hosokawa M, Kato M, Asaka M. Metachronous squamous cell carcinoma of the esophagus arising after endoscopic mucosal resection. Gastrointest Endosc 2001; 54:190–194.

25. Watanabe A, Hosokawa M, Taniguchi M, Sasaki S. Periodic pharyngolaryngoscopy detects early head and neck cancer and improves survival in esophageal cancer. Ann Thorac Surg 2003; 76:1699–1705.

26. Shimizu Y, Tukagoshi H, Fujita M, Hosokawa M, Kato M, Asaka M. Endoscopic screening for early esophageal cancer by iodine staining in patients with other current or prior primary cancers. Gastrointest Endosc 2001; 53:1–5.

27. Larsson LG, Sandstrom A, Westling P. Relationship of Plummer-Vinson disease to cancer of the upper alimentary tract in Sweden. Cancer Res 1975; 35:3308–3316.

28. Brown LM, Hoover RN, Silverman DT, et al. Excess Incidence of Squamous Cell Esophageal Cancer among US Black Men: Role of Social Class and Other Risk Factors. Am J Epidemiol 2001; 153:114–122.

29. Munoz N, Victora CG, Crespi M, Saul C, Braga NM, Correa P. Hot mate drinking and precancerous lesions of the esophagus: an endoscopic survey in southern Brazil. Int J Cancer 1987; 39:708–709.

30. Castelletto R, Castellsague X, Munoz N, Iscovich J, Chopita N, Jmelnitsky A. Alcohol, tobacco, diet, mate drinking, and esophageal cancer in Argentina. Cancer Epidemiol Biomarkers Prev 1994; 3:557–564.

31. Castellsague X, Munoz N, De Stefani E, Victora CG, Castelletto R, Rolon PA. Influence of mate drinking, hot beverages and diet on esophageal cancer risk in South America. Int J Cancer 2000; 88:658–664.

32. Meijssen MAC, Tilanus HW, van Blankenstein M, Hop WCJ, Ong GL. Achalasia compicated by oesophageal squamous cell carcinoma: a prospective study in 195 patients. Gut 1992; 33:155–158.

33. Sandler RS, Nyren O, Ekbom A, Eisen GM, Yuen J, Josefsson S. The risk of esophageal cancer in patients with achalasia: a population-based study. JAMA 1995; 274:1359–1362.

34. Risk JM, Field EA, Field JK, et al. Tylosis esophageal cancer mapped. Nat Genet 1994; 8:319–321 (Letter).

35. Lind L, Lundstrom A, Hofer PA, Holmgren G. The gene for diffuse palmoplantar keratoderma of the type found in northern Sweden is localized to chromosome 12q11-q13. Hum Mol Genet 1994; 3:1789–1793.

36. Maillefer RH, Greydanus MP. To B or not to B: is tylosis B truly benign? Am J Gastroenterol 1999; 94:829–834.

37. Clarke CA, Howel-Evans W, McConnell RB, Sheppard PM. Carcinoma of oesophagus in assocation with tylosis. Br Med J 1959; 2:1100.

38. Ahsan H, Neugut AI. Radiation Therapy for Breast Cancer and Increased Risk for Esophageal Carcinoma. Ann Intern Med 1998; 128:114–117.

39. Scully C, el-Kom M. Lichen planus: review and update on pathogenesis. J Oral Pathol 1985; 14:431–458.

40. Gumber SC, Chopra S. Hepatitis C: a multifaceted disease. Review of extrahepatic manifestations. Ann Intern Med 1995; 123:615–620.

41. Eisen D. The clinical features, malignant potential, and systemic associations of oral lichen planus: a study of 723 patients. J Am Acad Dermatol 2002; 46:207–214.

42. Calabrese C, Fabbri A, Marco B, et al. Squamous cell carcinoma arising in esophageal lichen planus. Gastrointest Endosc 2003; 57:596–599.

43. Jacobson BC, Hirota W, Baron TH, Leighton JA, Faigel DO. The role of endoscopy in the assessment and treatment of esophageal cancer. Gastrointest Endosc 2003; 57:817–822.

44. Winawer S, Sherlock P, Belladonna J, Melamed M, Beattie E. Endoscopic brush cytology in esophageal cancer. JAMA 1975; 232:1358.

45. Zargar S, Khuroo M, Jan G, Mahajan R, Shah P. Prospective comparison of the value of brushings before and after biopsy in the endoscopic diagnosis of gastroesophageal malignancy. Acta Cytol 1991; 35:549–552.

46. Anonymous. Technology status evaluation report. High resolution and high-magnification endoscopy. Gastrointest Endosc 2000; 52:864–866.

47. Stevens PD, Lightdale CJ, Green PH, Siegel LM, Garcia-Carrasquillo RJ, Rotterdam H. Combined magnification endoscopy with chromoendoscopy for the evaluation of Barrett's esophagus. Gastrointest Endosc 1994; 40:747–749.

48. Kiesslich R, Hahn M, Herrmann G, Jung M. Screening for specialized columnar epithelium with methylene blue: chromoendoscopy in patients with Barrett's esophagus and a normal control group. Gastrointest Endosc 2001; 53:47–52.

49. Siegel LM, Stevens PD, Lightdale CJ, et al. Combined magnification endoscopy with chromoendoscopy in the evaluation of patients with suspected malabsorption. Gastrointest Endosc 1997; 46:226–230.

50. Fleischer DE. Chromoendoscopy and magnification endoscopy in the colon. Gastrointest Endosc 1999; 49:S45–49.

51. Takayama T, Katsuki S, Takahashi Y, et al. Aberrant crypt foci of the colon as precursors of adenoma and cancer. N Engl J Med 1998; 339:1277–1284.

52. Inoue H, Rey J, Lightdale C. Lugol chromoendoscopy for esophageal squamous cell cancer. Endoscopy 2001; 33:75–79.

53. Sugimachi K, Kitamura K, Baba K, Ikebe M, Kuwano H. Endoscopic diagnosis of early carcinoma of the esophagus using Lugol's solution. Gastrointest Endosc 1992; 38:657–661.

54. Falk G, Rice T, Goldblum J, Richter J. Jumbo biopsy forceps protocol still misses unsuspected cancer in Barrett's esophagus with high-grade dysplasia. Gastrointest Endosc 1999; 49:170–176.

55. Montgomery E, Bronner M, Goldblum J, et al. Reproducibility of the diagnosis of dysplasia in Barrett's esophagus: a reaffirmation. Hum Pathol 2001; 32:368–378.

56. Alikhan M, Rex D, Khan A, Rahmani E, Cummings O, Ulbright T. Variable pathologic interpretation of columnar lined esophagus by general pathologists in community practice. Gastrointest Endosc 1999; 50:23–26.

57. Jacobson BC, Van Dam J. Endoscopic detection of esophageal dysplasia and neoplasia. In: Kelloff GJ, Hawk ET, Sigman CC, eds. Strategies for Cancer Prevention, vol. 2. Totowa: Humana Press, 2005; pp. 343–352.

58. Zuccaro G, Gladkova N, Vargo J, et al. Optical coherence tomography of the esophagus and proximal stomach in health and disease. Am J Gastroenterol 2001; 96:2633–2639.

59. Georgakoudi I, Jacobson BC, Van Dam J, et al. Fluorescence, reflectance, and light-scattering spectroscopy for evaluating dysplasia in patients with Barrett's esophagus. Gastroenterology 2001; 120: 1620–1629.

60. Poneros J, Brand S, Bouma B, Tearney G, Compton C, Nishioka N. Diagnosis of specialized intestinal metaplasia by optical coherence tomography. Gastroenterology 2001; 120:7–12.

61. Ban S, Toyonaga A, Harada H, Ikejiri N, Tanikawa K. Iodine staining for early endoscopic detection of esophageal cancer in alcoholics. Endoscopy 1998; 30:253–257.

62. Atabek U, Mohit-Tabatabai M, Rush BF, Ohanian M, Rovelli P. Impact of esophageal screening in patients with head and neck cancer. Am Surgeon 1990; 56:289–292.

63. Fagundes RB, de Barros SGS, Putten ACK, et al. Occult dysplasia is disclosed by Lugol chromoendoscopy in alcoholics at high risk for squamous cell carcinoma of the esophagus. Endoscopy 1999; 31:281–285.

64. Ina H, Shibuya H, Ohashi I, Kitagawa M. The frequency of a concomitant early esophageal cancer in male patients with oral and oropharyngeal cancer: Screening results using Lugol dye endoscopy. Cancer 1994; 73:2038–2041.

65. Muto M, Hironaka S, Nakane M, Boku N, Ohtsu A, Yoshida S. Association of multiple Lugol-voiding lesions with synchronous and metachronous esophageal squamous cell carcinoma in patients with head and neck cancer. Gastrointest Endosc 2002; 56:517–521.

66. Petit T, Georges C, Jung G-M, et al. Systematic esophageal endoscopy screening in patients previously treated for head and neck squamous-cell carcinoma. Ann Oncol 2001; 12:643–646.

67. Shiozaki H, Tahara H, Kobayashi K, et al. Endoscopic screening of early esophageal cancer with the Lugol dye method in patients with head and neck cancers. Cancer 1990; 66:2068–2071.

68. Scherubl H, von Lampe B, Faiss S, et al. Screening for oesophageal neoplasia in patients with head and neck cancer. Br J Cancer 2002; 86:239–243.

69. Meyer V, Burtin P, Bour B, et al. Endoscopic detection of early esophageal cancer in a high-risk population: does Lugol staining improve videoendoscopy? Gastrointest Endosc 1997; 45:480–484.

70. Tincani AJ, Brandalise N, Altemani A, et al. Diagnosis of superficial esophageal cancer and dysplasia using endoscopic screening with a 2% Lugol dye solution in patients with head and neck cancer. Head Neck 2000; 22:170–174.

71. Yokoyama A, Muramatsu T, Ohmori T, et al. Multiple primary esophageal and concurrent upper aerodigestive tract cancer and the aldehyde dehydrogenase-2 genotype of Japanese alcoholics. Cancer 1996; 77:1986–1990.

72. Soetikno RM, Gotoda T, Nakanishi Y, Soehendra N. Endoscopic mucosal resection. Gastrointest Endosc 1003; 57:567–579.

73. AJCC. AJCC Cancer Staging Manual, Sixth Edition. New York: Springer-Verlag; 2002.

3   Image Enhancement Endoscopy

Stephan M. Wildi, md and Michael B. Wallace, md, mph

Contents

1. INTRODUCTION TO ENHANCED ENDOSCOPY

1.1. BEYOND STANDARD WHITE LIGHT IMAGING

Endoscopy altered the practice of gastroenterology by providing nonoperative access to the gastrointestinal (GI) tract and the pancreaticobiliary system. The detection of microscopic and biochemical changes within the mucosa and submucosa, however, has remained beyond the realm of routine endoscopy. Distinguishing hyperplastic from neoplastic polyps, differentiating malignant from benign ulcers, and detecting mucosal dysplasia in patients with inflammatory bowel disease or Barrett's esophagus (BE) remains within the purview of the GI pathologist. In particular, endoscopic detection of dysplasia relies on the recognition of visible lesions (e.g., adenomatous polyps, dysplasia-associated lesion, or mass), or random sampling of tissue (biopsy). Endoscopy alone can neither reliably detect regions of invisible or flat dysplasia nor distinguish dysplasia from nondysplastic changes within visible lesions. Histological examination of the excised material is required to diagnose and locate dysplasia. Random biopsy techniques are subject to sampling errors and increased risk because of long procedure time and multiple biopsy sites. In patients with inflammatory bowel disease, it has been estimated that a total of 33 and 56 biopsy specimens are required for a 90 and 95% confidence to detect dysplasia or carcinoma (1). Although the microscopic examination of tissue remains the gold standard for pathological assessment, it is not without its limitations. Histopathological diagnosis of dysplasia often relies on the observation of particular features of the overall tissue morpho-logy and the morphometry of specific cellular organelles, such as the nucleus. Although the gross and microscopic appearance of dysplasia in different organs and different types of epithelium can vary

significantly, nuclear morphological features are common to all types of dysplasia. Based on these features, nonpolypoid lesions are categorized as nondysplastic, indefinite for dysplasia, or low- or high-grade dysplasia (2). Polypoid lesions are classified as nondysplastic lesions (hyperplastic and inflammatory) and dysplastic lesions (tubular, tubulovillous, villous adenoma, or invasive carcinoma) (3). The histopathological diagnosis of dysplasia is problematic because there is poor interobserver agreement on the classification of a particular specimen, even among expert GI pathologists (4,5). One reason for such variation may be the subjective nature of determining increased nuclear size, nuclear crowding, or architectural disorganization (2,6). The biochemical changes that take place during the development of neoplastic lesions are not typically considered during histopathological diagnosis, because cutting and processing of tissue before examination likely alters its biochemical state. As a result, potentially significant information is lost in this type of analysis.

New optically based endoscopic technologies have the potential to overcome many of these limitations by rapidly and safely evaluating wide regions for dysplasia or other pathological changes without requiring excision of the tissue. The term used for many of these techniques is "optical biopsy." This chapter reviews the different emerging technologies that hold the promise for an "optical biopsy."

1.2. OVERVIEW OF TECHNOLOGIES

"Image-enhanced endoscopy" encompasses different technologies exploiting previously unused properties of light and implies the ability to make clinical diagnoses without removing tissue.

1.2.1. Point-Probe Spectroscopic Technologies

Spectroscopy follows the same principle by objectively quantifying the color and brightness of light. Most spectroscopic techniques are initially developed and tested using optical-fiber probes. These probes have several advantages including ease of passage through the accessory channel of

From: *Endoscopic Oncology: Gastrointestinal Endoscopy and Cancer Management.* Edited by: D. O. Faigel and M. L. Kochman © Humana Press, Totowa, NJ

standard diagnostic endoscopes. Although many types of point-probe spectroscopy have been applied for examining GI disease, the three that have been used for examining dysplasia are *laser-induced fluorescence spectroscopy, reflectance spectroscopy*, and *light-scattering spectroscopy*.

1.2.2. Imaging Technologies

Imaging technologies enable the screening of larger surface areas of the mucosa and therefore allow taking optical-guided biopsies owing to selective characteristics of malignant tissue. The clinically most promising techniques are *chromoendoscopy, high-resolution and high-magnification endoscopy, fluorescence imaging with or without exogenous fluorophores*, and *narrow band making*.

1.2.3. Optical Coherence Tomography

Endoscopic optical coherence tomography (OCT) is a method that provides two-dimensional cross-sectional images of the GI tract. OCT measures the magnitude and echo time delay of single-scattered light waves. OCT is analogous to ultrasound imaging, but uses infrared light waves instead of acoustic waves. Compared with high-frequency ultrasonography, this results in 10-fold higher resolution.

1.2.4. Investigational Methods in Development

Preliminary reports of new techniques have been published recently. Some of them have been investigated in small number of patients. All of them need further investigation to demonstrate feasibility and diagnostic accuracy. The most promising developments are *activatable fluorescent imaging probes* (*molecular beacons*), *confocal microscopy, Raman spectroscopy*, and *immunoscopy*.

1.3. LIMITATIONS OF NEW IMAGING TECHNOLOGIES

A major question is whether these optical detection techniques will be good enough to be used in large-scale surveillance programs. Sensitivity should exceed 90%, and specificity, even in the presence of inflammation, should be high. These new imaging techniques have to be simple, fast, and easy to learn. Interobserver variability should be equal to or better than the current gold standard, the assessment of the histology by the pathologist. To date, none of the new techniques fulfills all of these requirements. Furthermore, in the increasingly restrictive reimbursement environment, it will be critical to establish the cost-effectiveness of these new technologies to integrate them into daily practice. In summary, there are as yet insufficient data to recommend the routine use of these new technologies. But all these new imaging technologies are still in their infancy, and there is room for improvement.

2. POINT-PROBE SPECTROSCOPIC METHODS

When performing endoscopy, light emitted from the endoscope's light source is reflected back from the luminal GI tract to optical fibers or charged-coupled devices (CCDs) and projected onto video monitors. During each procedure, the endoscopist can evaluate indirectly the color and brightness of the GI tract and thereby distinguish normal mucosa from abnormal tissue. Spectroscopy follows the same principle by objectively quantifying the color and brightness of light. This information can be used to detect changes that are too fine or outside the spectrum (UV or infrared) to be noticed by the normal eye. Many aspects of spectroscopy offer advantages over standard histopathology. By providing a more quantitative measure of features, such as nuclear size and number, or changes in collagen, porphyrin, or tryptophan concentrations, spectroscopy may enhance the current qualitative measures used in pathological diagnosis. Different spectroscopic techniques can be used to provide information about tissue biochemistry and oxygenation. Light of any source directed toward a mucosal surface may undergo one of the following interactions by the physical properties of light and tissue:

1. Reflection by the tissue, as it occurs when the endoscopist visualizes the mucosa by the fiberoptic or video endoscopy.
2. Absorption by the tissue and conversion to another form of energy such as heat.
3. Absorption by the tissue and re-emission as another wavelength (color) of light. This last property is referred to as fluorescence.

Finally, photons of light can be scattered within the tissue and return (termed "backscattering") or they can transmitted through the tissue.

Spectroscopic systems require an excitation light source and a detector or spectrometer to analyze the light that returns from the tissue. For reflectance spectroscopy and light-scattering spectroscopy, standard white light lamps such as Xenon flash lamps are used. For laser-induced autofluorescence spectroscopy, light of a single color (monochromatic light) is used to excite the tissue. Monochromatic light is best achieved by laser light, although light of a narrow range of wavelengths can also be produced by filtered white light.

Most spectroscopic techniques are initially developed and tested using optical-fiber probes. These probes have several advantages including ease of passage through the accessory channel of standard diagnostic endoscopes and highly predictable geometry between fibers that provide the source of light and those that deliver collected light to the detector. These factors make point probes highly suitable for research and technology development; however, they are limited by the small surface are they examine at the tip of the probe. Other spectroscopic methods, which use modified fiberoptic endoscopes or video-endoscopes to create fluorescence images of GI mucosa, are summarized later in this chapter.

Although many types of point-probe spectroscopy have been applied for examining GI disease, the three that have been used for examining dysplasia are laser-induced fluorescence spectroscopy, reflectance spectroscopy, and light-scattering spectroscopy.

2.1. DIFFUSE REFLECTANCE SPECTROSCOPY

Reflectance spectroscopy measures quantitatively the color and intensity of reflected light. Unlike autofluorescence spectroscopy, the reflected light always maintains the same wavelength, although different wavelengths are absorbed and reflected to different degrees. A typical example is provided by hemoglobin. When illuminated with white light, oxygenated hemoglobin absorbs much of the blue light, and reflects

Table 1
Common Fluorophores in GI Tissue

Fluorophores	Peak excitation (nm)	Peak emission (nm)
NADH	340	470
FAD	460	520
Collagen	335	390
Porphyrin	390	630–680
Elastin	285	350
Tryptophan	305	340

back only the red light, giving blood its characteristic color. Deoxygenated hemoglobin absorbs a higher degree of red light, thus appears bluer when illuminated with white light. Reflectance spectroscopy thus provides information about tissue hemoglobin concentrations and oxygenation status. Because of the property of malignant tissue to promote angiogenesis, reflectance spectroscopy may be capable of detecting neoplastic tissue based on hemoglobin absorption parameters.

2.2. LASER- OR LIGHT-INDUCED FLUORESCENCE SPECTROSCOPY

All tissues exhibit endogenous fluorescence (autofluorescence) when exposed to light of a certain wavelength. Fluorescence is based on the principle that certain molecules of GI cells, called fluorophores, emit light when stimulated by light (excitation). During this process energy is transferred to the molecule, hence the wavelength of the emitted light is longer (lower energy) than the excitation wavelength. Among the most relevant fluorophores in the GI tract are the reduced form of NADH, flavin adenine dinucleotide (FADH$_2$), collagen, porphyrins, and tryptophan. Each of these fluorophores has its characteristic excitation and emission spectrum (Table 1). The success of autofluorescence spectroscopy as a technique for detecting dysplastic changes is based on the observation that the development of dysplasia is accompanied by modification in the biochemical composition of tissue and consequently changes of the concentration of certain fluorophores. Autofluorescence of tissue is induced by monochromatic light, mostly generated by lasers, or by filtered white light. Typically, dye lasers or more recently less expensive diode lasers are used to induce tissue autofluorescence.

In contrast to endogenous fluorophores, exogenous fluorophores might give better results in discriminating tissue. Exogenous fluorophores are specifically retained in neoplastic tissue and exhibit an induced fluorescence signal of much higher intensity. Among different sensitizers the group of porphyrins has been best studied for application in fluorescence spectroscopy. The major limitation of exogenous sensitization with porphyrins is their photosensitizing property with prolonged skin photosensitivity. Newer agents with shorter half-life are more promising (e.g., 5-aminolaevulinic acid [5-ALA]).

One major difficulty in measuring fluorescence spectra is the background generated by scattering and absorption. To remove these distortions, some investigators analyzed the fluorescence spectra in combination with information from the corresponding reflectance spectra, which allows "subtraction" of this background to leave "intrinsic fluorescence."

2.3. MULTIEXCITATION FLUORESCENCE SPECTROSCOPY

Different fluorophores are excited by different wavelengths of light. The optimal excitation wavelength for detecting dysplasia and discriminating dysplasia from nondysplastic or normal mucosa remains unknown. A significant technical advance in fluorescence spectroscopy was made with the development of a fast multiexcitation system capable of exciting the tissue with up to 11 different wavelengths in less than 1 s (Fig. 1) (7,8). The excitation light source of this rapid multiexcitation system pumps 10 dye cuvets precisely mounted on a rapidly rotating wheel. In this manner, 11 different excitation wavelengths are obtained and delivered to the optical-fiber probe.

2.4. TIME-RESOLVED FLUORESCENCE SPECTROSCOPY

In addition to specific excitation and emission wavelengths, different fluorophores fade or decay their fluorescence at different rates. Hence, the difference between normal and abnormal tissue can be enhanced by measuring fluorescence at different times (often measured in nanoseconds) after excitation. This technique, termed "time-resolved fluorescence," has been used to increase the accuracy of detecting dysplasia in BE (9) and of distinguishing adenomas from nonadenomas in the colon (10).

2.5. LIGHT-SCATTERING SPECTROSCOPY

Light propagation in tissue is governed by elastic scattering and absorption. Light-scattering spectroscopy measures the extent to which the angular paths of the photons of light are altered by structures (scatterers) they encounter. Like a steel ball in a pinball machine, photons encounter many structures in their way and bounce forward, backward, up, down, and sideways. The scattering in tissue depends on the scatterer's size, the number of the scatterers, and on the wavelength of the incident light. The primary scattering centers are thought to be a collagen fiber network of the extracellular matrix, the mitochondria, cell nuclei, and other intracellular structures. By mathematical modeling, the number, size, and optical density of cellular structures (such as nuclei) can be determined by measuring the diffuse reflected light from epithelial surfaces (11). This phenomenon has been exploited during endoscopic procedures to determine the number of nuclei, the size of nuclei, and the degree of crowding of nuclei in patients with dysplastic changes in BE, colon polyps, bladder, and oral cavity (7,12,13). Unlike fluorescence, light-scattering spectroscopy uses a broad range of light, such as white light, to detect changes over the entire visible spectrum.

2.6. TRIMODAL SPECTROSCOPY

Reflectance spectroscopy, laser-induced autofluorescence spectroscopy, and light-scattering spectroscopy provide quantitative information that characterizes either biochemical or morphological aspects of tissue that can be significantly altered during development of neoplasia. The ability to characterize dysplastic and nondysplastic tissue is improved by combining the information provided by each of the spectroscopic techniques, obtained simultaneously with one system (Fig. 1), an approach that was named *trimodal spectroscopy*. When spectroscopic classification is consistent with at least two of the three analysis methods, high-grade dysplasia is identified with very high sensitivity and specificity.

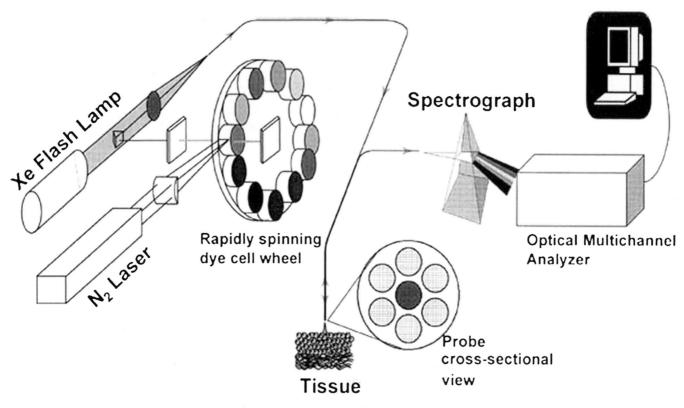

Fig. 1. Diagram of device for collection of trimodal spectroscopy (fluorescence, reflectance, and light scattering). The dye wheel allows for excitation at multiple wavelengths in order to stimulate fluorescence of a wide range of molecules. The Xenon (X2) flash lamp is use as a white light source for both reflectance and light scattering.

2.7. CLINICAL EXPERIENCE WITH POINT-PROBE SPECTROSCOPY

Different authors have investigated the use of spectroscopy in the detection of neoplastic changes in the esophagus (Table 2). Light-induced autofluorescence spectroscopy *(14,15)* and laser-induced autofluorescence spectroscopy *(16–19)*, laser-induced fluorescence spectroscopy with exogenous fluorophores *(20,21)*, light-scattering spectroscopy *(7,13)*, and trimodal spectroscopy *(7)* were evaluated. Light- and laser-induced fluorescence has been used for the detection of premalignant lesions in the colon (Table 3). Some authors investigated the role of spectroscopy in distinguishing between normal colonic mucosa and adenomatous tissue *(10,22–24)*, others included also dysplastic adenomas and adenocarcinoma in their evaluation *(25–27)*. There is very limited data regarding point-probe spectroscopy for the detection of dysplasia in inflammatory bowel disease. There are different GI tissues, which could be efficiently investigated by spectroscopy techniques. Screening or surveillance of other forms of dysplasia such as ampullary dysplasia in patients with familiar polyposis, intraductal papillary mucinous tumor (IPMT) of the pancreas, dysplasia in hereditary pancreatic cancer, may also be helpful. Thus far, there is only minimal data in patients with neoplastic changes in the stomach *(14)*.

3. IMAGING TECHNOLOGIES

Point-probe spectroscopy is limited in the way tissue is sampled by point measurement. Although theoretically, numerous samples can be taken, this seems unpractical, and sampling error is likely to occur. In contrast to the point-probe technologies, imaging technologies enables the screening of larger surface areas of the mucosa and therefore allows taking optical-guided biopsies owing to selective characteristics of malignant tissue. The clinically most promising techniques are *chromoendoscopy, high-resolution and high-magnification endoscopy, fluorescence imaging with or without exogenous fluorophores,* and *narrow band imaging (NBI)*.

3.1. CHROMOENDOSCOPY
3.1.1. Technology

Chromoendoscopy is a very simple and widely used technique for enhancing mucosal detail by spraying a variety of colored solutions. Agents used for chromoendoscopy are categorized according their working principle. The stains are mainly vital dyes (Lugol's solution, methylene blue, and toluidine blue) or contrast agents (indigo carmine and dilute acetic acid solution). Lugol's solution is absorbed by glycogen-containing, nonkeratinized squamous epithelium. Lugol's stained tissue will characteristically turn green-brown (Fig. 2). Any condition that depletes glycogen, including inflammation, dysplasia, and early-stage cancer, will result in an absence of uptake of the dye. The most widely accepted use of Lugol's solution currently involves detection of squamous cell dysplasia and carcinoma of the esophagus in high-risk patients. Methylene blue dye is taken up by the cytoplasm or absorptive cells such as the normal epithelial cells of the colon and small intestine. It also stains the intestinal metaplasia that is pathognomonic for BE (Fig. 3). It will not stain nonabsorptive

Table 2
Accuracy of Spectroscopy for Barrett's Dysplasia

Author	Setting	Patients (n)	Specimen (n)	Technique	Sensitivity	Specificity
Panjehpour et al. (16)	Normal esophagus vs esophageal cancer	32	134	Laser-induced autofluorescence spectroscopy	100%	98%
Von-Dinh et al. (18)	Normal esophagus vs esophageal cancer	48	>200	Laser-induced autofluorescence spectroscopy	n.c.	n.c.
Stael von Holstein et al. (20)	Normal esophagus vs BE vs esophageal cancer (in vitro)	7	145	Laser-induced fluorescence spectroscopy (Photofrin)	n.c.	n.c.
Mayinger et al. (14)	Normal esophagus vs esophageal cancer	11		Light-induced autofluorescence spectroscopy	n.c.	n.c.
Vo-Dinh et al. (19)	Normal esophagus vs BE or vs esophageal carcinoma	70	114	Laser-induced autofluorescence spectroscopy	n.c.	n.c.
Panjehpour et al. (17)	Nondysplastic BE vs BE with HGD	36	308	Laser-induced autofluorescence spectroscopy	n.c.	96%
	BE with LGD vs BE with HGD	36	308	Laser-induced autofluorescence spectroscopy	n.c.	100%
	Nondysplastic BE and LGD vs LGD with focal HGD	36	308	Laser-induced autofluorescence spectroscopy	28%	n.c.
	Non-dysplastic BE and LGD vs HGD	36	308	Laser-induced autofluorescence spectroscopy	90%	n.c.
Bourg-Heckly et al. (15)	Normal esophagus and BE vs dysplastic BE and cancer	24	218	Light-induced autofluorescence spectroscopy	86%	95%
Wallace et al. (13)	Nondysplastic BE vs dysplastic BE	13	76	Light-scattering	90%	90%
Georgakoudi et al. (7)	Nondysplastic BE vs dysplastic BE	16	40	Trimodal spectroscopy	93%	100%
	Nondysplastic BE and LGD vs BE with HGD	16	40	Trimodal spectroscopy	100%	100%
Brand et al. (21)	Nondysplastic BE vs BE with HGD	20	97	Laser-induced fluorescence spectroscopy (5-ALA)	77%	71%
Ortner et al. (9)	Nondysplastic BE vs dysplastic BE	53	141	Time-resolved fluorescence spectroscopy (5-ALA)	76%	63%

BE, Barrett's esophagus; HGD, high-grade dysplasia; LGD, low-grade dysplasia.

Table 3
Accuracy of Spectroscopy for Colonic Dysplasia

Author	Setting	Patients (n)	Specimen (n)	Technique	Sensitivity	Specificity
Kapadia et al. (22)	Normal colon vs nondysplastic adenoma (in vitro)		50	Laser-induced autofluorescence spectroscopy	100%	100%
Marchesini et al. (25)	Normal colon vs adenoma/carcinoma (in vitro)	45	78	Light-induced autofluorescence spectroscopy	81%	91%
	Normal colon vs adenoma (in vitro)	45	59	Light-induced autofluorescence spectroscopy	88%	95%
	Normal colon vs carcinoma (in vitro)	45	61	Light-induced autofluorescence spectroscopy	58%	93%
	Adenoma vs carcinoma (in vitro)	45	36	Light-induced autofluorescence spectroscopy	58%	77%
Cothren et al. (23)	Normal colon/hyperplastic polyps vs adenoma	20	67	Laser-induced autofluorescence spectroscopy	100%	97%
Schomacker et al. (24)	Hyperplastic polyp vs adenoma	49	84	Laser-induced autofluorescence spectroscopy	86%	80%
Cothren et al. (26)	Nondysplastic colon vs dysplastic adenoma	23	88	Laser-induced autofluorescence spectroscopy	90%	95%
Mycek et al. (10)	Nonadenomatous polyps vs adenoma	17	24	Time-resolved autofluorescence spectroscopy	85%	91%
Eker et al. (27)	Normal colon vs nondysplastic adenoma	40		Laser-induced autofluorescence spectroscopy and fluorescence spectroscopy (5-ALA) at 337 nm	100%	96%
	Normal colon vs nondysplastic adenoma		16	Laser-induced autofluorescence spectroscopy at 405 nm	20%	82%
	Normal colon vs nondysplastic adenoma		26	Laser-induced fluorescence spectroscopy (5-ALA) at 405 nm	89%	94%
	Normal colon vs nondysplastic adenoma		18	Laser-induced autofluorescence spectroscopy at 436 nm	50%	86%
	Normal colon vs nondysplastic adenoma		23	Laser-induced fluorescence spectroscopy (5-ALA) at 436 nm	86%	100%

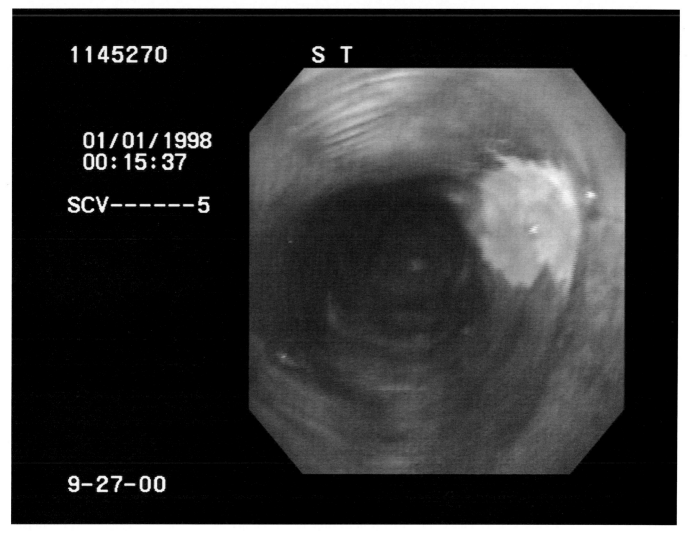

Fig. 2. Lugol's iodine staining of the esophagus showing a focus on nonstaining. Biopsies of the unstained area revealed squamous cell carcinoma. The normal squamous esophagus stains a rich chocolate brown-green color.

normal epithelium of the stomach as is found in the cardia and fundus, or normal squamous mucosa of the esophagus. Methylene blue has been successfully used to aid in the identification of gastricintestinal metaplasia and early gastric cancer, and to highlight subtle mucosal changes in the small intestine and colon. Contrast stains like indigo carmine are not absorbed but accumulate in pits and valleys between cells highlighting mucosal architecture. Most of its reported use has been to detect diminutive, flat and depressed lesions in the colon. All the stains are usually sprayed with specially designed catheters can be ingested or given as enemas. To prepare the mucosa for optimal staining and clear it from mucus it is first washed with a mucolytic agent (*N*-acetylcysteine). The effects of these stains can be visualized either by conventional white light endoscopes or by video endoscopes with image enhancement, or high-power magnification. Therefore, chromoendoscopy is often used in combination with high-resolution and high-magnification endoscopy. Chromoendoscopy has been used in several regions of the GI tract, including the esophagus, stomach, duodenum, and colon, to aid the characterization of multiple disease states.

3.1.2. Clinical Experience With Chromoendoscopy

Chromoendoscopy with Lugol's solution has been used to determine the extent of BE *(28–30)*, and to screen for squamous esophageal cancer in high-risk populations *(31–34)*. Lugol's solution has been shown to be effective to help delineate the squamocolumnar junction as well concerns in identifying residual areas of columnar epithelium after segments of Barrett's epithelium, which have been ablated *(30)*. It is particularly useful when techniques such as endoscopic mucosal resection are applied with curative intention *(29)*. Other investigators found that chromoendoscopy using Lugol's solution significantly increases the accuracy of the endoscopic diagnosis of BE *(28)*. Lugol's solution also has been used to detect endoscopy negative reflux disease in combination with high-resolution endoscopy *(35)*.

Chromoendoscopy with methylene blue has been used to screen for colonic neoplasia *(36,37)*, to diagnose BE *(38–41)*, and to screen for areas of precursor lesions and carcinoma in the stomach *(42,43)*. Chromoendoscopy utilizing methylene blue was first described for the diagnosis of early-stage cancer *(42)*. It was used to detect intestinal metaplasia within the

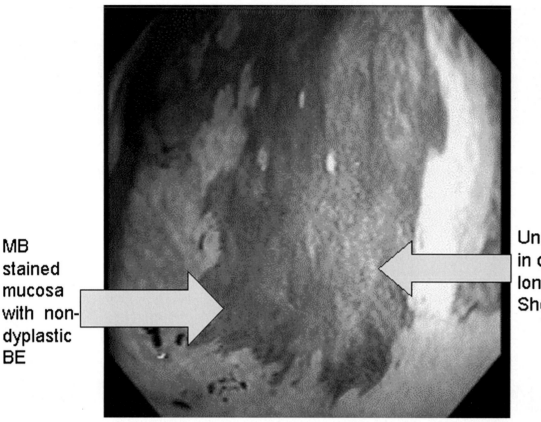

MB
stained
mucosa
with non-
dyplastic
BE

Unstained mucosa
in diffusely staining
long BE; biopsies
Showed HGD.

Fig. 3. Methylene blue staining of dysplastic BE. The nondysplastic columnar epithelium stains blue. Within the regions of blue are areas of relative nonstaining. Biopsies of these regions confirmed high-grade dysplasia. The squamous tissue is also unstained but readily distinguishable from the columnar tissue. (Kindly provided by Dr. Marcia Canto.)

stomach, which is considered to be a precursor lesion of gastric cancer (43). Several investigators found that staining with methylene blue has a sensitivity and specificity of 95–98% and 61–97%, respectively, to detect intestinal metaplasia in the distal esophagus (38,40). Other studies have not shown a significant benefit of methylene blue staining in the identification of intestinal metaplasia (44,45). Unfortunately, the staining of dysplastic epithelium, above all low-grade dysplasia, seems to be much more variable and operator-dependent. Methylene blue was also used to differentiate between small hyperplastic polyps and adenomas in the colon (36) and to diagnose flat adenomas and carcinomas of the colon (37).

Chromoendoscopy with indigo carmine has been used to diagnose BE (46,47), and to investigate polypoid and nonpolypoid lesions in the colon (48,49). Investigators found that by spraying with indigo carmine and the use of a conventional, nonmagnifying colonoscope the diagnosis of flat and depressed lesions increased by 65% (49). It has been shown that by using indigo carmine and magnification endoscopy, patterns are detected which may suggest the presence of intestinal metaplasia and/or dysplasia.

3.2. HIGH-RESOLUTION AND HIGH-MAGNIFICATION ENDOSCOPY

3.2.1. Technology

High-resolution imaging improves the ability to discriminate detail, whereas magnification enlarges the image. Resolution is

a function of pixel density, which is determined by the video chip, or CCD of the endoscope. By incorporating high-pixel CCDs, minute lesions will be more likely discriminated and detected. Conventional video-endoscopes are equipped with CCD chips of 100–400 K individual pixels. Endoscopes with 850 K pixel density are referred to as high-resolution endoscopes. Magnifying endoscopes incorporate a mechanism that allows the movement of a lens at the distal end of the insertion tube. Magnification ranges from ×1.5 to ×105, although instruments that magnify up to 35 times are satisfactory for clinical purposes. The position of the lens is changed using a knob or other device on the control section of the instrument. Both high-resolution and high-magnification endoscopes are commonly used in conjunction with chromoendoscopy.

3.2.2. Clinical Experience With High-Resolution and High-Magnification Endoscopy

In the upper GI tract, magnification and/or high-resolution endoscopy has been used to characterize BE with different staining dyes (46,47,50,51); or early gastric cancer (52,53). Different investigators have shown that specific patterns observed under magnification may help in identifying intestinal metaplasia (47,50,51). However, there are some indications that the good accuracy depends on the use of dyes (50). In the colon, magnification or high-resolution endoscopy has been used to differentiate hyperplastic from adenomatous polyps (36,48,54,55). The sensitivity and specificity was reported to be as high as 93

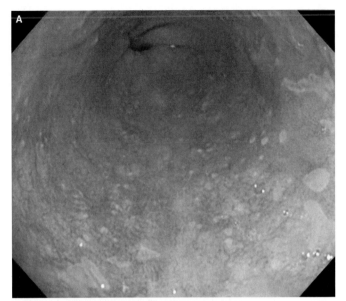

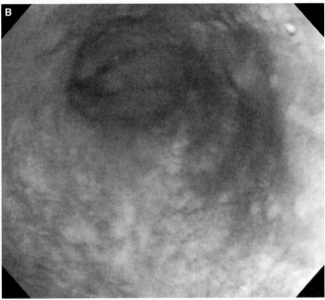

Fig. 4. **(A)** White light endoscopy view of BE with high-grade dysplasia. No over lesions are seen other than squamous islands. **(B)** Autofluorescence endoscopy (prototype endoscopy, Olympus Corp., Tokyo, Japan) showing regions of red fluorescence corresponding to histologically confirmed high grade dysplasia. (Kindly provided by Dr. Paul Fockens.)

and 95%, respectively *(36)*. A classification for the pit pattern was proposed, indicating the risk of neoplastic abnormality *(48)*. This classification has five grades. Types I and II correlate with non-neoplastic changes (e.g., hyperplastic polyps), types III and IV with adenoma and type V with invasive carcinoma. In a larger study comparing this pit pattern with histology, an accuracy of 75% was found for non-neoplastic lesions, 94% for adenomas, and 85% for carcinomas *(48)*.

3.3. FLUORESCENCE IMAGING
3.3.1. Technology
Analogous to point-probe spectroscopy, fluorescence imaging (or fluorescence endoscopy) can use the detection of autofluorescence or exogenous-induced fluorescence. But in

contrast to point-probe spectroscopy, fluorescence imaging permits full inspection of the area at risk. Fluorescence endoscopy is performed with special endoscopes, which are connected to a light source delivering white and blue light. The newer systems use blue-light excitation (400–450 nm) and two intensified CCD cameras to detect selected fluorescence emission bands in the green (490–560 nm) and in the red (630–750 nm). The two fluorescence images are combined to a composite image in real time, in which normal tissue typically appears green and abnormal tissue appears red (Fig. 4A,B). The systems can switch easily between standard white light and endoscopic fluorescence. In this way, large areas of tissue surface are screened in the blue light modus. Whenever selective fluorescence of abnormal tissue (red) appears optical-guided biopsies can be taken in the white-light modus.

Analogous to point-probe spectroscopy, fluorescence imaging can use the detection of autofluorescence or exogenously induced fluorescence. As described in the Subheading 2.2, several endogenous fluorophores can be used to detect specific autofluorescence of dysplastic or malignant tissue. The advantage of drug-induced fluorescence is that the fluorescent signal generated by these exogenous fluorophores is typically stronger than autofluorescence and can be detected by simpler and cheaper instruments. Among exogenous fluorophores, 5-ALA is the most interesting substance for fluorescence diagnosis. 5-ALA is converted intracellularly into the photoactive compound protoporphyrin IX (PPIX). PPIX is associated with a significantly higher tumor selectivity compared with other exogenous fluorophores used in fluorescence imaging (e.g., photophrin) *(56)*. Furthermore, compared with other exogenous fluorophores skin sensitivity is reduced to 24–48 h *(57,58)*.

3.3.2. Clinical Experience With Fluorescence Imaging
With the development of the fluorescence imaging systems, scientific interest concentrated mostly on the esophagus, not least because of the increasing clinical significance of BE. Other potential applications are diagnosis of dysplasia in patients with chronic inflammatory bowel disease or early recognition of preliminary stages of gastric cancer. Two different systems were used for the investigation of the GI tract: a laser-induced fluorescence endoscopy GI system (LIFE-GI and LIFE II), which uses fiber endoscopes, and a light-induced system based on the use of the exogenous fluorophores 5-ALA. Most of the studies dealing with fluorescence imaging in patients with BE investigated patients with long-segment BE. Studies of fluorescence imaging in patients with short-segment BE are lacking. Early reports showed the feasibility and usefulness of both fluorescence imaging systems in the detection of dysplasia and neoplasms in patients with BE and other GI diseases *(59,60)*. In a study of 47 patients with BE, high-grade dysplasia or carcinoma was found in 14 of 113 biopsies taken from areas that exhibited fluorescence *(58)*. High-grade dysplasia was found in only 3 of 130 fluorescence-negative biopsy specimens. Another study correctly diagnosed two cases of high-grade dysplasia and 20 cases of nondysplastic intestinal metaplasia *(61)*. However, out of eight cases with low-grade dysplasia, only five and three cases of low-grade dysplasia were correctly diagnosed by fluorescence imaging and standard white-light endoscopy, respectively. A recent study

demonstrated the good diagnostic performance of autofluorescence imaging in the detection of high-grade dysplasia in patients with known BE *(62)*. Different authors have shown conflicting results by fluorescence imaging in the detection neoplastic changes in patients with colonic neoplasms, inflammatory bowel disease and gastric cancer *(63–66)*.

3.4. NBI TECHNOLOGY

The application of filters is another, relatively simple possibility for improving image quality in endoscopy. NBI uses optical filters for red, green, and blue sequential lighting with a narrow bandwidth of spectral transmittance. Because light of shorter wavelength has very shallow penetration into the tissue and is highly absorbed by hemoglobin, blue light NBI emphasizes the image of capillary vessels on surface mucosa. The pattern produced is similar to using nonvital dyes (indigo carmine) but avoids the need for exogenous agents and variability in dose and washing techniques. The diagnosis of neoplastic changes is improved as the pit pattern of mucosa is reflected in the network pattern of capillary vessels (Fig. 5A–C). Special NBI endoscopic systems with a red-green-blue sequential illumination system are used. The light source consists of a xenon lamp and a rotation disk with three optical filters. The rotation disk and monochrome CCD are synchronized and sequentially generate images in three color bands (red, green, and blue). By using all three narrow-band images, a single color endoscopic image is synthesized by the videoprocessor.

3.4.1. Clinical Experience With NBI

This method is in its infancy and only few clinical data are available. In one study, the NBI system improved the accuracy of magnifying endoscopy for assessment of superficial esophageal lesions *(67)*. In particular, the depth of invasion was assessed more precisely by NBI. Another group has demonstrated the value of NBI in the assessment and diagnosis of BE *(68)*.

4. OPTICAL COHERENCE TOMOGRAPHY (OCT)

4.1. TECHNOLOGY

Endoscopic OCT is a method that provides two-dimensional cross-sectional images of the GI tract. OCT provides true anatomic images corresponding to the four layers of the GI tract (Fig. 6). Although the images are similar in orientation to radial endoscopic ultrasound, by using light instead of ultrasound waves, the resolution of OCT is increased to nearly 10-fold greater than high-frequency endoscopic ultrasound and approaches that of light microscopy. Like ultrasound, OCT uses an energy source to deliver a signal, light in this case, to an organ or tissue and a detector to collect the signal if or when it returns. Because light travels exponentially faster than ultrasound waves, most detectors are unable to determine precisely the time of flight of a photon. OCT overcomes this technical limitation by delivering a light signal via two separate pathways. One light beam is delivered to the tissue, and an identical light beam is delivered to a mirror, a known distance away from the detector. Using an interferometer and a property of light called coherence, only the light that returns from the tissue to the detector at the same time (and therefore the same distance) as the light delivered to the reference mirror creates an interference signal

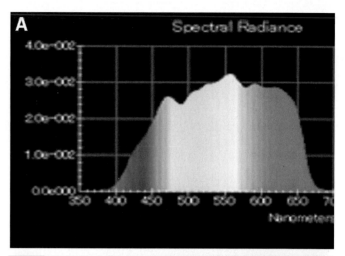

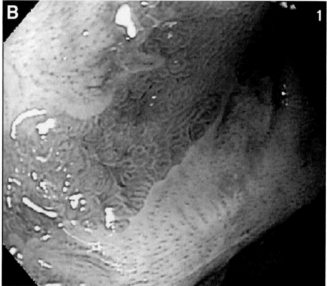

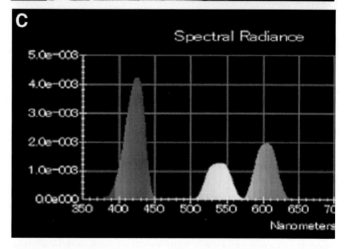

Fig. 5. In NBI, the broad-band white light (**A**) used to illuminate the tissue (**B**) is filtered into three narrow bands of light. The blue band in particular is used to image the surface pattern and blood vessels. (A color version of B appears in the color insert following p. 84.) (**C**) Image of BE with white light and NBI. Note the clear detection of mucosal cerebriform pattern suggestive of intestinal metaplasia. (Kindly provided by Hitoshi Mizuno, Olympus Corp. Japan.)

Intestinal Metaplasia

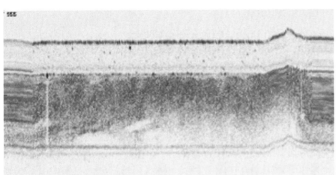 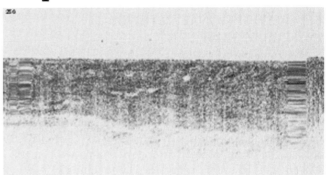

High Grade Dysplasia

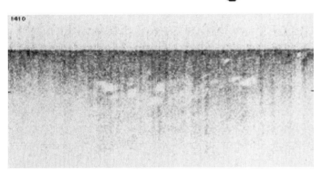 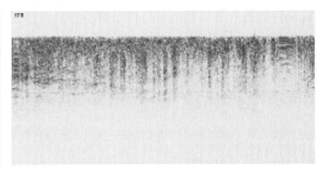

Fig. 6. OCT image of non-dysplastic and dysplastic BE. Note the homogeneity of the upper left sample. Similarly the top right sample has the homogeneity of light penetration but more irregular gland architecture. In contrast, the bottom two images have intense upper borders, irregular light penetration, high backreflection, and numerous glands. (Kindly provided by Drs. Norman Nishioka and John Evans.)

and thus is detected. By varying the distance of the reference mirror, structures of varying depth in the tissue can be imaged.

OCT is typically performed with near infrared light because tissue is relatively transparent at these frequencies. OCT uses catheters passed through the accessory channel of standard endoscopes. Radial scanning and linear scanning catheters have been described. Unlike endoscopic ultrasound, OCT can be performed through air so tissue contact or coupling is not required. Scanning depth is limited to 1–2 mm because of scattering of light by tissue. Most of the systems described achieve a resolution of about 20 μm, which is sufficient for visualizing mucosal glands, crypts, and villi but not cellular features such as nuclear dysplasia. In newer systems, a 512 by 512 pixel image can be acquired in 0.25 s; older systems required up to 45 s to scan an image.

4.2. CLINICAL EXPERIENCE WITH OCT

The first clinical publications of OCT reported on the use to image the coronary vasculature and retina (69). In the GI tract, catheter-based OCT systems were used in the endoscopic examination of the esophagus, the pancreatico-biliary tract, and the colon.

4.2.1. Esophagus

BE has been the focus of intense OCT research in the GI tract, because OCT is potentially an ideal imaging technique for endoscopic surveillance in patients with BE. A large-scale study formulated objective OCT criteria that are highly sensitive and specific for the diagnosis of specialized intestinal metaplasia (70). Loss of regular crypt-and-pit architecture of the esophageal mucosa was identified as the main OCT feature in the diagnosis of Barrett's epithelium. Two features seem to be characteristic for dysplasia and cancer: focal (dark) areas of decreased light scattering, and focal loss of mucosal structure and organization (71). Dysplasia was identified with an accuracy of 70% and a negative predictive value of 91%. Other preliminary data also suggest that OCT signals contain information that can be used to identify dysplasia within Barrett's epithelium with a high degree of accuracy (72).

4.2.2. Pancreaticobiliary Tract

OCT of the biliary system is feasible in patients with biliary pathology (73,74). Interpretable images are obtainable, but clinical use needs further assessment. As current OCT probes and processors do not yet provide optimal resolution, further generations of equipment with improved image quality are required.

4.2.3. Colon

OCT can visualize the mucosa, muscularis mucosa, and submucosa of the colon (75,76). Similar to the OCT data on esophageal cancer, the OCT image of colon cancer revealed complete loss of the normal tissue morphology (76). OCT has also the ability to differentiate adenoma from nonadenomatous polyps and normal colon mucosa (77). Other potential applications may be the surveillance of patients with longstanding inflammatory bowel disease or the diagnosis of microscopic colitis.

5. INVESTIGATIONAL METHODS IN DEVELOPMENT

5.1. CONFOCAL MICROSCOPY

Laser-scanning confocal microscopy (LCM) is a novel optical method that may be able to provide a microscopic image of mucosal surfaces. A special LCM instrument and a probe-type endomicroscope that can be passed through the working channel of an endoscope have been developed for LCM. They scan the mucosa using an argon laser beam with a wavelength of 488 nm and analyze the reflected light. An objective lens with a magnification of ×40 is mounted on the LCM instrument. Two studies have shown that the LCM images correspond well with the conventional hematoxylin–eosin light-microscopic images (78,79). Cell wall, nucleus, cytoplasm, and tissue structural elements were simultaneously visualized by LCM scanning. Further development of improved probe-type endomicroscopes is expected.

5.2. RAMAN SPECTROSCOPY

Raman spectroscopy is another form of image enhancement based on the principle that incident light can cause molecules within a tissue to vibrate and rotate. The charged molecules can resonate, emitting energy that can be measured by spectroscopy. The resulting resonance spectrum provides a molecular profile of a tissue. Raman scattering within tissue is more difficult to measure because the signal is much weaker relative to fluorescence or light scattering and is masked by a broad tissue autofluorescence background. There are only few preliminary reports for the GI tract (80,81). The prospect for a real-time endoscopic Raman imaging system remains uncertain because of the weak Raman signals and technological limitations.

5.3. IMMUNOSCOPY

Fluorescent dyes are routinely coupled to tumor-related or tumor-specific antigens for immunohistochemical staining of biopsied tissues. Recent studies in animals have demonstrated that fluorophore labeling of monoclonal antibodies produces adequate sensitivity and improved resolution (82,83). Preliminary work has been done in patients with Crohn's disease or colon cancer (84,85). To give this new technique a future, important issues need to be resolved, finding the optimal biomarkers, optimizing the relative tumor uptake, and cost and safety issues.

5.4. MOLECULAR IMAGING PROBES

One general limitation of all imaging methods is the need to increase the signal-to-noise ratio. Many of the spectroscopic and imaging methods discuss above have a relatively low signal with a large background signal (noise). One method of increasing this signal-to-noise ratio is to use contrast agents with are selectively taken up or activated by neoplastic tissue. One such example is the fluorescent molecular beacons. These agents generally contain one or two fluorescent moleculars, which are activated by a protease enzymes normally contained in neoplastic tissue. Because many neoplastic tissue have increased protease activity such as Cathepsins, there is increased activation at the site of dysplasia, and this fluorescence can be detected with simple endoscopic

imaging methods. Marten et al. (86) have demonstrated this technique to detect colon polyps in a mouse model of familial polyposis (86).

6. PRIORITIES FOR RESEARCH AND NEW DEVELOPMENT

Decades of background research and technology develop have recently led to major developments in enhanced endoscopic imaging technologies. Several of these are now nearing clinical applications, including NBI and fluorescence imaging. At the same time, many new tools are in the early stages of preclinical development, yet offer substantial promise toward the "ideal" imaging system. Key areas for active research include:

1. Clinical evaluation of NBI and autofluorescence imaging in BE and flat and polypoid colon neoplasia.
2. Development of highly sensitive, specific, and safe molecular imaging probes for GI neoplasia.
3. Improved technical performance of OCT systems for staging of early neoplasia.
4. Development of broad area imaging systems for light-scattering spectroscopy and combined modality spectroscopy techniques (light scattering, fluoresence, and reflectance).

7. CONCLUSIONS

For the past two decades, a new major advance has been developing; the ability to characterize the tissue with increasingly sophisticated technologies that provide full thickness images, biochemical characterization, and morphological images on a microscopic scale. Many of these technologies are early in development. Most are not in widespread use. None of them is yet perfected. As with fiberoptics, video imaging, and ultrasound, major advances often occur over a long period of time. It is very likely that we will continue to see major development in each of these areas of the next decade and it is predictable that 20 yr from now we look at our video-endoscopes with white light imaging, the way we now look at the first generation of fiberoptic endoscopes.

REFERENCES

1. Bachwich DR, Lichtenstein GR, Traber PG. Cancer in inflammatory bowel disease. Med Clin N Am 1994; 78:1399–1412.
2. Riddell R, Goldman H, Ransohoff DF, et al. Dysplasia in inflammatory bowel disease: Standardization classification with provisional clinical implications. Hum Pathol 1983; 14:931–968.
3. Jass JR, Sobin LH. World Health Organization: Histological typing of intestinal tumours, 2nd ed., New York: Springer-Verlag; 1989:29–41.
4. Reid BJ, Haggitt RC, Rubin CE, et al. Observer variation in the diagnosis of dysplasia in Barrett's esophagus. Hum Pathol 1988; 19:166–178.
5. Petras RE, Sivak MV, Rice TW. Barrett's esophagus. A review of the pathologists role in the diagnosis and management. Pathol Annu 1991; 26:1–232.
6. Haggit RC. Barrett's esophagus, dysplasia, and adenocarcinoma. Hum Pathol 1994; 25:982–993.
7. Georgakoudi I, Jacobson BC, Van Dam J, et al. Fluorescence, reflectance, and light-scattering spectroscopy for evaluation dysplasia in patients with Barrett's esophagus. Gastroenterology 2001; 120:1620–1629.
8. Zangaro R, Silveira L, Manoharan R. Rapid multiexcitation fluorescence spectroscopy for in vivo tissue diagnosis. Appl Optics 1996; 35:5211–5219.
9. Ortner MA, Ebert B, Hein E, et al. Time gated fluorescence spectroscopy in Barrett's esophagus. Gut 2003; 52:28–33.

10. Mycek MA, Schomacker KT, Nishioka NS. Colonic polyp differentiation using time-resolved autofluorescence spectroscopy. Gastrointest Endosc 1998; 48:390–394.

11. Perelman LT, Backman V, Wallace MB. Observation of periodic fine structure in reflectance from biological tissue: A new technique for measuring nuclear size distribution. Phys Rev Lett 1998; 80:627–630.

12. Backman V, Wallace MB, Perelman LT,MG, et al. Detection of preinvasive cancer cells. Nature 2000; 406:35–36.

13. Wallace MB, Perelman LT, Backman V, et al. Endoscopic detection of dysplasia in patients with Barrett's esophagus using light-scattering spectroscopy. Gastroenterology 2000; 119:677–682.

14. Mayinger B, Horner P, Jordan M, et al. Endoscopic fluorescence spectroscopy in the upper GI tract for the detection of GI cancer: initial experience. Am J Gastroenterol 2001; 96:2616–2621.

15. Bourg-Heckly G, Blais J, Padilla JJ, et al. Endoscopic ultraviolet-induced autofluorescence spectroscopy of the esophagus: tissue characterization and potential for early cancer diagnosis. Endoscopy 2000; 32:756–765.

16. Panjehpour M, Overholt BF, Schmidhammer JL, Farris C, Buckley PF, Vo-Dinh T. Spectroscopic diagnosis of esophageal cancer: new classification model, improved measurement system. Gastrointest Endosc 1995; 41:577–581.

17. Panjehpour M, Overholt BF, Vo-Dinh T, Haggitt RC, Edwards DH, Buckley FP. 3rd. Endoscopic fluorescence detection of high-grade dysplasia in Barrett's esophagus. Gastroenterology 1996; 111: 93–101.

18. Vo-Dinh T, Panjehpour M, Overholt BF, Farris C, Buckley FP. 3rd, Sneed R. In vivo cancer diagnosis of the esophagus using differential normalized fluorescence (DNF) indices. Lasers Surg Med 1995; 16:41–47.

19. Vo-Dinh T, Panjehpour M, Overholt BF. Laser-induced fluorescence for esophageal cancer and dysplasia diagnosis. Ann NY Acad Sci 1998; 838:116–122.

20. von Holstein CS, Nilsson AM, Andersson-Engels S, Willen R, Walther B, Svanberg K. Detection of adenocarcinoma in Barrett's oesophagus by means of laser induced fluorescence. Gut 1996; 39:711–716.

21. Brand S, Wang TD, Schomacker KT, et al. Detection of high-grade dysplasia in Barrett's esophagus by spectroscopy measurement of 5-aminolevulinic acid-induced protoporphyrin IX fluorescence. Gastrointest Endosc 2002; 56:479–487.

22. Kapadia CR, Cutruzzola FW, O'Brien KM, Stetz ML, Enriquez R, Deckelbaum LI. Laser-induced fluorescence spectroscopy of human colonic mucosa. Detection of adenomatous transformation. Gastroenterology 1990; 99:150–157.

23. Cothren RM, Richards-Kortum R, Sivak MV Jr, et al. Gastrointestinal tissue diagnosis by laser-induced fluorescence spectroscopy at endoscopy. Gastrointest Endosc 1990; 36:105–111.

24. Schomacker KT, Frisoli JK, Compton CC, et al. Ultraviolet laser-induced fluorescence of colonic polyps. Gastroenterology 1992; 102:1155–1160.

25. Marchesini R, Brambilla M, Pignoli E, et al. Light-induced fluorescence spectroscopy of adenomas, adenocarcinomas and non-neoplastic mucosa in human colon. J Photochem Photobiol B 1992; 14:219–230.

26. Cothren RM, Sivak MV Jr, Van Dam J, et al. Detection of dysplasia at colonoscopy using laser-induced fluorescence: a blinded study. Gastrointest Endosc 1996; 44:168–176.

27. Eker C, Montan S, Jaramillo E, et al. Clinical spectral characterisation of colonic mucosal lesions using autofluorescence and delta aminolevulinic acid sensitisation. Gut 1999; 44:511–518.

28. Woolf GM, Riddell RH, Irvine EJ, Hunt RH. A study to examine agreement between endoscopy and histology for the diagnosis of columnar lined (Barrett's) esophagus. Gastrointest Endosc 1989; 35:541–544.

29. Fleischer DE, Wang GQ, Dawsey S, et al. Tissue band ligation followed by snare resection (band and snare): a new technique for tissue acquisition in the esophagus. Gastrointest Endosc 1996; 44:68–72.

30. Overholt BF, Panjehpour M, Haydek JM. Photodynamic therapy for Barrett's esophagus: follow-up in 100 patients. Gastrointest Endosc 1999; 49:1–7.

31. Endo M, Sakakibara N, Suzuki H. Observation of esophageal lesions with the use of endoscopic dyes. Prog Dig Endosc 1972; 1:34.

32. Ina H, Shibuya H, Ohashi I, Kitagawa M. The frequency of a concomitant early esophageal cancer in male patients with oral and oropharyngeal cancer. Screening results using Lugol dye endoscopy. Cancer 1994; 73:2038–2041.

33. Yokoyama A, Ohmori T, Makuuchi H, et al. Successful screening for early esophageal cancer in alcoholics using endoscopy and mucosa iodine staining. Cancer 1995; 76:928–934.

34. Inoue H, Rey JF, Lightdale C. Lugol chromoendoscopy for esophageal squamous cell cancer. Endoscopy 2001; 33:75–79.

35. Tam W, Edebo A, Bruno M. Endoscopy negative reflux disease (ENRD): High-resolution endoscopic and histological signs. Gastroenterology 2002; 122:A74.

36. Axelrad AM, Fleischer DE, Geller AJ, et al. High-resolution chromoendoscopy for the diagnosis of diminutive colon polyps: implications for colon cancer screening. Gastroenterology 1996; 110:1253–1258.

37. Kudo S, Kashida H, Nakajima T, Tamura S, Nakajo K. Endoscopic diagnosis and treatment of early colorectal cancer. World J Surg 1997; 21:694–701.

38. Canto MI, Setrakian S, Petras RE, Blades E, Chak A, Sivak MV Jr. Methylene blue selectively stains intestinal metaplasia in Barrett's esophagus. Gastrointest Endosc 1996; 44:1–7.

39. Canto MI, Setrakian S, Willis J, et al. Methylene blue-directed biopsies improve detection of intestinal metaplasia and dysplasia in Barrett's esophagus. Gastrointest Endosc 2000; 51:560–568.

40. Kiesslich R, Hahn M, Herrmann G, Jung M. Screening for specialized columnar epithelium with methylene blue: chromoendoscopy in patients with Barrett's esophagus and a normal control group. Gastrointest Endosc 2001; 53:47–52.

41. Sharma P, Topalovski M, Mayo MS, Weston AP. Methylene blue chromoendoscopy for detection of short-segment Barrett's esophagus. Gastrointest Endosc 2001; 54:289–293.

42. Tatsuta M, Okuda S, Taniguchi H. Diagnosis of early gastric cancer by the endoscopic Congo red-methylene blue test. Endoscopy 1983; 15:252–256.

43. Fennerty MB, Sampliner RE, McGee DL, Hixson LJ, Garewal HS. Intestinal metaplasia of the stomach: identification by a selective mucosal staining technique. Gastrointest Endosc 1992; 38: 696–698.

44. Dave U, Shousha S, Westaby D. Methylene blue staining: is it really useful in Barrett's esophagus? Gastrointest Endosc 2001; 53: 333–355.

45. Wo JM, Ray MB, Mayfield-Stokes S, et al. Comparison of methylene blue-directed biopsies and conventional biopsies in the detection of intestinal metaplasia and dysplasia in Barrett's esophagus: a preliminary study. Gastrointest Endocs 2001; 54:294–301.

46. Stevens PD, Lightdale CJ, Green PH, Siegel LM, Garcia-Carrasquillo RJ, Rotterdam H. Combined magnification endoscopy with chromoendoscopy for the evaluation of Barrett's esophagus. Gastrointest Endosc 1994; 40:747–749.

47. Sharma P, Weston AP, Topalovski M, Cherian R, Bhattacharyya A, Sampliner RE. Magnification chromoendoscopy for the detection of intestinal metaplasia and dysplasia in Barrett's oesophagus. Gut 2003; 52:24–27.

48. Kudo S, Tamura S, Nakajima T, Yamano H, Kusaka H, Watanabe H. Diagnosis of colorectal tumorous lesions by magnifying endoscopy. Gastrointest Endosc 1996; 44:8–14.

49. Saitoh Y, Waxman I, West AB, Popnikolov NK, Gatalica Z, Watari J. Prevalence and distinctive biologic features of flat colorectal adenomas in a North American population. Gastroenterology 2001; 120: 1657–1665.

50. Guelrud M, Herrera I, Essenfeld H, Castro J. Enhanced magnification endoscopy: a new technique to identify specialized intestinal metaplasia in Barrett's esophagus. Gastrointest Endosc 2001; 53:559–565.

51. Endo T, Awakawa T, Takahashi H, et al. Classification of Barrett's epithelium by magnifying endoscopy. Gastrointest Endosc 2002; 55:641–647.

52. Tajiri H, Doi T, Endo H, et al. Routine endoscopy using a magnifying endoscope for gastric cancer diagnosis. Endoscopy 2002; 34: 772–777.

53. Dinis-Ribeiro M, da Costa-Pereira A, Lopes C, et al. Magnification chromoendoscopy for the diagnosis of gastric intestinal metaplasia and dysplasia. Gastrointest Endosc 2003; 57:498–504.

54. Togashi K, Konishi F, Ishizuka T, Sato T, Senba S, Kanazawa K. Efficacy of magnifying endoscopy in the differential diagnosis of neoplastic and non-neoplastic polyps of the large bowel. Dis Colon Rectum 1999; 42:1602–1608.

55. Kato S, Fujii T, Koba I, et al. Assessment of colorectal lesions using magnifying colonoscopy and mucosal dye spraying: can significant lesions be distinguished? Endoscopy 2001; 33:306–310.

56. el-Sharabasy MM, el-Waseef AM, Hafez MM, Salim SA. Porphyrin metabolism in some malignant diseases. Br J Cancer 1992; 65:409–412.

57. Regula J, MacRobert AJ, Gorchein A, et al. Photosensitisation and photodynamic therapy of oesophageal, duodenal, and colorectal tumours using 5 aminolaevulinic acid induced protoporphyrin IX—a pilot study. Gut 1995; 36:67–75.

58. Endlicher E, Knuechel R, Hauser T, Szeimies RM, Scholmerich J, Messmann H. Endoscopic fluorescence detection of low and high grade dysplasia in Barrett's oesophagus using systemic or local 5-aminolaevulinic acid sensitisation. Gut 2001; 48:314–319.

59. Messmann H, Knuechel R, Baeumler W, Holstege A, Schoelmerich J. Endoscopic fluorescence detection of dysplasia in patients with Barrett's esophagus, ulcerative colitis, or adenomatous polyps after 5-aminolevulinic acid-induced protoporphyrin IX sensitization. Gastrointest Endosc 1999; 49:97–101.

60. Haringsma J, Tytgat GNJ, Yano H, et al. Autofluorescence endoscopy: feasibility of detection of GI neoplasms unapparent to white light endoscopy with an evolving technology. Gastrointest Endosc 2001; 53:642–650.

61. Stepinac T, Felley C, Jornod P, et al. Endoscopic fluorescence detection of intraepithelial neoplasia in Barrett's esophagus after oral administration of aminolevulinic acid. Endoscopy 2003; 35:663–668.

62. Niepsuj K, Niepsuj G, Cebula W, et al. autofluorescence endoscopy for detection of high-grade dysplasia in short-segment Barrett's esophagus. Gastrointest Endsoc 2004; 58:715–719.

63. Izuishi K, Tajiri H, Fujii T, et al. The histological basis of detection of adenoma and cancer in the colon by autofluorescence endoscopic imaging. Endoscopy 1999; 31:511–516.

64. Messmann H, Endlicher E, Freunek G, Ruemmele P, Schoelmerich J, Knuechel R. Fluorescence endoscopy for the detection of low and high grade dysplasia in ulcerative colitis using systemic or local 5-aminolevulinic acid sensitization. Gut 2003; 52:1003–1007.

65. Abe S, Izuishi K, Tajiri H, Kinoshita T, Matsuoka T. Correlation of in vitro autofluorescence endoscopy images with histopathologic findings in stomach cancer. Endoscopy 2000; 32:281–286.

66. Kobayashi M, Tajiri H, Seike E, Shitaya M, Tounou S, Mine M, et al. detection of early gastric cancer by a real-time autofluorescence imaging system. Cancer Lett 2001; 165:155–159.

67. Yoshida T, Inoue H, Usui S, Satodate H, Fukami N, Kudo S. Narrow-band imaging system with magnifying endoscopy for superficial esophageal lesions. Gastrointest Endosc 2004; 59:288–295.

68. Hamamoto Y, Endo T, Nosho K, Arimura Y, Sato M, Imai K. Usefulness of narrow-band imaging endoscopy for diagnosis of Barrett's esophagus. J Gastroenterol 2004; 39:14–20.

69. Brezinski ME, Tearney GJ, Bouma BE, et al. Imaging of coronary artery microstructure (in vitro) with optical coherence tomography. Am J Cardiol 1996; 77:92–93.

70. Poneros JM, Brand S, Bouma BE, Tearney GJ, Compton CC, Nishioka NS. Diagnosis of specialized intestinal metaplasia by optical coherence tomography. Gastroenterology 2001; 120:7–12.

71. Isenberg G, Sivak MV. Gastrointestinal optical coherence tomography. Tech Gastrointest Endosc 2003; 5:94–101.

72. Poneros JM, Hishioka NS. Diagnosis of Barrett's esophagus using optical coherence tomography. Gastrointest Endosc Clin N Am 2003; 13:309–323.

73. Seitz U, Freund J, Jaeckle S, et al. First in vivo optical coherence tomography on the human bile duct. Endoscopy 2001; 33:1018–1021.

74. Poneros JM, Tearney GJ, Shiskov M, et al. Optical coherence tomography of the biliary tree during ERCP. Gastrointest Endosc 2002; 55:84–88.

75. Sivak MV Jr, Kobayashi K, Izatt JA, et al. High-resolution endoscopic imaging of the GI tract using optical coherence tomography. Gastrointest Endosc 2000; 51:474–479.

76. Jaeckle S, Gladkova N, Feldchtein, et al. In vivo endoscopic optical coherence tomography of the human gastrointestinal tract—toward optical biopsy. Endoscopy 2000; 32:743–749.

77. Pfau PR, Sivak MV, Chak A, et al. Criteria for the diagnosis of dysplasia by endoscopic optical coherence tomography. Gastrointest Endosc 2003; 58:196–202.

78. Inoue H, Igari T, Nishikage T, Ami K, Yoshida T, Iwai. A novel method of virtual histopathology using laser-scanning cofocal microscopy in-vitro with untreated fresh specimens from the gastrointestinal mucosa. Endoscopy 2000; 32:439–443.

79. Sakashita M, Inoue H, Kashida H, et al. Vitual histology of colorectal lesions using laser-scanning confocal microscopy. Endoscopy 2003; 35:1033–1038.

80. Shim MG, Song LM, Marcon NE, Wilson BC. In vivo near-infrared Raman spectroscopy: demonstration of feasibility during clinical gastrointestinal endoscopy. Photochem Photobiol 2000; 72:146–150.

81. Wong Kee Song LM, Marcon NE. Fluorescence and Raman spectroscopy. Gastrointest Endosc Clin N Am 2003; 13:279–296.

82. Pelegrin A, Folli S, Buchegger F, Mach JP, Wagnieres G, van den Bergh H. Antibody-fluorescein conjugates for photoimmunodiagnosis of human colon carcinoma in nude mice. Cancer 1991; 67:2529–2537.

83. Folli S, Westermann P, Braichotte D, Pelegrin A, Wagnieres G, van den Bergh H, et al. Antibody-indocyanin conjugates for immunophotodetection of human squamous cell carcinoma in nude mice. Cancer Res 1994; 54:2643–2649.

84. Maunoury V, Mordon S, Geboes K, et al. Early vascular changes in Crohn's disease: an endoscopic fluorescence study. Endoscopy 2000; 32:700–705.

85. Folli S, Wagnieres G, Pelegrin A, et al. Immunophotodiagnosis of colon carcinomas in patients injected with fluoresceinated chimeric antibodies against carcinoembryonic antigen. Proc Natl Acad Sci USA 1992; 89:7973–7977.

86. Marten K, Bremer C, Khazaie K, et al. Detection of dysplastic intestinal adenomas using enzyme-sensing molecular beacons in mice. Gastroenterology 2002; 122:406–414.

4 Staging of Esophageal Cancer

Jason Vollweiler, MD and Gregory Zuccaro, Jr., MD

Contents

1. INTRODUCTION

Esophageal carcinoma is the fifth most common gastrointestinal cancer, and the recent data suggests that it is rising in incidence faster than any other malignancy. Although esophageal carcinoma is generally felt to have a poor prognosis, this is largely owing to the heterogeneity of patients. As with any malignancy, the stage of the tumor predicts prognosis and determines treatment options. Stage of the tumor at diagnosis is the best predictor of long-term survival. Patients with early or localized disease may have excellent survival when treated surgically, whereas patients with more advanced disease may not. Multimodality chemoradiotherapy plus surgery may optimize survival. Patients with invasion into adjacent structures or distant metastatic disease are more appropriately treated with palliation alone. Every patient with esophageal carcinoma should be clinically staged to determine which treatment options are appropriate and to individualize management. Clinical stage can be accurately determined by a combination of modern staging techniques including computed tomography (CT), esophagogastroduodenoscopy (EGD), endoscopic ultrasonography (EUS), positron emission tomography (PET), and minimally invasive surgery.

2. DEFINITION OF STAGES IN ESOPHAGEAL CARCINOMA

Staging for esophageal carcinoma is based on the 2002 TNM staging system of the American Joint Committee on Cancer (Table 1) *(1)*. The system is based on depth of invasion of the primary tumor (T classification), the status of the regional lymph nodes (N classification), and presence or absence of distant metastases (M classification). With respect to T classification, pathological Tis tumors are intraepithelial malignancies without invasion of the basement membrane (also referred to by some as high-grade dysplasia). Pathological T1 tumors are confined to the submucosa. Although not an official designation, these T1 tumors are often subdivided into T1a tumors, which are limited to the mucosa and T1b tumors, which invade into the submucosa *(2)*. Pathological T2 tumors invade into, but do not breach, the muscularis propria. Pathological T3 tumors invade beyond the esophageal wall into the adventitia, but do not invade adjacent structures. Pathological T4 tumors directly invade adjacent structures in the vicinity of the esophagus, such as the aorta, pericardium, or airway. Regional lymph nodes are classified by the presence (N1) or absence (N0) of metastases. Likewise, distant sites (M) are characterized by the presence (M1) or absence (M0) of metastases. Distant metastases are subdivided into M1a, which are distant nonregional lymph node metastases, and M1b, which are other distant metastases.

The TNM classifications are then grouped into stages with similar prognosis (Table 1). Physical examination, diagnostic imaging, and endoscopic methods predict clinical stage preoperatively with variable degrees of accuracy. For those patients who are operative candidates, pathological stage is determined by histopathology at the time of esophagectomy.

2.1. RATIONALE FOR PRE-OPERATIVE TNM STAGING

There are a number of reasons to accurately classify esophageal cancer. This process in fact is essential to determine prognosis, guide therapy, and allow evaluation of treatment protocols. The prognosis for patients with esophageal cancer is strongly associated with stage. After 5 yr, survival rates worsen with increasing T classification; 46, 30, 22, and 7% for pathological T1, T2, T3, and T4, respectively *(3)*. The status of regional lymph nodes also has substantial prognostic value. Among patients with surgically resectable tumors, the 5-yr survival rate is 40% for N0 disease compared with only 17% for N1 status. After surgical resection of the tumor and complete surgical pathological stage, the 5-yr survival rate is more than 95% for stage 0 disease, is 50–80% for stage I disease, 30–40% for stage IIA disease, 10–30% for stage IIB disease, and 10–15% for stage III disease *(4)*. Patients who have

From: *Endoscopic Oncology: Gastrointestinal Endoscopy and Cancer Management.* Edited by: D. O. Faigel and M. L. Kochman © Humana Press, Totowa, NJ

Table 1
TNM Classification of Esophageal Carcinomas

T:	Primary tumor
TX	Tumor cannot be assessed
T0	No evidence of primary tumor
Tis	High-grade dysplasia (carcinoma-*in situ*)
T1	Tumor invades the lamina propria, muscularis mucosa submucosa, but does not breach the submucosa
T2	Tumor invades the muscularis propria, but does not breach muscularis propria
T3	Tumor invades the periesophageal tissue, but does not invade adjacent structures
T4	Tumor invades adjacent structures
N:	*Regional lymph nodes*
NX	Regional lymph nodes cannot be assessed
N0	No regional lymph node metastases
N1	Regional lymph node metastases
M:	*Distant metastasis*
MX	Presence of distant metastases cannot be assessed
M0	No distant metastasis
M1	Distant metastasis
M1a	Distant, nonregional lymph node metastases
	Lower thoracic esophagus: metastasis in celiac lymph nodes
	Upper thoracic esophagus: metastasis in cervical lymph nodes
M1b	Other distant metastasis

Stage grouping

Stage 0	Tis	N0	M0
Stage I	T1	N0	M0
Stage IIA	T2	N0	M0
	T3	N0	M0
Stage IIB	T1	N1	M0
	T2	N1	M0
Stage III	T3	N1	M0
	T4	Any N	M0
Stage IVA	Any T	Any N	M1a
Stage IVB	Any T	Any N	M1b

metastatic disease treated with palliative chemotherapy have a dismal median survival of less than 1 yr *(5)*.

The primary role of clinical staging is to provide stage-directed therapy (Table 2). Patients found to have distant metastases or invasion of adjacent structures are usually unresectable and are candidates for palliative treatment only. Common sites of distant metastases include the liver (35%), lung (20%), bone (9%), adrenal gland (2%), brain (2%), and pericardium, stomach, pancreas, and spleen (1%) *(6)*. Data from a large experience at the Cleveland Clinic suggest that patients with disease extending beyond the esophageal wall, such as carcinomas that have metastasized to the regional lymph nodes (any N1) and/or penetrating into the adventitia (T3 or T4), appear to benefit from a regimen of induction chemoradiotherapy followed by esophagectomy *(7)*. Patients with esophageal carcinoma limited to the esophageal wall (i.e., ≤T2, N0, and M0) have optimal survival when treated with esophagectomy alone; this classification specific response to pre-operative chemoradiotherapy is presumably owing to the toxicity of induction chemoradiotherapy. It should be noted that the several prospective randomized trials have differed in their conclusions regarding the efficacy of preoperative chemoradiotherapy *(8–16)*; whereas a randomized trial by Walsh et al. demonstrated a survival benefit, others have shown no benefit. A significant limitation in all these studies was that pathological classification was not predicted with EUS, and

therefore pretreatment staging may have been inaccurate. Thus, these studies very likely to group together as a mixture of stages with different prognoses. As stated earlier, the more accurate the clinical staging, the better we can interpret clinical studies evaluating neoadjuvant therapy or other methods of treatment for esophageal cancer.

3. STAGING MODALITIES

Clinical stage is determined pre-operatively by physical examination, diagnostic imaging, endoscopic methods, and/or minimally invasive surgery. A number of diagnostic techniques may be employed including CT scan, EGD, EUS, PET scan, laparoscopy, and thoracoscopy. Each technique has benefits and limitations, but by employing a combination of complimentary tests, clinical stage can be accurately determined.

3.1. COMPUTED TOMOGRAPHY

CT may provide information regarding T and N classification, but its role is primarily in detecting distant metastases. Asymmetric esophageal wall thickening is the primary CT finding of esophageal carcinoma. The normal esophageal wall is less than 3 mm thick, and any thickness greater than 5 mm is considered abnormal. However, CT scan does not accurately define the layers of esophageal wall and is unable to distinguish between Tis, T1, and T2 tumors. Invasion of the paraesophageal fat with an ill-defined abnormal soft tissue density may indicate T3 tumor by CT, but this finding is unreliable *(18)*. T4

Table 2
Cleveland Clinic Protocol for Stage-Directed Therapy

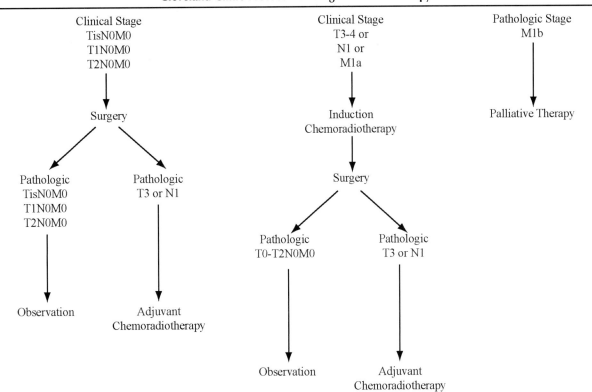

tumors can be demonstrated by the obliteration of fat planes between the esophagus and adjacent structures including the aorta, trachea, pericardium, and left mainstem bronchus.

Regional and nonregional lymph nodes are visualized by CT scan. Enlarged nodes are considered abnormal. The criteria for enlargement are based on the location of the node. Supraclavicular nodes greater than 0.5 cm, retrocrural nodes greater than 0.6 cm, and intrathoracic or abdominal nodes greater than 1 cm are generally called pathological (19). However, metastases can be found in normal-sized nodes, and not all enlarged nodes contain malignant metastases; enlarged lymph nodes may be caused by inflammation, leading to a false-positive interpretation of the CT scan. Reported accuracy of CT scan for nodal metastases has varied from 68 to 96%, with sensitivities of 8 to 75%, and specificities of 60 to 98%, depending on lymph node location (20).

Conventional contrast CT scans allow assessment of the common sites of metastases. Sensitivity for identifying hepatic metastases greater than 2 cm is 70–80% (21). Subcentimeter metastases are often not identified by CT scan and are the main cause of false-negative examinations. Adrenal metastases appear as heterogeneous enlargement of the gland, but this is a nonspecific finding. CT is also very sensitive for the detection of pulmonary nodules, but these findings are again nonspecific. Overall, CT has a sensitivity of 37–66% in screening for distant metastases in patients with esophageal cancer.

3.2. ESOPHAGOGASTRODUODENOSCOPY

EGD has an essential role in the diagnosis of esophageal cancer, and may provide some information regarding T classification as well. Most patients undergo EGD when symptoms such as dysphagia and odynophagia develop. Endoscopy allows identification of the location, length, and morphology of the tumor. Endoscopic biopsies confirm the diagnosis. Endoscopic evaluation of wall infiltration based on the macroscopic appearance of the tumor (Table 3), as defined by the Japanese Society for Esophageal Diseases and the Japanese Gastric Cancer Society, has been used to predict T classification (22,23). In the report by Dittler et al. (22), endoscopic classification predicted T class with an overall accuracy of 86%. Kienle and colleagues (24) prospectively compared staging by endoscopy alone, endoscopic ultrasound, and CT scan to postoperative histology in 117 patients. Interestingly, accuracy of endoscopy and endoscopic ultrasound was not significantly different for T classification, 72 vs 75%, respectively. Both were significantly better than CT scan, which was 50% accurate. Endosonography was more accurate than endoscopy for predicting lymph node metastases, 79 vs 68%. Patients were subjectively classified by EGD as lymph node positive if there were large ulcerations, high-grade stenosis, or wall rigidity over a long distance. In another study, the degree of luminal stenosis and length of esophageal cancer predicted T classification by EUS, with sensitivity of up to 89% and specificity of 92% accurately predicting pathological T3 (25). In conclusion, endoscopic macroscopic staging allows a reasonably accurate assessment of the T classification, but the macroscopic criteria are complicated and no objective assessment of lymph node status can be made.

Table 3
Macroscopic Tumor Stage Modified According to the Japanese Society for Esophageal Diseases
and the Japanese Gastric Cancer Society

EGD stage	T class	Criteria for evaluation
mT0	T1	Soft, polypoid, supple
mT1	T2	Polypoid, supple, but partly scirrhous, surface structure regular or superficial ulceration, if excavated only shallow depression, fold convergence without major stiffening, or interruptions, base of lesion <3 cm
mT2	T2	Moderately deep ulceration with stiffening and irregularly shaped nodules on the margin, interrupted and enlarged folds, lesion may be surrounded by a tumorous bank, Margins of lesion generally sharply demarcated, tumor involves not more than half of the circumference
mT3	T3	Lesion diameter >5 cm with deep ulceration and tumorous bank without definite limits, partially rigid esophagus
mT4	T4	Circular stenosis over longer distance (>5 cm), appearance is diffusely infiltrating, rigid esophagus, ulceration is not a marked feature

3.3. ENDOSCOPIC ULTRASOUND

A large body of literature has demonstrated that EUS is the most accurate clinical modality for regional staging of esophageal cancer. EUS allows a detailed view of the esophageal wall and is ideally suited for the evaluation of T classification. By EUS, $T1_{submucosal}$ tumors extend into, but not through, the third ultrasound layer. T2 tumors extend into, but not through, the fourth ultrasound layer, and T3 tumors extend beyond the fourth ultrasound layer (Figs. 1–3). Most published studies report accuracy of T classification (i.e., accuracy in prediction of pathological T) ranging between 75 and 92% (26–30). In a review of 21 series, EUS was 84% accurate for prediction of T classification (29). Most clinical series have used the radial scanning echoendoscopes with 7.5- and 12-MHz-frequency transducers, but a small number of studies have demonstrated comparable results with linear array echoendoscopes (31).

The accuracy of T classification varies somewhat for each pathological classification. The literature varies in the reported accuracy of EUS prediction of pathological T: 75–84% for T1, 64–85% for T2, 89–94% for T3, and 88–100% for T4 (32). Because the tumor is seen as hypoechoic, and the wall layers are readily apparent, why should errors in EUS prediction of pathological T occur at all? There are several potential reasons. One relates to technical factors of maneuvering the echoendoscope. If a tight tumor stricture is encountered, an examination of the entire length of the tumor may not be possible. Likewise, depending on the positioning of the transducer, wall layers may be compressed together and difficult to interpret images generated (Fig. 4). The greatest inaccuracy is reported for T2 tumors, and in most experiences overclassification is more frequent than underclassification. Often when a tumor appears to invade into but not through the fourth ultrasound layer, there is slight extension of hypoechoic material beyond the fourth ultrasound layer (Fig. 5). This can often lead to erroneous prediction of pathological T3, when in actuality this hypoechoic material may be peritumor inflammation or because of some other factors. The EUS anatomy may also account for specific difficulty predicting pathological T classification.

Studies have demonstrated that the third ultrasonographic layer is acually the submucosa and the acoustic interface between the submucosa and muscularis propria. The fourth ultrasonographic layer is the muscularis propria minus the acoustic interface between the submucosa and the muscularis propria (33,34). Because the ultrasound layers do not correspond exactly to the anatomic layers of the esophageal wall, it is not surprising that errors in T classification occur.

Because invasion beyond the esophageal wall is important in determining treatment, some investigators have examined the accuracy of EUS in determining T classification dichotomously (i.e., pathological Tis–T2 vs T3–T4). The reported accuracy of EUS in predicting pathological T (dichotomized) is 87%, with 82% sensitivity, 91% specificity, 89% positive predictive value, and 86% negative predictive value (35). A systemic review of 13 studies also confirmed that EUS is highly accurate in differentiating pathological T1/T2 tumors from T3/T4 tumors (36).

EUS also has advantages over other imaging modalities in the evaluation of regional lymph nodes. In addition to size, EUS evaluates nodal shape, border, and internal echo characteristics. Large (size > 1 cm), hypoechoic, round nodes with sharp borders are more likely to be malignant; small, hyperechoic, angular nodes with indistinct borders are more likely to be benign (37). However, no single feature independently predicts malignancy and these combined features are only present in 25% of malignant lymph nodes observed (38). Published experience with the assessment of lymph nodes reports overall accuracy in a wide range of 50–90% (26–29). In Rosch's review of 21 series, the accuracy of EUS was 77, 69, and 89% for overall N, N0, and N1 classes, respectively (29). The ability of EUS to diagnose nodal metastases varies with nodal location. It is better for the assessment of celiac nodes (accuracy of 95%) than for mediastinal nodes (73%) (39). It should be noted that the likelihood of N1 disease increases with deeper tumor invasion; 17% for T1 tumors, 55% for T2, 83% for T3, and 88% for T4 (40).

EUS-guided fine-needle aspiration (EUS-FNA) allows the addition of tissue sampling to endosonographic characteristics

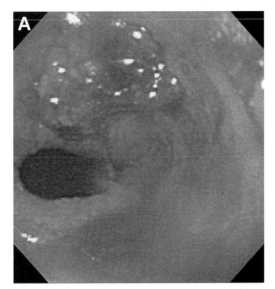

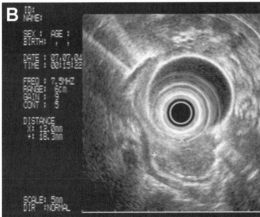

Fig. 1. (**A**) A discrete adenocarcinoma at the gastroesophageal junction arising in Barrett's. (**B**) The lesion invades into, but not through, the third ultrasound layer (bright line) at the level of the plus sign, as depicted using a standard radial echoendoscope at 7.5 mHz frequency. The fourth ultrasound layer, which is the dark line outside the third layer, is unaffected. This indicates $T1_{submucosal}$ classification.

(Figs. 6 and 7). This significantly improves the ability to confirm malignant adenopathy *(41–44)*. In a large multicenter study of upper GI lesions, 171 patients had EUS-FNA of 192 lymph nodes. The accuracy of EUS-FNA in determination of lymph node status was 92% with a sensitivity of 92%, specificity of 93%, positive predictive value 100%, and negative predictive value 86% *(41)*. In this study, FNA improved the accuracy of lymph node classification from 69% by EUS alone to 92%. Subsequent studies from Vazquez-Sequeiros have confirmed and extended these findings *(43,44)*. In the most recent report, the first prospective and blinded study, EUS-FNA was more accurate than EUS (87 vs 74%) when compared with surgical histopathology *(44)*. EUS-FNA was also found to change the tumor stage of 38% of the patient compared with CT scan, which significantly altered the treatment decision. In the published experiences with EUS-FNA, complications are extremely rare. Unfortunately, some lymph nodes cannot be aspirated because of their location with respect to the primary

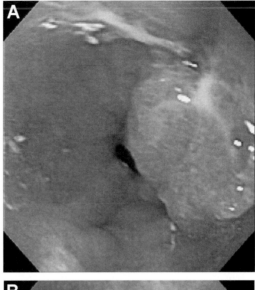

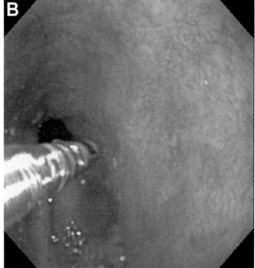

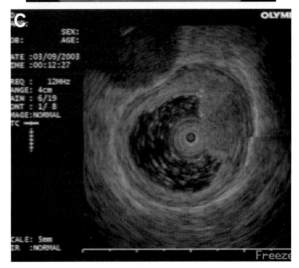

Fig. 2. (**A**) A larger nodular adenocarcinoma in Barrett's. (**B**) A high-frequency probe is passed into the esophagus via the operating channel. (**C**) EUS probe image shows the cancer (best seen from 12 to 3 o'clock) extending into but not through the third ultrasound layer, indicating $T1_{submucosal}$ classification.

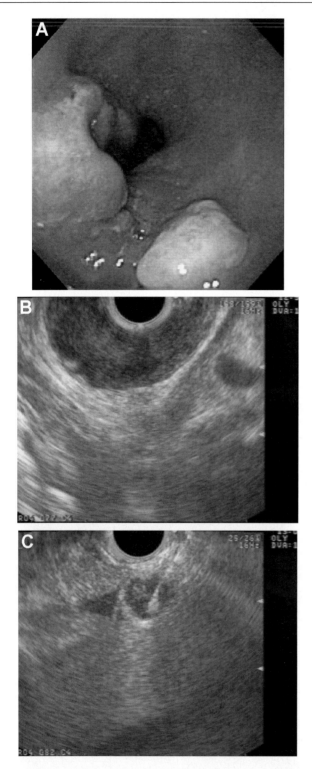

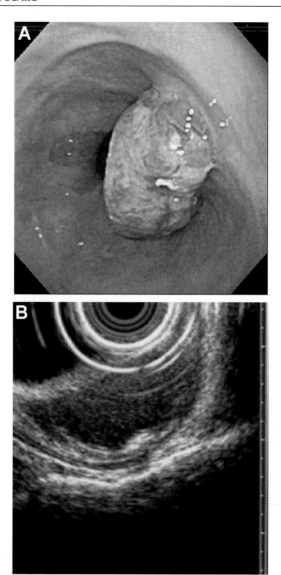

Fig. 4. **(A)** A pedunculated cancer in a tongue of Barrett's esophagus. (A color version of A appears in the color insert following p. 84.) **(B)** EUS image suggests $T1_{submucosal}$ along the majority of the tumor, but on the right side the layer structure is lost and the tumor appears to invade to the fourth ultrasound layer, suggesting T2.

EUS has limited value in the evaluation of distant metastases (M1b). Distant metastases may be serendipitously found in organs in direct contact with the upper gastrointestinal tract, such as the left lateral segment of the liver or the retroperitoneum. Celiac lymph nodes, which are considered M1a for cancers of the lower esophagus, can be identified accurately by EUS *(39,45,46)*. EUS-FNA has 98% accuracy in detecting malignant celiac lymph nodes.

3.3.1. Limitations of EUS

A study by Meining and colleagues *(47)* has questioned whether EUS staging in a truly blinded fashion is as accurate as previously reported. A blinded review of videotaped EUS examinations of 32 patients with esophageal cancer demonstrated a significantly decreased accuracy of 50% compared to 81% by routine analysis (retrospective review of EUS reports). When interpreters were unblinded and given endoscopy tapes, accuracy improved to 72%. The authors speculated that the

Fig. 3. **(A)** Multifocal adenocarcinoma in the distal esophagus. **(B)** As seen by linear ultrasound, the hypoechoic tumor extends into, but not through, the fourth ultrasound layer, indicating T2 classification. **(C)** Typical of multifocal adenocarcinoma, a search for involved regional lymph nodes reveals this enlarged node found to be involved with adenocarcinoma by FNA (depicted).

tumor (Fig. 8). Only those nodes to which the path of the needle avoids the primary cancer are appropriate for FNA, as false-positive results might otherwise be obtained.

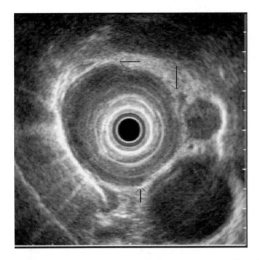

Fig. 5. EUS image showing hypoechoic tumor extending into the fourth ultrasound layer. There are small areas of hypoechoic foci that may extend beyond the fourth ultrasound layer (arrows). It is difficult to determine if these foci represent pathological T3 disease, hypoechoic non-neoplastic tissue, or artifact. A lymph node highly suspicious for malignant involvement is also seen at 3 o'clock.

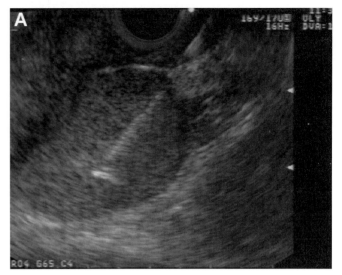

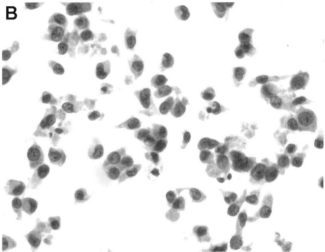

Fig. 6. **(A)** A large lymph node is seen by radial echoendoscope at the proximal aspect of a large malignant esophageal tumor. An FNA needles is seen within the lymph node. **(B)** Metastatic adenocarcinoma involving a lymph node: the entire FNA sample from this lymph node consists of metastatic poorly differentiated adenocarcinoma. The tumor cells are arranged singly and in small clusters with marked nuclear pleomorphism and prominent nucleoli. No normal lymphoid cells are seen. (Pap stain, ×40 magnification.)

better results with EUS obtained in a clinical setting are owing to additional sources of information, such as clinical history and previous imaging.

Another potential drawback of EUS is lack of widespread availability and utilization. Extensive experience is necessary for both examination technique and ultrasound interpretation. There is a significant learning curve with 75–100 examinations required before competence is obtained *(48)*. For these reasons, EUS should be performed at institutions in which there is a dedicated, experienced endoscopic ultrasonographer with equipment that allows specialty imaging and EUS-FNA. EUS has not been universally accepted as a principal tool in the evaluation of patients with esophageal cancer. In a study of 100 gastroenterologists, only 41% judged endosonography to be very useful or essential in staging esophageal cancer. Only 50% of the respondents had EUS available in their community *(49)*. As discussed earlier, most of the prospective, randomized trials evaluating treatment strategies for esophageal cancer did not employ EUS in pretreatment evaluation.

Esophageal obstruction caused by malignant high-grade stricture prohibits staging in a significant number of examinations. Some studies have suggested that EUS may be less reliable in nontransversable esophageal cancer *(50–51)*. Another study has shown that failure to pass an ultrasound probe beyond a malignant stricture is an accurate predictor of advanced stage with more than 90% of these patients have stage III or IV disease *(52)*. These disconcordant findings may be reconciled when viewed in the context of a study from Hordijk and colleagues *(53)*. In this study, the accuracy rates for prediction of pathological T were 87, 46, and 92% for nontransversable strictures, tight strictures that were difficult to pass, and easily transversable strictures, respectively. Options in the case of nontransversable strictures include limited examination of the proximal tumor margin, dilation, and subsequent complete EUS, and the use of miniprobes. Limited examination of the

tumor above the stricture has variable accuracy but may be useful in staging if T3 or N1 disease is seen. Dilation of malignant strictures may be associated with an increased incidence of perforation *(52)*, but allows complete examination in 42–85% of patients with high-grade strictures *(53–55)*. Several recent studies have not found a significant increased perforation rate with cautious stepwise dilation *(53–55)*. In the study by Wallace et al. *(55)* dilation directly resulted in detection of advanced disease in 19% of patients, mostly owing to detection of celiac nodes *(55)*. Passed through the biopsy channel of the endoscope and advanced through the stricture, miniprobes have accurately predicted T in 85–90% of patients *(56–59)*. Miniprobes may have limited depth of examination and therefore may not fully assess tumor extention into adjacent structures, and obviously FNA cannot be performed of suspicious regional lymph nodes.

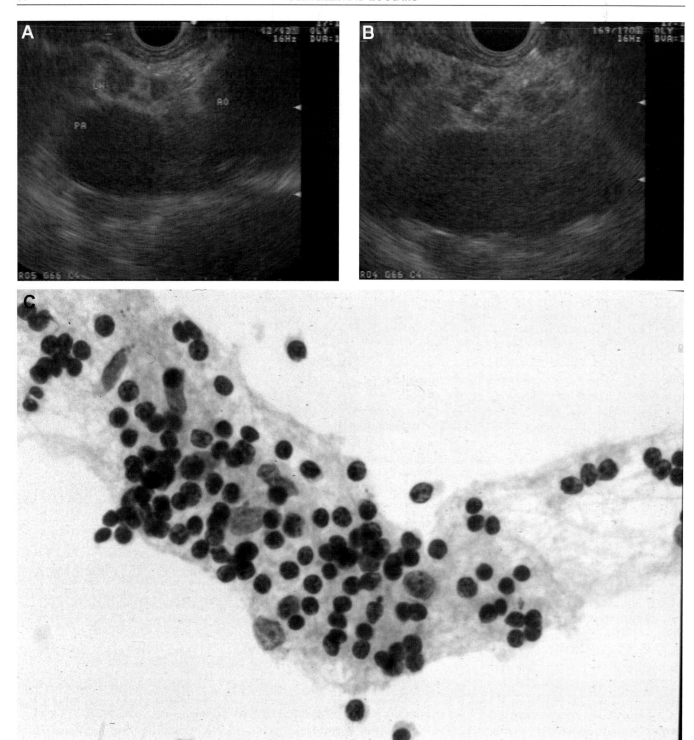

Fig. 7. **(A)** Small mediastinal lymph nodes visualized by radial echoendoscope. **(B)** Fine-needle aspiration (FNA) of lymph node. **(C)** Benign lymph-node: this FNA from a benign lymph node shows a predominance of small mature lymphocytes with round, dark nuclei, and inconspicuous nucleoli. The small lymphocytes are admixed with larger histiocytes with abundant basophilic cytoplasm. The pictured aggregate likely represents a fragment from a germinal center. No tumor cells are seen. (Pap stain, ×40 magnification.)

Clinical staging after neoadjuvant therapy has proven problematic because of inability to distinguish peritumoral inflammatory or fibrous reactions from residual tumor (Fig. 9). Patients with advanced tumors whose disease is downstaged to pathological T2N0 or less with induction therapy will derive maximum survival benefit *(7,17)*. Because EUS is not capable of distinguishing inflammation from viable residual tumor, it is not accurate in determining which patients are free of disease *(60–62)*. Zuccaro et al. *(60)* found that EUS correctly predicted a complete response to chemotherapy in only 3 of 17

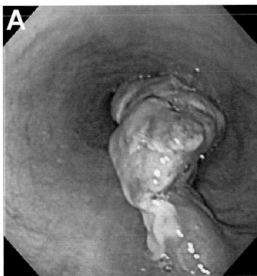

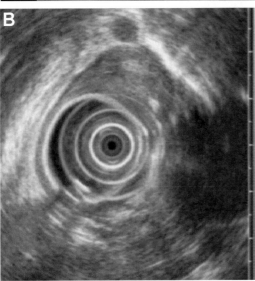

Fig. 8. **(A)** A pedunculated cancer in the distal esophagus. **(B)** A small lymph node is visualized outside the primary tumor; it is possible that no clear needle path may exist to such nodes without passing through the primary tumor. In such cases, morphological criteria must be employed to classify the node.

patients (17%) who had no residual tumor demonstrated in the resection specimen. Measuring the change in maximal cross-sectional area pre- and post-chemoradiotherapy appears to be a more useful measure to assess the response of esophageal cancer to pre-operative chemoradiation *(63,64)*. A single case report of EUS-FNA of residual lymph nodes after chemoradiation has been reported *(65)*. In this case study, FNA documented nodal response and correlated with the surgical specimen.

3.4. COMPARISON OF CT SCAN AND EUS

CT scan and EUS have been compared head-to-head in a number of clinical trials *(26–28,66)*. In all studies, endoscopic ultrasound was superior to CT scan in the accurate prediction of T and N classification. Botet et al. found improved accuracy for EUS, 92 vs 60% for T classification, and 88 vs 74% for N classification. In the same study, CT was more accurate, 90 vs

70% for distant metastasis *(26)*. Similarly, in 74 patients, Tio et al., found T classification accuracy of 89% for EUS vs 59% for CT; and N classification accuracy of 80% for EUS vs 51% for CT. In practice, CT and EUS are complimentary rather than competitive. EUS is used for regional staging and CT scan is used for identification of distant metastases. Most centers perform a CT scan first; if no distant metastases are identified then EUS is performed for regional staging. It should be noted that EUS can detect advanced disease such as T4 tumors and celiac node disease better than CT scan *(28,45)*. This has brought into question the practice of performing an initial CT, as patients with advanced disease by EUS would be treated with palliation and no further staging. Hadzijahic and colleagues *(67)* have addressed this issue with a cost-minimization analysis. Initial CT remained the least costly strategy in most clinical settings. However, if the probability of finding advanced disease by EUS was greater than 30% or was less than 20% by CT (a condition met in their referral population), initial EUS was reasonable.

3.5. POSITRON EMISSION TOMOGRAPHY SCAN

Whole-body PET scan, acquired after injection of flude oxyglucose F18 (FDG) is increasingly being used to identify tumor involvement of regional nodes and distant sites. FDG accumulates in cells with active glucose metabolism and PET can detect degradation of this radioactive material. The increased glycolytic activity of malignancies can be used to stage cancer. FDG-PET has been reported to accumulate in nearly 100% of esophageal cancers *(68,69)*. However, FDG-PET provides no definition of the esophageal wall and has no value in determination of T classification. The accuracy of FDG-PET for the detection of lymph node metastases is variable, ranging from 37 to 90% *(69–72)*. This may be partially owing to the fact that FDG-PET lacks anatomical definition and cannot differentiate primary tumor from adjacent regional nodal disease.

In screening for distant metastases FDG-PET is the most accurate radiological examination, being superior to CT scan. In a study of 91 patients, FDG-PET detected metastatic disease with 84% accuracy compared with 63% accuracy of CT scanning *(73)*. It should be noted that the overall sensitivity for FDG-PET in this study was only 69% (vs 46% for CT scan) with all missed metastases being smaller than 1 cm. Similar findings have been demonstrated in several other studies with PET scan detecting metastatic disease in 10–20% of patients who were thought to have localized disease based on conventional imaging *(71,73,74)*. The combination of PET and CT has a diagnostic accuracy of 80–92% *(70,71)* and unnecessary surgery can be avoided in 90% *(71)*.

3.6. MINIMALLY INVASIVE SURGERY (LAPAROSCOPY/THORACOSCOPY)

Minimally invasive surgery with laparoscopy and/or thoracoscopy has also been evaluated in the staging of esophageal carcinoma. Although more invasive and costly, these procedures have the potential benefit of direct nodal dissection and sampling. In addition, laparoscopy can detect peritoneal metastases.

Thoracoscopy has been reported to correctly stage 88% of patients undergoing resection of esophageal carcinomas.

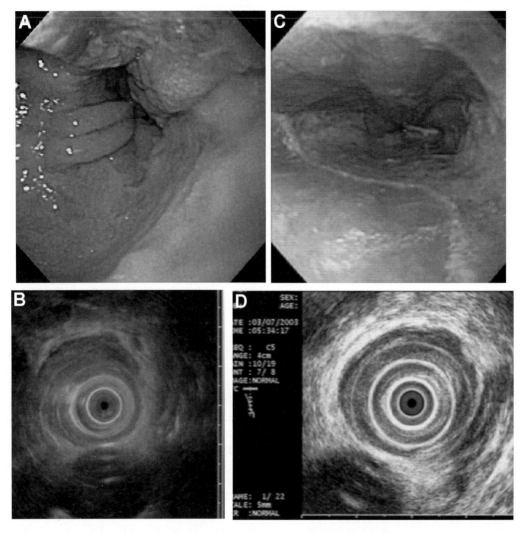

Fig. 9. **(A)** Endoscopic view of distal adenocarcinoma prechemoradiation. **(B)** Radial EUS image of this tumor. **(C)** Endoscopic view after chemoradiotherapy suggesting a significant response. **(D)** EUS image after chemoradiation is unchanged from pretreatment image. EUS does not always adequately distinguish peritumor inflammation from residual tumor.

Accurate in defining N, it is less accurate in the assessment of T *(75)*. Laparoscopic ultrasound has been reported to have TMN assessment equivalent to published results for EUS *(76)*. In a comparative trial, Luketich et al. *(77)* reported improved accuracy of combined laparoscopy and thoracoscopy compared with conventional imaging with CT scan and EUS. In 32% of patients, minimally invasive surgery changed the original stage assigned by conventional imaging. However, this study had several limitations. Patients who had definitive non-resectable disease by conventional imaging were excluded. This exaggerates the benefit of surgical staging. This study was also performed without EUS-FNA, which has been shown to improve the sensitivity and specificity of EUS for lymph node metastases. At this time, laparoscopy and thoracoscopy are not routinely performed at most institutions but do have a role in patients with equivocal findings on conventional imaging, especially if management will be changed.

3.7. COMPLEMENTARY STUDIES

In patients with carcinoma of the cervical esophagus, EUS does not always define the presence or absence of airway inva-

sion *(78)*. For this reason, bronchoscopy is performed at the time of EUS staging for all carcinomas of the cervical and upper or middle thoracic esophagus.

4. CONCLUSION

Esophageal cancer staging is important for prognosis, clinical trials, but most importantly, to guide therapy. All patients should be clinically staged before undergoing treatment. Staging is best accomplished with a combination of modalities including physical examination, endoscopy with biopsy, endoscopic ultrasound with FNA, CT scan, FDG-PET, and thoracoscopy/laparoscopy.

The optimal staging strategy is not entirely clear; however, CT scan and EUS-FNA form the foundation for clinical staging in esophageal cancer and should be routinely performed. When possible, FDG-PET should be added to CT scan to increase the detection of non-nodal M1b disease. In addition, bronchoscopy should be utilized for proximal tumors, and thoracoscopy/laparoscopy in patients with equivocal studies. This strategy is supported by a decision analysis from

Wallace and colleagues *(79)*. This study compared six different staging strategies for health care costs and effectiveness. CT scan plus EUS-FNA was the least expensive strategy and offered more quality-adjusted life years than all other strategies with the exception of FDG-PET plus EUS-FNA. FDG-PET plus EUS-FNA was slightly more effective but also more expensive with the marginal cost-effectiveness ratio of $60,544 for quality-adjusted life-year. In the future, studies are needed to assess if more accurate staging improves patient outcomes. Oncological studies should include EUS-FNA staging in their protocols to better determine optimal therapy based on more precise staging.

REFERENCES

1. American Joint Committee on Cancer. AJCC cancer staging handbook. 6th ed. Philadelphia: Lippincott-Raven; 2002. p 3–8, 91–103.
2. Rice TW, Blackstone EH, Rybicki LA, et al. Refining esophageal cancer staging. J Thorac Cardiovasc Surg 2003; 125:1103–1113.
3. American Joint Committee on Cancer: Esophagus. In Beahrs OH, Hansen DE, Hutter RVP, et al. (eds.): Manual for Staging of Cancer, 4th ed. Philadelphia, JB: Lippincott, 1992:57.
4. Reed CE. Surgical management of esophageal carcinoma. Oncologist 1999; 4:95–105.
5. Enzinger PC, Ilson DH, Kelsen DP. Chemotherapy in esophageal cancer. Semin Oncol 1999; 26 Suppl 15:12–20.
6. Quint LE, Hepburn LM, Francis IR, et al. Incidence and distribution of distant metastases in newly diagnosed esophageal carcinoma. Cancer 76; 1995:1120–1125.
7. Rice TW, Blackstone EH, Adenstein DJ, et al. N1 Esophageal carcinoma: The importance of staging and downstaging. J Thorac Cardiovasc Surg 2001; 121:454–464.
8. Le Prise E, Etienne PL, Meunier B, et al. A randomized study of chemotherapy, radiation therapy, and surgery versus surgery for localized squamous cell carcinoma of the esophagus. Cancer 1994; 73:1779–1784.
9. Apinop C, Puttisak P, Preecha N. A prospective study of combined therapy in esophageal cancer. Hepatogastroenterology 1994; 41:391–393.
10. Bosset J-F, Gignoux M, Triboulet J-P, et al. Chemoradiotherapy followed by surgery with surgery alone in squamous cell cancer of the esophagus. N Engl J Med 1997; 337:161–167.
11. Burmeister BH, Smithers BM, Fitzgerald L, et al. A randomized phase III trial of preoperative chemoradiation followed by surgery (CR-S) versus surgery alone (S) for localized resectable cancer of the esophagus. Prog Proc Am Soc Clin Oncol 2002; 21:130a (abstract).
12. Urba SG, Orringer MB, Turrisi A, et al. Randomized trial of preoperative chemoradiation versus surgery alone in patients with locoregional esophageal carcinoma. J Clin Oncol 2001; 19:305–313.
13. Law S, Kwong D, Tung H, et al. Preoperative chemoradiation for squamous cell esophageal cancer: a prospective randomized trial. Can J Gastroenterol 1998; 12 Suppl B:56B (abstract).
14. Enzinger PC, Mayer RJ. Medical progress: Esophageal cancer. N Engl J Med 2003; 349:2241–2252.
15. Nygaard K, Hagen S, Hansen HS, et al. Preoperative radiotherapy prolongs survival in operable esophageal cancer: a randomized, multicenter study of preoperative radiotherapy and chemotherapy. The second Scandinavian trial in esophageal cancer. World J Surg 1992; 16:1104–1110.
16. Walsh T, Noonan N, Hollywood D, et al. A comparison of multimodal therapy and surgery for esophageal adenocarcinoma. N Engl J Med 1996; 335:462–467.
17. Refaely Y, Krasna MJ. Multimodality therapy for esophageal cancer. Surg Clin North Am 2002; 82:729–746.
18. Rice TW. Clinical Staging of Esophageal Carcinoma. Chest Surg Clin North Am 2000; 10:471–485.
19. van Overhagen H, Becker CD. Diagnosis and Staging of Carcinoma of the Esophagus and Gastroesophageal Junction, and the Detection of Postoperative Recurrence, by Computed Tomography. In: Meyers MA. (ed.) Neoplasms of the Digestive Tract. Imaging, Staging, and Management. Philadelphia: Lippincott-Raven; 1998:31–48.
20. Chandawarkar RY, Kakegawa T, Fujita H, et al. Comparative analysis of imaging modalities in the preoperative assessment of nodal metastases in esophageal cancer. J Surg Oncol 1996; 61:214–217.
21. Wernecke K, Rummeny E, Bongartz G, et al. Detection of hepatic metastases in patients with carcinoma: Comparative sensitivities of sonography, CT and MR imaging. Am J Roentgenol 1991; 157: 731–739.
22. Dittler HJ, Pesarini AC, Siewert JR. Endoscopic classification of esophageal cancer: Correlation with the T stage. Gastrointest Endosc 1992; 38:662–668.
23. Caletti GC, Ferrari A, Fiorino S, et al. Staging of esophageal carcinoma by endoscopy. Endoscopy 1993; 25:2–9.
24. Kienle P, Buhl K, Kuntz C, et al. Prospective comparison of endoscopy, endosonography and computed tomography fro staging tumours of the oesophagus and gastric cardia. Digestion 2002; 66:230–236.
25. Bhutani MS, Barde CJ, Markert RJ, et al. Length of esophageal cancer and degree of luminal stenosis during upper endoscopy predict T stage by endoscopic ultrasound. Endoscopy 2002; 34:457–460.
26. Botet JF, Lightdale CJ, Zauber AG, et al. Preoperative staging of esophageal cancer: Comparison of endoscopic US and dynamic CT. Radiology 1991; 181:419–425.
27. Heintz A, Hohne U, Schweden F, et al. Preoperative detection of intrathoracic tumor spread of esophageal cancer: Endosonography versus computer tomography. Surg Endosc 1991; 5:75–78.
28. Tio TL, Cohen P, Coene PP, et al. Endosonography and Computed Tomography of Esophageal Carcinoma: Preoperative classification compared to the new (1987) TNM system. Gastroenterol 1989; 96:1478–1486.
29. Rosch T. Endosonographic staging of esophageal cancer: a review of the literature results. Gastrointest Endosc Clin N Am 1995; 5:537–547.
30. Heidemann J, Schilling MK, Schmassman A, et al. Accuracy of endoscopic ultrasonography in preoperative staging of esophageal carcinoma. Dig Surg 2000; 17:219–224.
31. Vilmann P, Khattar S, Hancke S. Endoscopic ultrasound examination of the upper gastrointestinal tract using a curved array transducer: A preliminary report. Surg Endosc 1991; 5:79–82.
32. Saunders HS, Wolfman NT, Ott DJ. Esophageal cancer. Radiologic staging. Radiol Clin North Am 1997; 35:281–294.
33. Kimmey MB, Martin RW, Haggitt RC, et al. Histologic correlates of gastrointestinal ultrasound images. Gastroenterology 1989; 96:433–441.
34. Bolondi L, Casenova P, Santi V, et al. The sonographic appearance of the normal gastric wall: an in vivo study. Ultrasound Med Biol 1986; 12:991–998.
35. Rice TW, Blackstone EH, Adelstein DJ, Zuccaro G, et al. Role of clinically determined depth of tumor invasion in the treatment of esophageal carcinoma. J Thorac Cardiovasc Surg 2003; 125: 1091–1102.
36. Kelly S, Harris KM, Berry E, et al. A systemic review of the staging performance of endoscopic ultrasound in gastro-oesophageal carcinoma. Gut 2001; 49:534–539.
37. Catalano MF, Sivak MV Jr, Rice TW, et al. Endosonographic features predictive of lymph node metastases. Gastrointest Endosc 1994; 40:442–446.
38. Bhutani MS, Hawes RH, Hoffman BJ. A comparison of the accuracy of echo features during endoscopic ultrasound and EUS guided fine needle aspiration for diagnosis of malignant lymph node invasion. Gastrointest Endosc 1997; 45:474–479.
39. Catalano MF, Alcocer E, Chak A, et al. Evaluation of metastatic celiac lymph nodes in patients with esophageal carcinoma: accuracy of EUS. Gastrointest Endosc 1999; 50:352–356.
40. Rice TW, Zuccaro G Jr., Adelstein DJ, et al. Esophageal carcinoma: Depth of tumor invasion is predictive of regional lymph node status. Ann Thorac Surg 1998; 65:787–792.

41. Wiersema MJ, Vilmann P, Giovannini M, et al. Endosonography-guided fine-needle aspiration biopsy: diagnostic accuracy and complication assessment. Gastroenterol 1997; 112:1087–1095.

42. Mortensen MB, Pless T, Durup J, et al. Clinical impact of endoscopic ultrasound-guided fine needle aspiration biopsy in patients with upper gastrointestinal tract malignancies. A prospective study. Endoscopy 2001; 33:478–483.

43. Vazquez-Sequeiros E, Norton IA, Clain JE, et al. Impact of EUS-guided fine-needle aspiration on lymph node staging in patients with esophageal carcinoma. Gastrointest Endosc 2001; 53:751–757.

44. Vazquez-Sequeiros E, Wiersema M, Clain JE, et al. Impact of lymph node staging on therapy of esophageal carcinoma. Gastroenterol 2003; 125:1626–1635.

45. Reed CE, Mishra G, Sahai AV, et al. Esophageal cancer staging: improved accuracy by endoscopic ultrasound of celiac lymph nodes. Ann Thorac Surg 1999; 67:319–321.

46. Eloubeidi MA, Wallace MB, Reed CE, et al. The utility of EUS and EUS-guided fine needle aspiration in detecting celiac lymph node metastasis in patients with esophageal cancer: a single-center experience. Gastrointest Endosc 2001; 54:714–719.

47. Meining A, Dittler HJ, Wolf A, et al. You get what you expect? A critical appraisal of imaging methodology in endosonographic cancer staging. Gut 2002; 50:599–603.

48. Fockens P, van den Brande JHM, van Dullemen HM, et al. Endosonographic T-staging of esophageal carcinoma: A learning curve. Gastrointest Endosc 1996; 44:58–62.

49. Kim LS, Koch J. Do we practice what we preach? Clinical decision making and utilization of endoscopic ultrasound for staging esophageal cancer. Am J Gastoenterol 1999; 94:1847–1852.

50. Vilgrain V, Mompoint D, Palazzo L, et al. Staging of oesophageal carcinoma: Comparison of results with endoscopic sonography and CT. AJR 1990; 155:277–281.

51. Catalano MF, Van Dam J, Sivak Jr MV. Malignant esophageal strictures: Staging accuracy of endoscopic ultrasonography. Gastrointest Endosc 1995; 41:535–539.

52. Van Dam J, Rice TW, Catalano MF, et al. High-grade malignant stricture is predictive of esophagel stage. Cancer 1993; 71:2910–2917.

53. Pfau PR, Ginsberg GG, Lew RJ, et al. Esophageal dilation for endosonographic evaluation of malignant esophageal strictures is safe and effective. Am J Gastroenterol 2000; 95:2813–2815.

54. Kallemanis GE, Gupta PK, al-Kawas FH, et al. Endoscopic ultrasound for staging esophageal cancer, with and without dilation, is clinically important and safe. Gastrointest Endosc 1995; 41:540–546.

55. Wallace MB, Hawes RH, Sahai AV, et al. Dilation of malignant esophageal stenosis to allow EUS guide fine-needle aspiration: safety and effect on patient managment. Gastrointest Endosc 2000; 51:309–313.

56. Menzel J, Hoepffner N, Nottberg H, et al. Preoperative staging of esophageal carcinoma: Miniprobe sonography versus conventional endoscopic ultrasound in a prospective histopathologically verified study. Endoscopy 1999; 31:329–332.

57. McLoughlin RF, Cooperberg PL, Mathieson JR, et al. High resolution endoluminal ultrasonography in the staging of esophageal carcinoma. J Ultrasound Med 1995; 14:725–730.

58. Hunerbein M, Ghadimi BM, Haensch W, et al. Transendoscopic ultrasound of esophageal and gastric cancer using miniaturized ultrasound catheter probes. Gastrointest Endosc 1998; 48:371–375.

59. Menzel J, Hoepffner N, Nottberg H, et al. Preoperative staging of esophageal carcinoma: Miniprobe sonography versus conventional endoscopic ultrasound in a prospective histopathologically verified study. Endoscopy 1999; 31:291–297.

60. Zuccaro G, Rice TW, Goldblum J, et al. Endoscopic ultrasound cannot determine suitability for esophagectomy after aggressive chemoradiotherapy for esophageal cancer. Am J Gastroenterol 1999; 94:906.

61. Isenberg G, Chak A, Canto MI, et al. Endoscopic ultrasound in restaging of esophageal cancer after neoadjuvant chemoradiation. Gastrointest Endosc 1998; 48: 158–163.

62. Laterza E, de Manzoni G, Guglielmi A, et al. Endoscopic ultrasonography in the staging of esophageal carcinoma after preoperative radiotherapy and chemotherapy. Ann Thorac Surg 1999; 67:1466–1469.

63. Isenberg G, Chak A, Canto MI, et al. Endoscopic ultrasound in restaging of esophageal cancer after neoadjuvant chemoradiation. Gastrointest Endosc 1998; 48:158.

64. Chak A, Canto MI, Cooper GS, et al. Endosonographic assessment of multimodality therapy predicts survival of esophageal carcinoma patients. Cancer 2000; 88:1788–1795.

65. Penman ID, Williams DB, Sahai AV, et al. Ability of EUS with fine-needle aspiration to document nodal staging and response to neoadjuvant chemoradiotherapy in locally advanced esophageal cancer: a case report. Gastrointest Endosc 1999; 49:783–786.

66. Kienle P, Buhl K, Kuntz C, et al. Prospective comparison of endoscopy, endosonography and computed tomography for staging of tumours of the oesophagus and gastric cardia. Digestion 2002; 66:230–236.

67. Hadzijahic N, Wallace MB, Hawes RH, et al. CT or EUS for the initial staging of esophageal cancer? A cost minimization analysis. Gastrointest Endosc 2000; 52:715–720.

68. Flanagan FL, Dehdashti F, Siegel BA, et al. Staging of esophageal cancer with ^{18}F-flurodeoxyglucose positron emission tomography. Am J Roentgenol 1997; 168:417–424.

69. Rankin SC, Taylor H, Cook GJ, et al. Computed tomography and positron emission tomography in the pre-operative staging of esophageal carcinoma. Clin Radiol 1998; 53:659–665.

70. Block MI, Patterson GA, Sundaresan RS, et al. Improvement in staging of esophageal cancer with the addition of positron emission tomography. Ann Thorac Surg 1997; 64:770–777.

71. Kole AC, Plukker JT, Nieweg OE, et al. Positron emission tomography for staging of oesophageal and gastroesophageal malignancy. Br J Cancer 1998; 78:521–527.

72. Luketich JD, Schauer PR, Meltzer CC, et al. Role of positron emission tomography in staging esophageal cancer. Ann Thorac Surg 1997; 64:765–769.

73. Luketich JD, Friedman DM, Weigel TL, et al. Evaluation of distant metastases in esophageal cancer: 100 consecutive positron emission tomography scans. Ann Thorac Surg 1999; 68:1133–1137.

74. Flamen P, Lerut A, Van Cutsem E, et al. Utility of positron emission tomography for the staging of patients with potentially operable esophageal carcinoma. J Clin Oncol 2000; 18:3202–3210.

75. Krasna MJ, Reed CE, Jaklitsch MT, et al. Thoracoscopic staging of esophageal cancer: A prospective, multiinstitutional trial. Cancer and Leukemia Group B Thoracic Surgeons. Ann Thorac Surg 1995; 60:1337–1340.

76. Finch MD, John TG, Garden OG, et al. Laparoscopic ultrasonography for staging gastroesophageal cancer. Surgery 1997; 121:10–17.

77. Luketich JD, Meehan M, Nguyen NT, et al. Minimally invasive surgical staging for esophageal cancer. Surg Endosc 2000; 14:700–702.

78. Di Simone P, Mattioli S, Caletti GC, et al. Role of computed tomography, endoscopic ultrasound and bronchoscopy in the preoperative study of cancer of the thoracic esophagus. 1992; 53 (abstract).

79. Wallace MB, Nietert PJ, Earle C, et al. An analysis of multiple staging management strategies for carcinoma of the esophagus: Computed tomography, endoscopic ultrasound, positron emission tomography, and thoracoscopy/laparoscopy. Ann Thorac Surg 2002; 74:1026–1032.

5 Endoscopic Therapy for Early Esophageal Cancer and Premalignant Lesions in Barrett's Esophagus

GANAPATHY A. PRASAD, MD AND KENNETH K. WANG, MD

CONTENTS

1. INTRODUCTION

The major medical consequence of Barrett's esophagus (BE) is the potential risk of development of esophageal adenocarcinoma. It is the management of this cancer risk and early cancers that is the focus of endoscopic therapies. As the risk of cancer increases, the types of endoscopic therapies that can be applied become more invasive. These therapies involve removal of the esophageal mucosa and portions of the submucosa, thermal therapies to cauterize the neoplastic tissue, and the use of photochemical therapies that cause localized tissue necrosis. Case series suggest that these treatments are effective and in selected patients can be used in lieu of surgery or in patients who are not surgical candidates. However, randomized controlled trials are lacking.

2. BE AND CANCER RISK

BE is defined by the presence of specialized intestinal metaplasia (SIM) in the distal esophagus. Endoscopically this appears as pink salmon colored mucosa proximal to the gastroesophageal junction (GEJ). Histological confirmation of incomplete intestinal metaplasia above the GEJ is essential to confirming the diagnosis of BE. Incomplete intestinal metaplasia is characterized by the presence of mucin-secreting goblet cells in the columnar lining epithelium. This incomplete metaplasia is thought to occur as a result of chronic gastroesophageal reflux. BE has been classified on the basis of its length above the GEJ, i.e., long segment Barrett's (>3 cm), short segment Barrett's (<3 cm), and BE at the GEJ (1). In general,

patients with short segment BE are better candidates for ablative therapies because less mucosal area need to be destroyed and therapies are better tolerated in this group of patients.

The risk of cancer in BE correlates to the degree of dysplasia present in the mucosa. The relative risk of developing adenocarcinoma in any BE is thought to be 30–40 times higher than the general population, with a lifetime risk of 5% (5). The higher the degree of dysplasia found in the BE, the greater the risk of adenocarcinoma (2). It is generally felt that adenocarcinoma within BE arises as the final step of a gradual and sequential change in the metaplastic epithelium, progressing from nondysplastic mucosa, to low-grade dysplasia (LGD), then to high-grade dysplasia (HGD) and finally carcinoma. This has also been corroborated in animal models with surgically created jejunesophageal reflux (3). Nondysplastic Barrett's mucosa has a very low risk of cancer and current therapies in these patients have not been felt to be clinically beneficial. HGD, which carries a 30% risk of cancer, has been a condition to which ablative therapy has been directed because of the potentially greater clinical benefit. Early stage adenocarcinoma can also be treated endoscopically, provided that accurate staging is available. Unfortunately, esophageal adenocarcinoma is characterized by a proclivity to spread via the lymphatics. This has ramifications for endoscopic therapy because invasion of the submucosa by an early staged cancer may be associated with lymphatic or distant metastases.

2.1. RATIONALE FOR TREATMENT OF HGD

HGD would seem to be a logical treatment point of patients with BE. Adenocarcinoma of the esophagus has the most rapidly rising incidence of all carcinomas in the United States and western Europe (4). In order to impact this rate of adenocarcinoma, it would be sensible to treat the highest risk lesions for

From: Endoscopic Oncology: Gastrointestinal Endoscopy and Cancer Management. Edited by: D. O. Faigel and M. L. Kochman © Humana Press, Totowa, NJ

adenocarcinoma. There is some debate over the cancer risk with HGD within BE. Some studies have found that invasive adenocarcinoma may often be found in patients with HGD undergoing esophagectomy (up to 40% in some series) (8). Studies that have followed cohorts of patients with HGD provide estimates of the incidence rate for adenocarcinoma (9). Levine et al. followed 58 patients over 10 yr. They found that 26% of patients developed HGD/invasive cancer over a mean of 27 mo and 27% displayed a regression of HGD over a mean of 40 mo (10). A cohort of 75 patients followed at the Hines VA Hospital found evolution to cancer from HGD in 16% after the first year of surveillance. A retrospective cohort study by Buttar et al. (11) found that diffuse HGD (defined as the involvement of more than five crypts in a single biopsy, or the presence of HGD in more than one biopsy specimen) predicted a 3.7-fold increase in the risk of esophageal cancer, compared with focal HGD (defined as the presence of HGD in one focus, involving up to five crypts). Although the risk of cancer development does vary, the risk in each of the published series is substantial and identifies this group for potential prophylactic therapy.

2.2. STAGING OF EARLY ESOPHAGEAL CANCER

Esophageal cancer is staged according to the TNM classification proposed by the American Joint Commission on Cancer Staging and the International Union against Cancer. Tis, refers to carcinoma *in situ* and T1 refers to tumor invading the lamina propria (T1a) and submucosa (T1b).

The Japanese Classification of intramucosal carcinoma further classifies esophageal cancer in to the following subgroups:

- m1: involving the epithelium (Tis or intramucosal carcinoma).
- m2: involving the lamina propria.
- m3: involving the muscularis mucosa.
- sm1: involving the upper one-third of the submucosa.
- sm2: involving the middle one-third of the submucosa.
- sm3: involving the deepest one-third of the submucosa.

T2, T3, and T4 refer to tumor invading into the muscularis propria, through the muscularis propria into the adventitia and invasion of adjacent organs, respectively. Superficial esophageal cancers are defined as Tis and T1a (tumor involving the epithelium and lamina propria: m1 + m2 + m3). The clinical significance of this classification is the direct correlation of the depth of invasion of the tumor with the presence of lymph node metastasis in patients with squamous cell cancer. Presence of lymph node metastasis is uncommon in patients with intramucosal cancer, i.e., 1–3%, which increases up to 30% when the tumor invades into the submucosa (12,13). Kodama et al. (14) reported for squamous cell carcinoma that the incidence of lymph node metastasis was 0% for an m1 cancer, 3.3% for an m2 cancer, 12.2% for an m3 cancer, 26.5% for an sm1 cancer, 35.8% for an sm2 cancer, and 45.9% for an sm3 cancer. Although there is no comparable data from patients with early adenocarcinoma, it is generally accepted that the depth of invasion for adenocarcinoma likely correlates well with risk of metastasis. Endoscopic treatment of adenocarcinomas should be reserved for earlier stage tumors In asymptomatic patients because once symptoms arise in late-stage tumors, survival is limited (6,7).

3. MODALITIES FOR THE TREATMENT OF HGD IN BE

3.1. SURVEILLANCE ENDOSCOPY AND TREATMENT OF REFLUX

Despite the elevated cancer risk, the majority of patients with HGD will not develop adenocarcinoma. For this reason, many surveillance protocols have been proposed with the aim of detecting patients with early cancer for treatment although there still is a high likelihood of cure (10,15). Typically, surveillance involves obtaining four quadrant biopsies every 1–2 cm, along the BE, with additional biopsies at sites with visible mucosal abnormalities. In addition, patients are placed on higher dosages of proton pump inhibitors (PPIs) to eliminate symptoms of acid reflux. These results have been shown to lead to reasonable results in expert centers in which large numbers of biopsies can be obtained. In expert hands, surveillance can be performed with minimal morbidity or mortality. One group of 75 patients had only one cancer-related death during a mean of 7 yr of follow-up (15a). Although this strategy has been demonstrated to be effective in tertiary centers, there are some problems with the implementation of these techniques in clinical practice. The surveillance required is very time and labor intensive. In a group of 22 patients who underwent surveillance endoscopy, the mean number of biopsies obtained was 133 (10). Others calculated that a biopsy rate of more than 60 biopsies/cm^2 of Barrett's mucosa was obtained during surveillance (16). This degree of surveillance is intensive and costly because the specimens must be processed and histological interpretation obtained. In addition, there is considerable inter- and intraobserver variation in the interpretation of these biopsies among pathologists. Most of the studies have used single or small groups of very experienced pathologists that have special interests in the in BE. Although obtaining second opinions in biopsy interpretation is routine in the management of HGD, the cost of sending multiple biopsies for second opinion may be prohibitive in a managed care environment. Finally, patients who chose to undergo this approach must be aware there is a small chance that significant lesions might not be detected. This risk exists for any of these endoscopic therapies but is probably the greatest with surveillance because the risk of cancer development is the highest.

3.2. ESOPHAGECTOMY

Although esophagectomy is not an endoscopic therapy, it is important to discuss this option with patients before any endoscopic therapy. In many centers esophagectomy is the standard of care for patients with HGD. The primary advantage of this therapy is the ability to assure the patient about the elimination of the problem mucosa. For patients who are most concerned about possible cancer-related mortality, this represents the option with the least risk of cancer development. Unfortunately, this operation is very invasive and although mortality following esophagectomy has declined from 40 yr ago, it is still 5–10% in recent reports (17,18). The mortality has been shown to be inversely proportional to the volume of surgery at a particular center. Mortality rates as low as 2.6% have been obtained in specialized expert centers *(19)*. Despite the reduction in the mortality, morbidity in the postoperative phase, both immediate and delayed continues to be substantial. Muller et al. *(17)* found an overall early complication rate of 36% for 46,692 patients *(17)*. These complications include anastomotic strictures, leaks, postvagotomy symptoms, respiratory, and cardiac insufficiency. Many patients with HGD are elderly, with multiple comorbidities, which further increases the likelihood of complications and mortality. Although new methods of esophagectomy are being performed such as vagal sparing esophagectomy and laparoscopic esophagectomy, there have not been any studies prospectively comparing these techniques to traditional esophagectomy.

3.3. ENDOSCOPIC MUCOSAL ABLATION

Efforts at inducing "reversal" of BE with medical therapies have been successful *(20,21)*. The dogma that BE, once formed, is irreversible was disproved by Sampliner *(22)* and Berenson et al. *(23)* who demonstrated that once BE was ablated by thermal energy from either multipolar probe or laser, squamous epithelium could replace BE if acid reflux is controlled. It appears that any technique that can destroy the metaplastic epithelium can induce squamous re-epithelialization. Multiple techniques have been developed and these include photodynamic therapy (PDT), thermal therapy, and mucosal resection.

3.3.1. Photodynamic Therapy

PDT is a novel therapeutic method that uses nondestructive light to destroy tissue. PDT was first described in BE by the research group at Roswell Park in 1990, who used PDT to treat two patients with early-stage cancer in the esophagus with underlying BE.

3.3.1.1. Mechanism of Action

PDT involves the use of three major components: a photosensitizing drug, light of a specific wavelength that can activate the drug, and oxygen that can mediate the photodynamic process. All three components are essential to the success of this procedure. Several photosensitizing drugs have been studied including chlorophyll, chlorines, and porphyrins. All can be modified to produce photosensitizers that are selective for specific tissues. In addition, different wavelengths of light activation can be selected, which can lead to greater depths of tissue penetration and increased tissue destruction. Photosensitizers available in the United States include sodium porfimer (Photofrin II, Axcan Pharma, Montreal, Quebec, Canada) or topical amino levulinic acid (Levulan, DUSA Pharmaceuticals, Wilmington, MA) for dermatological applications.

Sodium porfimer is a porphyrin derivative that is preferentially delivered to areas with leaky vasculature, such as those around tumors. The compound then infiltrates into the interstitial space and binds to tumor tissues. The drug is administered intravenously at a dose of 2 mg/kg at 48 h before intended photoradiation of the esophagus. The photosensitizer is then activated by the proper wavelength of light. Lasers provide the light source to activate the photosensitizer. New generation sources include the Diomed 630 PDT laser Model T2USA (Cambridge, UK) that can provide up to 2 W of total power at

630 nm. A cylindrical diffuser delivers the light produced by the laser, which is available in sizes of 1, 2.5, and 5 cm. Balloon diffusers have also been created that now can treat segment lengths of 3, 5, and 7 cm (Fig. 1).

The larger balloon diffusers can be best utilized by the use of high-energy laser systems that can produce at least 3 W of power. Unfortunately, these systems are not currently available. Previously, a potassium titanyl phosphate (KTP)-YAG pumped tunable dye laser was available but currently the company only manufactures the KTP-YAG (Laserscope Series 800 KTP-YAG laser, San Jose, CA). These diffuser lengths represent the length of the BE that can be treated in a single application of light. If the segment to be treated is longer than 7 cm then multiple sessions may be needed, which increases the chance of complications such as strictures. The diffuser is placed in the center of the esophageal lumen for ideal photoradiation. The balloons must be placed orally and positioned with endoscopic guidance. A total of 200 J/cm of fiber is used to treat BE with HGD using a bare diffuser, although higher dosages of 300 J/cm of fiber are needed for treating nodular esophageal cancer. The balloon diffusers require less energy because the ends of the balloons are capped with a reflective surface to prevent loss of light. Light dosages with the diffusing balloon are recommended to be 130 J/cm of fiber.

The lack of a commercially available of a high-powered laser system has been a limitation. The diode laser that is available cannot power more than a 5-cm long fiber that can only deliver sufficient light for a 3-cm window balloon. The diode laser does not claim to be usable for the new balloon diffusers. Although longer fibers can be used with this system, some of the automated features make it difficult to actually use these longer fibers because fibers greater than 5 cm cannot be calibrated in the diode laser. These issues can be partially overcome by adjusting the software with the laser but this should only be done by well-trained individuals.

3.3.1.2. Efficacy and Results

Multiple studies have been done in the United States and Europe evaluating the use of PDT in BE. PDT is a well-suited treatment for this setting as it is able to treat a large amount of tissue with a single application. Before treatment, patients should be assessed for the presence of cancer. Endoscopic ultrasound (EUS) should be used to further evaluate any visible mucosal irregularity or nodule. If histology confirms the presence of a cancer, EUS is used to determine the depth of invasion of the tumor.

Table 1 lists the results of the most current studies in BE with HGD. Some studies have used PDT in combination with other adjuvant therapies such as argon plasma coagulation, electrocoagulation, and laser ablation. As is seen in Table 1, PDT can eliminate HGD from 88 to 100% of cases. However, cancer can appear in 4–5% of patients after the elimination of BE macroscopically, emphasizing the need for close surveillance of this population with endoscopy and biopsies.

Long-term results were recently reported by Overholt et al. *(24)*. They followed 103 patients treated by PDT using Porfimer sodium, followed by Nd:YAG laser to ablate residual areas of

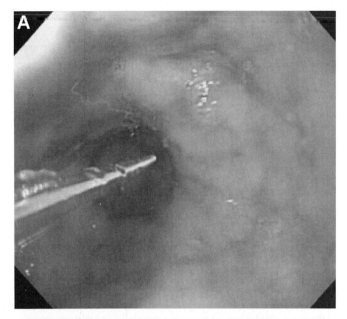

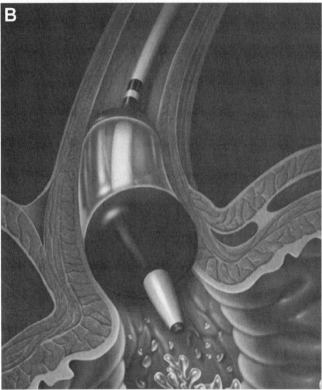

Fig. 1. The illustration (A) shows a cylindrical diffuser fiber in the esophagus. This is placed through the therapeutic channel of the endoscope. In (B), a cartoon is shown of a balloon diffuser placed orally into the stomach over a wire into the distal esophagus.

specialized intestinal metaplasia less than 2 cm in size. Acid suppression was maintained in all patients with twice a day PPI therapy. Indication for treatment was BE with LGD (14), HGD (80), and early-stage adenocarcinoma—T1N0 (9). After PDT, the length of BE decreased by a mean of 6.9 cm and 94% of patients with HGD had elimination of the dysplastic mucosa, whereas 4.6% of patients had developed subsquamous adenocarcinoma. Subsquamous nondysplastic metaplastic epithelium

was found in four patients (4,9%). Intention to treat success rates were 92.9, 77.5, and 44.4%, respectively, for HGD, LGD, and early-stage adenocarcinoma. Mean follow-up was close to 5 yr. All participants in the trial were patients who had refused surgery or were poor surgical candidates, out of which 7.5% of patients developed adenocarcinoma despite PDT. This was felt to be a reduction from the 25–50% of patients who would be expected to have or develop adenocarcinoma with HGD as reported in previous studies. However, this study lacked a control group making it impossible to draw firm conclusions regarding the potential benefits of PDT. Esophageal strictures developed in 30% of patients overall, with a higher proportion (50%) in patients who received two sessions of PDT.

More recently, a phase III randomized trial of porfirmer sodium PDT vs omeprazole alone for the treatment of HGD has been published (25). Two hundred and eight patients were randomized 2:1 to the two groups. Only the pathologists were blinded to treatment assignment. This study reported a significantly lower incidence of cancer in the treatment group (13 vs 28%, $p < 0.006$) with a mean follow-up of approx 1 yr. There was also a higher rate of ablation of HGD in the PDT group (77 vs 39%, $p < 0.0001$).

3.3.1.3. Complications

Short-term complications after PDT include cutaneous photosensitivity, which may persist for 30–90 d after drug administration, chest pain, odynophagia, and dysphagia (26). Patient education regarding measures to avoid phototoxicity, and close monitoring and early intervention for dehydration are important. Pain control is usually provided by narcotic patches, which provide long-term pain relief and bypass the oral route, avoiding esophageal mucosal irritation.

The most common long-term complication is stricture formation. Strictures are most likely to occur in patients with multiple treatments, those requiring more than one application of the light owing to a long length of the BE, and those with preexisting luminal narrowing. Rates of stricture formation range from 16 to 30%. Patients are managed with stricture dilations and may need one or multiple dilations (27). Oral steroids do not seem to have any effect on stricture development rates (28).

3.3.1.4. Limitations of PDT

Subsquamous islands of metaplastic or dysplastic Barrett's tissue can persist in patients after PDT, but may be minimized if additional thermal techniques are used. One patient developed cancer arising under squamous mucosa during follow-up after therapy, emphasizing the need for continued close surveillance (29). Genetic abnormalities also persist in the mucosa after PDT (30). This raises the possibility that genetic changes produce clones of cells in BE that are resistant to PDT. Effective treatment of patients with coexisting early adenocarcinoma needs the addition of another modality, such as endoscopic mucosal resection (EMR). In such patients, PDT may serve as an important adjunct, eliminating the at risk mucosa, potentially reducing rates of recurrence.

3.3.2. Argon Beam Plasma Coagulation

Argon beam plasma coagulation (ABPC) is a noncontact technique of electrocautery to achieve mucosal ablation, wherein argon gas is delivered through a catheter to which a

Table 1
Studies of PDT of BE With HGD and Early Esophageal Cancer

Reference	N	Photosensitizer	Adjuvant therapy	Elimination of HGD/Ca	Cancers after photoablation	Follow-up (months)
25	208	Photophrin	No	PDT: 106/138 (77%) Control: 27/70 (39%) $p < 0.0001$	PDT: 18/138 (13%) Control: 20/70 (28%) $p < 0.006$	12
24	HGD = 80 Early Ca = 9	Photofrin	Yes	62/80 = 77.6% 4/9 = 44.4%	3/62 = 5%	50
30	56	Photofrin	None	100%	3/56 = 5%	46
48	4	MTHPC	None	100%	0	27
15a	208	Photofrin	None	80%	9%	6
28	43	Photofrin	Yes	96%	0	12
49	10	ALA	No	100%	0	5.4
50	5	ALA	No	100%	0	26–44

HGD, high-grade dysplasia; Ca, cancer.

voltage is applied generating a plasma that transmits the electrical energy to the mucosal surface. Attwood et al. from the United Kingdom have reported their experience of treating 29 patients with BE and HGD with ABPC (31). These patients were either unfit for or had refused esophagectomy. Eighty three percent of patients had macroscopically evident areas of mucosal abnormality, i.e., nodules or ulcers. None of these lesions were subjected to EMR. Treatment was stopped after no dysplasia was found on surveillance biopsies taken every 1–2 cm in the distal esophagus. Mean follow-up was approx 3 yr. Of 29 patients, 25 had no residual HGD and 22 had no residual BE present. Four patients (14%) developed esophageal adenocarcinoma and three of these patients continue to receive ablation therapy with ABPC. One perforation occurred followed by esophagectomy but the patient expired owing to postoperative complications. Patients needed a median of two treatments for resolution of the HGD. No strictures occurred in this series.

Although ABPC was felt to be successful in decreasing the risk of cancer, this decrease rate of progression is questioned by many investigators who believe that the earlier reports of progression to adenocarcinoma in patients with HGD were biased and overestimated (32). No randomized controlled trials evaluating ABPC have been published.

3.3.3. Electrocoagulation

In multipolar electrocoagulation (MPEC), electric current flows between the electrodes in the tip of the probe. The maximum temperature achieved is 100°C. MPEC has been used in combination with high-dose PPI therapy. In 54 BE patients without dysplasia, MPEC achieved complete endoscopic reversal in 85% and complete histological reversal in 78% with a mean of 3.5 treatments (range 1–6) (33). MPEC has been performed after anti-reflux surgery followed and lead to the reversal of BE in 14 patients (34).

Dulai et al. have recently reported the results of a randomized trial comparing thermoablation by ABPC and MPEC. All

patients had 2–7 cm of BE without HGD or cancer. The primary outcome was the number of treatment sessions to endoscopic ablation and 52 patients were randomized. The mean number of treatments to ablation were 2.9 for MPEC and 3.8 for argon plasma coagulation ($p = 0.04$). The mean time for the first session was 6 min for MPEC vs 10 min for argon plasma coagulation. No serious adverse events were noted and transient upper gastrointestinal symptoms occurred in 8–13% of patients.

3.3.4. Other Methods

Other methods of thermal mucosal ablation include Laser (light amplication by stimulated emission of radiation) and Heater Probe. Various lasers including the Nd:YAG laser, and the KTP:YAG laser have been used to ablate HGD and early adenocarcinoma (35,36). Small case series have reported success in eradicating BE and also adenocarcinoma. All series have also used PPIs to maintain a relatively anacid environment to promote reepithelialization with squamous epithelium. Cryoablation using liquid CO_2 has also been reported in small series with promising preliminary results.

4. ENDOSCOPIC TREATMENT OF EARLY ESOPHAGEAL CANCER

4.1. ENDOSCOPIC MUCOSAL RESECTION

EMR is useful for providing accurate tissue diagnoses of macroscopic esophageal lesions and for treatment of early esophageal cancer. EMR techniques have evolved significantly because the introduction of the "big particle biopsy" concept in the 1970s. The largest experience with EMR is found in the Japanese literature, with its use beginning primarily in the treatment of superficial gastric neoplasms (37).

Suggested criteria for esophageal neoplasms suitable for EMR include:

- Diameter of less than 2 cm.
- Involvement of less than one-third the circumference of the esophageal wall.
- Disease limited to the mucosa on EUS.

Table 2
Macroscopic Types of Early Carcinoma (Japanese Classification)

Type	Definition
I	Polypoid type
II	Flat type
II a	Flat raised
II b	At the mucosal level
II c	Slightly depressed
III	Ulcerated type

4.1.1. Techniques of EMR

Different EMR techniques can be adapted to the kind of lesion being targeted (Table 2).

4.1.1.1. Strip Biopsy Technique

In this technique, a diathermy loop is introduced through the working channel of the endoscope and is positioned over a polypoid lesion. The loop is then tightened and the lesion is slowly resected using electric cutting current. This is suitable for polypoid tumors (type 1), but is difficult for flat lesions. Submucosal injection of a solution can lift flat or depressed lesions and make them easier to resect (the lift and cut technique). Injection of a saline–epinephrine solution into the submucosa lifts the early carcinoma, potentially reducing the risk of perforation. The epinephrine also provides better hemostasis.

4.1.1.2. Suck-and-Cut Technique

Inoue et al. *(38)* developed the cap technique, improving the effectiveness of EMR compared with the strip biopsy. In this technique, a specially developed transparent plastic cap is attached to the end of the endoscope. After submucosal injection under the target lesion, the lesion is sucked into the cap and resected with a diathermy loop that was previously loaded into the specially designed groove on the lower edge of the cap. Marking the perimeter of the lesion before resection is recommended, as the margins become indistinct after the submucosal injection.

The suck-and-cut technique may also be performed by using a ligation device. In this technique, the target lesion is sucked into the ligation device cylinder and a polyp is created by releasing a rubber band around the lesion. The polyp can then be resected at its base, either above or below the band. This technique may necessitate the withdrawal of the endoscope and reintroduction to resect the polyp with the diathermy loop.

4.1.1.3. Grasping Technique

The grasping technique for EMR uses a double-channel endoscope. In this technique, a grasping forcep is used to pull the target lesion through a diathermy loop, which is introduced through the second channel. This procedure is technically demanding especially at the GEJ, in which retroflexion may be needed, and the large diameter of the endoscope makes this difficult *(39)*.

4.1.2. Efficacy and Results

May et al. *(40)* compared the suck-and-ligate technique without submucosal injection to the cap technique with submucosal injection, in a prospective fashion. They included 70 patients who needed 100 resections; 82% of patients had early-stage esophageal cancers. Fifty resections were performed with the ligation device and 50 were performed using the cap technique, with submucosal saline–epinephrine injection. The primary end point of the study was the maximum diameter of the resection specimen, the resection area, and the complication rate. No significant difference was noted between the groups in terms of the maximum diameter of the resected specimens and the resection area at 24 h. One minor bleed occurred in each group, but no severe complications occurred.

May et al. *(41)* have also reported their experience in treating more than 350 patients with HGD or early-stage esophageal cancers with more than 800 EMRs. Complete resection was accomplished in 82.5% of patients. During the mean follow-up period of 12 mo, recurrences or metachronous cancers were seen in 14% of patients, and they underwent successful repeat endoscopic treatment. The overall rate of complications was 12.5%.

Other investigators have also reported on smaller series of patients with HGD and BE or adenocarcinoma of the esophagus, who have been treated with either EMR alone or a combination of EMR and a mucosal ablative technique such as PDT or ABPC. Nijhawan and Wang *(42)* reported their results with treatment of 25 patients with HGD and intramucosal carcinoma of the esophagus. EMR was performed because of a nodule or polyp within BE in 11 patients (44%) or because of endoscopic features that raised a suspicion of superficial cancer or HGD in 14 patients (56%). The latter included areas endoscopically recognizable by the presence of mucosa that was irregular, friable, ulcerated, or villous appearing. They used the lift-and-cut EMR technique in most cases, and the ligation device (the suck-and-cut technique) in two patients. EMR resulted in a significant change in the diagnosis in 11 patients (44%). Eight patients were diagnosed with adenocarcinoma after the pathologists reviewed the EMR specimen, two patients underwent esophagectomies, and the remainder were managed endoscopically. Four patients with adenocarcinoma underwent PDT as an adjunctive treatment. No deaths or recurrent HGD/cancer were reported after a mean follow-up of 14 mo.

Ahmad et al. *(43)* reported on a heterogenous group of 101 patients who underwent EMR for lesions throughout the gastrointestinal tract. This series included 12 patients with HGD *(6)* and adenocarcinoma *(6)* in the esophagus. Complete resection was obtained in almost 90% of these lesions.

Fujita et al. *(44)* attempted to define the optimal treatment strategy for superficial squamous esophageal cancer. They retrospectively evaluated the morbidity and mortality rates, survival rates, and recurrence rates for patients with superficial esophageal cancer: 72 patients with mucosal esophageal cancer who underwent either esophagectomy or EMR and 78 patients with submucosal esophageal cancer who underwent extended radical esophagectomy or less radical esophagectomy. Patients with mucosal esophageal cancer were comparable in terms of demographics and tumor stage. Fourteen patients had positive margins after EMR and underwent repeat EMR. Hospital mortality was 14% in the surgical group and 0% in the EMR group. Morbidity was also significantly lower in the EMR group (7%)

compared with the surgical group (69%). There was no significant difference in the overall survival rates between the EMR and surgery groups. No difference was seen in the disease-specific survival rates. Lymph node metastasis was seen in only one patient in the surgical group and in none of the patients who underwent EMR. Multivariate analysis did not find treatment modality to be a prognostic factor in patients with mucosal esophageal cancer, leading the authors to conclude that EMR was the treatment of choice in patients with mucosal esophageal cancer.

4.1.3. Complications

Immediate complications include bleeding and perforation. These are reported to be relatively infrequent, with no perforations or major bleeding reported in the large series reported by May et al. *(45)*. Minor bleeding (hemoglobin drop of <2 g/dL) and esophageal stenosis occurred in a small portion of patients: 5 and 3 patients out of 112, respectively. Delayed complications have included esophageal stenosis.

4.1.4. Limitations

In current practice, EMR is limited by its application to visible areas of mucosal abnormality, which are then targeted. Its utility in patients with long segments of BE and HGD without any mucosal abnormality remains to be defined. The applicability of this specialized technique to general endoscopy and gastroenterology practice in the United States is unclear. Piecemeal resection of neoplastic lesions has also been shown to be associated with a higher chance of residual tumor as opposed to *en-bloc* resections. New techniques toward this end are being explored and are discussed in the following paragraphs. Resection of malignant lesions by EMR does not obviate the need for close endoscopic surveillance as demonstrated by the significant rates, up to 14%, of tumor or dysplasia recurrence.

4.2. COMBINED MODALITY TREATMENT

The rationale for a multiple modality treatment approach to HGD in BE or early adenocarcinoma lies in the ability of EMR to target only macroscopically abnormal areas of mucosa: providing effective treatment, but leaving a background of at risk mucosa. This correlates to the significant number of metachronous lesions seen in series in which EMR has been the sole modality of treatment. Mucosal ablative techniques, such as PDT or ABPC complement EMR, by targeting not only the residual dysplastic mucosa, but also eliminating the surrounding BE. This should potentially eliminate the source of future cancer formation. EMR complements mucosal ablative techniques by treating elevated lesions, which may not be addressed by PDT or ABPC owing to inadequate penetration.

Buttar et al. *(46)* described the use of EMR with PDT in 17 consecutive nonsurgical patients with early esophageal ACA. The EMR margins were involved by cancer in three cases. EMR improved staging in eight patients (47%). Ninety-four percent of patients remained in remission at a median follow-up of 13 mo. Complications included bleeding in one patient, stricture in five (30%), and cutaneous phototoxicity in two (12%).

More recently, Pacifico et al. *(47)* reported the results of their retrospective review of 24 patients with early-stage ACA,

who underwent EMR and PDT and 64 concurrent patients who underwent esophagectomy for the same diagnosis. All patients underwent EUS to define the depth of cancer involvement and assess for lymph node involvement. Early esophageal adenocarcinoma was defined as intramucosal carcinoma (uT1m) and cancers with submucosal involvement (uT1sm). Patients who underwent EMR and PDT were either poor surgical candidates or had refused surgery. EMR was performed by the ligation technique and the cap technique. PDT was performed a mean of 4 wk after the EMR to allow for healing of the mucosa. Both groups were largely comparable. Patients were followed for a mean of 12–19 mo.

Of 24 patients, 4 (17%) in the EMR/PDT group failed treatment, as defined by the persistence of cancer on the first surveillance biopsy after treatment. One of these patients underwent esophagectomy, and another underwent chemoradiation therapy. Both were alive at the end of the study. The remaining two died of unrelated causes before alternative treatment could be considered. In the surgical group, one patient died from a surgical complication and another died of unknown causes. Complications included photosensitivity and strictures in 8% of patients in the EMR/PDT group and strictures and anastomotic leaks in 16 and 8% of patients, respectively, in the surgical group.

This study highlights the need to take the important next step in defining the treatment of HGD in BE and early ACA: comparing the current standard of treatment, surgery, with less invasive techniques which eliminate treatment related mortality and reduce treatment related morbidity, in a prospective randomized manner, with long-term follow-up, in an adequately powered study.

5. CONCLUSION

A number of techniques are now available to treat HGD in BE and early-stage adenocarcinoma of the esophagus. A combination of EMR-guided by EUS to target visible lesions and mucosal ablation of the surrounding BE to treat the premalignant surrounding mucosa seems to be the most logical method of treating dysplasia and neoplasia in the esophagus. The advent of widespread tissue removal may be in the future for ablation therapy although many modalities appear to be still in evolution. The depth and breadth of subsurface mucosal ablation remains to be defined. The gains of anatomical preservation with endoluminal therapy need to be weighed against the costs of the repeated procedures, which many patients need during and after ablation, as well as the costs of the drugs and therapies. The risk of metachronous lesions developing during follow-up, needing more therapy, and the continued need for intense acid suppression also needs to be factored in. Although these techniques appear to be safe and effective, long-term follow-up data and comparison with the current gold standard, esophagectomy, in a randomized trial is required before endoluminal therapy can be offered to all patients as an alternative to esophagectomy. Hence, endoluminal therapy for BE and early esophageal cancer remains a reasonable option for patients who are poor surgical candidates, or those who refuse surgery with full understanding of their options.

ACKNOWLEDGMENTS

The authors would like to acknowledge the support of NIH grants CA85992-01 and R01CA097048-01 and the Mayo Foundation.

REFERENCES

1. Sharma P, Morales TG, Sampliner RE. Short segment Barrett's esophagus—the need for standardization of the definition and of endoscopic criteria. Am J Gastroenterol 1998; 93(7):1033–1036.

2. Hamilton SR, Smith RR. The relationship between columnar epithelial dysplasia and invasive adenocarcinoma arising in Barrett's esophagus. Am J Clin Pathol 1987; 87(3):301–312.

3. Pera M, Trastek VF, Carpenter HA, et al. Influence of pancreatic and biliary reflux on the development of esophageal carcinoma. Ann Thor Surg 1993; 55(6):1386–1392; discussion 1392–1393.

4. Devesa SS, Blot WJ, Fraumeni JF Jr. Changing patterns in the incidence of esophageal and gastric carcinoma in the United States. Cancer 1998; 83(10):2049–2053.

5. Li H. Malignant Barrett's oesophagus. Eur J Cancer Prevention 1993; 2(1):47–52.

6. Streitz JM Jr, Andrews CW Jr, Ellis FH Jr. Endoscopic surveillance of Barrett's esophagus. Does it help? J Thor Cardiovasc Surg 1993; 105(3):383–387, discussion 387–388.

7. Clark GW, Smyrk TC, Burdiles P, et al. Is Barrett's metaplasia the source of adenocarcinomas of the cardia? Arch Surg 1994; 129(6):609–614.

8. Spechler SJ. Clinical practice. Barrett's Esophagus. N Eng J Med 2002; 346(11):836–842.

9. Hameeteman W, Tytgat GN, Houthoff HJ, van den Tweel JG. Barrett's esophagus: development of dysplasia and adenocarcinoma. Gastroenterology 1989; 96(5 Part 1):1249–1256 (see comment).

10. Levine DS, Haggitt RC, Blount PL, Rabinovitch PS, Rusch VW, Reid BJ. An endoscopic biopsy protocol can differentiate high-grade dysplasia from early adenocarcinoma in Barrett's esophagus. Gastroenterology 1993; 105(1):40–50 (see comment).

11. Buttar NS, Wang KK, Sebo TJ, et al. Extent of high-grade dysplasia in Barrett's esophagus correlates with risk of adenocarcinoma. Gastroenterology 2001; 120(7):1630–1639 (see comment).

12. Nigro JJ, Hagen JA, DeMeester TR, et al. Prevalence and location of nodal metastases in distal esophageal adenocarcinoma confined to the wall: implications for therapy. J Thor Cardiovasc Surg 1999; 117(1):16–23 discussion 23–25 (see comment).

13. Stein HJ, Feith M, Mueller J, Werner M, Siewert JR. Limited resection for early adenocarcinoma in Barrett's esophagus. Ann Surg 2000; 232(6):733–742.

14. Kodama M, Kakegawa T. Treatment of superficial cancer of the esophagus: a summary of responses to a questionnaire on superficial cancer of the esophagus in Japan. Surgery 1998; 123(4):432–439.

15. Reid BJ, Weinstein WM, Lewin KJ, et al. Endoscopic biopsy can detect high-grade dysplasia or early adenocarcinoma in Barrett's esophagus without grossly recognizable neoplastic lesions. Gastroenterology 1988; 94(1):81–90.

15a. Schnell TG, Sontag SJ, Chijfec G, et al. Long-term nonsurgical management of Barrett's esophagus with high-grade dysplasia. Gastroenterology 2001; 120(7):1607–1619 (see comment).

16. Spechler SJ, Goyal RK. Cancer surveillance in Barrett's esophagus: what is the end point? Gastroenterology 1994; 106(1):275–277 (comment).

17. Muller JM, Erasmi H, Stelzner M, Zieren U, Pichlmaier H. Surgical therapy of oesophageal carcinoma. Br J Surg 1990; 77(8):845–857.

18. Orringer MB, Marshall B Stirling MC. Transhiatal esophagectomy for benign and malignant disease. J Thor Cardiovasc Surg 1993; 105(2):265–276 discussion 276–277.

19. Korst RJ, Altorki NK. High grade dysplasia: surveillance, mucosal ablation, or resection? World J Surg 2003; 27(9):1030–1034.

20. Sampliner RE. Effect of up to 3 years of high-dose lansoprazole on Barrett's esophagus. Am J Gastroenterol 1994; 89(10):1844–1848 (see comment).

21. Sharma P, Sampliner RE, Camargo E. Normalization of esophageal pH with high-dose proton pump inhibitor therapy does not result in regression of Barrett's esophagus. Am J Gastroenterol 1997; 92(4):582–585 (see comment).

22. Sampliner RE, Hixson LJ, Fennerty MB, Garewal HS. Regression of Barrett's esophagus by laser ablation in an anacid environment. Digestive Diseases and Sciences 1993; 38(2):365–368.

23. Berenson MM, Johnson TD, Markowitz NR, Buchi KN, Samowitz WS. Restoration of squamous mucosa after ablation of Barrett's esophageal epithelium. Gastroenterology 1993; 104(6):1686–1691.

24. Overholt BF, Panjehpour M, Halberg DL. Photodynamic therapy for Barrett's esophagus with dysplasia and/or early stage carcinoma: long-term results. Gastrointest Endosc 2003; 8(2):183–188.

25. Overholt BE, Lightdale CJ, Wang KF, et al. Photodynamic therapy with porfirmer sodium for ablation of high-grade dysplasia in Barrett's esophagus: international, partially blinded, randomized phase III trial. Gastrointest Endosc 2005; 68:488–498.

26. Wolfsen HC, Ng CS. Cutaneous consequences of photodynamic therapy. Cutis 2002; 69(2):140–142.

27. Wang KK, Nijhawan PK. Complications of photodynamic therapy in gastrointestinal disease. Gastrointest Endosc Clin North Am 2000; 10(3):487–495.

28. Panjehpour M, Overholt BF, Haydek JM, Lee SG. Results of photodynamic therapy for ablation of dysplasia and early cancer in Barrett's esophagus and effect of oral steroids on stricture formation. Am J Gastroenterol 2000; 95(9):2177–2184.

29. Overholt BF, Panjehpour M, Haydek JM. Photodynamic therapy for Barrett's esophagus: follow-up in 100 patients. Gastrointest Endosc 1999; 49(1):1–7 (see comment).

30. Krishnadath KK, Wang K, Liu W, et al. Persistent genetic abnormalities in Barrett's esophagus after photodynamic therapy. Gastroenterology 2000; 119(3):624–630 (see comment).

31. Attwood SE, Lewis CJ, Caplin S, Hemming K, Armstrong G. Argon beam plasma coagulation as therapy for high-grade dysplasia in Barrett's esophagus. Clin Gastroenterol and Hepatol 2003; 1(4):258–263 (see comment).

32. Fennerty MB. Endoscopic ablation of Barrett's related neoplasia: what is the evidence supporting its use? Gastrointest Endosc 2003; 58(2):246–249 (comment).

33. Sampliner RE, Faigel DO, Fennerty MB, et al. Effective and safe endoscopic reversal of non-dysplastic Barrett's esophagus with thermal electrocoagulation combined with high-dose acid inhibition: a multicenter study. Gastrointest Endosc 2001; 53:554–558.

34. Montes CG, Brandalise NA, Deliza R, Novais de Magalhaes AF, Ferraz JG. Antireflux surgery followed by bipolar electrocoagulation in the treatment of Barrett's esophagus. Gastrointestinal Endoscopy 1999; 50(2):173–177.

35. Sharma P, Jaffe PE, Bhattacharyya A, Sampliner RE. Laser and multipolar electrocoagulation ablation of early Barrett's adenocarcinoma: long-term follow-up. Gastrointestinal Endoscopy 1999; 49(4 Part 1):442–446.

36. Barham CP, Jones RL, Biddlestone LR, Hardwick RH, Shepherd NA, Barr H. Photothermal laser ablation of Barrett's oesophagus: endoscopic and histological evidence of squamous re-epithelialisation. Gut 1997; 41(3):281–284.

37. Kojima T, Parra-Blanco A, Takahashi H, Fujita R. Outcome of endoscopic mucosal resection for early gastric cancer: review of the Japanese literature. Gastrointest Endosc 1998; 48(5):550–554, discussion 554–555.

38. Inoue H, Takeshita K, Hori H, Muraoka Y, Yoneshima H, Endo M. Endoscopic mucosal resection with a cap-fitted panendoscope for esophagus, stomach, and colon mucosal lesions. Gastrointest Endosc 1993; 39(1):58–62 (see comment).

39. Noda M, Kobayashi N, Kanemasa H, et al. Endoscopic mucosal resection using a partial transparent hood for lesions located tangentially to the endoscope. Gastrointest Endosc 2000; 51(3): 338–343.

40. May A, Gossner L, Behrens A, et al. A prospective randomized trial of two different endoscopic resection techniques for early stage cancer of the esophagus. Gastrointest Endosc 2003; 58(2):167–175 (*see* comment).

41. Ell C, May A, Gossner L, et al. Endoscopic mucosal resection of early cancer and high-grade dysplasia in Barrett's esophagus. Gastroenterology 2000; 118(4):670–677.

42. Nijhawan PK, Wang KK. Endoscopic mucosal resection for lesions with endoscopic features suggestive of malignancy and high-grade dysplasia within Barrett's esophagus. Gastrointest Endosc 2000; 52(3):328–332 (*see* comment).

43. Ahmad NA, Kochman ML, Long WB, Furth EE, Ginsberg GG. Efficacy, safety, and clinical outcomes of endoscopic mucosal resection: a study of 101 cases. Gastrointest Endosc 2002; 55(3): 390–396.

44. Fujita H, Sueyoshi S, Yamana H, et al. Optimum treatment strategy for superficial esophageal cancer: endoscopic mucosal resection versus radical esophagectomy. World J Surg 2001; 25(4): 424–431.

45. May A, Gossner L, Pech O, et al. Local endoscopic therapy for intraepithelial high-grade neoplasia and early adenocarcinoma in Barrett's oesophagus: acute-phase and intermediate results of a new treatment approach. Eur J Gastroenterol and Hepatology 2002; 14(10):1085–1091 (*see* comment).

46. Buttar NS, Wang KK, Lutzke LS, Krishnadath KK, Anderson MA. Combined endoscopic mucosal resection and photodynamic therapy for esophageal neoplasia within Barrett's esophagus. Gastrointest Endosc 2001; 54(6):682–688.

47. Pacifico RJ, Wang KK, Wongkeesong LM, Buttar NS, Lutzke LS. Combined endoscopic mucosal resection and photodynamic therapy versus esophagectomy for management of early adenocarcinoma in Barrett's esophagus. Clin Gastroenterol Hepatol 2003; 1(4):252–257 (see comment).

48. Javaid B. Photodynamic therapy (PDT) for oesophageal dysplasia and early carcinoma with mTHPC (m-Tetrahidroxyphenyl chlorin): a preliminary study. Lasers Med Sci 2002; 17(2):135 (comment).

49. Gossner L, May A, Sroka R, Stolte M, Hahn EG, Ell C. Photodynamic destruction of high grade dysplasia and early carcinoma of the esophagus after the oral administration of 5-aminolevulinic acid. Cancer 1999; 86(10):1921–1928.

50. Barr H, Shephard NA, Dix A, Robers DJ, Tan WC, Krasner N. Eradication of high-grade dysplasia in columnar-lined (Barrett's) oesophagus by photodynamic therapy with endogenously generated protoporphyrin IX. Lancet 1996; 348(9027): 584–585 (*see* comment).

6 Endoscopic Therapy for Advanced Esophageal Cancer

SANJAY JAGANNATH, MD AND MARCIA I. CANTO, MD, MHS

CONTENTS

1. BACKGROUND

Esophageal cancer is currently the ninth leading cause of cancer death in the United States, and since the 1970s, the incidence of esophageal adenocarcinoma has been rising at an alarming rate *(1)*. The National Cancer Institutes estimates 14,250 new cases of esophageal cancer and 13,300 deaths owing to esophageal cancer in 2004. The estimated 5-yr mortality rate remains at 5–10% *(1)*.

Unfortunately, the majority of patients present with advanced disease that is not curative by surgery *(2)*. Palliative surgery is associated with a relatively high morbidity (20–60%) and mortality (10–33%), and approximately one-third of these patients will develop anastomotic strictures or local tumor recurrence necessitating further intervention *(3)*. Because the median survival of such patients is less than 6 mo, palliative surgery has been replaced by nonsurgical techniques, primarily chemoradiation, brachytherapy, and/or endoscopic therapy *(4)*. This chapter summarizes the goals, safety and efficacy, and techniques for endoscopic palliation of advanced esophageal cancer, focusing primarily on techniques for treatment of malignant dysphagia but also including treatment options for esophageal fistulas and bleeding tumors.

2. TREATMENT OF DYSPHAGIA

2.1. GOALS OF PALLIATIVE ENDOSCOPIC THERAPY FOR DYSPHAGIA

Malignant dysphagia is defined as difficulty swallowing owing to malignancy and usually results from a partially or completely occluded esophageal lumen. It might present as intraluminal disease, extraluminal compression, tumor encroachment on esophageal innervation, or a combination of these mechanisms. In general, bulky, short, and nonangulated strictures in the mid or distal esophagus are the easiest to palliate. Treatment goals in the management of malignant dysphagia include (1) maintaining esophageal lumen patency, (2) minimizing hospitalization, (3) providing pain relief, and (4) elimination of reflux and regurgitation. Choosing the appropriate technique(s) depends on the patient's clinical factors, physician's experience, and tumor characteristics. Occasionally, palliative treatment can result in adverse effects that diminish a patient's quality of life.

Table 1 is an overview of the currently available endoscopic techniques for the palliation of advanced esophageal cancer. In general, these techniques are safe, effective, and ideal for patients who present with advanced disease or severe comorbid conditions that preclude more aggressive surgical treatment. These techniques are often performed on an outpatient basis. They also do not require prolonged treatment periods, unlike external beam radiation therapy. Furthermore, endoscopic palliation allows patients to resume eating earlier than compared with other nonendoscopic palliative techniques *(5)*.

2.2. ESOPHAGEAL DILATION

Endoscopic dilation of obstructing esophageal tumors can provide excellent, safe, and immediate albeit temporary relief of dysphagia (Fig. 1). It is most often used in preparation for endoscopic ultrasound staging *(6)* of the tumor or before esophageal stenting or laser therapy. Dilation is also a safe and effective palliative method for dysphagia, whereas waiting for tumor shrinkage to occur after chemoradiation, which can take up to 6 wk *(7)*. There are two techniques for endoscopic dilation of the esophagus: one that uses bougies and the other uses balloons. Bougies exert both a shearing and radial force and dilate progressively from the proximal to the distal extent of the tumor. The most commonly used bougies are the thermoplastic Savary-type (Savary-Gillard, Wilson Cook, Winston-Salem, NC; American Endoscopy Dilators, Bard Interventional

From: *Endoscopic Oncology: Gastrointestinal Endoscopy and Cancer Management.* Edited by: D. O. Faigel and M. L. Kochman © Humana Press, Totowa, NJ

Table 1
Endoscopic Modalities for the Management of Malignant Dysphagia

Injection therapy
    Chemicals: alcohol
    Chemotherapeutic agents
Dilation
Thermal ablation
    Laser therapy (Nd:YAG or Diode)
    Bipolar cautery
    Argon plasma coagulator (APC)
    Monopolar snare cautery
Photodynamic therapy (PDT)
Self-expanding metal stents (SEMS)
Enteral feeding (e.g., percutaneous endoscopic gastrostomy)

Products, Billerica, MA) dilators, which are tapering polyvinyl flexible bougies of various widths that allow guidewire passage. On the other hand, balloons deliver the entire dilating force radially and simultaneously over the entire length of the stricture, thereby reducing the shearing force on the tumor. There are two types of dilating balloons: the through-the-scope (TTS) balloon (multiple manufacturers), and the wire-guided balloons (Boston Scientific Corp, Natick, MA). Newer TTS balloons provide the added convenience of expansion to a range of three different diameters without the need for changing balloons.

The choice of dilation technique is influenced by the accurate identification of tumor borders, the stricture width and complexity, the relationship of the tumor to the gastroesophageal junction (GEJ) and to the cricopharyngeal muscle, and the resiliency of the tumor. The best method to assess these factors is a combination of barium esophagram and endoscopy; patients with advanced esophageal cancer can present with tortuous and narrow lumens that preclude safe passage of the endoscope and therefore dilation technique using a guidewire and fluoroscopic assistance may be necessary.

To partially relieve solid food dysphagia, the residual luminal diameter should be at least 12 mm. Savary dilation is successful in approx 90% of patients, and published studies suggesting that dilation is safe and effective when performed with a conservative approach (6–9). If the stricture is traversable by the endoscope, Savary dilation involves passage of a spring-tipped guidewire into the antrum via the working channel of the endoscope, followed by withdrawal of the endoscope to leave the guidewire in place. The use of a very small caliber pediatric endoscope with a standard diagnostic channel facilitates use of this technique for dilation as well as initial endoscopic examination. Otherwise, if the stricture is not traversable, the guidewire is advanced under fluoroscopic observation through the stricture, whereas the tip of the endoscope is positioned just above the stricture, until the guidewire tip is in the antrum. The initial dilator selected is of the next size larger than the estimated stricture diameter; for example, if the stricture was thought to be 10 mm in diameter, a 33F (11 mm diameter) dilator would be selected. The "rule of 3" is the use of no more than three dilators successively larger than the first dilator to meet moderate resistance when passed (10). Because

Savary dilators are inexpensive, readily available, and most endoscopists are well trained in its use, Savary dilation is an excellent initial method to temporarily palliate malignant dysphagia.

The potential complications of esophageal dilation include perforation (11), pain (11), hemorrhage (11), and bacteremia (12) or sepsis (11). The overall incidence of perforation following dilation of malignant esophageal strictures is 10% (11). Perforation occurs owing to transmural disruption or the creation of a false track (1,16). Transmural disruption may occur when axial or radial forces exceed the structural integrity limits of the wall. A false track occurs when the fixed diameter dilator directly penetrates the wall, such as blind dilation of a complex stricture with a Maloney dilator, a bougie, which does not accept a guidewire (13); the risk is minimized if a wire-guided bougie is used. There are insufficient data to substantiate a difference in perforation rates with fixed-diameter vs balloon dilators (15). Antibiotic prophylaxis should be considered for patients at high risk for bacterial endocarditis (14,15).

2.3. ALCOHOL INJECTION THERAPY

Endoscopic injection therapy of 95–100% alcohol is rarely used as the primary modality for achieving palliation of malignant dysphagia. However, it can be a valuable adjunct given that it is inexpensive, readily available, and easy to use. Most published studies are case series that report an improvement in dysphagia scores in approx 75–100% of patients with malignant dysphagia (16–20). The alcohol results in tissue fixation, ulceration, and necrosis, and is ideal for treating bulky, exophytic lesions (21). The endoscopic technique most commonly used is to inject aliquots of 0.5–1.0 cc of alcohol from the distal to the proximal margin of the tumor. Total volumes injected vary with stricture length, however, most studies report between 10 and 20 cc (18,19). Because there are no clearly defined endoscopic end points to assess the adequacy of the injection, this is a drawback in evaluating success and safety.

Tracking of sclerosant along tissue planes can lead to perforation (11). One study reported mediastinitis and tracheoesophageal fistulas (TEFs) as complications in 3 of the 36 patients treated (19). The dysphagia-free period after treatment lasts approx 1 mo, and ethanol injection can be applied as needed when symptoms recur (16–18). As a result of increasing popularity of other palliative endoscopic modalities, such as laser, stents, or photodynamic therapy (PDT), alcohol injection is rarely used in the United States. One clinical scenario in which alcohol injection therapy may be particularly beneficial is when there is complete or near complete obstruction of the esophageal lumen, making it impossible for a stent or a PDT fiber to traverse the esophageal stricture. Injection of alcohol may open the esophageal lumen enough so that one of the other modalities can subsequently be used to more definitively palliate dysphagia.

2.4. LASER THERAPY

Laser therapy has been used for decades in the palliation of malignant dysphagia. It is a well-established form of treatment for esophageal and gastric cardia tumors (22). This modality uses the direct application of high-energy laser light to burn and vaporize tissue under endoscopic visualization. The greatest

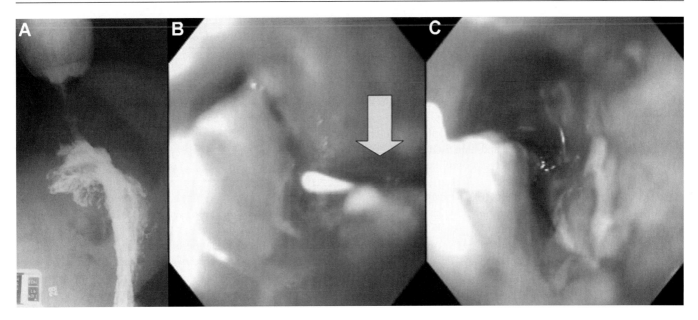

Fig. 1. (**A**) Barium radiograph of high-grade distal esophageal cancer. (**B**) Endoscopic image of nontraversable malignant stricture with guidewire in place across it (arrow). (**C**) Endoscopic image of malignant esophageal stricture following Savary dilation with flouoroscopic assistance. There was moderate improvement in the luminal diameter owing to compression of tumor tissue and minimal bleeding but the stricture became traversable.

amount of experience exists with the neodymium:yttrium-aluminum-garnet (Nd:YAG) laser which uses a wavelength of 1064 nm *(21)*.

Factors that influence the success of laser therapy include the degree of obstruction, the length of the tumor (<5 cm), its circumferential extension, the course of the residual lumen, and the baseline performance status of the patient *(23)*. Malignant dysphagia owing to exophytic lesions, short-segment tumors, noncircumferential or discrete strictures are particularly amenable to laser treatment, which is superior to dilation or other methods of thermal destruction. Laser therapy is well suited for the management of proximal esophageal lesions that are difficult to treat with stents.

The overall success rate with laser therapy varies from 69 to 95% *(24–26)*. Advantages for laser therapy include the prompt relief of dysphagia, the long duration of dysphagia relief (2–4 mo), and the relatively low complication rate (4–20%) *(27)*. A distinct disadvantage of laser therapy is that multiple treatment sessions (two to three sessions) are often required to fully palliate dysphagia. The dysphagia-free interval can be prolonged further when combined with percutaneous *(28)* or intracavitary radiotherapy. However, like other endoscopic therapies, recurrent dysphagia is a problem despite initial success; in one randomized using laser therapy plus percutaneous radiotherapy *(28)*, the restenosis rate was 43%.

Functional success may not always be associated with technical success; radiation-induced pharyngeal dysphagia, anorexia, painful tumor load and debility, and treatment complications can cause problems with ingestion of necessary calories and adequate palliation of symptoms *(29)*. Complications of endoscopic laser therapy include TEF formation (0.7–6.3%), bleeding *(28)*, and perforation (1–5.8%), with a procedure-related 30-d mortality of 1–5% *(27)*. The mean survival of

patients treated with laser therapy ranges from 12 to 22 wk, which is comparable with other treatment modalities for malignant dysphagia *(24–26,30)*.

2.5. ESOPHAGEAL STENTS

There are two general types of esophageal stents: conventional plastic and expandable metal. In the past, nonexpandable, semi-rigid plastic esophageal stents were used to palliate malignant dysphagia. These conventional plastic stents contained a fixed external and internal diameter requiring aggressive dilation before stent placement, and resulting in a relatively high esophageal perforation rate of up to 17%. In one retrospective study comparing plastic with metal stents, the death rate was significantly higher with the latter (4.4% plastic vs 0% for metal stents) *(31)*. The risk was particularly elevated in tight, angulated malignant strictures *(32,33)*. Additionally, if the residual fixed internal diameter of the plastic stent was less than 12 mm, optimal dysphagia relief was not achieved. A recent study described a ratively high technical success rate of 100% for conventional plastic stent placement in 169 patients with inoperable cancer *(34)*; there was one intramural perforation and a high incidence of bleeding (42.6%).

The advent of self-expanding metal stents (SEMS) in the 1990s was an important development in the management of malignant esophageal strictures. Although metal stents are more expensive than plastic ones, they have become the most commonly used type of esophageal stent and the standard for comparison for other endoscopic therapies for palliation. SEMS are made up of tightly wound wire coils or mesh (made of either stainless steel or nickel–titanium alloy) that is wrapped around a small delivery device, making endoscopic placement simple and obviating the need for aggressive dilation (the recommended maximal Savary dilation is to 12.8 mm). On successful deployment, the radial expansive force allows the stent to expand to its final shape and diameter, and the stent coils or mesh embed into the esophageal mucosa and/or submucosa and trigger a mild inflammatory response reducing the risk of stent migration (35).

Both conventional plastic and SEMS stents can be successfully placed in more than 90% of cases, and both are equally effective in palliating dysphagia (31). However, conventional plastic stents are associated with increased complication rates, increased length of hospitalization, and increased cost (primarily owing to the increased number of complications) when compared with SEMS (31–33,36,37). Hence, rigid plastic stents are now rarely used in current clinical practice. A recent randomized study comparing rigid plastic with SEMS concluded that SEMS improved patient's quality of life, and although the initial placement cost for SEMS was higher than plastic stents, the difference in cost was eliminated after 4 wk of follow-up (38).

2.5.1. Types of SEMS: When to Use?

The timing of SEMS placement in the spectrum on one's illness and dysphagia is critical. It is inappropriate to palliate patients at either end of the two extremes of their disease (39). Placement of SEMS for mild dysphagia does not result in significant clinical improvement, and other therapeutic palliative modalities should be employed first (40). In addition, it is inappropriate to place SEMS in patients with only a few weeks to live; because they are better served with hospice placement (39).

An esophageal stent is indicated when dilation becomes either ineffective, too risky, or when the frequency of dilation is too great to justify the risk of perforation. Table 2 describes lesions that are amenable to SEMS placement. Relative contraindications are soft or noncircumferential stenoses or markedly angulated strictures that may prevent adequate anchoring of the SEMS.

2.5.2. Types of SEMS: Which Stent to Use?

Several commercially manufactured SEMS are available; however, each differs with respect to their physical properties and characteristics (rigidity, radial expansive force, absence or presence of shortening during expansion, radiological markers, and the type of introducer). An awareness of each stent's distinguishing properties allows the physician to choose the most appropriate stent based on the characteristics of the malignant stricture.

Of the metal stents, the Z stent (Wilson Cook Medical, Winston-Salem, NC) is the only fully covered stent currently available, whereas the Ultraflex (Microvasive, Boston Scientific, Inc., Natick, MA) and esophageal Wallstent (Flamingo®, Microvasive, Boston Scientific, Inc., Natick, MA) are partially covered.

In addition to the rigid, nonexpandable conventional plastic stent and expanding metal stents, there is a plastic expandable esophageal stent (Polyflex, Microvasive, Boston Scientific, Inc., Natick, MA) that has been used for malignant esophageal obstruction. Experience with esophageal cancer palliation is very limited. Two small pilot studies describe good technical success with using an expandable plastic stent made of polyester netting lined with silicone (41), with a low cost ($400) (42). The Polyflex stent has potential advantages compared

Table 2
Lesions Amenable to Esophageal Stenting

Long, circumferential stenoses
Rapidly growing tumors
Extraluminal neoplasms resulting in compression
  of the esophageal lumen
Recurrent stenosis following:
  Chemoradiotherapy
  Laser photocoagulation
  Surgery
Esophagotracheal fistula (requires placement of a covered SEMS)

with the metal stents because it causes less trauma to surrounding tissues (which may lessen tissue hyperplasia and/or the development of a fistula), and is removable.

The Wallstent is made up of a cross hatched stainless steel wire in a double wall configuration with an occluding material between the two layers of the stent (Fig. 2). Wallstents, which have a high radial force, tend to provide better relief from dysphagia, but are associated with pain and occasional perforation. They are the ideal stent for advanced lesions, and have been used successfully for patients with associated bronchial or tracheal fistulas. Wallstents are now always coated with polyurethane. Following deployment, they are not removable.

Esophageal Z-stents are built from interconnecting rows of open stainless steel wires configured in a Z pattern in 2-cm long coated cylinders; the cylinders are connected to achieve the desired length. Originally plagued by tumor ingrowth, they are now coated by a polyethylene film, which greatly reduces tumor ingrowth, and facilitates removal, if needed. The end cylinders are flared and have small barbs in the center (or with uncovered flanges at each end) to reduce the chance of stent migration. The delivery catheter is quite rigid and requires a relatively complicated loading process before fitting over a guidewire for stenting.

A Z-stent with a "Dua" antireflux valve has been introduced to palliate lesions that extend across the GEJ to prevent reflux of gastric contents. This device consists of a coated Z-stent with a distal "windsock" design that consists of a 7-cm compressible valve on the distal end of the stent.

Ultraflex stents are built from a single layer of braided, knitted flexible nitinol (nickel–titanium alloy) wire covered with a thin, occluding material. They are deployed from a compressed state by gradually removing a suture that secures the stent. These stents exert less radial force than Wallstents; hence, they may produce less relief from dysphagia. They also may need to be dilated following deployment because of incomplete expansion against a rigid tumor. Compared with the Wallstent, the Ultraflex stents have no bare metal ends, so they are less traumatic to the mucosa and theoretically removable. Because of their flexibility, Ultraflex stents are the best choice for stenting proximal lesions. Ultraflex stents are available both coated and uncoated, but the uncoated stent is susceptible to tissue ingrowth.

A prospective study randomized 100 patients with malignant dysphagia to receive one of three models of expandable

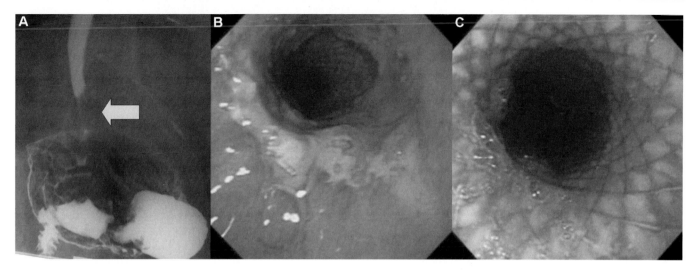

Fig. 2. (**A**) Barium X-ray image of a patient with adenocarcinoma of the distal esophagus and gastric cardia. (**B**) Endoscopic images of the proximal and (**C**) distal esophagus following placement of an expandable esophageal metal stent (Wallstent).

metal stents (Ultraflex, Flamingo Wallstent, or Gianturco-Z stent). Twenty-nine of the tumors involved the GEJ. Dysphagia improved in all patients regardless of the type of stent placed, and the complication rates ranged from 18 to 36%, but there was no statistical difference between the three groups (43). In another comparative study of the Wallstent, Ultraflex, and Z stents (44), reintervention rates were 43, 35, and 21%, respectively. With respect to stent diameter, large diameter stents are associated with less stent migration. In a prospective study of three different types of stents, stent migration was associated almost uniformly (12/13 cases) with smaller diameter stents (45).

2.5.3. Technique of SEMS Placement

The technique for placement of an expandable metal stent involves endoscopy, dilation, and fluoroscopy. All three types of SEMS are deployed by advancing the stent introducer with the constrained stent over a guidewire following dilation to no more than 12 mm to minimize stent migration. Then, the proximal and distal borders of the tumor are marked, using either external radio-opaque markers, endoscopic clips, or contrast injection with sclerotherapy needle. It is important to have the patient in the supine position when the markers are placed and to deploy the stent with the patient in the same position. The endoscope is backed out, leaving the guidewire in place. The stent introducer is then advanced over the guidewire until the tip is in the stomach and then withdrawn with fluoroscopic assistance so that the markings on the stent indicate that placement will be with a 2 cm or more margin proximal and distal to marked tumor borders. Most malignant strictures can be completely covered with a 10- or 15-cm stent, but rarely a second stent may be needed for very long tumors that also involve the GEJ. Finally, with fluoroscopic assistance, the stent is deployed althuogh minor adjustments are made in the position of the stent, depending on the degree of stent shortening. It is important not to leave an excessive length of stent within the stomach because the stent may contact the opposite gastric wall leading to ulceration (Fig. 3). Wallstents are deployed by

pulling back the constraining plastic catheter; deployment is facilitated by the ability to reconstrain the stent up to a "point-of-no-return" when the stent is 50% deployed. Ultraflex stents are deployed by pulling back on a securing suture that unravels either from proximal to distal or distal to proximal. Repeat passage of the endoscope is not necessary and discouraged because of the risk of causing stent migration. However, in certain situations, the stent may need to be dilated with a TTS balloon (particularly the Ultraflex stent) when deployment is suboptimal based on the fluoroscopic appearance (Fig. 4).

Patients should routinely be instructed regarding poststent complications (see Complications of Esophageal SEMS section). Pain medication should be prescribed before discharge. Patients should be also advised to have liquids for the first 24 h because the stent has not fully deployed, and then to consume a liquid/soft mechanical diet to avoid food impaction. They should chew their food properly and avoid dense and fibrous foods (such as large pieces of meat) taking all oral intake in a fully upright position. Patients with stents bridging the GEJ should be advised to raise the head of the bed to at least 30° and should be prescribed proton pump inhibitor therapy.

2.5.4. Efficacy of SEMS

There are numerous case reports and case series in the medical literature describing the success and complications of SEMS placement for palliation of malignant dysphagia secondary to primary esophageal and GE malignancies, mediastinal malignancies (primarily lung cancer), and for management of esophago-respiratory fistulas. A few comparative trials evaluating the different SEMS models have been performed. To summarize more than a decade's worth of literature, SEMS can be placed successfully in approx 85–100% of patients with primary or secondary esophageal obstruction, and all types of SEMS are highly and equally effective in palliating dysphagia. Treatment efficacy is assessed using a dysphagia scoring system ranging from zero (no dysphagia) to four (aphagia), with virtually every study demonstrating a statistically significant and a clinically relevant improvement in dysphagia (43,46–56).

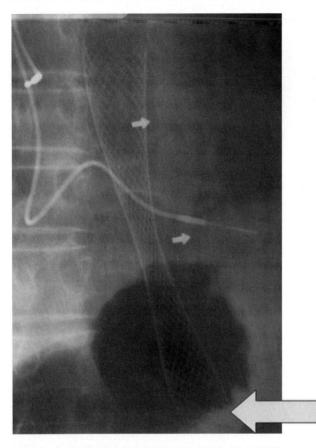

Fig. 3. Radiograph of esophageal metal stent (Wallstent) that migrated distally into the stomach, impacting on the greater curvature (arrow). Note the radio-opaque markers taped to the patient's chest that mark the proximal and distal borders of the tumor.

A recent study by Tomaselli et al. *(48)* reflects the therapeutic benefits and risks of SEMS placement. The covered Ultraflex (Microvasive/Boston Scientific, Natick, MA) stent was used to palliate dysphagia is 41 patients who had difficulty swallowing liquids and saliva, 5 patients with TEFs, and 1 patient with persistent tumor bleeding. Nearly one-third of patients had been treated by prior therapeutic modalities without success. Improvement in dysphagia was reported in all patients, but 17% suffered major complications on follow-up. Investigators were unable to identify any risk factors that predicted a stent-related complication *(48)*.

2.5.5. Complications of Esophageal SEMS

SEMS are highly effective but they are associated with significant serious life-threatening complications. Table 3 lists many of these complications. Complications are loosely classified as early (within 30 d) vs late (after 30 d) in relation to the timing of the stent placement, but these complications can occur at almost any time following placement. Complications such as chest pain, stent migration (Figs. 3 and 4), hemorrhage, food impaction, tumor ingrowth or overgrowth, fistulization, and tracheal compression complicate 20–40% of cases *(11)*. Stent obstruction and recurrent dysphagia may be caused by impacted food, tumor ingrowth, or benign hyperplasia (Fig. 5). Furthermore, death can occur in 3% owing to exsanguinating bleeding *(57)*, aspiration, and perforation *(58)*. In the review of

Bartelsman et al. of 153 patients who underwent SEMS for palliation of malignant dysphagia, the overall early complication rate was 29.9%, consisting primarily of stent migration, stent obstruction, aspiration pneumonia, bleeding, perforation, and pain. Late complications occurred in 27.8% of patients, and included many of the same complications. The 30-d mortality rate was 26, and 3.3% of patients died as a direct complication of stent placement *(59)* Higher mortality rates from SEMS placement have been reported *(53,60)*. Physicians must comprehend the comorbidities associated with esophageal stent placement, and engage in open and honest discussion with patients and their families regarding the risks, benefits, and timing of SEMS placement.

Recent changes in the design of SEMS have been made to minimize the complications of tumor ingrowth, stent migration, and persistent dysphagia owing to incomplete expansion. SEMS have been improved to contain a polyurethane or silicone coating ("covered SEMS") to prevent tumor ingrowth, to have larger proximal and distal flanges to minimize migration, and to have larger internal diameters to improve dysphagia.

Covered SEMS are just as effective as uncovered SEMS in treatment of dysphagia *(61)*. However, the drawback of an uncovered SEMS is the development of tumor ingrowth between exposed wire mesh, whereas the drawback of a covered SEMS is the increased rate of stent migration *(61)*. In one prospective study, patients randomized to receive covered vs uncovered SEMS were followed monthly to assess dysphagia relief and complications for 6 mo. Rates for stent migration and survival were similar in both groups *(47)*. However, patients with uncovered stents had a higher incidence of obstructing tumor ingrowth (30 vs 3%, *p* < 0.001) and a higher endoscopic reintervention rate (27 vs 0%, *p* = 0.002). Hence, covered SEMS are more commonly used for malignant strictures of the esophagus and GEJ.

The risk of migration of the covered stents can be reduced by several methods including use of larger diameter stents *(45)*, the addition of barbs, an enlarged proximal flange, and uncovering of the proximal and distal ends of the stent (i.e., partially covered stents). A modification of the SEMS design was made to resist distal migration; the Flamingo stent was developed (Boston Scientific, Inc., Watertown, MA) so that it is partially covered (inside-out covering), has a conical shape, and a varying braiding angle of the mesh along its length. In a prospective randomized controlled trial of 40 patients, major complications (bleeding *[4]*, perforation *[1]*, fever *[1]*, and fistula *[1]*) occurred in seven (18%) patients but there was only one stent migration and no tumor ingrowth. The Flamingo stent was compared with the covered Ultraflex stent (Boston Scientific Inc, Watertown, MD) in a randomized trial and no differences were found in stent migration rates *(50)*.

With the rising incidence of carcinoma involving the GEJ and the gastric cardia, SEMS are increasingly being placed across the lower esophageal sphincter. This can predispose patients to serious GE reflux that may diminish their quality of life. Aggressive measures to be taken to ensure an anacid environment (high-dose proton pump inhibitors), consider using promotility agents such as metoclopramide, and patients should

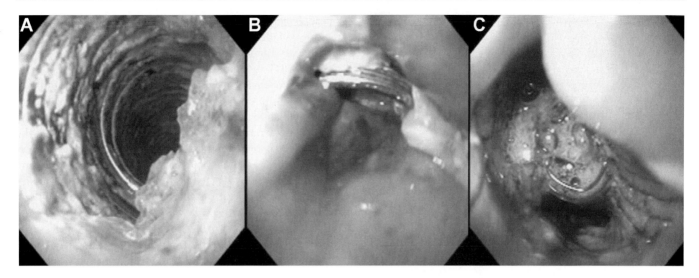

Fig. 4. Endoscopic images from a patient with severe dysphagia from a high-grade stricture. **(A)** Necrotic cervical esophageal tumor with a metal stent (Esopahacoil) following chemoradiation therapy. **(B)** The patient did well for a 1 mo but suffered recurrent dysphagia; the Esophacoil stent had buckled and recoiled distally. **(C)** The patient was treated with an Ultraflex stent, which was deployed to overlap the Esophacoil but have the proximal stent border distal to the cricopharyngeus. The proximal tip of the Ultraflex stent is located just a few millimeters distal to the cricopharyngeus; the patient did not experience any throat pain or discomfort from the stent wires. Note that incomplete expansion of the proximal tip of the Ultraflex stent, necessitating TTS-balloon dilation.

Table 3
Complications Associated With Self-Expanding Metal Stents

Stent migration	Tumor ingrowth or overgrowth
Esophageal perforation	Tracheal compression
Stent obstruction	Granulomatous obstruction
Stent-induced hemorrhage	Reflux
Aspiration pneumonia	Food impaction
Chronic pain-, often narcotic-requiring	Death
Tracheoesophageal fistula	Esophago-aortic fistula

be routinely advised to sleep in an upright position. Attempts have been made to devise SEMS with antireflux mechanisms. The only commercially available SEMS product with an anti-reflux valve is the Dua-Z stent (Wilson-Cook Medical®, Bloomington, IN), which has been shown in a randomized trial to significantly reduce symptomatic reflux in patients with distal esophageal tumors with cardia extension (96% Wallstent vs 12% Dua-Z stent). There were no differences in thevsurvival, complication, or reintervention rates *(62)*.

Of esophageal tumors, 7 to 10% involve the cervical esophagus, and palliative resection, radiation, and laser therapy are often associated with treatment failure. SEMS placement within 2 cm of the cricopharyngeal muscle has been considered a relative contraindication because of the concerns over increased risk of perforation, pulmonary aspiration, stent migration into the hypopharynx, and an intolerable sensation of a foreign body (reported by up to 28% of patients) *(63,64)*. With modifications to existing SEMS, it may be possible to reliably and successfully place SEMS near the upper esophageal sphincter *(65)*. One point of concern is that although a SEMS can be placed successfully, the swallowing mechanism may subsequently become impaired owing to submucosal tumor infiltration of the upper esophageal sphincter *(66)*.

Occasionally, patients may develop dyspnea or stridor following placement of an upper esophageal SEMS, and this may be owing to external tracheal compression. Such scenarios are treated with placement of a tracheal stent, and some medical centers will electively perform a bronchoscopy to rule out extension of an upper esophageal tumor into the trachea; especially, if suggested by CT scan or endoscopic ultrasound. Patients with both esophageal and tracheal stenosis have benefited from double stenting of both anatomic lumens *(67)*. The tracheal stent should be placed first in this scenario *(67–70)*.

2.5.6. SEMS Complications Associated With Radiation or Chemoradiation Therapy

Patients treated with SEMS before or during radiation therapy *(71–73)* or chemoradiation therapy *(74)* may have a higher rate of complications. In particular, massive hemorrage (21%) *(71–73)*, formation or worsening of esophageal perforation *(73)* and esophageal fistulas (28%) *(71)* have been noted, and the development of a vertebral body and mediastinal abscesses have also been described *(74)*. Hence, some physicians recommend delaying SEMS placement until after radiotherapy or chemotherapy have failed *(71)*. One study suggested that prior radiation and/or chemotherapy appears to have no effect on the outcome of SEMS *(75)*, whereas other studies have found a significantly higher incidence of stent-related complications *(76,77)*. Siersema et al. *(76)* found that poststent pain is more common in those with prior radiation therapy. Kinsman et al. *(77)* performed a multivariate analysis in 59 patients with SEMS, and noted a significant increase in life-threatening complications (36.4 vs 2.5%) and stent-related mortality (23 vs 0%) in patients who had undergone chemotherapy and/or radiation compared with those who had no prior history. This increased risk is unrelated to the patient's age, length of stricture, dysphagia grade, or prior history of surgery *(77)*. Postmortem examinations confirm SEMS-induced pressure necrosis on the esophageal wall

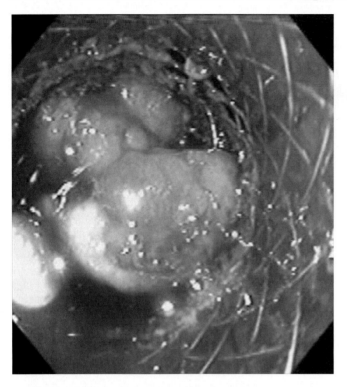

Fig. 5. Endoscopic image of benign gastric hyperplastic tissue partially obstructing the distal lumen of the esophageal Wallstent. Note the pill that is stuck just inside the distal edge of the stent.

resulting in subsequent fibrosis, thinning of the esophageal wall, and occasional wall rupture *(78)*. It appears that tissue integrity is compromised with administration of chemotherapy and/or radiation therapy.

Identifying patients with T4 esophageal cancer (invasion into adjacent structures) is important when considering SEMS placement. Several studies have reported a high incidence of fatal bleeding or perforation in patients with tumor encroachment of the trachea or aorta *(73,79)*. However, these patients also had a history of chemotherapy and/or radiation, and further investigation is required to understand true risks or benefits of stenting in extensive locally invasive disease.

2.6. PHOTODYNAMIC THERAPY

2.6.1. PDT Indications and Contraindications

PDT is a nonthermal ablative technique resulting in local necrosis of malignant esophageal tissue. PDT is indicated for the palliative management of malignant esophageal strictures and ablation of Barrett's esophagus with high-grade dysplasia in non-surgical candidates. In this chapter, the focus is solely on palliation of malignant dysphagia. When considering PDT for palliation, most esophageal cancer patients have either failed, refused, or are ineligible for surgery or systemic therapy owing to stage IV disease or associated comorbidity. Tumor characteristics amenable to PDT include length greater than 8–10 cm, circumferential lesions, tumor location in the upper third of the esophagus or at the GEJ, and flat, recurrent anastomotic tumors *(21)*. Clinical contraindications to PDT include known porphyria (or hypersensitivity to porphyrins), tumor infiltration into the respiratory tract, and the presence of

an esophagopulmonary fistula. Relative contraindications may include symptomatic pleural or pericardial effusions and unstable arrythmias *(80)*.

2.6.2. PDT Technique

A photosensitizing compound (Porfimer sodium or Δ-aminolevulinic acid [ALA]) is administered to the patient before activation using endoscopically applied laser light. The laser generates a monochromatic beam, which activates the photosensitive compound and generates cytotoxic singlet oxygen radicals resulting in rapid vascular stasis, hemorrhage, and an acute inflammatory reaction, followed by direct and anoxia-induced tumor cell death. Only Porfimer sodium is available in the United States at this time *(80)*.

The localized effect of PDT is based on several factors: the relative specificity of the photosensitizer for malignant tissue, the directed application of light, the transmission depth of the wavelength of light, and the oxygen content of the tissue *(21)*. The remaining tissue heals with little cumulative or systemic toxicity; therefore PDT can be repeated, and does not interfere with or preclude other forms of therapy. Approximately 48 h after the first light treatment session, a second endoscopy is performed to assess the necrotic effect, measure the luminal diameter, and to debride residual tumor. Any remaining visible tumor is retreated in the same manner without re-injection of the photosensitive compound.

2.6.3. Efficacy of PDT

PDT is an excellent option for palliation of malignant dysphagia (Fig. 6). A large retrospective review of 215 PDT patients treated for malignant dysphagia showed an improvement in dysphagia scores and severity of obstruction in 85% of patients *(81)*. This study reflects the success of PDT in various other smaller studies, ranging from 80 to 100% *(82–88)*.

2.6.4. Complications of PDT

After PDT, patients may develop transient substernal or epigastric pain, odynophagia, or worsening dysphagia. Fever, leukocytosis, and asymptomatic pleural effusions may be present, and often resolve after several days without any intervention. Major complications include perforation, aspiration, fistulae, and stricture formation with rates varying between 2 and 10% *(81–83, 88)*. Photosensitivity occurs in approx 60% of patients treated with PDT *(89)*. Photofrin is primarily retained by the reticuloendothelial system of the liver, spleen, and kidney and redistributed into the skin. Given that the longest half-life of photofrin is 36 d, skin photosensitivity can occur for up to 3 mo. Patients are cautioned to avoid direct sunlight, strong fluorescent or incandescent light, strong residential indoor lights, and radiant heat for at least 30 d. Skin photosensitivity can vary from mild erythema and pruritus, to severe erythema and edema, to blisters with skin desquamation. Topical suncreens are not beneficial because they block ultraviolet light, not infrared light. Most patients should be cautioned that they would develop at least a tan *(90,91)*. Different photosensitizers have been tested, including ALA, which may carry a lower rate of skin photosensitivity. However, the efficacy of these photosensitizers may be less effective than polyhematoporphyrin in treating malignant dysphagia *(92)*.

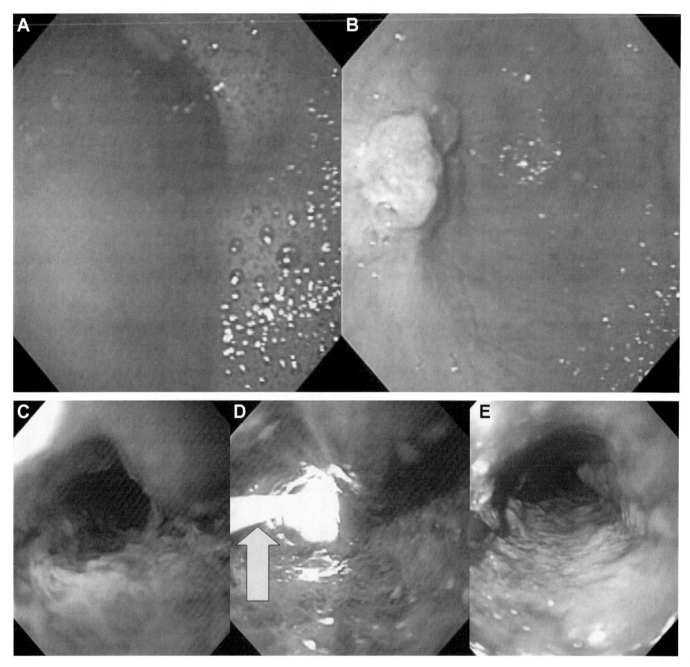

Fig. 6. High-grade stricture from adenocarcinoma involving the distal esophagus and gastroesophageal junction. The obstruction was near total, resulting in difficulty with swallowing liquids and saliva. Note the patient's secretions pooling in the distal esophagus above the stricture (**A**). After suctioning the secretions, the high stricture diameter was found to be no more than 1–2 mm (**B**). The patient was treated with photodynamic therapy. After one laser light session (24 h after injection of the photosensitizer) and debridement of necrotic tumor, the stricture diameter was increased to 6 mm (**C**). A second laser light session was performed 48 h after photosensitizer injection (**B**). Note the laser fiber within the stricture (arrow). (**D**) After 7 d of initiation photodynamic therapy and repeat tumor debridement, the stricture diameter was increased to 12 mm. The patient was able to eat soft solid food for the remainder of his life (**E**).

The reported complications of PDT include esophageal perforation (about 2%) *(81,82)* fistulae formation (about 5%) *(93)*; symptomatic pleural effusions (~3–6%) *(81–83);* and severe "sunburn" or photosensitivity reactions (~4–13%) *(81–83,94).* Bleeding is also associated with PDT, and the risk is higher in patients who have had radiation therapy *(95).*

2.6.5. PDT vs Other Endoscopic Modalities

Various comparative studies of laser therapy, PDT, and SEMS have been performed to evaluate their efficacy in managing malignant dysphagia. It is important to remember that many patients undergo multiple modalities to manage malignant dysphagia during the course of their illness. In general, PDT is equivalent to the other modalities, and is excellent for treatment of tumor ingrowth in uncovered stents and tumor overgrowth in covered stents *(81).* The mean dysphagia-free interval is reported to be as long as 92 d. The nonthermal nature of PDT obviates concerns about damaging the metal frame or plastic coverings of stents as observed with Nd:YAG laser, monopolar electrocoagulation, and argon plasma coagulation (90). Another scenario in which PDT is particularly advantageous is in treating tumors adjacent to or involving the upper esophageal sphincter (88).

A minority of patients in several studies will fail PDT as a first option, and are often treated with SEMS subsequently. The survival rate reported in PDT studies varies between 4 and 17 mo. (81,83,87,93,94). This is equivalent to other endoscopic modalities, and likely reflects the underlying condition of these terminally ill patients, and less so the modality of treatment. Patients with higher Karnofsky Performance Status (>70) with stages III and IV esophageal cancer who received PDT survived longer than those with lower scores (94).

A randomized, controlled trial comparing PDT vs SEMS in the palliation of malignant dysphagia evaluated the efficacy, quality of life, and cost-effectiveness of each modality (96). Both modalities were equivalent in palliating dysphagia, but only patients with SEMS had improved health-related quality of life. Both PDT and SEMS were expensive methods for palliation malignant dysphagia, but SEMS was a more cost-effective than performing PDT.

PDT is effective at reducing tumor bulk and is comparable in efficacy to Nd:YAG laser but safer. A prospective, randomized study of 236 PDT patients and 218 Nd:YAG laser patients showed that both modalities were equivalent in improving dysphagia at 1 wk; however, at 1 mo, PDT-treated patients exhibit significantly greater improvements in tumor response (32% PDT group vs 20% laser group). The median survival was 4.5 mo. Subgroup analysis revealed that PDT was a better option compared to laser for tumors localized to the upper or lower one-third of the esophagus, in long tumors, and in patients with prior treatment for malignant dysphagia. Nineteen percent of PDT patients had phototoxicity reactions and 7% of laser patients suffered from acute perforation, compared with 3% with PDT (97). The equivalent efficacy of PDT and laser therapy was confirmed in another comparative trial. However, PDT was noted to be associated with improved dietary performance, and credited with improving the Karnofsky performance status at 1 mo. In addition, the number of endoscopic treatment sessions required was equivalent between the two modalities, but the duration of response was longer with PDT-treated patients (84 vs 53 d) (98). In summary, PDT appears to be equivalent to Nd-YAG laser therapy for palliating dysphagia, but has fewer side effects and improves patient performance status.

3. TREATMENT OF MALIGNANT ESOPHAGO-RESPIRATORY FISTULAE

TEFs occur in approx 5–15% of patients with esophageal cancer or other mediastinal malignancies. Primary esophageal cancer and lung cancer constitute more than 90% of all malignant TEF, with the vast majority of TEF owing to cervical esophageal cancer (99). Once a TEF develops, the general condition of a patient declines rapidly owing to recurrent aspiration, life-threatening pneumonia, and severe malnutrition. The goal in managing such patients is to achieve rapid and successful palliation whereas minimizing inpatient hospitalization, cost, and complication rates (64).

Covered SEMS successfully palliate esophago-respiratory fistulas between 67 and 100% of cases, with a mean closure rate of approx 90% (51,54,69,79,100–103). Uncovered SEMS are not suitable options for management of TEF, because esophageal lumen contents will easily travel through the uncoated wires and into the respiratory tract. In one of the few studies dedicated to managing patients with TEF, six patients were treated with a covered SEMS. A contrast radiograph obtained 2 h after successful stent placement revealed closure of the fistula, and all patients were able to eat a normal diet. Dysphagia scores improved in all patients from a median of 4 to 1, and Karnofsky performance status improved from a median of 40 to 65. One patient suffered from chronic post-stent pain, and one patient died of massive hematemesis 5 d poststent placement. All patients were followed to death, and their fistulas remained closed, demonstrating that covered SEMS were effective in palliation of TEFs (35). A more recent study demonstrated successful fistula closure (tracheo-esophageal and esophagopleural) in 87.5%, with an overall complication rate of 26.8%. Two patients suffered procedure-related deaths, and two patients died because the fistula could not be closed. The remainder of the patients exhibited a median survival time of 94 d (53).

4. TREATMENT OF BLEEDING FROM ESOPHAGEAL CANCER

Few studies specifically address the use of endoscopic therapy for bleeding from advanced cancers of the esophagus and esophagogastric junction. Nd:YAG laser therapy has been used successfully in achieving hemostasis in bleeding tumors (104), with high success rates (90%) (105), comparable with thermal and injection treatments for peptic ulcer bleeding. PDT has been used to treat bleeding esophageal cancers with good success but the experience is limited (81). In a large study of 215 patients, 31 were treated with PDT for bleeding with or without obstruction. Bleeding was controlled in 29/31 patients (93%) with one course of PDT (81). One patient required three courses of PDT to control bleeding and obstruction. The other patient failed PDT and was treated with an esophageal stent, primarily for obstruction. Rarely, patients with bleeding tumors have been treated with a covered esophageal stent (48) in an attempt to exert pressure on exposed superficial bleeding tumor vessels.

5. CONCLUSION

Although the overall prognosis of advanced esophageal cancer remains poor, the spectrum of available therapeutic modalities for palliation of symptoms and the chances for possible improvement in quality of life after treatment have substantially improved. Endoscopic therapeutic options such as laser therapy, PDT, and stenting are complementary, and it is important to understand the advantages, disadvantages, and indications for each type of modality. With a lack of randomized controlled studies to guide decision making, the choice concerning, which modality is most appropriate relies on the clinical scenario, patient comorbidities, tumor characteristics, and physician's experience.

REFERENCES

1. Ries L, Eisner M, Kosary C, et al. SEER Cancer Stat Rev 1975–2001. http://seer.cancer.gov/csr/1975_2001/ 2004; National Cancer Institute. Bethesda, MD. Accessed 2004.

2. Krasna MJ. Surgical staging and surgical treatment in esophageal cancer. Semin Oncol 1999; 26:9–11.

3. Siersema PD, Dees J, van Blankenstein M. Palliation of malignant dysphagia from oesophageal cancer. Rotterdam Oesophageal Tumor Study Group. Scand J Gastroenterol Suppl 1998; 225:75–84.

4. Segalin A, Little AG, Ruol A, et al. Surgical and endoscopic palliation of esophageal carcinoma. Ann Thorac Surg 1989; 48:267–71.

5. Kimmey M, Ponec R. Primary malignant and metastatic tumors of the esophagus. In: DiMarino Jr A, Benjamin S, eds. Gastrointestinal Disease: An Endoscopic Approach. 2nd ed. Thorofare: Slack, 2002:275–297.

6. Pfau PR, Ginsberg GG, Lew RJ, Faigel DO, Smith DB, Kochman ML. Esophageal dilation for endosonographic evaluation of malignant esophageal strictures is safe and effective. Am J Gastroenterol 2000; 95:2813–2815.

7. Boyce HW, Jr. Palliation of Dysphagia of Esophageal Cancer by Endoscopic Lumen Restoration Techniques. Cancer Control 1999; 6:73–83.

8. Lew RJ, Kochman ML. A review of endoscopic methods of esophageal dilation. J Clin Gastroenterol 2002; 35:117–126.

9. Wallace MB, Hawes RH, Sahai AV, Van Velse A, Hoffman BJ. Dilation of malignant esophageal stenosis to allow EUS guided fine-needle aspiration: safety and effect on patient management. Gastrointest Endosc 2000; 51:309–313.

10. Tulman AB, Boyce HW, Jr. Complications of esophageal dilation and guidelines for their prevention. Gastrointest Endosc 1981; 27: 229–234.

11. Eisen GM, Baron TH, Dominitz JA, et al. Complications of upper GI endoscopy. Gastrointest Endosc 2002; 55:784–793.

12. Nelson DB, Sanderson SJ, Azar MM. Bacteremia with esophageal dilation. Gastrointest Endosc 1998; 48:563–567.

13. Hernandez LV, Jacobson JW, Harris MS, Hernandez LJ. Comparison among the perforation rates of Maloney, balloon, and savary dilation of esophageal strictures. Gastrointest Endosc 2000; 51:460–462.

14. Antibiotic prophylaxis for gastrointestinal endoscopy. American Society for Gastrointestinal Endoscopy. Gastrointest Endosc 1995; 42:630–635.

15. Hirota WK, Petersen K, Baron TH, et al. Wheeler-Harbough J, Faigel DO. Guidelines for antibiotic prophylaxis for GI endoscopy. Gastrointest Endosc 2003; 58:475–482.

16. Payne-James JJ, Spiller RC, Misiewicz JJ, Silk DB. Use of ethanol-induced tumor necrosis to palliate dysphagia in patients with esophagogastric cancer. Gastrointest Endosc 1990; 36:43–46.

17. Moreira LS, Coelho RC, Sadala RU, Dani R. The use of ethanol injection under endoscopic control to palliate dysphagia caused by esophagogastric cancer. Endoscopy 1994; 26:311–314.

18. Nwokolo CU, Payne-James JJ, Silk DB, Misiewicz JJ, Loft DE. Palliation of malignant dysphagia by ethanol induced tumour necrosis. Gut 1994; 35:299–303.

19. Chung SC, Leong HT, Choi CY, Leung JW, Li AK. Palliation of malignant oesophageal obstruction by endoscopic alcohol injection. Endoscopy 1994; 26:275–277.

20. Carazzone A, Bonavina L, Segalin A, Ceriani C, Peracchia A. Endoscopic palliation of oesophageal cancer: results of a prospective comparison of Nd:YAG laser and ethanol injection. Eur J Surg 1999; 165:351–356.

21. Adler DG, Baron TH. Endoscopic palliation of malignant dysphagia. Mayo Clin Proc 2001; 76:731–738.

22. Fleischer D, Kessler F, Haye O. Endoscopic Nd: YAG laser therapy for carcinoma of the esophagus: a new palliative approach. Am J Surg 1982; 143:280–283.

23. Low D, Kozarek R. Esophageal endoscopy, dilation and intra-esophageal prosthetic devices. In: Hill L, Kozarek R, McCullum R, Mercer D, eds. The esophagus. Medical and surgical management. New York: W.B. Saunders, 1988; 47–59.

24. Lightdale CJ, Zimbalist E, Winawer SJ. Outpatient management of esophageal cancer with endoscopic Nd:YAG laser. Am J Gastroenterol 1987; 82:46–50.

25. Naveau S, Chiesa A, Poynard T, Chaput JC. Endoscopic Nd-YAG laser therapy as palliative treatment for esophageal and cardial cancer. Parameters affecting long-term outcome. Dig Dis Sci 1990; 35:294–301.

26. Sander RR, Poesl H. Cancer of the oesophagus—palliation—laser treatment and combined procedures. Endoscopy 1993; 25:679–682.

27. Gevers AM, Macken E, Hiele M, Rutgeerts P. A comparison of laser therapy, plastic stents, and expandable metal stents for palliation of malignant dysphagia in patients without a fistula. Gastrointest Endosc 1998; 48:383–388.

28. Konigsrainer A, Riedmann B, De Vries A, et al. Expandable metal stents versus laser combined with radiotherapy for palliation of unresectable esophageal cancer: a prospective randomized trial. Hepatogastroenterology 2000; 47:724–727.

29. Mellow MH, Pinkas H. Endoscopic laser therapy for malignancies affecting the esophagus and gastroesophageal junction. Analysis of technical and functional efficacy. Arch Intern Med 1985; 145:1443–1446.

30. Spinelli P, Cerrai FG, Dal Fante M, Mancini A, Meroni E, Pizzetti P. Endoscopic treatment of upper gastrointestinal tract malignancies. Endoscopy 1993; 25:675–678.

31. Mosca F, Consoli A, Stracqualursi A, Persi A, Portale TR. Comparative retrospective study on the use of plastic prostheses and self-expanding metal stents in the palliative treatment of malignant strictures of the esophagus and cardia. Dis Esophagus 2003; 16:119–125.

32. Davies N, Thomas HG, Eyre-Brook IA. Palliation of dysphagia from inoperable oesophageal carcinoma using Atkinson tubes or self-expanding metal stents. Ann R Coll Surg Engl 1998; 80:394–397.

33. Birch JF, White SA, Berry DP, Veitch PS. A cost-benefit comparison of self-expanding metal stents and Atkinson tubes for the palliation of obstructing esophageal tumors. Dis Esophagus 1998; 11:172–176.

34. Szentpali K, Palotas A, Lazar G, Paszt A, Balogh A. Endoscopic intubation with conventional plastic stents: a safe and cost-effective palliation for inoperable esophageal cancer. Dysphagia 2004; 19:22–27.

35. Bethge N, Sommer A, Gross U, von Kleist D, Vakil N. Human tissue responses to metal stents implanted in vivo for the palliation of malignant stenoses. Gastrointest Endosc 1996; 43:596–602.

36. De Palma GD, di Matteo E, Romano G, Fimmano A, Rondinone G, Catanzano C. Plastic prosthesis versus expandable metal stents for palliation of inoperable esophageal thoracic carcinoma: a controlled prospective study. Gastrointest Endosc 1996; 43:478–482.

37. Siersema PD, Hop WC, Dees J, Tilanus HW, van Blankenstein M. Coated self-expanding metal stents versus latex prostheses for esophagogastric cancer with special reference to prior radiation and chemotherapy: a controlled, prospective study. Gastrointest Endosc 1998; 47:113–120.

38. O'Donnell CA, Fullarton GM, Watt E, Lennon K, Murray GD, Moss JG. Randomized clinical trial comparing self-expanding metallic stents with plastic endoprostheses in the palliation of oesophageal cancer. Br J Surg 2002; 89:985–992.

39. Kozarek RA. Endoscopic palliation of esophageal malignancy. Endoscopy 2003; 35:S9–S13.

40. Kostopoulos PP, Zissis MI, Polydorou AA, et al. Are metal stents effective for palliation of malignant dysphagia and fistulas? Dig Liver Dis 2003; 35:275–282.

41. Decker P, Lippler J, Decker D, Hirner A. Use of the Polyflex stent in the palliative therapy of esophageal carcinoma: results in 14 cases and review of the literature. Surg Endosc 2001; 15:1444–1447.

42. Bethge N, Vakil N. A prospective trial of a new self-expanding plastic stent for malignant esophageal obstruction. Am J Gastroenterol 2001; 96:1350–1354.

43. Siersema PD, Hop WC, van Blankenstein M, et al. A comparison of 3 types of covered metal stents for the palliation of patients with dysphagia caused by esophagogastric carcinoma: a prospective, randomized study. Gastrointest Endosc 2001; 54:145–153.

44. May A, Hahn EG, Ell C. Self-expanding metal stents for palliation of malignant obstruction in the upper gastrointestinal tract. Comparative assessment of three stent types implemented in 96 implantations. J Clin Gastroenterol 1996; 22:261–266.

45. Siersema PD, Hop WC, van Blankenstein M, et al. A comparison of 3 types of covered metal stents for the palliation of patients with dysphagia caused by esophagogastric carcinoma: a prospective, randomized study. Gastrointest Endosc 2001; 54:145–153.

46. May A, Hahn EG, Ell C. Self-expanding metal stents for palliation of malignant obstruction in the upper gastrointestinal tract. Comparative assessment of three stent types implemented in 96 implantations. J Clin Gastroenterol 1996; 22:261–266.

47. Vakil N, Morris AI, Marcon N, et al. A prospective, randomized, controlled trial of covered expandable metal stents in the palliation of malignant esophageal obstruction at the gastroesophageal junction. Am J Gastroenterol 2001; 96:1791–1796.

48. Tomaselli F, Maier A, Sankin O, Pinter H, Smolle J, Smolle-Juttner FM. Ultraflex stent—benefits and risks in ultimate palliation of advanced, malignant stenosis in the esophagus. Hepatogastroenterology 2004; 51:1021–1026.

49. Siersema PD, Schrauwen SL, van Blankenstein M, et al. Self-expanding metal stents for complicated and recurrent esophagogastric cancer. Gastrointest Endosc 2001; 54:579–586.

50. Sabharwal T, Hamady MS, Chui S, Atkinson S, Mason R, Adam A. A randomised prospective comparison of the Flamingo Wallstent and Ultraflex stent for palliation of dysphagia associated with lower third oesophageal carcinoma. Gut 2003; 52:922–926.

51. Rozanes I, Poyanli A, Acunas B. Palliative treatment of inoperable malignant esophageal strictures with metal stents: one center's experience with four different stents. Eur J Radiol 2002; 43:196–203.

52. Riccioni ME, Shah SK, Tringali A, et al. Endoscopic palliation of unresectable malignant oesophageal strictures with self-expanding metal stents: comparing Ultraflex and Esophacoil stents. Dig Liver Dis 2002; 34:356–363.

53. Sarper A, Oz N, Cihangir C, Demircan A, Isin E. The efficacy of self-expanding metal stents for palliation of malignant esophageal strictures and fistulas. Eur J Cardiothorac Surg 2003; 23:794–798.

54. Raijman I, Siddique I, Ajani J, Lynch P. Palliation of malignant dysphagia and fistulae with coated expandable metal stents: experience with 101 patients. Gastrointest Endosc 1998; 48:172–179.

55. Kozarek RA, Raltz S, Brugge WR, et al. Prospective multicenter trial of esophageal Z-stent placement for malignant dysphagia and tracheoesophageal fistula. Gastrointest Endosc 1996; 44:562–567.

56. Christie NA, Buenaventura PO, Fernando HC, et al. Results of expandable metal stents for malignant esophageal obstruction in 100 patients: short-term and long-term follow-up. Ann Thorac Surg 2001; 71:1797–1801; discussion 1801,1802.

57. Allgaier HP, Schwacha H, Technau K, Blum HE. Fatal esophago-aortic fistula after placement of a self-expanding metal stent in a patient with esophageal carcinoma. N Engl J Med 1997; 337:1778.

58. Faigel DO. Endoscopy for the diagnosis and management of esophageal cancer. ASGE Clinical Update 2000; 8:1–4.

59. Bartelsman JF, Bruno MJ, Jensema AJ, Haringsma J, Reeders JW, Tytgat GN. Palliation of patients with esophagogastric neoplasms by insertion of a covered expandable modified Gianturco-Z endoprosthesis: experiences in 153 patients. Gastrointest Endosc 2000; 51:134–138.

60. Neale JC, Goulden JW, Allan SG, Dixon PD, Isaacs RJ. Esophageal stents in malignant dysphagia: a two-edged sword? J Palliat Care 2004; 20:28–31.

61. Vakil N, Morris AI, Marcon N, et al. A prospective, randomized, controlled trial of covered expandable metal stents in the palliation of malignant esophageal obstruction at the gastroesophageal junction. Am J Gastroenterol 2001; 96:1791–1796.

62. Laasch HU, Marriott A, Wilbraham L, Tunnah S, England RE, Martin DF. Effectiveness of open versus antireflux stents for palliation of distal esophageal carcinoma and prevention of symptomatic gastroesophageal reflux. Radiology 2002; 225:359–365.

63. Macdonald S, Edwards RD, Moss JG. Patient tolerance of cervical esophageal metallic stents. J Vasc Interv Radiol 2000; 11:891–898.

64. Shim CS. Esophageal stenting in unusual situations. Endoscopy 2003; 35:S14–S18.

65. Shim CS, Jung IS, Bhandari S, et al. Management of malignant strictures of the cervical esophagus with a newly-designed self-expanding metal stent. Endoscopy 2004; 36:554–557.

66. Conio M, Caroli-Bosc F, Demarquay JF, et al. Self-expanding metal stents in the palliation of neoplasms of the cervical esophagus. Hepatogastroenterology 1999; 46:272–277.

67. Yamamoto R, Tada H, Kishi A, Tojo T, Asada H. Double stent for malignant combined esophago-airway lesions. Jpn J Thorac Cardiovasc Surg 2002; 50:1–5.

68. Han YM, Song HY, Lee JM, Cho SI, Chung GH, Kim CS, Sohn MH, Choi KC. Esophagorespiratory fistulae due to esophageal carcinoma: palliation with a covered Gianturco stent. Radiology 1996; 199:65–70.

69. Lam YH, Chan A, Lau J, Lee D, Ng E, Wong S, Chung S. Self-expandable metal stents for malignant dysphagia. Aust N Z J Surg 1999; 69:668–671.

70. Nomori H, Horio H, Imazu Y, Suemasu K. Double stenting for esophageal and tracheobronchial stenoses. Ann Thorac Surg 2000; 70:1803–1807.

71. Nishimura Y, Nagata K, Katano S, et al. Severe complications in advanced esophageal cancer treated with radiotherapy after intubation of esophageal stents: a questionnaire survey of the Japanese Society for Esophageal Diseases. Int J Radiat Oncol Biol Phys 2003; 56:1327–1332.

72. Nemoto K, Takai Y, Ogawa Y, et al. Fatal hemorrhage in irradiated esophageal cancer patients. Acta Oncol 1998; 37:259–262.

73. Yakami M, Mitsumori M, Sai H, Nagata Y, Hiraoka M, Nishimura Y. Development of severe complications caused by stent placement followed by definitive radiation therapy for T4 esophageal cancer. Int J Clin Oncol 2003; 8:395–398.

74. Christie NA, Buenaventura PO, Fernando HC, et al. Results of expandable metal stents for malignant esophageal obstruction in 100 patients: short-term and long-term follow-up. Ann Thorac Surg 2001; 71:1797–1801; discussion 1801,1802.

75. Homs MY, Hansen BE, van Blankenstein M, Haringsma J, Kuipers EJ, Siersema PD. Prior radiation and/or chemotherapy has no effect on the outcome of metal stent placement for oesophagogastric carcinoma. Eur J Gastroenterol Hepatol 2004; 16:163–70.

76. Siersema PD, Hop WC, van Blankenstein M, Dees J. A new design metal stent (Flamingo stent) for palliation of malignant dysphagia: a prospective study. The Rotterdam Esophageal Tumor Study Group. Gastrointest Endosc 2000; 51:139–145.

77. Kinsman KJ, DeGregorio BT, Katon RM, et al. Prior radiation and chemotherapy increase the risk of life-threatening complications after insertion of metallic stents for esophagogastric malignancy. Gastrointest Endosc 1996; 43:196–203.

78. Maier A, Pinter H, Friehs GB, Renner H, Smolle-Juttner FM. Self-expandable coated stent after intraluminal treatment of esophageal cancer: a risky procedure? Ann Thorac Surg 1999; 67:781–784.

79. Sumiyoshi T, Gotoda T, Muro K, et al. Morbidity and mortality after self-expandable metallic stent placement in patients with progressive or recurrent esophageal cancer after chemoradiotherapy. Gastrointest Endosc 2003; 57:882–885.

80. Overholt BF. Laser and photodynamic therapy of esophageal cancer. Semin Surg Oncol 1992; 8:191–203.

81. Litle VR, Luketich JD, Christie NA, et al. Photodynamic therapy as palliation for esophageal cancer: experience in 215 patients. Ann Thorac Surg 2003; 76:1687–1692; discussion 1692,1693.

82. Luketich JD, Nguyen NT, Weigel TL, Keenan RJ, Ferson PF, Belani CP. Photodynamic therapy for treatment of malignant dysphagia. Surg Laparosc Endosc Percutan Tech 1999; 9:171–175.

83. Luketich JD, Christie NA, Buenaventura PO, Weigel TL, Keenan RJ, Nguyen NT. Endoscopic photodynamic therapy for obstructing esophageal cancer: 77 cases over a 2-year period. Surg Endosc 2000; 14:653–657.

84. McCaughan JS, Jr, Williams TE, Jr, Bethel BH. Palliation of esophageal malignancy with photodynamic therapy. Ann Thorac Surg 1985; 40:113–120.

85. Okunaka T, Kato H, Conaka C, Yamamoto H, Bonaminio A, Eckhauser ML. Photodynamic therapy of esophageal carcinoma. Surg Endosc 1990; 4:150–153.

86. Kashtan H, Konikoff F, Haddad R, Skornick Y. Photodynamic therapy of cancer of the esophagus using systemic aminolevulinic acid and a non laser light source: a phase I/II study. Gastrointest Endosc 1999; 49:760–764.

87. Maier A, Anegg U, Fell B, et al. Effect of photodynamic therapy in a multimodal approach for advanced carcinoma of the gastro-esophageal junction. Lasers Surg Med 2000; 26:461–466.

88. Moghissi K, Dixon K. Photodynamic therapy (PDT) in esophageal cancer: a surgical view of its indications based on 14 years experience. Technol Cancer Res Treat 2003; 2:319–326.

89. Webber J, Herman M, Kessel D, Fromm D. Current concepts in gastrointestinal photodynamic therapy. Ann Surg 1999; 230:12–23.

90. Saidi RF, Marcon NE. Nonthermal ablation of malignant esophageal strictures. Photodynamic therapy, endoscopic intratumoral injections, and novel modalities. Gastrointest Endosc Clin N Am 1998; 8:465–491.

91. Marcon NE. Photodynamic therapy and cancer of the esophagus. Semin Oncol 1994; 21:20–23.

92. Maier A, Tomaselli F, Matzi V, Rehak P, Pinter H, Smolle-Juttner FM. Does new photosensitizer improve photodynamic therapy in advanced esophageal carcinoma? Lasers Surg Med 2001; 29:323–327.

93. McCaughan JS, Jr, Ellison EC, Guy JT, et al. Photodynamic therapy for esophageal malignancy: a prospective twelve-year study. Ann Thorac Surg 1996; 62:1005–1009; discussion 1009,1010.

94. Moghissi K, Dixon K, Thorpe JA, Stringer M, Moore PJ. The role of photodynamic therapy (PDT) in inoperable oesophageal cancer. Eur J Cardiothorac Surg 2000; 17:95–100.

95. Sanfilippo NJ, Hsi A, DeNittis AS, et al. Toxicity of photodynamic therapy after combined external beam radiotherapy and intraluminal brachytherapy for carcinoma of the upper aerodigestive tract. Lasers Surg Med 2001; 28:278–281.

96. Canto M, Smith C, McClelland L, Heath E, Powe N. Randomized trial of PDT vs. stent for palliation of malignant dysphagia: cost-effectiveness and quality of life. Gastrointest Endosc 2002; 55:AB100 abstract.

97. Lightdale CJ, Heier SK, Marcon NE, et al. Photodynamic therapy with porfimer sodium versus thermal ablation therapy with Nd:YAG laser for palliation of esophageal cancer: a multicenter randomized trial. Gastrointest Endosc 1995; 42:507–512.

98. Heier SK, Rothman KA, Heier LM, Rosenthal WS. Photodynamic therapy for obstructing esophageal cancer: light dosimetry and randomized comparison with Nd:YAG laser therapy. Gastroenterology 1995; 109:63–72.

99. Burt M, Diehl W, Martini N, et al. Malignant esophagorespiratory fistula: management options and survival. Ann Thorac Surg 1991; 52:1222–1228; discussion 1228,1229.

100. Tomaselli F, Maier A, Sankin O, Woltsche M, Pinter H, Smolle-Juttner FM. Successful endoscopical sealing of malignant esophageotracheal fistulae by using a covered self-expandable stenting system. Eur J Cardiothorac Surg 2001; 20:734–738.

101. Nelson DB, Axelrad AM, Fleischer DE, et al. Silicone-covered Wallstent prototypes for palliation of malignant esophageal obstruction and digestive-respiratory fistulas. Gastrointest Endosc 1997; 45:31–37.

102. Bethge N, Sommer A, Vakil N. Treatment of esophageal fistulas with a new polyurethane-covered, self-expanding mesh stent: a prospective study. Am J Gastroenterol 1995; 90:2143–2146.

103. Chauhan SS, Long JD. Management of Tracheoesophageal Fistulas in Adults. Curr Treat Options Gastroenterol 2004; 7:31–40.

104. Norberto L, Ranzato R, Marino S, et al. Endoscopic palliation of esophageal and cardial cancer: neodymium-yttrium aluminum garnet laser therapy. Dis Esophagus 1999; 12:294–296.

105. Suzuki H, Miho O, Watanabe Y, Kohyama M, Nagao F. Endoscopic laser therapy in the curative and palliative treatment of upper gastrointestinal cancer. World J Surg 1989; 13:158–164.

7 Radiological Imaging of the Upper Gastrointestinal Tract

Marc S. Levine, MD

Contents

1. BACKGROUND

Radiological imaging of the upper gastrointestinal (GI) tract provides useful diagnostic information regarding a wide variety of benign and malignant tumors. Whereas computed tomography (CT) scanning may detect larger invasive tumors and provide information regarding lymphatic and distant metastases, properly done barium studies provide more detail regarding mucosally based or intramural lesions. This chapter reviews the radiological findings of the various benign and malignant tumors of the esophagus and stomach.

2. ESOPHAGUS

2.1. BENIGN TUMORS

Benign tumors of the esophagus constitute only about 20% of all esophageal neoplasms (1). Often they are small, asymptomatic lesions that are detected fortuitously on barium studies or endoscopy. However, some patients may exhibit dysphagia, bleeding, or other symptoms. Depending on the site of origin in the esophageal wall, benign tumors may be classified as *mucosal* or *submucosal*. These lesions have typical radiographic features that are discussed separately in the following sections.

2.1.1. Mucosal Lesions

2.1.1.1. Papilloma

Squamous papillomas are uncommon benign tumors, constituting less than 5% of all esophageal neoplasms. These lesions consist of a fibrovascular core with multiple finger-like projections covered by hyperplastic squamous epithelium. They usually occur as solitary lesions ranging from 0.5 to 1.5 cm in size. Most patients are asymptomatic, but some with larger polyps may present with dysphagia. Multiple papillomas may be present in patients with a rare condition known as esophageal papillomatosis (2).

From: *Endoscopic Oncology: Gastrointestinal Endoscopy and Cancer Management*. Edited by: D. O. Faigel and M. L. Kochman © Humana Press, Totowa, NJ

Papillomas may be recognized on double-contrast esophagrams as small, sessile polyps with a smooth or slightly lobulated contour (Fig. 1) (3). Occasionally, papillomas may be larger and more lobulated, or they may have a bubbly appearance as a result of trapping of barium between the frond-like projections of the tumor (4). Although papillomas are always benign, they cannot be differentiated with certainty from early esophageal cancers on radiographic criteria. Endoscopic biopsy or resection of the lesion therefore is required when a papilloma is suspected on barium studies.

2.1.1.2. Adenoma

Adenomas are rarely found in the esophagus because this structure is lined by squamous rather than columnar epithelium. However, esophageal adenomas may develop in metaplastic columnar epithelium associated with Barrett's esophagus (5,6). These lesions are important because they can undergo malignant transformation via an adenoma–carcinoma sequence similar to that found in the colon (5,6). Endoscopic or surgical resection therefore is warranted.

Adenomas typically appear on barium studies as sessile or pedunculated polyps in the distal esophagus (Fig. 2) (6). Lesions that are larger or more lobulated have a greater risk of harboring cancer. Because of their location, adenomatous polyps sometimes can be mistaken for inflammatory esophagogastric polyps on the basis of the radiographic findings. When an adenoma is suspected on barium studies, endoscopy and biopsy therefore are required for a definitive diagnosis.

2.1.1.3. Inflammatory Esophagogastric Polyp

Although inflammatory esophagogastric polyps are not true neoplasms, they may be manifested on esophagography by polypoid lesions in the distal esophagus at or near the gastroesophageal junction (GEJ) (7–9). These lesions consist of inflammatory and granulation tissue and are presumed to develop as a sequela of reflux esophagitis (8).

Inflammatory esophagogastric polyps usually are manifested on barium studies by a single prominent fold that arises at the cardia and extends upward into the distal esophagus as a smooth

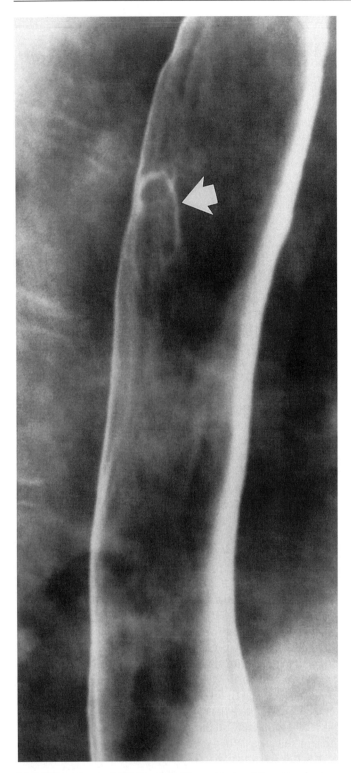

Fig. 1. Squamous papilloma. Double-contrast esophagram shows a small, slightly lobulated papilloma etched in white (arrow) in the mid-esophagus. Early esophageal cancer could produce similar findings, so endoscopic biopsy specimens are required for a definitive diagnosis. (Reproduced with permission from ref. *16*.)

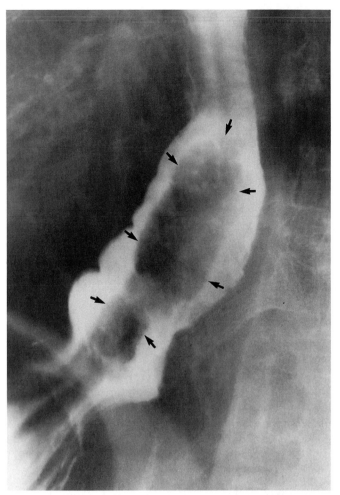

Fig. 2. Adenomatous polyp in Barrett's esophagus. Prone single-contrast esophagram shows a pedunculated polyp (arrows) extending from the gastroesophageal junction into the distal esophagus. The resected specimen revealed Barrett's mucosa, with an adenomatous polyp containing a solitary focus of adenocarcinoma. (Reproduced with permission from ref. *6*.)

should be performed to exclude an adenomatous polyp in Barrett's esophagus.

2.1.1.4. Glycogenic Acanthosis

Glycogenic acanthosis is a benign condition in which there is accumulation of cytoplasmic glycogen in squamous epithelial cells lining the esophagus, causing plaque-like thickening of the mucosa *(10,11)*. It is a degenerative condition that occurs primarily in the elderly *(10)*. This condition rarely causes esophageal symptoms and is not associated with any risk of malignant degeneration. As a result, it usually is discovered as an incidental finding on radiological or endoscopic examinations.

Glycogenic acanthosis is manifested on double-contrast esophagrams by multiple small, rounded nodules or plaques in the mid or, less commonly, distal esophagus (Fig. 4) *(12,13)*. The nodules usually range from 1 to 3 mm in size, but occasional plaques can be as large as several centimeters *(12,13)*. The major consideration in the differential diagnosis is *Candida* esophagitis. However, the plaques of candidiasis tend to be more linear and typically develop in immunocompro-

and polypoid protuberance (Fig. 3) *(7–9)*. Because of its characteristic appearance and location, endoscopy is not warranted when a typical inflammatory esophagogastric polyp is detected on barium studies. If the polyp has a lobulated contour or other atypical radiographic features, however, endoscopy and biopsy

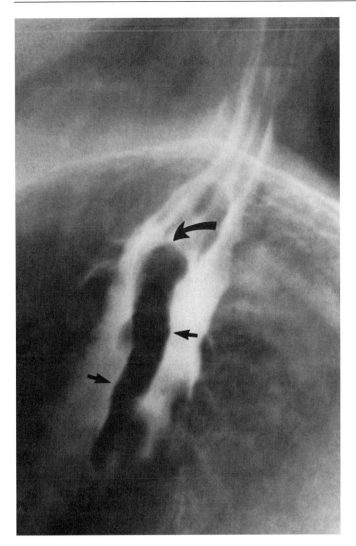

Fig. 3. Inflammatory esophagogastric polyp. Prone single-contrast esophagram shows a prominent fold (straight arrows) extending from the gastroesophageal junction into the distal esophagus as a smooth polypoid protuberance (curved arrow). This lesion has the typical appearance of an inflammatory esophagogastric polyp.

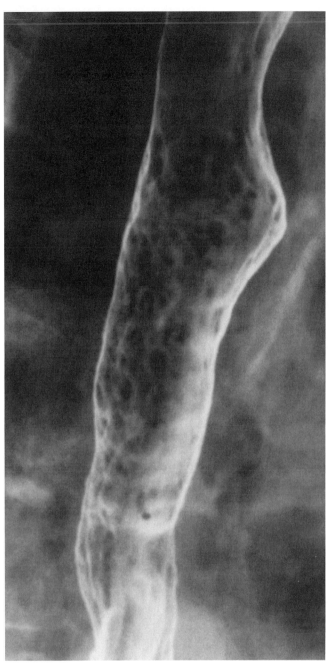

Fig. 4. Glycogenic acanthosis. Double-contrast esophagram shows multiple small, rounded nodules in the mid-esophagus. This was an elderly patient who had no esophageal symptoms. (Reproduced with permission from ref. *84*.)

mised patients with odynophagia, whereas glycogenic acanthosis occurs in older individuals who are not immunocompromised and have no esophageal symptoms. Thus, it usually is possible to differentiate these conditions on the basis of the clinical and radiographic findings

2.1.2. Submucosal Lesions

By definition, all submucosal lesions arising in the wall of the esophagus are intramural. Not all intramural lesions are submucosal, however, as they can also arise from the muscularis propria or even the subserosa. Despite this distinction, the terms *submucosal* and *intramural* are used interchangeably based on long-standing convention.

2.1.2.1. Leiomyoma

Leiomyomas are by far the most common benign submucosal tumors in the esophagus *(14)*. These lesions consist of intersecting bands of smooth muscle surrounded by a well-defined capsule. Esophageal leiomyomas are rarely located above the level of the aortic arch because of the presence of striated rather than

smooth muscle in this portion of the esophagus. They usually occur as solitary lesions, but multiple leiomyomas are present in 3–4% of cases *(15)*. Most esophageal leiomyomas cause no symptoms, but some patients may present with dysphagia, depending on the size of the tumor and how much it encroaches on the lumen. In contrast, GI bleeding rarely occurs because leiomyomas in the esophagus, unlike those in the stomach, are almost never ulcerated *(16)*. Unlike other GI stromal tumors (GISTs), esophageal leiomyomas virtually never undergo sarcomatous degeneration. Thus, surgical removal of small lesions in asymptomatic patients probably is not warranted.

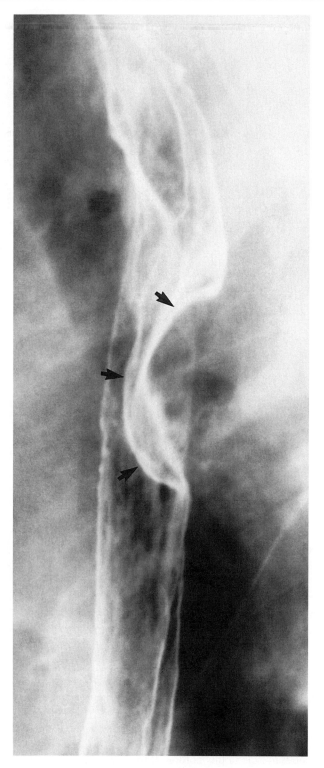

Fig. 5. Leiomyoma. Double-contrast esophagram shows a smooth-surfaced mass (arrows) in the mid-esophagus. Note how this lesion has the typical radiographic features of a submucosal mass, forming slightly obtuse angles with the adjacent esophageal wall.

When leiomyomas grow exophytically into the mediastinum, they sometimes can be recognized on chest radiographs by the presence of a mediastinal mass (17). Rarely, these tumors may contain punctate areas of calcification (18). Leiomyomas usually appear on barium studies as smooth-sur-

faced submucosal masses that form right angles or slightly obtuse angles with the adjacent esophageal wall when viewed in profile (Fig. 5) (14,16). These tumors typically range from 2 to 8 cm in size but occasionally can be giant masses as large as 20 cm in size (19). Leiomyomas typically appear on CT as homogeneous soft tissue masses, but differentiation from other benign or malignant esophageal tumors is difficult on the basis of the CT findings (20).

2.1.2.2. Fibrovascular Polyp

Fibrovascular polyps are rare, benign mesenchymal tumors characterized by the development of pedunculated intraluminal masses that can grow to enormous sizes in the esophagus. These lesions consist of varying amounts of fibrovascular and adipose tissue covered by normal squamous epithelium (21). Depending on the predominant histological components, these tumors variously have been called hamartomas, fibromas, lipomas, and fibrolipomas. More recently, however, the lesions have all been classified together by the World Health Organization as fibrovascular polyps (22).

Fibrovascular polyps almost always arise on a pedicle or pseudo-pedicle in the cervical esophagus near the level of the cricopharyngeus (23). The lesions gradually elongate over a period of years as they are dragged inferiorly by esophageal peristalsis until the inferior tip has reached the mid- or even distal esophagus, occasionally prolapsing through the cardia into the gastric fundus (23).

Fibrovascular polyps most commonly occur in elderly men who present with long-standing dysphagia (23). Rarely, these individuals may have a spectacular clinical presentation with regurgitation of a fleshy mass into the pharynx or mouth or even asphyxia and sudden death if the regurgitated polyp occludes the larynx (23,24). Although malignant degeneration of fibrovascular polyps is extremely rare, removal of these lesions is recommended because of the inexorable progression of symptoms and the theoretical risk of asphyxia and sudden death.

Fibrovascular polyps usually are manifested on barium studies by a smooth, expansile, sausage-shaped mass in the upper or upper and mid-esophagus (Fig. 6A) (23,25). Fibrovascular polyps that contain a large amount of adipose tissue classically appear on CT as fat density lesions that expand the lumen of the esophagus, with a thin rim of contrast surrounding the polyp, confirming its intraluminal location (Fig. 6B) (23,26). However, polyps that contain varying amounts of fibrovascular and adipose tissue may appear on CT as heterogeneous lesions, and polyps that contain an abundance of fibrovascular tissue may appear on CT as soft tissue density lesions with a paucity of fat (23).

2.1.2.3. Duplication Cyst

Duplication cysts are developmental anomalies in which large nests of cells are sequestered from the primitive foregut. These cysts contain all layers of the bowel wall, including a mucosa, submucosa, and muscularis propria and are lined by a ciliated columnar epithelium (27). Affected individuals are almost always asymptomatic, but symptoms occasionally may be caused by bleeding or infection of the cysts (28). Although most duplication cysts are noncommunicating, some may communicate directly with the esophageal lumen.

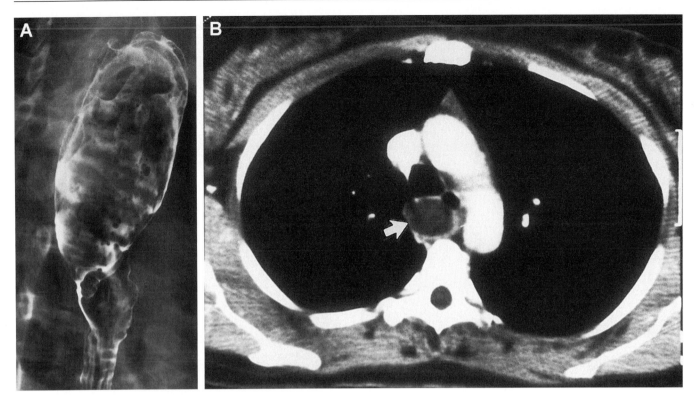

Fig. 6. Fibrovascular polyp. (**A**) Double-contrast esophagram shows a smooth, expansile, sausage-shaped mass in the upper third of the thoracic esophagus. This lesion has the classic features of a fibrovascular polyp on barium studies. (**B**) CT scan shows an expansile intraluminal mass (arrow) in the upper third of the thoracic esophagus. Note how a peripheral rim of contrast material surrounds the polyp, confirming its intraluminal location. Also note the predominant fat density of the lesion at this level. (Reproduced with permission from ref. *23*.)

Duplications cysts tend to be located in the right lower mediastinum, so they sometimes can be recognized on frontal chest radiographs by the presence of a mediastinal mass *(16)*. The cysts typically appear on barium studies as smooth submucosal masses indistinguishable from other more common mesenchymal lesions such as leiomyomas (Fig. 7) *(16)*. These fluid-filled cysts usually have characteristic findings on cross-sectional imaging studies, appearing as low-attenuation structures on CT and as high-signal intensity structures on T2-weighted magnetic resonance images *(29,30)*. When duplication cysts do communicate with the esophageal lumen, they occasionally may be recognized as tubular, branching outpouchings from the esophagus that fill with barium *(16)*. Endoscopic ultrasound may be useful when there is diagnostic uncertainty.

2.2. MALIGNANT TUMORS
2.2.1. Squamous Cell Carcinoma

Patients with esophageal cancer usually develop symptoms only after the tumor has invaded adjacent mediastinal structures *(31)*. As a result, most patients have advanced disease at the time of diagnosis, with 5-yr survival rates of less than 10% *(32)*. Occasionally, however, early esophageal cancers can be detected by serendipity or by screening of asymptomatic patients in high-risk groups.

2.2.1.1. Early Esophageal Cancer

Early esophageal cancers may be manifested on double-contrast barium studies by small polypoid lesions, plaque-like lesions, focal irregularity of the wall, or superficial spreading lesions *(32–34)*. Some early cancers may appear as small, sessile polyps with a smooth or slightly lobulated contour (Fig. 8). Other early cancers may appear as plaque-lesions, often containing a flat central ulcer. Still other lesions may be manifested by puckering or deformity of the esophageal wall, so the radiographic findings can be extremely subtle *(32)*. Finally, some early cancers may be superficial spreading lesions, manifested by a cluster of poorly defined nodules, producing a confluent area of disease (Fig. 9) *(32,34,35)*. When early esophageal cancer or superficial spreading cancer is suspected on barium studies, endoscopy and biopsy should be performed for a definitive diagnosis, as patients with early esophageal cancer have 5-yr survival rates as high as 95% *(32)*.

2.2.1.2. Advanced Esophageal Cancer

Advanced squamous cell carcinomas of the esophagus may be manifested on chest films by a widened mediastinum, anterior tracheal bowing, or a dilated, obstructed esophagus *(36)*. Barium studies may reveal infiltrating, polypoid, ulcerative, or varicoid lesions that tend to be located in the upper or mid-esophagus *(32)*. Regardless of the morphology of the tumor, CT typically reveals marked circumferential thickening of the esophageal wall. Infiltrating carcinomas usually are manifested on barium studies by irregular luminal narrowing with mucosal nodularity, ulceration, and abrupt, shelf-like proximal and distal borders (Fig. 10) *(32)*. Unfortunately, by the time these tumors cause dysphagia, they are almost always advanced, lesions with poor prognoses.

Other cancers may be polypoid masses (Fig. 11), often containing irregular areas of ulceration *(32)*. Polypoid carcinomas

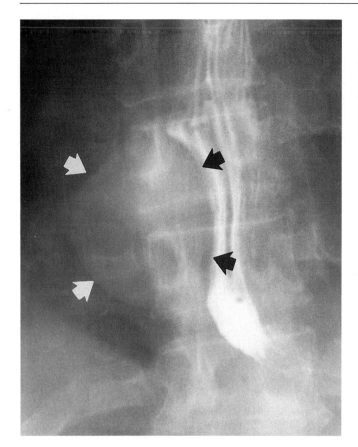

Fig. 7. Duplication cyst. Double-contrast esophagram shows a smooth, submucosal-appearing mass (black arrows) on the right lateral wall of the distal esophagus. Note how the lateral portion of the cyst is visible where it interfaces with the adjacent lung (white arrows). (Reproduced with permission from ref. *84*.)

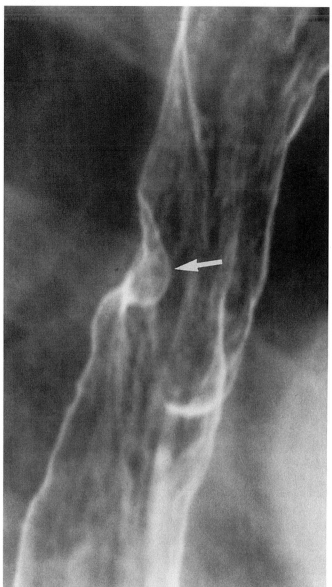

Fig. 8. Early squamous cell carcinoma. Double-contrast esophagram shows a small, sessile polyp (arrow) in the mid-esophagus. A benign squamous papilloma could produce similar findings (*see* Fig. 1). (Courtesy of Seth N. Glick, MD, Philadelphia, PA.)

of the cervical esophagus are more likely to be missed on barium studies than polypoid carcinomas of the thoracic esophagus because barium passes so rapidly through the cervical esophagus that it often is difficult to obtain adequate spot films of this region. Fortunately, most squamous cell carcinomas are located in the thoracic esophagus. Other esophageal carcinomas may be primary ulcerative lesions, with a giant meniscoid ulcer surrounded by a radiolucent rind of tumor (Fig. 12) *(37)*. Such lesions occasionally may be mistaken for benign ulcers with a surrounding mound of edema, but the tumor mass surrounding these ulcers usually is larger than the pencil-thin rim of edema adjacent to benign ulcers.

Less commonly, squamous cell carcinomas of the esophagus may appear as varicoid lesions, manifested by submucosal defects that can resemble varices on a single radiograph (Fig. 13) *(38)*. However, these defects have a fixed, unchanging appearance, whereas varices would be expected to change in size and shape with varying esophageal distention and peristalsis. Patients with varicoid carcinoma may also present with dysphagia, a rare finding in patients with varices. Other esophageal cancers that infiltrate the submucosa may cause narrowing, occasionally resembling benign strictures *(32)*. However, malignant strictures tend to be more asymmetric and have a more irregular contour than benign strictures. Thus, any strictures that have suspicious

or atypical features should be evaluated by endoscopy and biopsy to rule out malignant tumor.

2.2.2. Adenocarcinoma

Almost all esophageal adenocarcinomas are found to arise in patients with underlying Barrett's esophagus. These tumors predominantly are located in the distal esophagus and have a marked tendency to invade the gastric cardia and fundus *(6,39)*. At one time, esophageal adenocarcinomas were thought to be rare lesions, in part because these tumors invading the cardia and fundus were incorrectly classified as primary gastric carcinomas invading the esophagus. Currently, however, adenocarcinomas arising in Barrett's mucosa are thought to constitute as many as 20–50% of all esophageal cancers *(40,41)*, so this is a much more common tumor than previously has been recognized. Most patients with

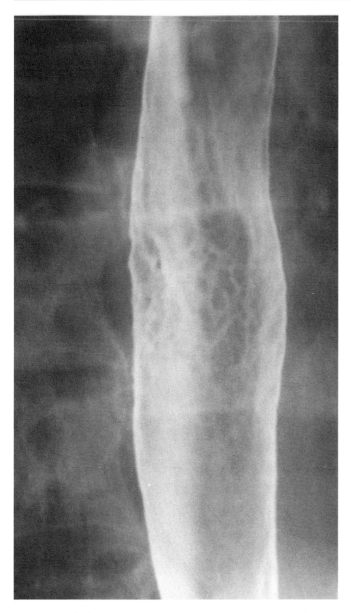

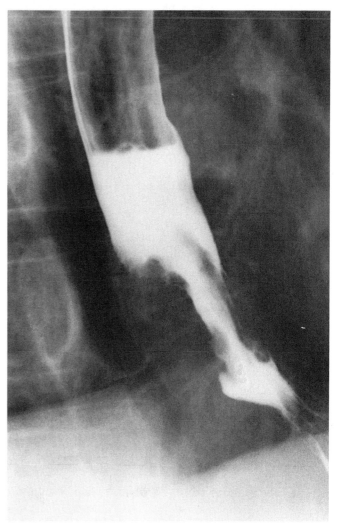

Fig. 10. Infiltrating squamous cell carcinoma. Double-contrast esophagram shows a circumferentially infiltrating tumor in the distal esophagus. Note how this lesion has abrupt, shelf-like borders.

Fig. 9. Superficial spreading carcinoma. Double-contrast esophagram shows focal nodularity in the mid-esophagus with tiny, coalescent nodules and plaques. (Reproduced with permission from ref. *85.*)

esophageal adenocarcinomas have advanced tumors at the time of diagnosis, but early cancers occasionally may be detected in patients who present because of their underlying reflux disease or in asymptomatic patients who undergo surveillance for known Barrett's esophagus.

2.2.2.1. Early Esophageal Cancer

Early adenocarcinomas may be manifested on double-contrast barium studies by small sessile polyps, plaque-like lesions, or superficial spreading lesions that cause focal nodularity of the mucosa without a discrete mass *(6,32,34).* Occasionally, these early cancers can also be recognized by focal irregularity, flattening, or nodularity within a pre-existing peptic stricture (Fig. 14) *(6).* The presence of any suspicious features in the region of a peptic stricture therefore should lead to early endoscopy and biopsy to rule out a superimposed adenocarcinoma.

2.2.2.2. Advanced Esophageal Cancer

Advanced adenocarcinomas may appear on barium studies as infiltrating, polypoid, ulcerative, or varicoid lesions *(6,39).* CT typically reveals marked circumferential thickening of the esophageal wall by tumor. These lesions therefore have the same radiographic features as squamous cell carcinomas. However, squamous cell carcinomas tend to be located in the upper or mid-esophagus, whereas adenocarcinomas predominantly are located in the distal esophagus and have a marked tendency to invade the gastric cardia and fundus (Fig. 15).

Gastric involvement by esophageal adenocarcinoma sometimes is recognized by the presence of a polypoid, ulcerated mass in the gastric fundus. However, other tumors may be manifested by relatively subtle findings, with distortion or obliteration of the normal cardiac rosette *(32).* When the cardia is involved by tumor, it may be difficult or impossible to differentiate an esophageal adenocarcinoma invading the cardia from a cardiac carcinoma invading the distal esophagus on the basis of the radiographic findings.

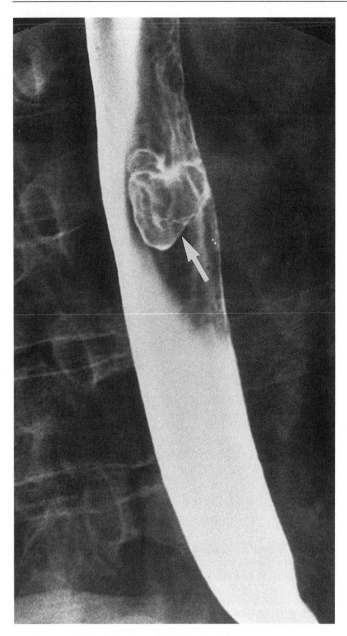

Fig. 11. Polypoid squamous cell carcinoma. Double-contrast esophagram shows a polypoid mass (arrow) in the mid-esophagus.

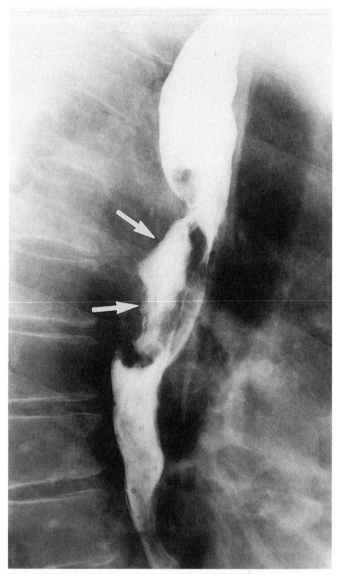

Fig. 12. Primary ulcerative squamous cell carcinoma. Double-contrast esophagram shows a giant, meniscoid ulcer (arrows) in the mid-esophagus. Note the radiolucent rim of tumor surrounding the ulcer. (Reproduced with permission from ref. 85.)

2.2.3. Spindle Cell Carcinoma

Spindle cell carcinoma is an unusual malignant tumor that consists pathologically of innumerable tumor-like spindle cells with islands or nests of carcinomatous cells interspersed throughout the lesion (42). These tumors typically appear on barium studies as bulky, polypoid intraluminal masses that characteristically expand or dilate the esophagus without causing obstruction (Fig. 16) (42). The differential diagnosis for an expansile intraluminal mass includes malignant melanoma, another rare malignant tumor of the esophagus.

2.2.4. Kaposi's Sarcoma

Kaposi's sarcoma is a malignant tumor that has been encountered with increased frequency in patients with AIDS. About 30% of AIDS patients have Kaposi's sarcoma, and 50% with Kaposi's sarcoma have GI involvement (43), usually the stomach or small bowel but occasionally the esophagus. GI involvement by Kaposi's sarcoma almost always occurs in patients who have concomitant skin lesions. Kaposi's sarcoma may be manifested on barium studies by submucosal masses or polypoid lesions in the esophagus (43). In patients with AIDS, esophageal involvement by lymphoma should be the major consideration in the differential diagnosis.

2.2.5. Malignant Melanoma

Malignant melanoma is a rare primary malignant tumor of the esophagus (44). In fact, melanocytes are found in the basement membrane of the esophagus in about 4–8% of patients (45). Malignant degeneration of these cells subsequently can result in the development of an esophageal melanoma. These patients have an extremely poor prognosis, with an average survival of only 7 mo (44). Esophageal melanomas usually appear on barium studies as bulky, polypoid intraluminal masses

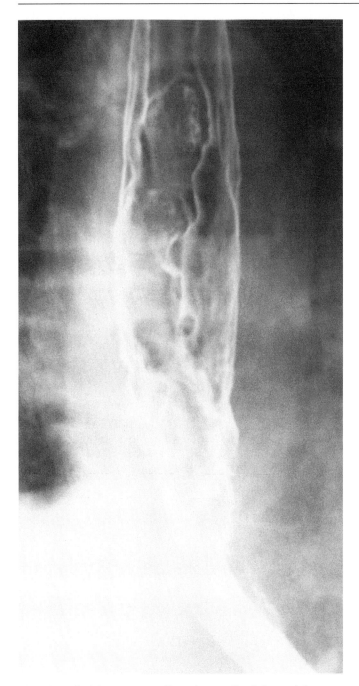

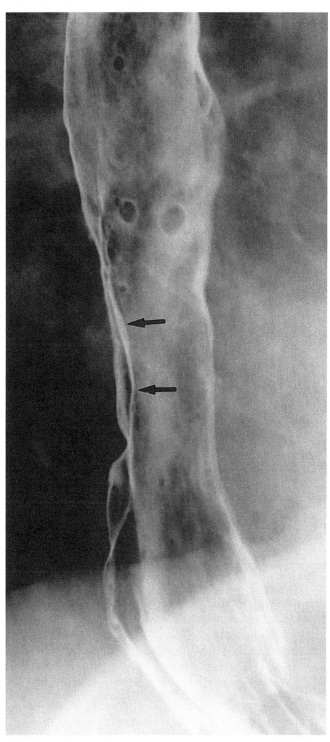

Fig. 13. Varicoid squamous cell carcinoma. Serpiginous defects are seen in the distal third of the esophagus owing to submucosal spread of tumor. This type of lesion could be mistaken for varices on a single radiograph. (Courtesy of Robert A. Goren, MD, Philadelphia, PA.)

Fig. 14. Early adenocarcinoma in Barrett's esophagus. Double-contrast esophagram shows a relatively long peptic stricture in the distal esophagus with slight flattening and stiffening of one wall of the stricture (arrows) owing to pathologically proven carcinoma *in situ* arising in Barrett's mucosa. (Reproduced with permission from ref. *6*.)

indistinguishable from spindle cell carcinomas (Fig. 17) *(44)*. However, the correct diagnosis should be suggested by the presence of a darkly pigmented mass in the esophagus at endoscopy.

3. STOMACH

3.1. BENIGN TUMORS

Benign gastric tumors can either be mucosal or submucosal in origin. Mucosa lesions consist primarily of hyperplastic and adenomatous polyps, whereas submucosal lesions include GI stromal tumors, lipomas, and ectopic pancreatic rests.

3.1.1. Mucosal Lesions
3.1.1.1. Hyperplastic Polyp

Hyperplastic polyps are by far the most common benign mucosal lesions in the stomach, constituting as many as 75–90% of all gastric polyps. These lesions have no malignant

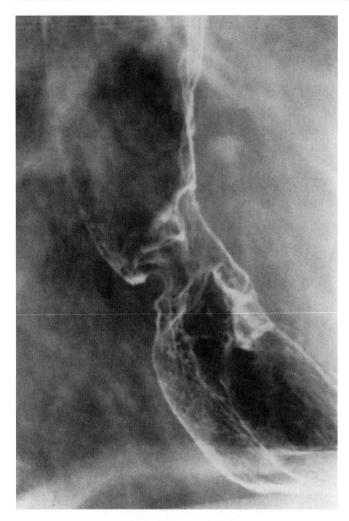

Fig. 15. Infiltrating adenocarcinoma in Barrett's esophagus. Double-contrast esophagram shows a relatively short area of irregular narrowing that extends from the distal esophagus into an adjacent hiatal hernia. Note the abrupt, shelf-like borders of the lesion.

potential. Hyperplastic polyps usually appear on barium studies as multiple smooth, rounded nodules (<1 cm in size) in the gastric body and fundus (Fig. 18) *(46)*. Some patients may have innumerable polyps filling the stomach, whereas others may have a conglomerate mass of hyperplastic polyps, mimicking the findings of a polypoid carcinoma (Fig. 19) *(47)*.

3.1.1.2. Adenomatous Polyp

Adenomatous polyps are premalignant lesions that may degenerate into invasive adenocarcinoma via an adenoma–carcinoma sequence similar to that found in the colon. Adenomatous polyps usually appear on barium studies as solitary, sessile, lobulated, or pedunculated lesions (>1 cm in size) in the gastric antrum (Fig. 20) *(48)*. When an adenomatous polyp is suspected on barium studies, endoscopy should be performed for biopsy or removal of the lesion.

3.1.2. Submucosal Lesions

3.1.2.1. Benign GIST

Benign GISTs are common benign submucosal lesions found in the stomach *(49)*. Benign GISTs typically appear on barium studies as smooth, round or ovoid submucosal masses that form

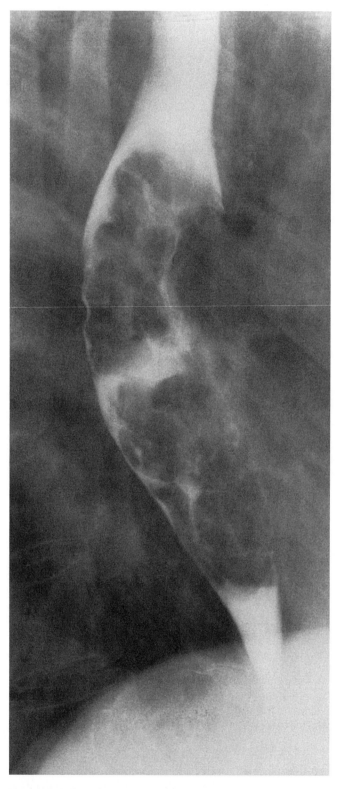

Fig. 16. Spindle cell carcinoma. Single-contrast esophagram shows a large polypoid intraluminal mass expanding the distal esophagus without causing obstruction. These findings are characteristic of spindle cell carcinomas. (Reproduced with permission from ref. *86*.)

right angles or slightly obtuse angles with the adjacent gastric wall when viewed in profile (Fig. 21). These lesions may be difficult to differentiate from other mesenchymal tumors on the basis of the radiographic findings, except for the fact that benign

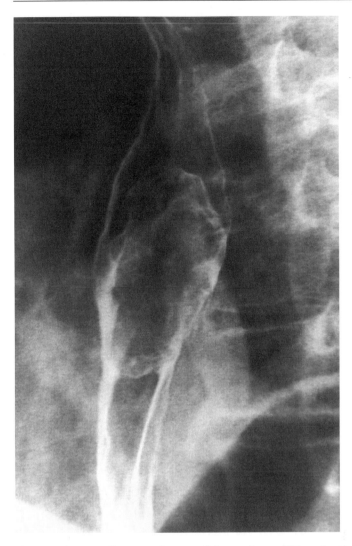

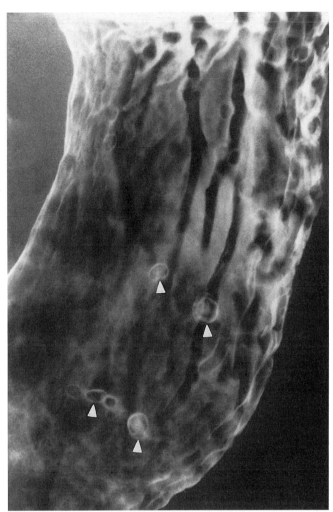

Fig. 17. Primary malignant melanoma of the esophagus. This patient has a polypoid intraluminal mass expanding the lumen of the distal esophagus. Spindle cell carcinoma could produce similar findings (*see* Fig. 16). (Reproduced with permission from ref. *44.*)

Fig. 18. Hyperplastic polyps. Double-contrast view of the stomach shows multiple small, sessile polyps etched in white (arrowheads) in the gastric body. These lesions have the typical radiographic features of hyperplastic polyps.

GISTs are more common on empirical grounds. Frequently, these tumors outgrow their blood supply with central ischemia and necrosis, resulting in the development of a centrally ulcerated submucosal mass, also known as a bull's eye or target lesion. Rarely, benign GISTs may contain areas of calcification that are visible on barium studies or even abdominal plain films *(50)*.

3.1.2.2. Lipoma

Gastric lipomas are rare benign tumors of the stomach. Most patients are asymptomatic, but GI bleeding can occur if the lesion is ulcerated. Lipomas typically appear on barium studies as smooth, round or ovoid submucosal masses. Unlike GISTs, these lesions may change dramatically in size and shape at fluoroscopy because of their soft consistency *(51)*. Gastric lipomas can be definitively diagnosed on CT by their characteristic fat density *(52)*.

3.1.2.3. Ectopic Pancreatic Rest

Ectopic pancreatic rests usually occur in the stomach, duodenum, or proximal jejunum. In the stomach, these lesions typically appear as discrete submucosal masses, almost always

located on the greater curvature of the distal antrum within 1–6 cm from the pylorus (Fig. 22) *(53)*. Occasionally, they may contain a central umbilication or ulceration and, rarely, barium can even be seen to enter a vestigial ductal system.

3.2. MALIGNANT TUMORS

3.2.1. Adenocarcinoma

Although the incidence of gastric carcinoma has declined during the past 50 yr, it continues to be a deadly disease, with overall 5-yr survival rates of less than 20% *(54)*. There also has been a gradual shift in the distribution of gastric cancer from the antrum proximally to the fundus and cardia *(55)*. As a result, 30–40% of all gastric cancers are located in the fundus or cardiac region *(55)*. The gastric cardia and fundus therefore should be carefully evaluated in all patients with suspected gastric tumors.

3.2.1.1. Early Gastric Cancer

By definition, early gastric cancers are confined to the mucosa or submucosa, regardless of the presence or absence of lymph node metastases. Unlike advanced carcinomas, which have a dismal prognosis, early gastric cancers are curable

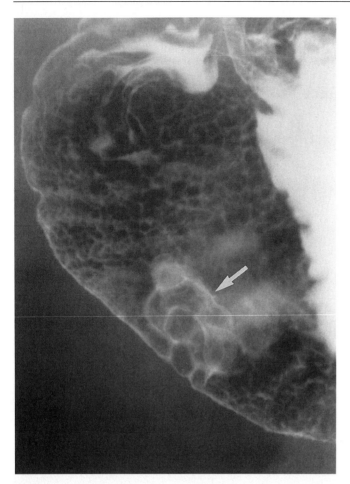

Fig. 19. Giant hyperplastic polyp. Double-contrast view of the stomach shows a large, multilobulated mass (arrow) on the greater curvature of the antrum. A gastric carcinoma could produce similar findings.

lesions, with 5-yr survival rates of more than 90% (56,57). Whereas these cancers often are detected in Japan, they rarely are diagnosed in the United States or other countries in the West. This discrepancy can be attributed to mass screening of the adult population in Japan because of the high prevalence of gastric carcinoma in that country (58). The Japanese Endoscopic Society has divided early gastric cancers into three types (see Table 1) (59). Type I cancers are elevated lesions that protrude more than 5 mm into the lumen. Type II cancers are superficial lesions that are further subdivided into three groups (types IIa, IIb, and IIc) depending on the morphological features of the tumor. Type IIa lesions protrude less than 5 mm into the lumen. Type IIb lesions are relatively flat. Type IIc lesions are slightly depressed but do not penetrate beyond the muscularis mucosae. Finally, type III lesions are true mucosal ulcers, with the ulcer penetrating beyond the muscularis mucosae into the submucosa but not the muscularis propria.

Type I early gastric cancers typically appear on double-contrast studies as small, protruded lesions (see Fig. 20) (60). Because adenomatous polyps sometimes undergo malignant degeneration, the possibility of early gastric cancer should be suspected for any polyps larger than 1 cm in size. Other larger polypoid lesions that protrude considerably into the lumen may still be

classified histologically as early gastric cancers (60). Thus, polypoid carcinomas cannot be definitively diagnosed as early or advanced lesions on the basis of the radiographic findings.

Type II early gastric cancers are relatively flat lesions with elevated, superficial, or protruded components. These lesions may be manifested on double-contrast studies by plaque-like elevations, mucosal nodularity, shallow ulcers, or some combination of these findings (61). Occasionally, these lesions can be quite extensive, involving a considerable surface area of the stomach without invading beyond the submucosa. Type III early gastric cancers usually appear on double-contrast studies as shallow ulcer craters with nodularity of the adjacent mucosa and clubbing or fusion of radiating folds resulting from infiltration of the folds by tumor (60). Careful analysis usually permits differentiation from benign gastric ulcers, which have different radiographic features (62). Although some lesions with a suspicious appearance are found to be benign, endoscopy is required for all lesions with equivocal radiographic findings in order to avoid missing early cancers (62).

3.2.1.2. Advanced Gastric Cancer

Concern about missing gastric cancer on barium studies has often been used as a rationale for performing endoscopy as the initial diagnostic test in patients with upper GI symptoms. In a recent study, however, double-contrast examinations showed the lesion in 99% of patients with gastric carcinoma, and malignant tumor was diagnosed or suspected on the basis of the radiographic findings in 96% (63). In the same study, endoscopy was recommended to rule out malignant tumor in less than 5% of all patients who underwent double-contrast examinations. Thus, a high sensitivity can be achieved in the radiographic diagnosis of gastric carcinoma without exposing an inordinate number of patients to unnecessary endoscopy. Advanced gastric carcinomas usually appear on barium studies as polypoid, ulcerative, or infiltrative lesions. Polypoid carcinomas often contain irregular areas of ulceration resulting from necrosis of tumor. Occasionally, polypoid carcinomas of the antrum may prolapse through the pylorus into the duodenal bulb, appearing as mass lesions at the base of the bulb.

Ulcerated carcinomas are those in which the bulk of the tumor has been replaced by ulceration. These lesions are often called "malignant ulcers," but the term is a misnomer, as it is not the ulcer but the surrounding tumor that is malignant. Malignant ulcers classically appear en face as irregular ulcer craters eccentrically located within a tumor mass (62). There may be distortion or even obliteration of surrounding areae gastricae resulting from infiltration of the adjacent mucosa by tumor. Malignant ulcers often have scalloped, irregular borders, with thickened, lobulated, or clubbed folds abutting the ulcers resulting from infiltration of the folds by tumor (62). When viewed in profile, malignant ulcers are located within a discrete tumor mass that forms acute angles with the adjacent gastric wall rather than the obtuse angles expected for a benign mound of edema (Fig. 23) (62).

Some authors believe that all gastric ulcers should be evaluated by endoscopy and biopsy to rule out gastric carcinoma. However, studies have shown that ulcers with an unequivocally

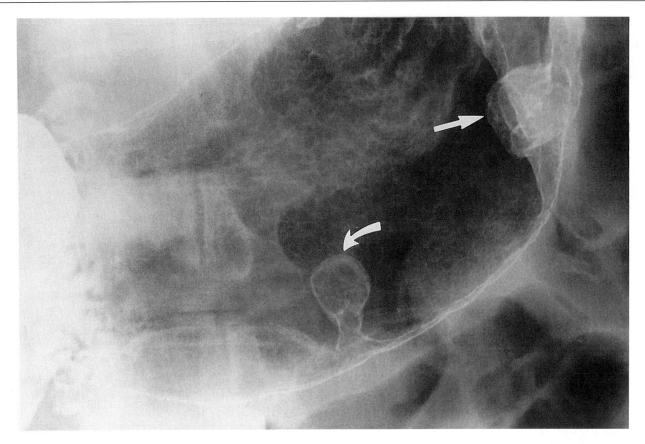

Fig. 20. Adenomatous polyp and polypoid early gastric cancer. Double-contrast view of the stomach shows a small polypoid carcinoma (straight arrow) on the greater curvature of the gastric body and a pedunculated adenomatous polyp (curved arrow) more distally on the greater curvature. (Reproduced with permission from ref. *63*.)

benign appearance on double-contrast examinations invariably are benign lesions *(62,64)*. In these studies, about two-thirds of all radiographically diagnosed ulcers have had a benign appearance *(62,64)*. Unnecessary endoscopy and biopsy therefore can be avoided in the majority of patients with ulcers detected on double-contrast barium studies. However, any ulcers with an equivocal or suspicious appearance must be evaluated by endoscopy and biopsy to rule out an ulcerated gastric carcinoma.

Infiltrative carcinomas are circumferential tumors that encase the stomach, causing marked luminal narrowing, often associated with polypoid, ulcerated components and a nodular, spiculated contour. Eventually, these lesions may cause gastric outlet obstruction.

3.2.1.3. Scirrhous Carcinoma

Scirrhous gastric carcinomas traditionally are thought to arise in the distal half of the stomach, gradually extending from the antrum proximally into the gastric body and fundus. In advanced cases, the entire stomach may be encased by tumor. These scirrhous carcinomas classically are manifested on barium studies by irregular narrowing and rigidity of the stomach, producing a linitis plastica or "leather bottle" appearance as a result of a marked desmoplastic response incited by the tumor (Fig. 24) *(65)*. However, some scirrhous carcinomas may be confined to the prepyloric antrum, appearing as short, annular lesions with shelf-like proximal borders *(66)*.

Despite the classic teaching that scirrhous carcinomas involve the gastric antrum, recent literature suggests that 40% of scirrhous tumors diagnosed on double-contrast studies are confined to the gastric fundus or body with sparing of the antrum (Fig. 25) *(65)*. Also, some lesions cause only minimal loss of distensibility and are recognized primarily by distortion of the normal surface pattern of the stomach, with thickened folds and mucosal nodularity or ulceration *(65)*. As a result, these lesions can be missed if the radiologist relies too heavily on gastric narrowing as the major criterion for diagnosing these tumors. It is important to be aware of the limitations of endoscopy in diagnosing scirrhous carcinomas. Because the tumor cells often are separated by sheets of fibrosis, endoscopic brushings and biopsies have a sensitivity of less than 50% in detecting these lesions *(65)*. Thus, repeat endoscopy, endoscopic ultrasound or even surgery may be required for some patients without a pre-operative histological diagnosis.

Although most cases of malignant linitis plastica are caused by primary scirrhous gastric carcinoma, metastatic breast cancer, and non-Hodgkin's lymphoma involving the stomach may occasionally produce identical findings on barium studies as a result of a dense infiltrate of metastatic tumor or lymphomatous tissue in the gastric wall *(67,68)*.

3.2.1.4. Carcinoma of the Cardia

The incidence of carcinoma of the cardia gradually has increased during the past 50 yr; these tumors currently constitute as many as 30–40% of all gastric cancers *(55)*. Carcinoma

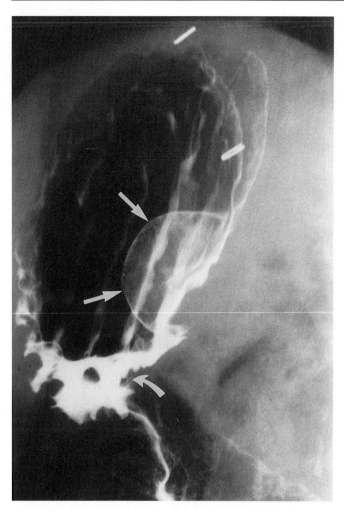

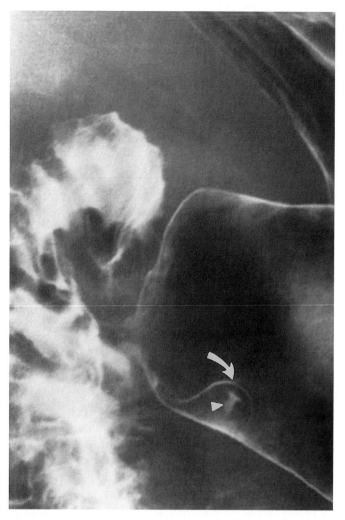

Fig. 21. Benign gastrointestinal stromal tumor (leiomyoma). Double-contrast view of the stomach shows a smooth submucosal mass (straight arrows) on the posterior wall of the gastric fundus. This patient had a partial gastrectomy and gastrojejunostomy (curved arrow) (Billroth II).

Fig. 22. Ectopic pancreatic rest. Double-contrast view of the stomach shows a small submucosal mass (curved arrow) on the greater curvature of the antrum near the pylorus. Note barium collecting in a central umbilication (arrowhead).

of the cardia has a marked predilection for men (7:1), and a small but significant percentage of patients are less than 40 yr of age (69). Affected individuals may have referred dysphagia to the upper chest or even the pharynx, so the gastric cardia and fundus should be carefully evaluated in all patients with dysphagia, regardless of its subjective localization.

Carcinoma of the cardia is notoriously difficult to diagnose on single-contrast barium studies because this area is inaccessible to manual palpation. With double-contrast technique, however, it is possible to evaluate the normal anatomic landmarks at the cardia for radiographic signs of malignancy. The normal cardia often can be recognized on double-contrast views by four or five stellate folds that radiate to a central point at the GEJ, also known as the cardiac rosette (70). Some tumors at the cardia may be recognized only by distortion or obliteration of these normal landmarks, with relatively subtle nodularity, mass effect, or ulceration in this region (Fig. 26) (69–71). Advanced carcinomas of the gastric cardia usually appear on barium studies as polypoid, ulcerated, or infiltrative lesions. Polypoid

tumors may be recognized as lobulated or fungating intraluminal masses, often containing irregular areas of ulceration. In contrast, infiltrative lesions may be manifested by thickened, nodular folds or decreased distensibility of the fundus as a result of tumor encasing the gastric wall.

Patients with carcinoma of the cardia usually have associated esophageal involvement by tumor, manifested by a polypoid mass, thickened folds, or irregular narrowing of the distal esophagus. Submucosal spread of tumor can also result in the development of secondary achalasia, with tapered, beak-like narrowing of the distal esophagus at or just above the GEJ (72). However, certain morphological features such as asymmetry, abrupt transitions, and mucosal nodularity or ulceration should suggest an underlying malignancy. Secondary achalasia should also be suspected when the narrowed segment extends proximally a considerable distance from the GEJ (72). In such cases, careful radiological evaluation of the fundus is essential to rule out an underlying carcinoma of the cardia as the cause of these findings.

Table 1
Japanese Endoscopy Society Classification
of Early Gastric Cancer

I. Protruded type	Elevated exophytic lesions protruding more than 5 mm
II. Superficial type	Flat spreading lesions
IIa. Elevated type	a. Elevated less than 5 mm
IIb. Flat type	b. Flat
IIc. Depressed type	c. Depressed but not ulcerated past the muscularis mucosae
III. Excavated type	Ulcerated through the muscularis mucosae

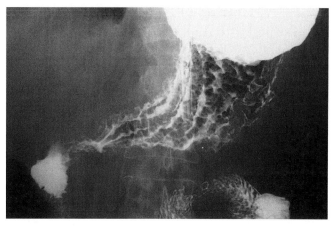

Fig. 24. Scirrhous carcinoma. Double-contrast view of the stomach shows a linitis plastic appearance with marked luminal narrowing, nodular folds, and an irregular contour in the gastric antrum and body owing to a primary scirrhous carcinoma of the stomach.

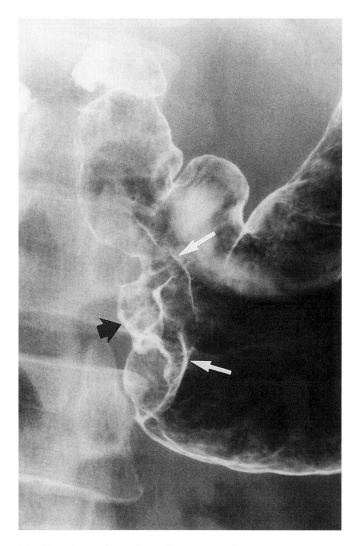

Fig. 23. Advanced gastric carcinoma. Double-contrast view of the stomach shows a polypoid mass etched in white (white arrows) with a large central area of ulceration (black arrow) on the greater curvature of the gastric antrum.

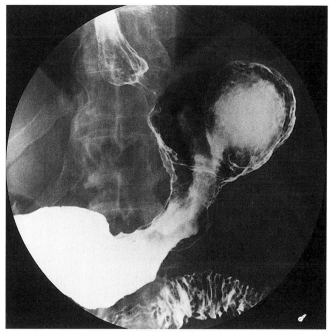

Fig. 25. Scirrhous carcinoma. Double-contrast view of the stomach shows irregular narrowing of the gastric body with sparing of the antrum and fundus in another patient with a primary scirrhous carcinoma of the stomach.

3.2.2. Gastric Lymphoma

The stomach is the most frequent site of GI involvement by non-Hodgkin's lymphoma *(73)*. Gastric lymphoma may be manifested on barium studies by a spectrum of findings, including thickened folds, ulcers, nodules, submucosal, or polypoid masses, bull's-eye lesions, and even a linitis plastica appearance *(68,73,74)*. When lymphoma involves the stomach on barium studies, it classically results in thickened folds without affecting gastric distensibility or pliability *(74)*. Occasionally, however, non-Hodgkin's lymphoma may produce a linitis plastica appearance indistinguishable from that of a primary scirrhous carcinoma or metastatic breast cancer involving the stomach *(68)*.

In recent years, an association has been recognized between *Helicobacter pylori* and gastric lymphoma. It has been shown that patients with chronic *H. pylori* gastritis gradually acquire lymphoid tissue in the gastric mucosa, also known as mucosa-associated lymphoid tissue (MALT). These monoclonal populations of B-cells may proliferate autonomously, resulting in the development of low-grade B-cell lymphomas, also known as MALT lymphomas (MALTOMAS), which have characteristic

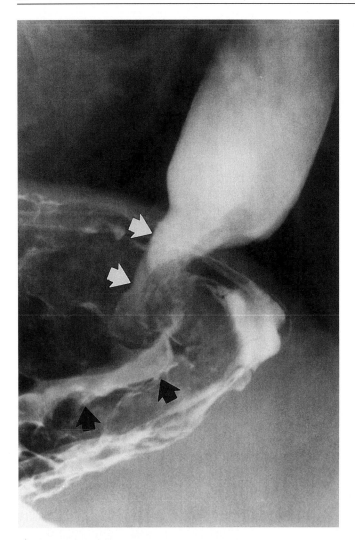

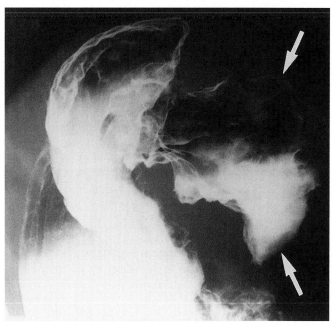

Fig. 28. Malignant gastrointestinal stromal tumor (leiomyosarcoma). Double-contrast view of the stomach shows a giant cavitated lesion containing a large extraluminal collection of barium (arrows). (Reproduced with permission from ref. *80*.)

Fig. 26. Carcinoma of the cardia. Double-contrast view of the gastric fundus shows how the normal anatomic landmarks at the cardia have been obliterated and replaced by an irregular area of ulceration (black arrows). Also note irregular narrowing (white arrows) of the distal esophagus owing to proximal extension of tumor.

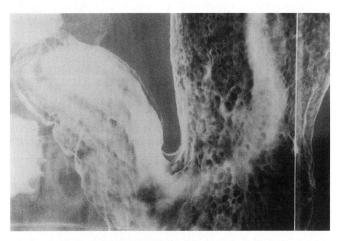

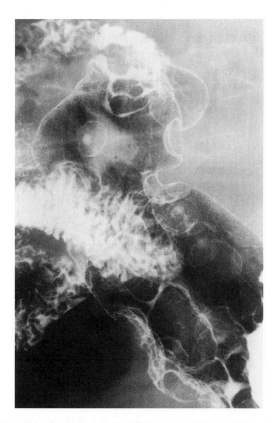

Fig. 27. Low-grade MALT lymphoma. Double-contrast view of the stomach shows confluent nodules of varying sizes in the gastric body owing to a low-grade, B-cell MALT lymphoma. (Reproduced with permission from ref. *78*.)

Fig. 29. Kaposi's sarcoma. Double-contrast view of the stomach shows multiple submucosal masses in the stomach. This patient had additional lesions in the small bowel.

pathological features *(75)*. Studies have shown that these low-grade MALT lymphomas may undergo complete regression in 70–80% of cases on treatment with antibiotics alone without need for surgery, radiation, or chemotherapy *(76,77)*. If untreated, however, MALTOMAS may undergo blastic transformation to more high-grade gastric lymphomas that have a much worse prognosis. Our goal therefore should be to detect these treatable MALTOMAS before they progress to more advanced lesions.

Gastric MALT lymphomas sometimes are manifested on double-contrast studies by multiple, rounded nodules of varying sizes that merge with one another, producing a confluent area of disease (Fig. 27) *(78)*. However, focal gastritis, intestinal metaplasia, or even enlarged areae gastricae caused by underlying infection with *H. pylori* may produce similar findings, so endoscopic biopsy specimens are required for a definitive diagnosis.

3.2.3. Malignant GISTs

Malignant GISTs (formerly known as leiomyosarcomas) are rare malignant neoplasms of the stomach. When they occur, 90% are located in the gastric fundus or body *(79)*. These tumors may be manifested on barium studies by a discrete submucosal mass that tends to be larger and more lobulated than benign GISTs. Not infrequently, these tumors may undergo extensive necrosis and liquefaction, resulting in the development of a giant, cavitated lesion on barium study and CT (Fig. 28) *(80,81)*. The differential diagnosis for these lesions includes cavitated metastases (particularly from malignant melanoma) and lymphoma.

3.2.4. Kaposi's Sarcoma

An aggressive form of Kaposi's sarcoma has been encountered with increasing frequency in patients with AIDS, primarily homosexuals. About 35% of AIDS patients are found to have Kaposi's sarcoma, and 50% with Kaposi's sarcoma are found to have GI involvement *(82)*. When the GI tract is involved, there is almost always associated involvement of the skin. Kaposi's sarcoma may be manifested on barium studies by one or more submucosal masses or centrally ulcerated bull's-eye lesions in the stomach (Fig. 29) *(83)*. The differential diagnosis for these bull's-eye lesions includes lymphoma and metastases, especially from malignant melanoma.

REFERENCES

1. Ming SC. Tumors of the esophagus and stomach. In: Ming SC, ed. Atlas of Tumor Pathology, Fascicle 7. Washington, DC: Armed Forces Institute of Pathology; 1973:16–23.
2. Sandvik AK, Aase S, Kveberg KH, Dalen A, Folvik M, Naess O. Papillomatosis of the esophagus. J Clin Gastroenterol 1996; 22:35–37.
3. Montesi A, Pesaresi A, Graziani L, Salmistraro D, Dini L, Beazi I. Small benign tumors of the esophagus: radiological diagnosis with double-contrast examination. Gastrointest Radiol 1983; 8:207–212.
4. Walker JH: Giant papilloma of the thoracic esophagus. AJR 1978; 131:519–520.
5. McDonald GB, Brand DL, Thorning DR. Multiple adenomatous neoplasms arising in columnar-lined (Barrett's) esophagus. Gastroenterology 1977; 72:1317–1321.
6. Levine MS, Caroline D, Thompson JJ, Kressel HY, Laufer I, Herlinger H. Adenocarcinoma of the esophagus: relationship to Barrett mucosa. Radiology 1984; 150:305–309.
7. Bleshman MH, Banner MP, Johnson RC, DeFord JW. The inflammatory esophagogastric polyp and fold. Radiology 1978; 128:589–593.
8. Staples DC, Knodell RG, Johnson LF. Inflammatory pseudotumor of the esophagus: a complication of gastroesophageal reflux disease. Gastrointest Endosc 1978; 24:175–176.
9. Styles RA, Gibb SP, Tarshis A, Silverman ML, Scholz FJ. Esophagogastric polyps: radiographic and endoscopic findings. Radiology 1985; 154:307–311.
10. Ghahremani GG, Rushovich AM. Glycogenic acanthosis of the esophagus: radiographic and pathologic features. Gastrointest Radiol 1984; 9:93–98.
11. Rose D, Furth EE, Rubesin SE: Glycogenic acanthosis. AJR 1995; 164:96.
12. Glick SN, Teplick SK, Goldstein J, Stead JA, Zitomer N. Glycogenic acanthosis of the esophagus. AJR 1982; 139:683–688.
13. Berliner L, Redmond P, Horowitz L, Ruoff M. Glycogen plaques (glycogenic acanthosis) of the esophagus. Radiology 1981; 141: 607–610.
14. Goldstein HM, Zornoza J, Hopens T. Intrinsic diseases of the adult esophagus: benign and malignant tumors. Semin Roentgenol 1981; 16:183–197.
15. Shaffer HA. Multiple leiomyomas of the esophagus. Radiology 1976; 118:29–34.
16. Levine MS. Benign tumors of the esophagus. In: Gore RM, Levine MS, eds. Textbook of Gastrointestinal Radiology, 2nd ed. Philadelphia: Saunders, 2000; 387–402.
17. Griff LC, Cooper J. Leiomyoma of the esophagus presenting as a mediastinal mass. AJR 1967; 101:472–481.
18. Gutman E. Posterior mediastinal calcification due to esophageal leiomyoma. Gastroenterology 1972; 63:665–666.
19. Tsuzuki T, Kakegawa T, Arimori M, Ueda M, Watanabe H. Giant leiomyoma of the esophagus and cardia weighing more than 1000 grams. Chest 1971; 60:396–399.
20. Megibow AJ, Balthazar EJ, Hulnick DH, Naidich DP, Bosniak MA. CT evaluation of gastrointestinal leiomyomas and leiomyosarcomas. AJR 1985; 144:727–731.
21. Avezzano EA, Fleischer DE, Merida MA, Anderson DL. Giant fibrovascular polyps of the esophagus. Am J Gastroenterol 1990; 85:299–302.
22. Watanabe H, Jass JR, Sobin LH. World Health Organization: Histological Typing of Oesophageal and Gastric Tumors, 2nd ed. Berlin: Springer-Verlag, 1990.
23. Levine MS, Buck JL, Pantongrag-Brown L, Buetow PC, Hallman JR, Sobin LH. Fibrovascular polyps of the esophagus: clinical, radiographic, and pathologic findings in 16 patients. AJR 1996; 166:781–787.
24. Cochet B, Hohl P, Sans M, Cox JN. Asphyxia caused by laryngeal impaction of an esophageal polyp. Arch Otolaryngol 1980; 106: 176–178.
25. Carter MM, Kulkarni MV. Giant fibrovascular polyp of the esophagus. Gastrointest Radiol 1984; 9:301–303.
26. Whitman GJ, Borkowski GP. Giant fibrovascular polyp of the esophagus: CT and MR findings. AJR 1989; 152:518–520.
27. Vithespongse P, Blank S. Ciliated epithelial esophageal cyst. Am J Gastroenterol 1971; 56:436–440.
28. Whitaker JA, Deffenbaugh LD, Cooke AR. Esophageal duplication cyst. Am J Gastroenterol 1980; 73:329–332.
29. Bondestam S, Salo JA, Salonen OL, Lamminen AE. Imaging of congenital esophageal cysts in adults. Gastrointest Radiol 1990; 15: 279–281.
30. Rafal RB, Markisz JA. Magnetic resonance imaging of an esophageal duplication cyst. Am J Gastroenterol 1991; 86:1809–1811.
31. Mannell A. Carcinoma of the esophagus. Curr Probl Surg 1982; 19:553–647.
32. Levine MS, Halvorsen RA. Esophageal carcinoma. In: Gore RM, Levine MS, eds. Textbook of Gastrointestinal Radiology, 2nd ed. Philadelphia: Saunders, 2000, pp. 403–433.
33. Koehler RE, Moss AA, Margulis AR: Early radiographic manifestations of carcinoma of the esophagus. Radiology 1976; 119;1–5.

34. Levine MS, Dillon EC, Saul SH, Laufer I. Early esophageal cancer. AJR 1986; 146:507–512.

35. Itai Y, Kogure T, Okuyama Y, Akiyama H. Superficial esophageal carcinoma: radiological findings in double-contrast studies. Radiology 1978; 126:597–601.

36. Lindell MM, Hill CA, Libshitz HI. Esophageal cancer: radiographic chest findings and their prognostic significance. AJR 1979; 133:461–465.

37. Gloyna RE, Zornoza J, Goldstein HM. Primary ulcerative carcinoma of the esophagus. AJR 1977; 129:599–600.

38. Yates CW, LeVine MA, Jensen KM. Varicoid carcinoma of the esophagus. Radiology 1977; 122:605–608.

39. Keen SJ, Dodd GD, Smith JL. Adenocarcinoma arising in Barrett's esophagus: pathologic and radiologic features. Mt Sinai J Med 1984; 51:442–450.

40. Hesketh PJ, Clapp RW, Doos WG, Spechler SJ. The increasing frequency of adenocarcinoma of the esophagus. Cancer 1989; 64:526–530.

41. Pera M, Cameron AJ, Trastek VF, Carpenter HA, Zinsmeister AR. Increasing incidence of adenocarcinoma of the esophagus and esophagogastric junction. Gastroenterology 1993; 104:510–513.

42. Agha FP, Keren DF. Spindle-cell squamous carcinoma of the esophagus: a tumor with biphasic morphology. AJR 1985; 145:541–545.

43. Rose HS, Balthazar EJ, Megibow AJ, Horowitz L, Laubenstein LJ. Alimentary tract involvement in Kaposi sarcoma: radiographic and endoscopic findings in 25 homosexual men. AJR 1982; 139:661–666.

44. Yoo CC, Levine MS, McLarney JK, Lowry MA. Primary malignant melanoma of the esophagus: radiographic findings in seven patients. Radiology 1998; 209:455–459.

45. Tateishi R, Taniguchi H, Wada A, Horai T, Taniguchi K. Argyrophil cells and melanocytes in esophageal mucosa. Arch Pathol Lab Med 1974; 98:87–89.

46. Gordon R, Laufer I, Kressel HY. Gastric polyps on routine double-contrast examination of the stomach. Radiology 1980; 134:27–29.

47. Cherukuri R, Levine MS, Furth EE, Rubesin SE, Laufer I. Giant hyperplastic polyps in the stomach: radiographic findings in seven patients. AJR 2000; 175:1445–1448.

48. Op den Orth JO, Dekker W. Gastric adenomas. Radiology 1981; 141:289–293.

49. Delikaris P, Golematis B, Missitzis G, Bang L, Nakopoulou L, Poulsen J. Smooth muscle neoplasms of the stomach. South Med J 1983; 76:440–442.

50. Crummy AB, Juhl JH. Calcified gastric leiomyoma. AJR 1962; 87:727–728.

51. Culver GJ, Toffolo RR. Criteria for roentgen diagnosis of submucosal gastric lipoma. Radiology 1964; 82:254–257.

52. Megibow AJ, Redmond PE, Bosniak MA, Horowitz L. Diagnosis of gastrointestinal lipomas by CT. AJR 1979; 133:743–745.

53. Kilman WJ, Berk RN. The spectrum of radiographic features of aberrant pancreatic rests involving the stomach. Radiology 1977; 123:291–296.

54. Fuchs CS, Mayer RJ. Gastric carcinoma. N Engl J Med 1995; 333:32–41.

55. Antonioli DA, Goldman H. Changes in the location and type of gastric adenocarcinoma. Cancer 1982; 50:775–781.

56. Green PH, O'Toole KM, Slonim D, Wang T, Weg A. Increasing incidence and excellent survival of patients with early gastric cancer: experience in a United States medical center. Am J Med 1988; 85:658–661.

57. Everett SM, Axon AT. Early gastric cancer in Europe. Gut 1997; 41:142–150.

58. White RM, Levine MS, Enterline HT, Laufer I. Early gastric cancer: recent experience. Radiology 1985; 155:25–27.

59. Murakami T. Pathomorphological diagnosis. In: Murakami T, ed. Early Gastric Cancer. Tokyo: University of Tokyo Press, 1971, pp. 53–55.

60. Gold RP, Green PH, O'Toole KM, Seaman WB. Early gastric cancer: radiographic experience. Radiology 1984; 152:283–290.

61. Koga M, Nakata H, Kiyonari H, Inakura M, Tanaka M. Roentgen features of the superficial depressed type of early gastric carcinoma. Radiology 1975; 115:289–292.

62. Levine MS, Creteur V, Kressel HY, Laufer I, Herlinger H. Benign gastric ulcers: diagnosis and follow-up with double-contrast radiography. Radiology 1987; 164:9–13.

63. Low VH, Levine MS, Rubesin SE, Laufer I, Herlinger H. Diagnosis of gastric carcinoma: sensitivity of double-contrast barium studies. AJR 1994; 162:329–334.

64. Thompson G, Somers S, Stevenson GW. Benign gastric ulcer: a reliable radiologic diagnosis? AJR 1983; 141:331–333.

65. Levine MS, Kong V, Rubesin SE, Laufer I, Herlinger H. Scirrhous carcinoma of the stomach: radiologic and endoscopic diagnosis. Radiology 1990; 175:151–154.

66. Balthazar EJ, Rosenberg H, Davidian MM. Scirrhous carcinoma of the pyloric channel and distal antrum. AJR 1980; 134:669–673.

67. Joffe N. Metastatic involvement of the stomach secondary to breast carcinoma. AJR 1975; 123:512–521.

68. Levine MS, Pantongrag-Brown L, Aguilera NS, Buck JL, Buetow PC. Non-Hodgkin lymphoma of the stomach: a cause of linitis plastica. Radiology 1996; 201:375–378.

69. Levine MS, Laufer I, Thompson JJ. Carcinoma of the gastric cardia in young people. AJR 1983; 140:69–72.

70. Herlinger H, Grossman R, Laufer I, Kressel HY, Ochs RH. The gastric cardia in double-contrast study: its dynamic image. AJR 1980; 135:21–29.

71. Freeny PC, Marks WM. Adenocarcinoma of the gastroesophageal junction: barium and CT examination. AJR 1982; 138:1077–1084.

72. Woodfield CA, Levine MS, Rubesin SE, Langlotz CP, Laufer I. Diagnosis of primary versus secondary achalasia: reassessment of clinical and radiographic criteria. AJR 2000; 175:727–731.

73. Levine MS, Rubesin SE, Pantongrag-Brown L, Buck JL, Herlinger H. Non-Hodgkin's lymphoma of the gastrointestinal tract: radiographic findings. AJR 1997; 168:165–172.

74. Menuck LS. Gastric lymphoma: a radiologic diagnosis. Gastrointest Radiol 1976; 1:157–161.

75. Wotherspoon AC, Ortiz-Hidalgo C, Falzon MR, Isaacson PG. Helicobacter pylori-associated gastritis and primary B-cell gastric lymphoma. Lancet 1991; 338:1175–1176.

76. Roggero E, Zucca E, Pinotti G, et al. Eradication of Helicobacter pylori infection in primary low-grade gastric lymphoma of mucosa-associated lymphoid tissue. Ann Intern Med 1995; 122:767–769.

77. Bayerdorffer E, Neubauer A, Rudolph B, et al. Regression of primary gastric lymphoma of mucosa-associated lymphoid tissue after cure of Helicobacter pylori infection. MALT Lymphoma Study Group. Lancet 1995; 345:1591–1594.

78. Yoo CC, Levine MS, Furth EE, et al. Gastric mucosa-associated lymphoid tissue lymphoma: radiographic findings in six patients. Radiology 1998; 208:239–243.

79. Bedikian AY, Khankhanian N, Valdivieso M, et al. Sarcoma of the stomach: clinicopathologic study of 43 cases. J Surg Oncol 1980; 13:121–127.

80. Levine MS, Megibow AJ. Other malignant tumors of the stomach and duodenum. In: Gore RM, Levine MS, eds. Textbook of Gastrointestinal Radiology, 2nd ed. Philadelphia: Saunders; 2000:627–657.

81. Scatarige JC, Fishman EK, Jones B, Cameron JL, Sanders RC, Siegelman SS. Gastric leiomyosarcoma: CT observations. J Comput Assist Tomogr 1985; 9:320–327.

82. Wall SD, Friedman SL, Margulis AR. Gastrointestinal Kaposi's sarcoma in AIDS: radiographic manifestations. J Clin Gastroenterol 1984; 6:165–171.

83. Falcone S, Murphy BJ, Weinfeld A. Gastric manifestations of AIDS: radiographic findings on upper gastrointestinal examination. Gastrointest Radiol 1991; 16:95–98.

84. Levine MS. Benign tumors. In: Levine MS, Radiology of the Esophagus. Philadelphia: Saunders; 1989:113–130.

85. Levine MS. Esophageal carcinoma. In: Radiology of the Esophagus. Philadelphia: Saunders; 1989:131–168.

86. Levine MS. Other malignant tumors. In: Radiology of the Esophagus. Philadelphia: Saunders; 1989:169–192.

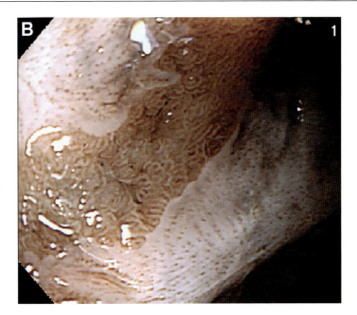

Color Plate 1. *Fig. 5B, Chapter 3:* In NBI, the broad-band white light used to illuminate the tissue is filtered into three narrow bands of light. The blue band in particular is used to image the surface pattern and blood vessels. (*See* complete caption and discussion on p. 26.)

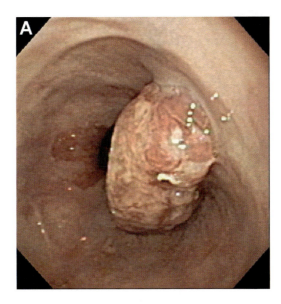

Color Plate 1. *Fig. 4A, Chapter 4:* A pedunculated cancer in a tongue of Barrett's esophagus. (*See* complete caption on p. 36 and discussion on p. 34.)

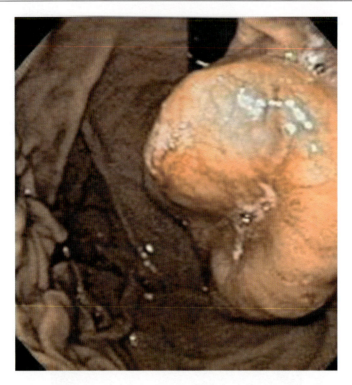

Color Plate 2. *Fig. 2, Chapter 13:* Gastric cardia MALT lymphoma. Exophytic, polypoid lesion with central ulceration in the cardia of the stomach. FNA cytology obtained during EUS revealed MALT lymphoma. (*See* complete caption on p. 143 and discussion on p. 142.)

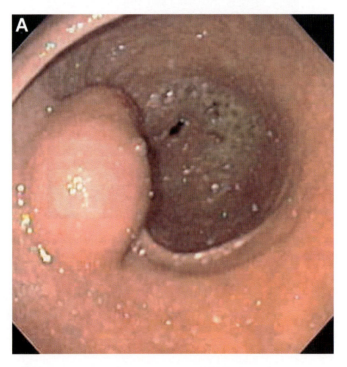

Color Plate 2. *Fig. 4A, Chapter 14:* Endoscopic image of a large gastric gastrointestinal stromal tumor (GIST) in the antrum appearing as a submucosal lesion with normal overlying mucosa. (*See* complete caption and discussion on p. 155.)

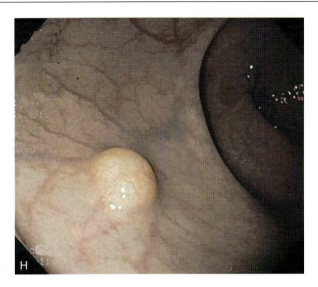

Color Plate 3. *Fig. 5H, Chapter 21:* Endoscopic view of a subepithelial lesion in the colon. (*See* complete caption on p. 246 and discussion on p. 244.)

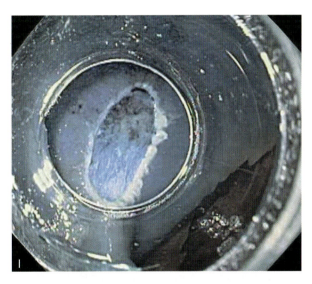

Color Plate 3. *Fig. 5I, Chapter 21:* Endoscopic view after cap-assisted EMR showing exposed submucosa and muscularis propria. Note the bluish discoloration of the colon from methylene blue stain. Histolopathologic examination revealed a carcinoid tumor. (*See* complete caption on p. 246 and discussion on p. 244.)

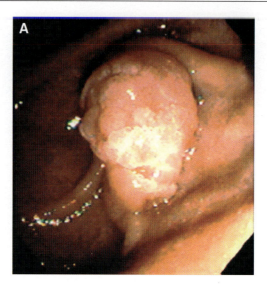

Color Plate 4. *Fig. 6A, Chapter 29:* Steps in snare ampullectomy: ampullary adenoma. (*See* complete caption on p. 340 and discussion on p. 342.)

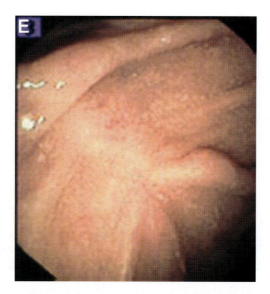

Color Plate 4. *Fig. 6E, Chapter 29:* Steps in snare ampullectomy: final result 3 mo later. (*See* complete caption on p. 340 and discussion on p. 342.)

8 Esophageal Cancer Therapy
Surgery, Radiation, and Chemotherapy

JOHN M. HOLLAND, MD AND CHRISTOPHER A. CANNING, MD

CONTENTS

1. BACKGROUND

Despite therapy, most patients diagnosed with esophageal cancer in 2004 will die from their disease. Surgery and radiation have been the historical treatments of choice for esophageal cancer. However, in an effort to improve outcome, combination therapies have emerged with concurrent chemoradiotherapy, neoadjuvant chemotherapy and chemoradiotherapy, and adjuvant chemotherapy and chemoradiotherapy. Strong proponents for specific individual therapeutic approaches exist, as does controversy because no optimal treatment plan for esophageal cancer has clearly emerged.

Therapy also continues to evolve with the development of new chemotherapeutic agents and chemotherapy combinations. Future work will hopefully reduce the morbidity of therapy and increase survival in patients treated with esophageal cancer.

2. INTRODUCTION

Esophageal cancer is a relatively uncommon cancer in the United States. Of the estimated 1,368,030 new cases of cancer that were diagnosed in the United States in 2004, only 14,250 of these were esophagus cancer. This represents only 1% of all cancers. Still esophagus cancer is a lethal disease with an estimated 13,300 deaths occurring in 2004 (1). Over the last century, various surgical, radiotherapeutic, and chemotherapeutic options have evolved to treat esophageal cancer for cure and relief of symptoms.

From: *Endoscopic Oncology: Gastrointestinal Endoscopy and Cancer Management*. Edited by: D. O. Faigel and M. L. Kochman © Humana Press, Totowa, NJ

3. SURGERY FOR ESOPHAGUS CANCER

3.1. HISTORICAL PERSPECTIVE

In 1871, Theodor Billroth pioneered surgical therapy for the cervical esophagus by performing experimental resections in dogs. He performed the first resection of the cervical esophagus on a human in 1872. The distal esophagus was first successfully resected in the early 1900s through an abdominal route.

The development of improved ventilatory support and positive pressure anesthesia made possible a transthoracic approach to resection of the intrathoracic esophagus. Patients undergoing this procedure in its early days had a very high mortality rate, most commonly from pneumothoraces. Franz Torek performed the first successful transthoracic esophageal excision in 1913. He excised a mid-esophageal carcinoma by a left thoracotomy. Torek had planned to perform an esophageal reconstruction but the patient refused. Instead, the cervical esophagostomy and gastrostomy were connected by an external rubber tube that allowed the patient to swallow liquids and semiliquid food. This 67-yr-old patient lived without recurrence for 13 yr.

Still, mortality from this transthoracic procedure continued to be very high for the next two decades, largely owing to sepsis caused by intrathoracic anastomotic failure. Surgical results began to improve after 1938 when multi-stage operations were abandoned in favor of single-stage procedures. Adams and Phemister performed a successful one-stage resection of a thoracic esophageal cancer with an intrathoracic esophagogastrostomy. Marshall in the United States and Oksawa in Japan also performed single stage transthoracic esophagectomies with reconstruction in the 1930s. With the improvement in preoperative and postoperative care, better anesthetic techniques,

Table 1
Comparison of Surgical Techniques for Resection
of Esophageal Cancer

Technique	Advantages	Disadvantages
Transhiatal esophagectomy	Avoids the morbidity of a thoracotomy, less pulmonary morbidity, extrathoracic anastamosis	Difficult to perform a full thoracic lymphadenectomy, poor visualization of the midthoracic dissection
Ivor Lewis (transthoracic) esophagectomy	Allows direct visualization of the thoracic esophagus and full lymphadenectomy	Toxicity of thoracotomy, greater pulmonary morbidity
Esophagectomy via left thoracotomy	Good exposure of lower esophagus	Same disadvantages as Ivor Lewis technique
Thoracoscopic esophagectomy	Less invasive, may be less morbid with quicker recovery	Unproven as an oncological surgery, lower morbidity is controversial
En-bloc esophagectomy	More comprehensive cancer surgery	Invasive, controversy regarding improved outcomes, increased morbidity

greater availability of antibiotics and increasing surgical experience, the success rate with transthoracic esophagectomies continued to improve.

In 1946, Ivor Lewis described a new approach for cancers of the mid-esophagus. His technique used both a right thoracotomy incision and a laparotomy incision to approach mid-esophageal tumors. This allowed direct visualization for lymph node dissection and complete resection and staging of the tumor. This operation, with some minor technical refinements, is still commonly employed today.

Another commonly utilized approach is the transhiatal esophagectomy. This technique was innovated by Denk in 1913 in animal experiments. It was first performed successfully in a human in 1936 by Turner. In this procedure, the incisions are made in the neck and abdomen *(2)*. The stomach is pulled up and anastomosed with the cervical esophagus. More recently, Orringer has become a major advocate for this technique and has reported his experience in 583 patients *(3)*. Historically, some surgeons have advocated more extensive surgical resections, such as the so-called "*en bloc*" resection. Recently, there has been interest in performing esophagectomy using less invasive techniques such as video assisted thoracoscopic surgery or laparoscopy.

3.2. SURGICAL TECHNIQUES

Many different surgical techniques have been developed to resect esophageal cancers. Several common surgical approaches are listed in Table 1. Radical or *en bloc* resection involves removal of the esophagus with 10 cm proximal and distal margins if possible as well as total resection of periesophageal tissues including the vascular and lymphatic supply. This includes removal of the pleura, part of the pericardium, the thoracic duct, and the azygous vein in the chest, and, for tumors of the distal esophagus, resection of the spleen, part of the stomach, and

diaphragm as well as the superior retroperitoneal lymph nodes. Skinner has long been a proponent of this surgical procedure *(4)*. He has argued that this procedure improves outcome. In a retrospective review of 128 patients, with 78 patients undergoing *en bloc* resection and 50 undergoing "standard" resection, Altorki and Skinner report a 4-yr survival of 34.5% and median survival of 27 mo after *en bloc* resection compared with 11% and 12 mo, respectively, after standard surgery ($p = 0.007$). Improved outcoume is felt to be related to the more extensive nodal resection seen in the *en bloc* surgery *(5)*. In a more recent review of *en bloc* resection for esophageal cancer performed on 111 patients, Altorki and Skinner report 5-yr survival rates of 78, 72, 0, 39, and 27% for stages I, IIA, IIB, III, and IV, respectively. Node-negative patients have a 5-yr survival of 75%. Lymph node-positive patients have a 5-yr survival of 26%. Overall local recurrence rate is only 8% *(6)*. Demonstrating the controversies that exist in surgery for esophagus cancer, others have argued that such aggressive surgery does not improve survival and may be associated with increased peri-operative morbidity and mortality, especially in less experience hands.

Transthoracic esophagectomy using a right-sided thoracotomy is often used for midthoracic esophageal tumors. The thoracic incision is usually made in the fifth intercostal space. The stomach is anastomosed either to the upper thoracic esophageal remnant or to the cervical esophagus. An abdominal incision may be used to mobilize the stomach (Fig. 1). The right-sided approach is preferred for mid to upper esophageal tumors to avoid the aortic arch.

The Ivor Lewis esophagectomy involves separate incisions for the right thoracotomy and laparotomy. Transthoracic resection using a left thoracotomy is utilized for tumors of the lower half of the esophagus or tumors of the gastroesophageal junction (GEJ) (Fig. 2) *(7)*. Transhiatal esophagectomy has been performed as an alternative procedure avoiding the morbidities seen with thoracotomy. This approach uses a combination of cervical and abdominal incisions to obtain access to and mobilize the esophagus and stomach (Fig. 3). The thoracic esophagus is freed via blunt manual dissection with the surgeon's hand coming up into the mediastinum from the abdominal incision. The stomach is pulled up into the chest with anastomosis in the neck. Extensive mediastinal exploration is not possible with the transhiatal approach, but there is less pulmonary morbidity because the procedure omits thoracotomy.

Recently, laparoscopic and thoracoscopic approaches have been utilized to resect malignant esophageal disease attempting to limit operative and peri-operative morbidity *(8)*. The use of a particular surgical technique depends on several factors including tumor location, the functional status of the patient (especially pulmonary function) and even individual surgeon expertise and preference. The use of thoracotomy clearly increases postoperative pulmonary morbidity. The best location for the surgical anastomosis is somewhat controversial. Some feel anastomosis within the chest is associated with increased morbidity/mortality from mediastinitis caused by anastomotic leak. Walther actually randomized 83 patients to undergo esophagogastric anastomosis either in the neck (41 patients) or in the chest (42 patients). These authors found

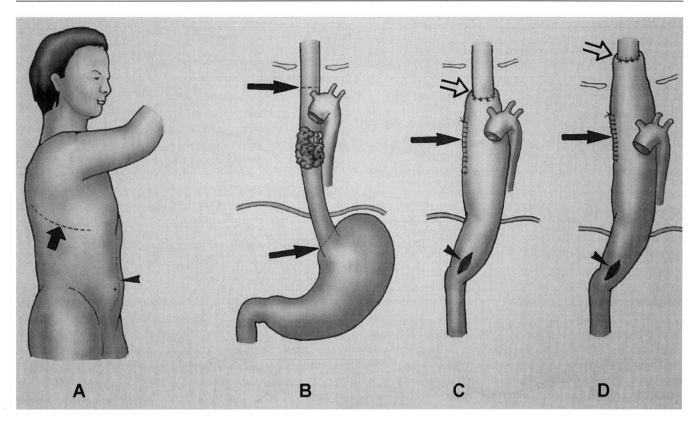

Fig. 1. Transthoracic esophagectomy through a right-sided thoracotomy. (Reproduced with permission from ref. 7.)

no difference in 5-yr survival (29 vs 30%) or anastomotic leak rate (1.8% overall). Furthermore, there was no difference in the anastomotic diameter on endoscopic follow-up or any difference in body weight development between the two anastomotic sites (9).

The specific type of surgery to resect esophageal carcinoma is controversial with strong proponents for particular techniques. Hulscher et al. (10) compared extended transthoracic resection with limited transhiatal resection for adenocarcinoma of the esophagus. This study randomized 220 patients with tumors of the mid-to-distal esophagus or adenocarcinoma of the gastric cardia. Transthoracic esophagectomy included an extended "en bloc" lymph node dissection. Surgery was performed at Dutch academic centers performing at least 50 esophagectomies per year. Transhiatal resection was associated with less morbidity and cost less than transthoracic resection. Patients undergoing transhiatal resection had fewer pulmonary complications (27 vs 57%) and chylous leakage (2 vs 10%). Transhiatal resection patients also had shorter durations of mechanical ventilation and shorter stays in the ICU. In-hospital mortality was 2% after transhiatal resection compared with 4% after extended transthoracic resection (p = 0.45). At a median follow-up of 4.7 yr, there is a trend, although not significant, toward improved overall 5-yr survival (39 vs 27%) in the group undergoing transthoracic esophagectomy. Transthoracic esophagectomy was associated with a 56% increased cost: $45,034.40 vs $28,901.70 for transhiatal surgery. The authors estimate a cost of $50,414.40 per "quality-adjusted life span" when using the extended transthoracic approach.

3.3. OUTCOMES AFTER SURGERY ALONE

Surgical resection of esophageal cancer is curative for patients with disease limited to the mucosa and submucosa without spread to regional lymph nodes. King reports a 5-yr survival rate of 86% after Ivor Lewis esophagogastrectomy for stage I disease (11). Unfortunately, such lesions are uncommon, accounting for only 7–10% of esophageal cancers (12). In the United States, patients are generally diagnosed with more advanced-stage disease. As stage increases, 5-yr survival rates fall after esophagectomy: 34% for stage II, 15% for stage III. In an early review of outcome following surgical resection of esophageal squamous cell carcinomas, Earlam finds a dismal 5-yr survival rate of only 10% with only 39 of 100 patients resectable and only 4 alive at 5 yr (13). These results may seem unduly pessimistic; still, even in academic centers with significant esophageal cancer surgery experience, most report overall 5-yr survival rates of only 22–39% (10,12).

3.4. ADJUVANT THERAPY FOR ESOPHAGUS CANCER

Given the relatively poor results using surgery alone to treat carcinoma of the esophagus, it is reasonable to consider combining other cancer modalities to try to improve outcome.

3.4.1. Adjuvant Radiation Alone for Esophagus Cancer: Pre-Operative Radiation

There have been five randomized trials evaluating the benefit of pre-operative radiation in resectable esophageal cancer (14–18). Most patients in these studies had squamous cell histology. Pre-operative radiation therapy was not shown to improve respectability. Gignoux did show a decrease in local

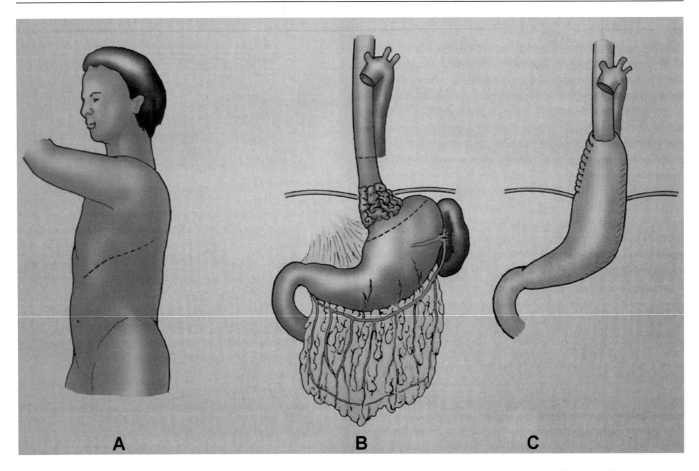

Fig. 2. Transthoracic esophagectomy through a left-sided thoracotomy. (Reproduced with permission from ref. 7.)

failure rate with the addition of 33 Gy pre-operative radiation: 67% after surgery alone vs 46% after combined therapy *(15)*. Nygaard reported an improvement in overall survival in patients receiving pre-operative radiation *(18)*. These results are tempered by the fact that this was a four-arm study: pre-operative chemotherapy, pre-operative radiation, pre-operative chemoradiation, or surgery alone. Three-year survival was significantly higher in the "pooled" groups receiving pre-operative radiotherapy with or without chemotherapy: 18 vs 5% ($p = 0.009$). In this series, 48 patients received pre-operative radiation alone and had a 20% survival rate at 3 yr. Still, this apparent benefit did not reach statistical significance for the pre-operative radiation alone arm. Arnott reported the results of a meta-analysis evaluating pre-operative radiotherapy in esophagus cancer from the Oesophageal Cancer Collaborative Group *(19)*. This analysis of five randomized trials included 1147 patients. With a median follow-up of 9 yr, hazard ratio analysis "suggests an overall reduction in the risk of death of 11% and an absolute survival benefit of 3% at 2 yr and 4% at 5 yr." This apparent benefit, though, did not reach statistical significance ($p = 0.062$). The authors, therefore, concluded that "there was no clear evidence that pre-operative radiotherapy improves the survival of patients with potentially resectable esophageal cancer." If such a benefit did exist, it would be "modest with an absolute improvement in survival of around 3–4%." The authors concluded:

"pre-operative radiotherapy cannot currently be routinely recommended outside of controlled clinical trials."

3.4.2. Adjuvant Radiation Alone for Esophagus Cancer: Postoperative Radiation

There have been two randomized trials evaluating postoperative radiation for esophagus cancer. Teniere reported the outcome of a French study of 221 patients with resected squamous cell carcinoma of the mid-to-distal esophagus *(20)*. Patients were randomized to undergo surgical resection followed by 45–55 Gy or surgery alone. Postoperative radiation did not improve survival: 5-yr survival was 19%. Locoregional failure was decreased after radiation (30–15%) but this benefit was only significant in lymph node negative patients (35 vs 10%). Fok and colleagues evaluated 130 patients with both squamous and adenocarcinoma histologies *(21)*. This study evaluated postoperative radiation in patients undergoing both curative and palliative resections. Postoperative radiotherapy was associated with increased complications of the intrathoracic stomach including four deaths from bleeding ulcers. The overall median survival was actually decreased in those patients receiving postoperative radiation: 8.7 vs 15.2 mo ($p = 0.02$). Radiotherapy did decrease intrathoracic recurrence with a particular benefit seen in patients with residual tumor having a decreased risk of dying from obstruction of the tracheobronchial tree (7 vs 33%, $p = 0.03$). The

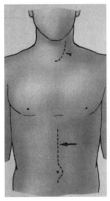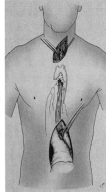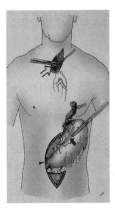

Fig. 3. Transhiatal esophagectomy. (Reproduced with permission from ref. 7.)

authors concluded that postoperative radiotherapy should be limited to those patients with residual mediastinal tumor after resection in an attempt to reduce recurrent disease obstructing the airway. Accordingly, postoperative radiation has generally been reserved for those patients left with positive surgical margins or gross residual tumor after resection.

3.4.3. Pre-Operative Chemotherapy

Three randomized studies give conflicting results regarding the benefit of pre-operative chemotherapy. Kelsen reported the results of a multi-institutional United States Intergroup trial involving 440 patients (22). Patients randomized to chemotherapy received three cycles of cisplatin and 5-FU before surgery followed by two more cycles after resection. With a median follow-up of 55.4 mo, there was no difference in survival: 16.1 mo after surgery alone vs 14.9 mo after surgery and peri-operative chemotherapy. Three-year survival rate was 26% after surgery alone vs 23% after chemotherapy plus surgery. The addition of chemotherapy did not improve resectability but it also did not increase operative morbidity or mortality. Chemotherapy did not affect locoregional or distant recurrence rates.

Kok has reported in abstract form the results of a phase III Dutch trial evaluating neoadjuvant cisplatin and etoposide in 160 operable squamous cell tumors (23). After two cycles of chemotherapy, tumor response was evaluated. Patients with a "major response" received two additional cycles of chemotherapy followed by transhiatal resection. Nonresponders proceeded directly to surgery. Those patients receiving pre-operative chemotherapy had improved median survival compared with patients undergoing surgery alone: 18.5 vs 11 mo ($p = 0.002$).

The largest randomized trial evaluating pre-operative chemotherapy for resectable esophagus cancer comes from the Medical Research Council Oesophageal Cancer Working Party (24). This study randomized 802 patients to surgery alone or two cycles of pre-operative cisplatin and 5-FU. Chemotherapy increased the percentage of complete resections (54 vs 60%, $p < 0.0001$) without increasing postoperative complications. Overall survival was improved with the addition of chemotherapy. Median survival increased from 13.3 to 16.8 mo; 2-yr survival rates were 43% after chemotherapy plus surgery compared with 34% after surgery alone. These three randomized trials are summarized in Table 2.

Table 2
Randomized Trials Evaluating Pre-Operative Chemotherapy for Esophageal Cancer

Variable	Kelson (22)	Kok (23)	MRC (35)
No. of patients	467	160	802
Histology	54% adeno	100% squamous	66% adeno
Chemotheraphy regimen	Cycles: three pre-op, two post-op, given every 4 wk	Cycles: two; two additional for responders	Two 40d cycles every 3 wk
Chemotherapy dose	Cisplatin: 100 mg/m²; 5-FU: 1000 mg/m² d	Cisplatin: 80 mg/m²; Etoposide: 100 mg iv/d 1 + 2; 200 mg po/d 3 + 5	Cisplatin: 80 mg/m²; 5-FU: 1000 mg/m² continuous inf × 4 d
Chemotherapy patients undergoing complete resection (%)	62%	More R0 resection in group receiving chemo	60%
Median survival with chemotherapy	14.9 mo	18.5 mo	16.8 mo
Survival benefit	None	7.5 mo	3.5 mo
Increased morbidity after chemotherapy	No	One toxic death	No

3.4.4. Postoperative Chemotherapy

There is little data regarding the use of postoperative chemotherapy alone for esophageal cancer. The Japan Clinical Oncology Group performed a multicenter randomized trial evaluating two cycles of adjuvant cisplatin and 5-FU after transthoracic esophagectomy with lymphadenectomy in 242 patients with squamous cell histology (25). Most patients (75%) received both full cycles of chemotherapy. Five-year disease-free survival was improved with the addition of chemotherapy: 55 vs 45% ($p = 0.037$). This benefit was most pronounced in the lymph node positive patients: 5-yr disease-free survival 52 vs 38% ($p = 0.041$). Overall survival after chemotherapy was 61% compared with 52% after surgery alone but this failed to reach statistical significance ($p = 0.13$).

3.4.5. Pre-Operative Chemoradiation

The concept of combining radiation with radiosensitizing chemotherapy before surgical resection now dates back over 20 yr. Leichman and colleagues at Wayne State University treated 21 patients with squamous cell carcinoma with two cycles of cisplatin and 5-FU combined with 30 Gy external beam radiation (26). Of these patients, 15 (71%) underwent resection and 7 of the 15 (47%) had no viable tumor in the resected specimen. Overall median survival was 18 mo; 24 mo in those with a complete pathological response. This approach was associated with a peri-operative mortality rate of 27%. Because of this work, several phase III studies have been completed with conflicting results making this treatment approach one of the most controversial in cancer care. Le Prise combined low-dose radiation (20 Gy) with two cycles of cisplatin and 5-FU and compared pre-operative chemoradiation with surgery alone for

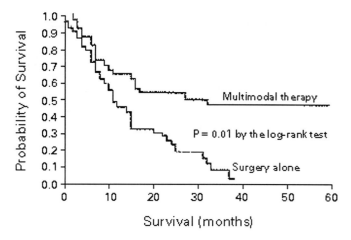

Fig. 4. Kaplan–Meier actuarial survival of patients with esophageal adenocarcinoma treated with pre-operative chemoradiation or surgery alone. (Reproduced with permission from ref. *29.*)

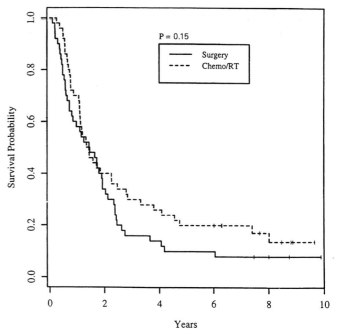

Fig. 5. Actuarial survival after pre-operative chemoradiation vs surgery alone for carcinoma of the esophagus. (Reproduced with permission from ref. *30.*)

86 patients with squamous cell histology *(27)*. Therapy was well tolerated with operative mortality of 8.5% after combined therapy and 7% after surgery alone. Unfortunately, long-term survival was also unaffected by the addition of neoadjuvant chemotherapy. Both groups had a 47% survival rate at 1 yr. Three-year survival was 19% in the multimodal group compared with 14% after surgery alone but this difference was not significant. Bosset reported another larger French trial of chemoradiation followed by surgery vs surgery alone for squamous cell tumors *(28)*. Most of these patients had early-stage (T1T2N0) disease. Radiation was delivered in an unusual split-course manner: two 1-wk courses of 3.7 Gy × 5 separated from each other by a 2-wk break, thereby delivering a total dose of 37 Gy over 4 wk. Cisplatin (80 mg/m^2) was administered 0–2 d before each round of radiation. Curative resection was more likely in the combined modality arm: 81 vs 69% ($p = 0.017$). A complete pathological response was seen in 26% with an additional 18% having a "major pathological response." Combined therapy was also associated with an increased postoperative mortality rate: 12.3 vs 3.6% ($p = 0.012$). With a median follow-up of 55 mo, the median survival is 18.6 mo for both treatment arms. There were fewer deaths from esophagus cancer in the combined arm (68 vs 86%, $p = 0.002$) but this benefit was lost owing to the increased postoperative mortality. The authors concluded: "Future efforts should aim to improve the efficacy of the treatment whereas reducing its toxicity."

A relatively small, single-institution trial from St. James' Hospital in Dublin, Ireland has had a significant impact on clinical practice, especially in the United States. Walsh and colleagues compared esophagectomy alone with pre-operative chemoradiation with 5-FU and cisplatin during 1–6 wk combined with 40 Gy external beam radiation delivered over 3 wk beginning with the first dose of chemotherapy *(29)*. This randomized trial included 113 patients with adenocarcinoma of the esophagus. Chemoradiation was well tolerated with a 13% rate of grade 3/4 toxicity and no increase in the frequency or grade of postoperative complications. Pre-operative chemoradiation resulted in a 25% complete pathological response rate

and a decrease in pathological lymph node positivity: 42 vs 82% after surgery alone ($p < 0.001$). Survival was improved in the multimodality arm with a median survival of 16 vs 11 mo after surgery alone ($p = 0.01$). Three-year survival was also improved in patients receiving pre-operative chemoradiation: 32 vs 6% ($p = 0.01$) (Fig. 4). A criticism of this study has been the poorer-than-expected survival seen after surgery alone.

Based on encouraging results of a pilot study, Urba et al. *(30)* designed a phase III trial comparing transhiatal esophagectomy alone with the same surgery after concurrent cisplatin, 5-FU and vinblastine chemotherapy combined with accelerated, hyperfractionated external beam irradiation (1.5 Gy BID to 45 Gy over 3 wk). One hundred patients were randomized: 25% had squamous histology, 75% had adenocarcinomas. With a median follow-up of 8.2 yr, there is no significant difference in median survival: 17.6 mo after surgery vs 16.9 mo after trimodality therapy. Three-year survival appears to favor the combined therapy arm: 30 vs 16% but this difference did not reach statistical significance ($p = 0.15$) (Fig. 5). Criticism of this study has focused on whether it had adequate patient numbers. The study was powered to detect "a relatively large increase in median survival from 1 to 2.2 yr."

These studies have failed to conclusively answer the question about the role of neoadjuvant chemoradiation for resectable esophagus cancer. The single positive study included only adenocarcinoma. A subsequent Intergroup trial comparing surgery alone vs pre-operative cisplatin and 5-FU combined with 50.4 Gy hoped to enroll 620 patients. Unfortunately, this study closed prematurely when only 75 patients had been enrolled in the first 2.5 yr, leaving the role of neoadjuvant chemoradiation unsettled *(31)*.

3.4.6. Postoperative Chemoradiation

There is little data on the use of combination chemotherapy together with radiation after resection of esophageal cancer. There exists the general perception that these patients are too frail after surgery to tolerate the morbidity of such aggressive adjuvant therapy.

Noting that "neither postoperative radiotherapy nor chemotherapy alone provide a survival benefit after curative esophagectomy for esophageal squamous cell carcinoma," Tachibana and colleagues devised a prospective randomized trial to compare postoperative chemotherapy with chemoradiotherapy (32). Patients were randomized to receive cisplatin and 5-FU chemotherapy alone or together with 50 Gy to the mediastinum after surgery. The 5-yr survival rates were 50% after chemoradiation vs 38% after chemotherapy alone but this was not significant ($p = 0.97$). Further, locoregional failure rate was not affected by mediastinal irradiation: 18 vs 17%. The authors concluded: "postoperative radiotherapy administered concurrently with chemotherapy does not provide a survival benefit compared with chemotherapy alone."

Although generally remembered as a gastric cancer study, MacDonald et al. (33) compared chemoradiotherapy after surgery with surgery alone for both adenocarcinoma of the stomach and the GEJ. In this study, 556 patients with resected adenocarcinomas of the stomach or GEJ were randomized to receive postoperative chemoradiation (5-FU and leucovorin and 45 Gy over 5 wk) or observation. Approximately 20% of the patients had tumors of the GEJ. Overall, the median survival was increased in those patients receiving adjuvant chemoradiation: 36 vs 27 mo($p = 0.005$). Three-year survival rates were also increased after chemoradiation: 50 vs 41% ($p = 0.005$). Local recurrence rates appeared to be less after chemoradiation as well (19 vs 29%) but because documentation only recorded the site of first relapse, statistical assessment was not felt reliable and potentially biased owing to a lack of complete reporting of sites of failure. Although these numbers apply to the entire set of 556 patients, most with gastric cancer, the authors "were unable to detect differences in the effects of treatment according to … location of the primary tumor." Therefore, it may be reasonable to apply this data accrued from approx 100 patients to the general management of resectable adenocarcinomas of the GEJ.

4. DEFINITIVE RADIATION ALONE FOR ESOPHAGUS CANCER

Radiation oncologists often complain that definitive radiation for esophageal cancer is limited only to the patients the surgeons do not want—either because the tumors are too locally advanced or the patients are felt too frail to tolerate surgery. Whether this is true or not, what is true is radiation therapy alone is rarely curative in the treatment of esophageal cancer. In his review of radiotherapy in the management of squamous cell carcinoma of the esophagus, the British surgeon Earlam reported a 1-yr survival rate of 18% and a 5-yr survival of 6% after radiation (34). Interestingly, Earlam was a strong proponent of an MRC trial comparing surgery alone

with radiotherapy alone. This trial closed early because it failed to enroll patients (35).

Radiotherapy alone has been used for early-stage esophageal cancer including patients medically unfit for surgery. Sykes reported on the use of "radical" radiation of 45–52.5 Gy in 15 or 16 fractions over 3 wk in 101 patients with tumors "no longer" than 5 cm. In this series of relatively favorable tumors, the median survival was 15 mo; 3-yr survival was 25%; 5-yr survival was 17% (36). Okawa reported an overall 9% 5-yr survival rate for 288 patients with squamous cell carcinomas treated with radiotherapy alone (37). Within this group, patients with tumors 5 cm long or less had a 17.7% 5-yr survival. Patients with stage I disease had a 20.2% 5-yr survival but this fell to 9.9% for patients with stage II disease. Hyden reviewed a less optimistic experience at the University of Southern California (38). Here, 46 patients with inoperable esophagus cancer were treated with a combination of external beam radiation and endoluminal brachytherapy. Even with this combination radiation therapy, the 5-yr actuarial survival for 28 patients with stages I or II disease was only 12%. Maingon and colleagues have used high-dose rate (HDR) brachytherapy alone or in combination with external beam radiotherapy to treat either primary or recurrent superficial esophageal cancers (39). This series included eleven patients without invasion of the basal membrane (Tis) and 14 patients with tumors involving the submucosa without spread into the muscle (T1). Overall survival was 24% for Tis patients and 20% for T1 disease. Those select patients treated with HDR brachytherapy alone had a survival rate of 43%. Complications included four patients with stenosis and one developing a fistula. Nemoto et al. (40) treated 78 select patients with superficial esophageal cancer using external beam radiotherapy alone. All patients had T1 biopsy-proven squamous cell carcinomas. Endoscopic ultrasound was used to confirm the depth of invasion in 34 patients. Patients undergoing endoscopic mucosal resection were excluded. Mean radiation dose was 65.5 Gy. Overall, the 5-yr survival was 45% with a local control rate of 66%. Late complications included esophageal stricture and radiation pneumonitis developing in two patients each.

4.1. ACCELERATED HYPERFRACTIONATED RADIOTHERAPY ALONE FOR ESOPHAGUS CANCER

During a fractionated course of radiotherapy, surviving cancer cells can continue to divide. In fact, radiobiologists and clinicians have observed tumor clonogens actually begin dividing at an increased rate during the course of radiotherapy. This "accelerated repopulation" can occur around the fourth week of standard once-a-day fractionated radiotherapy (41). In an attempt to deal with this tumor regrowth, clinicians have attempted to shorten or accelerate the course of radiation. Decreasing total treatment time by using hyperfractionated (more than one treatment per day) radiation may improve results when using radiation alone for esophagus cancer (42). Institut Gustave Roussy has used this approach delivering 65 Gy over 4–5 wk (median treatment duration 32 d) for 88 patients ineligible for surgery. Of these patients, 64% did receive neoadjuvant chemotherapy before radiation. Three-year

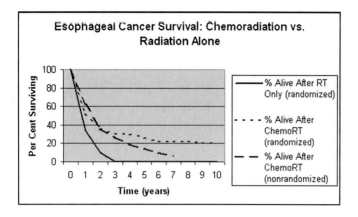

Fig. 6. Long-term survival benefit of chemoradiation over radiation alone for esophagus cancer (log-rank test of randomized patients *p* < 0.001). Survival curve created using data from ref. *47*.

cause-specific survival was 40, 22, and 6% for T1, T2, and T3 tumors, respectively. Grade 3 esophagitis was seen in 16%. Late toxicity included esophageal stenosis in 8% and pulmonary fibrosis in 9% *(43)*. Shi tested accelerated fractionation in a small randomized study *(44)*. Eighty-five patients with esophageal cancer were randomized to receive conventional once-a-day fractionation with 1.8 Gy delivered 5 d a week to a total dose of 68.4 Gy over 7–8 wk or late course-accelerated hyperfractionated (LCAF) radiation. This group received the same once-a-day radiation as the conventional group for the first two-thirds of the treatment (41.4 Gy/23 fractions over 4–5 wk). Accelerated hyperfractionation was then delivered as a boost to a reduced volume with 1.5 Gy fractions twice-a-day to 27 Gy. This delivered a total dose of 68.4 Gy as in the conventional arm but the LCAF therapy was completed sooner: 6.4 vs 7–8 wk. These authors found that the LCAF group achieved greater local control at 5 yr: 55 vs 21% (*p* = 0.003). Five-year actuarial survival was 34% after LCAF compared with 15% after conventional fractionation, but this difference did not reach statistical significance. Acute morbidity was "increased but acceptable." Late toxicity at 5 yr after LCAF was "not increased."

4.2. CONCURRENT CHEMOTHERAPY AND RADIATION

Radiation alone has been compared with radiation with concurrent cisplatin and 5-FU chemotherapy in an Intergroup study enrolling 129 patients with carcinoma of the thoracic esophagus *(45)*. Eighty-eight percent had squamous histology, 12% had adenocarcinomas. The total radiation dose was 64 Gy for radiation alone and decreased to 50 Gy when delivered with concurrent chemotherapy. The chemotherapy consisted of cisplatin at 75 mg/m^2 on the first day with continuous infusion 5-FU at 1 gm/m^2 on days 1–4. Two cycles of chemotherapy were delivered with thoracic radiation during weeks 1 and 5. Two additional cycles were then delivered after radiation during weeks 8 and 11. Concurrent chemoradiation was morbid with 44% "severe" and 20% "life-threatening" side effects. Hematological side effects were the most common: 33% severe, 13% life-threatening. Mucositis of the oral cavity, pharynx, and esophagus was severe in 26%, life-threatening in 13%.

Although chemoradiation was difficult, it also improved survival. Median survival was increased from 8.9 mo after radiation alone to 12.5 mo after chemoradiation. Two-year survival was 38% after chemoradiation vs 10% after radiation alone. By 5 yr, 27% were alive after chemoradiation compared with no survivors after radiation alone *(46)*. An additional group of 69 patients were treated with chemoradiation confirming these improved results with a median survival of 17.2 months and a 3-yr survival rate of 30%. Further long-term analysis found there were no further deaths from esophageal cancer in the chemoradiation arm after 8 yr with a 22% rate surviving "at least 8 yr" *(47)* (Fig. 6). Locoregional failure was decreased after concurrent chemoradiation but was still common. After completing chemoradiation, 27% had persistent disease and 16% suffered local failure as the first site of recurrence (43% total). At 12 mo, 22% of the chemoradiation patients had developed distant metastases compared with 38% after radiation alone. Late toxicity after chemoradiation was infrequent with no significant increase seen over radiation alone.

4.2.1. Concurrent Chemoradiation: Radiation Dose Escalation

Seeking to improve outcome in the use of chemoradiation for esophagus cancer and recognizing the greater than 40% local failure rate seen with its prior chemoradiation regimen, the Radiation Therapy Oncology Group (RTOG) developed two studies evaluating the benefit of increasing local therapy by increasing the radiation dose. RTOG 9207 was a phase I/II trial adding endoluminal brachytherapy to boost the site of the tumor in addition to the 50 Gy external beam dose used in the prior trial. Here, patients could receive boost with either HDR brachytherapy with three fractions of 5 Gy each or low-dose rate brachytherapy with a single boost fraction of 20 Gy. This study enrolled 49 patients (92% squamous, 6% adenocarcinomas). With a median follow-up of 29 mo, 3-yr survival was 29% but toxicity was felt to be unacceptably high with 6% "life-threatening" strictures and 12% fistulas. The authors concluded with the following advice: "use caution in employing esophageal brachytherapy when used in conjunction with chemotherapy" *(48)*. Finding that brachytherapy as a boost was associated with unacceptable morbidity, RTOG next tried to dose-escalate radiation by increasing external beam therapy. RTOG 9405 randomized patients to receive either: 50.4 Gy with 1.8 Gy daily fractions or 64.8 Gy with 1.8 Gy fractions. This phase III trial hoped to enroll 298 patients. However, the RTOG Data Monitoring Committee performed an interim analysis after enrollment of 230 patients (77% of the target number) and found "the survival associated with the assigned higher total dose (64.8 Gy) arm was worse than the control (50.4 Gy) arm" *(49)*. Two-year survival in the higher dose arm was 31 vs 40% after the standard dose. The decrease in survival was attributed to 11 treatment-related deaths in the high-dose arm compared with only two such deaths in the standard-dose arm. Interestingly, 7 of these 11 deaths occurred in patients receiving 50.4 Gy or less, and, therefore could not be attributed to the increased dose of radiation. Still, with these results RTOG was left to conclude "standard dose for patients receiving concurrent cisplatin/5-FU is 5040 cGy."

4.2.2. Concurrent Chemoradiation: New Chemotherapy Combinations

Current phase II studies combining radiation with concurrent chemotherapy tend to focus more on modification of the chemotherapeutic component rather than radiation. RTOG E-0113 adds paclitaxel to cisplatin and 5-FU. Ilson and colleagues have combined cisplatin with the topoisomerase I inhibitor irinotecan together with concurrent radiotherapy for locally advanced esophageal cancer *(50)*.

4.3. CHEMORADIATION VS CHEMORADIATION PLUS SURGERY FOR LOCALLY ADVANCED ESOPHAGEAL
4.3.1. Cancer

The best therapy for locally advanced esophageal cancer is far from established. Two recent European phase III trials question the value of adding surgical resection after chemoradiation for esophagus cancer. Bedenne reported the results of the French trial FFCD 9102 which evaluated induction chemoradiation with 5-FU and cisplatin combined with protracted (46 Gy over 4.5 wk) or split-course (3 Gy × 5 on days 1–5 and 22–26 for a total dose of 30 Gy) *(51)*. Patients experiencing at least a partial response were then randomized to receive either surgical resection or more chemoradiation with three cycles of 5-FU and cisplatin with radiation (protracted 20 Gy or split-course 15 Gy). This study enrolled 455 patients to receive the induction chemotherapy but only 259 (57%) were randomized. Two-year survival rate was 34% after surgery vs 40% after chemoradiation ($p = 0.56$). Median survival was 17.7 mo after surgery compared with 19.3 mo after chemoradiation. The 3-mo death rate was higher after surgery (9 vs 1% [$p = 0.002$]) but the patients with chemoradiation alone had a significantly greater likelihood of ultimately needing stent placement or dilatation for recurrent dysphagia. Interestingly, patients receiving continuous course radiotherapy needed less palliative intervention than those patients receiving the split-course radiotherapy.

At ASCO 2003, Stahl reported a similar German phase III study with induction chemoradiation (three cycles of 5-FU/leucovorin/etoposide/cisplatin followed by concurrent cisplatin/etoposide plus 40 Gy) *(52)*. A total of 177 patients with squamous histology were then randomized to receive either surgery via transthoracic esophagectomy with two-field lymphadenectomy or more chemoradiation with cisplatin/etoposide and radiation to doses ">60 Gy." Treatment related mortality was 10% after surgery vs 3.5% after chemoradiation. There was a "strong trend" toward improved local control after surgery. First site of tumor progression was observed locally in 64% after surgery compared with 81% after chemoradiation alone ($p = 0.08$). Still, there was no difference in median or 3-yr survival rate: 16 mo, 28% after surgery vs 15 mo, 20% after chemoradiation alone (log rank $p = 0.22$). Nonresponders to induction chemoradiation appeared to benefit from "complete tumor resection" with a 3-yr survival of 35% compared with 11% for nonresponders continuing with more chemoradiation. These two European studies strongly question the benefit of adding surgery to chemoradiation for esophagus cancer.

5. CARCINOMA OF THE CERVICAL ESOPHAGUS

Carcinoma of the cervical esophagus presents distinct problems in management. The cervical esophagus begins below the cricopharyngeus muscle (just below the level of the cricoid cartilage) at about 15 cm and extends down to the thoracic inlet at approx 20 cm measured from the upper incisors. These tumors are almost always squamous cell tumors and are often difficult to distinguish from primary tumors that originate in the hypopharynx. In fact, the narrow cricopharyngeus muscle is all that separates the postcricoid area of the hypopharynx from the cervical esophagus.

Surgical resection of cervical esophagus cancer is extensive. Most patients require total laryngoesophagectomy. Paratracheal lymphadenopathy is common and together with radial tumor growth, surgery often needs to include thyroidectomy and bilateral paratracheal lymph node dissection. Alimentary reconstruction may require gastric transposition or interposition of bowel. Overall, results of therapy are disappointing. Kakegawa reported outcome after surgical resection of 64 patients with cervical esophagus cancer *(53)*. In this series, most patients underwent "visceral replacement" using the stomach. Twelve patients underwent cervical esophagectomy with 33% peri-operative mortality and a 5-yr survival rate of 16.7%. Most patients (81%) were resected with total esophagectomy and fared better with a 5.8% operative mortality and a 5-yr survival rate of 30%. Therefore, these authors recommended total esophagectomy with stomach replacement for cervical esophagus cancer. Peracchia et al. at the University of Padua have resected 169 patients with cervical esophagus cancer *(54)*. Resection was complete in 85% and with palliative intent in 15%. Most patients (61%) underwent laryngopharyngo-total esophagectomy. Digestive tract reconstruction was with pharyngo-gastrostomy in 85 patients and pharyngo-colostomy in 16 patients. Operative mortality was 13–18%. Overall 5-yr actuarial survival, excluding operative mortality, was 15.8%.

Radiotherapy alone has also been used to treat carcinoma of the cervical esophagus. Mendenhall reported the University of Florida experience treating 34 patients *(55)*. With a minimum follow-up of 2 yr, only 26% of these patients maintained local control. Five-year survival was only 14%.

Concurrent chemoradiation has also been used for cervical esophagus cancer. Iop and colleagues reported a small series of 23 patients treated with concurrent cisplatin, 5-FU and radiation using a combination of external beam radiotherapy and endoluminal brachytherapy to a mean dose of 60 Gy *(56)*. With a short median follow-up of 14 mo, the actuarial 4-yr survival was estimated to be 30.4%. Locoregional failure as the first site of failure was also 30.4%. There were no toxic deaths; acute and late toxicity were "moderate." Two long-term survivors did develop stenosis requiring dilatation.

6. PALLIATIVE THERAPY FOR ESOPHAGUS CANCER: SURGERY AND RADIATION

Recognizing that all esophagus cancer patients are not good candidates for curative therapy, surgery still has a long-established history for providing effective palliation of dysphagia with either bypass surgery or esophagectomy. Mannel performed bypass surgery on 124 patients with unresectable esophagus cancer *(57)*. Peri-operative mortality was 11% and was increased in patients undergoing colonic bypass and patients with "large tumor load." Of those surviving surgery, 89% could eat a "normal, unrestricted" diet on discharge and 82% of survivors had complete and durable dysphagia relief. The most common complication was sepsis due to anastomotic leakage in the neck. Median survival after surgery was only 5 mo. Segalin et al. *(58)* reviewed their experience of surgery for palliation of advanced esophageal cancer. Resection was performed in 156 patients. Successful palliation was achieved in 78%: 41% were able to eat an unrestricted diet (scored as excellent) and 37% were able to eat a normal diet with occasional dysphagia (scored as good). In-hospital mortality was 9.6% with a median survival of 7.8 mo. Evaluating an additional 49 patients treated with bypass surgery, excellent or good palliation was achieved in 71% of operative survivors. In-hospital mortality was high at 20.2% with a median survival of only 6.2 mo.

Surgery, therefore, can provide effective palliation to relieve dysphagia but at the cost of significant peri-operative mortality and morbidity in a patient population with a very limited expected length of survival.

Radiation alone or in combination with chemotherapy has also been used for palliation of advanced esophageal cancer. Rosenberg has described the use of palliative radiation to relieve both dysphagia and pain in up to 80% *(59)*. Wara reviewed the University of California, San Francisco experience of radiation alone for 169 patients with squamous cell carcinoma of the esophagus *(60)*. In this group of patients, 66% achieved "significant relief" of dysphagia for 2 mo or longer. Median length of survival was 7 mo. Similar palliative response rates were seen for tumors of the upper, middle, and lower esophagus. Coia evaluated swallowing function in 120 patients receiving concurrent chemoradiation *(61)*. He found an improvement in dysphagia occurring by a median of 2 wk in 88%. There was no difference in dysphagia relief between patients with squamous cell or adenocarcinoma histologies. Patients with distal third tumors had both earlier and greater frequency of initial dysphagia relief than patients with tumors of the upper two-thirds of the esophagus: 95 vs 79%. In patients with advanced disease treated with palliative intent, 91% had an initial improvement in swallowing and 67% had dysphagia relief until death.

Endoluminal brachytherapy can also be useful in palliation especially in recurrent tumors. Sharma has used HDR Iridium-192 brachytherapy in 58 patients with advanced or recurrent esophageal carcinoma *(62)*. Improvement in swallowing was seen in 48% with median "dysphagia-free survival" of 10 mo. This benefit was at the expense of a 30% complication rate including strictures in 15%, ulceration in 10% and tracheoesophageal fistulas in 5%. Sur and colleagues have also used HDR brachytherapy as sole palliative therapy in 232 patients with inoperable advanced esophageal tumors. Patients received either 18 Gy in three fractions or 16 Gy in two fractions. The length of dysphagia-free survival for the entire group was 7.1

Table 3
Chemotherapeutic Agents Used for Esophageal Cancer: Response Rates and Mechanisms of Action

Agent	Response rate (%)	Mechanism of action
Bleomycin	15	Antibiotic
Mitomycin	35	Antibiotic
Methotrexate	13	Antimetabolite
5-FU	15–18	Antimetabolite
Cisplatin	19	DNA crosslink formation
Carboplatin	5	DNA crosslink formation
Paclitaxel	15–32	Prevents microtubule depolymerization
Docetaxel	33	Prevents microtubule depolymerization
Inrinotecan	15	Topoisomerase I inhibitor
Vinorelbine	6–20	Prevents microtubule assembly
Vindesine	22	Prevents microtubule assembly

mo with an overall survival of 7.9 mo. There was no significant outcome difference (dysphagia relief or complication rate) between the two fractionation regimens *(63)*. Using patient interviews, Stoller evaluated palliative outcome in a series of 82 patients and compared radiation alone (65%) with esophagectomy with reconstruction (35%). Level of palliation was based on scores for swallowing ability, sleep, leisure activity, and pain control in this nonrandomized study *(64)*. The authors found no significant differences between surgery or radiation in ability to provide palliation.

Clearly, surgery and radiation remain viable options for palliation in esophageal cancer. Still, over the last 20 yr, there has been rapid development of other palliative tools beyond the scope of this chapter including esophageal stents, Nd-Yag thermal ablation laser and photodynamic therapy.

7. CHEMOTHERAPY FOR ESOPHAGEAL CANCER

The use of chemotherapy combined with surgery and/or radiation for locoregional disease has been discussed. Still, as many as 50% of patients with esophagus cancer will present with metastatic disease. Further, most patients treated with curative intent will ultimately develop locoregionally recurrent or metastatic disease.

Most single agents of chemotherapy have response rates of 15–25% against esophagus cancer (Table 3) *(65)*. The use of chemotherapy in this population is palliative with most patients receiving therapy living less than 1 yr. Any hoped for benefit from therapy, therefore, must be weighed against the potential morbidity of side effects in these patients with limited life spans. Certainly patients with good performance status and limited weight loss are the best candidates for further therapy. Combination chemotherapy generally has higher response rates but may have greater toxicity. In a randomized phase II trial, the combination of cisplatin plus continuous infusion 5-FU was compared with cisplatin alone *(66)*. Ninety-two patients were randomized to receive cisplatin 100 mg/m^2 plus continuous infusion 5-FU 1000 mg/m^2 on days 1–5 or cisplatin alone with cycles

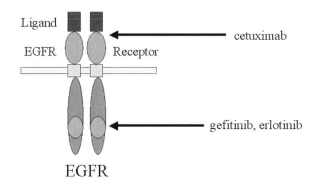

Fig. 7. Targeted therapy against the epidermal growth factor receptor.

repeated every 3 wk. Response rate was 35% in the combination arm with a 33-wk median survival compared with 19% and 28 wk, respectively, in the cisplatin alone arm. Still, these differences did not reach statistical significance. Toxicity, however, was greater in the combination arm with grade 4 hematological morbidity predominating. There were 16% treatment-related deaths in the combination arm compared with none in the cisplatin-only arm. The authors concluded "no standard chemotherapy can be recommended."

Petrasch and colleagues evaluated the combination of cisplatin with the taxane paclitaxel in a small phase II study of 20 patients (67). Patients received paclitaxel 90 mg/m^2 over 3 h followed by cisplatin 50 mg/m^2 with cycles of chemotherapy repeated every 2 wk. The overall response rate was 40% including 15% complete responders. Hematological morbidity was limited to 10% grade 3 neutropenia. Only 5% developed grade 4 neurotoxicity. Relief of dysphagia and/or significant weight gain occurred in 70%.

Ilson has studied the combination of cisplatin with irinotecan (68). Thirty-five patients with both adenocarcinoma (66%) and squamous cell (34%) cancers received weekly cisplatin 30 mg/m^2 and irinotecan 65 mg/m^2 for 4 wk followed by a 2 wk "rest." This therapy was "recycled every 6 wk." Major objective responses were seen in 57% with 6% complete responders. Response rates were similar for both adenocarcinomas (52%) and squamous tumors (66%). Median duration of response was 4.2 mo with a 14.6 mo median actuarial survival. Most impressively, of 20 patients with assessable dysphagia at baseline, 90% noted improvement or resolution with therapy. Toxicity was mild with 9% grade 4 neutropenia and 11% grade 3 diarrhea. There were no treatment-related deaths.

8. FUTURE DIRECTIONS

Clearly, given the current state of therapy for esophagus cancer, there is much room for improvement both in increasing survival and decreasing morbidity of therapy. Future directions in surgery may include the greater use of laparoscopic or thoracoscopic surgery. Perhaps, radiation dose can safely be escalated using newer treatment planning approaches such as intensity-modulated radiation therapy. The radioprotectant amifostine may prove useful in decreasing the morbidity of esophagitis and radiation pneumonitis in increasingly aggressive combination chemoradiation (69).

Inhibition of cyclooxygenase isoform 2, an enzyme involved in the conversion of arachidonic acid to prostaglandins involved in carcinogenesis, may have a role in the prevention and treatment of esophageal cancer (70,71).

Targeted therapy is also being investigated and may prove to play an important role in esophagus cancer therapy (72). The antibody cetuximab targets the extracellular component of the epidermal growth factor receptor. Other agents including gefitinib (iressa) and erlotinib (tarceva) target the intracellular component of the epidermal growth factor receptor by competing with adenosine triphosphate for binding with the catalytic domain of the tyrosine kinase enzyme (Fig. 7). Bevacizumab (avastin), a recombinant antibody to vascular epidermal growth factor, which inhibits tumor angiogenesis, also may play a future role in therapy for esophageal cancer.

REFERENCES

1. Jemal A, Tiwari RC, Murray T, et al. Cancer statistics, 2004. CA Cancer J Clin 2004; 54:8–29.
2. Townsend C. Sabiston Textbook of Surgery. Vol. 16th edition. Philadelphia: WB Saunders Company, 2001.
3. Whyte RI, Orringer MB. Surgery for Carcinoma of the Esophagus: The Case for Transhiatal Esophagectomy. Semin Radiat Oncol 1994; 4:146–156.
4. Skinner DB. En bloc resection for neoplasms of the esophagus and cardia. J Thorac Cardiovasc Surg 1983; 85:59–71.
5. Altorki NK, Girardi L, Skinner DB. En bloc esophagectomy improves survival for stage III esophageal cancer. J Thorac Cardiovasc Surg 1997; 114:948–955; discussion 955–956.
6. Altorki N, Skinner D. Should en bloc esophagectomy be the standard of care for esophageal carcinoma? Ann Surg 2001; 234:581–587.
7. Kim SH, Shim YM, Kim K, Yang PS, Kim TS. Esophageal Resection: Indications, Techniques, and Radiologic Assessment. Radiographics 2001; 21:1119–1140.
8. Nguyen NT, Roberts P, Follette DM, Rivers R, Wolfe BM. Thoracoscopic and laparoscopic esophagectomy for benign and malignant disease: lessons learned from 46 consecutive procedures. J Am Coll Surg 2003; 197:902–913.
9. Walther B, Johansson J, Johnsson F, Von Holstein CS, Zilling T. Cervical or thoracic anastomosis after esophageal resection and gastric tube reconstruction: a prospective randomized trial comparing sutured neck anastomosis with stapled intrathoracic anastomosis. Ann Surg 2003; 238:803–812; discussion 812–814.
10. Hulscher JB, van Sandick JW, de Boer AG, et al. Extended transthoracic resection compared with limited transhiatal resection for adenocarcinoma of the esophagus. N Engl J Med 2002; 347:1662–1669.
11. King RM, Pairolero PC, Trastek VF, Payne WS, Bernatz PE. Ivor Lewis esophagogastrectomy for carcinoma of the esophagus: early and late functional results. Ann Thorac Surg 1987; 44:119–122.
12. Orringer MB. Transthoracic versus transhiatal esophagectomy: what difference does it make? Ann Thorac Surg 1987; 44:116–118.
13. Earlam R, Cunha-Melo JR. Oesophageal squamous cell carcinoma: I. A critical review of surgery. Br J Surg 1980; 67:381–390.
14. Launois B, Delarue D, Campion JP, Kerbaol M. Preoperative radiotherapy for carcinoma of the esophagus. Surg Gynecol Obstet 1981; 153:690–692.
15. Gignoux M, Roussel A, Paillot B, et al. The value of preoperative radiotherapy in esophageal cancer: results of a study by the EORTC. Recent Results Cancer Res 1988; 110:1–13.
16. Wang M, Gu XZ, Yin WB, Huang GJ, Wang LJ, Zhang DW. Randomized clinical trial on the combination of preoperative irradiation and surgery in the treatment of esophageal carcinoma: report on 206 patients. Int J Radiat Oncol Biol Phys 1989; 16:325–327.
17. Arnott SJ, Duncan W, Kerr GR, et al. Low dose preoperative radiotherapy for carcinoma of the oesophagus: results of a randomized clinical trial. Radiother Oncol 1992; 24:108–113.

18 Nygaard K, Hagen S, Hansen HS, et al. Pre-operative radiotherapy prolongs survival in operable esophageal carcinoma: a randomized, multicenter study of pre-operative radiotherapy and chemotherapy. The second Scandinavian trial in esophageal cancer. World J Surg 1992; 16:1104–1109; discussion 1110.

19 Arnott SJ, Duncan W, Gignoux M, et al. Preoperative radiotherapy in esophageal carcinoma: a meta-analysis using individual patient data (Oesophageal Cancer Collaborative Group). Int J Radiat Oncol Biol Phys 1998; 41:579–583.

20 Teniere P, Hay JM, Fingerhut A, Fagniez PL. Postoperative radiation therapy does not increase survival after curative resection for squamous cell carcinoma of the middle and lower esophagus as shown by a multicenter controlled trial. French University Association for Surgical Research. Surg Gynecol Obstet 1991; 173:123–130.

21 Fok M, Sham JS, Choy D, Cheng SW, Wong J. Postoperative radiotherapy for carcinoma of the esophagus: a prospective, randomized controlled study. Surgery 1993; 113:138–147.

22 Kelsen DP, Ginsberg R, Pajak TF, et al. Chemotherapy followed by surgery compared with surgery alone for localized esophageal cancer. N Engl J Med 1998; 339:1979–1984.

23 Kok TC LJ, Siersema PD, Overhagen HV, Tilanus HW. Neoadjuvant Chemotherapy in Operable Esophageal Squamous Cell Cancer: Final Report of a Phase III Multicenter Randomized Controlled Trial (Meeting Abstract). Proc Am Soc Clin Oncol 1997; 16:277 (abtr 984).

24 Bancewicz J CP, Smith DB, Donnelly RJ, Fayers PM, Weeden S et al. Surgical Resection With or Without Preoperative Chemotherapy in Oesophageal Cancer: A Randomised Controlled Trial. The Lancet 2002; 359:1727–1733.

25 Ando N, Iizuka T, Ide H, et al. Surgery plus chemotherapy compared with surgery alone for localized squamous cell carcinoma of the thoracic esophagus: a Japan Clinical Oncology Group Study— JCOG9204. J Clin Oncol 2003; 21:4592–4596.

26 Leichman L, Steiger Z, Seydel HG, et al. Preoperative chemotherapy and radiation therapy for patients with cancer of the esophagus: a potentially curative approach. J Clin Oncol 1984; 2:75–79.

27 Le Prise E, Etienne PL, Meunier B, et al. A randomized study of chemotherapy, radiation therapy, and surgery versus surgery for localized squamous cell carcinoma of the esophagus. Cancer 1994; 73:1779–1784.

28 Bosset JF, Gignoux M, Triboulet JP, et al. Chemoradiotherapy followed by surgery compared with surgery alone in squamous-cell cancer of the esophagus. N Engl J Med 1997; 337:161–167.

29 Walsh TN, Noonan N, Hollywood D, Kelly A, Keeling N, Hennessy TP. A comparison of multimodal therapy and surgery for esophageal adenocarcinoma. N Engl J Med 1996; 335:462–467.

30 Urba SG, Orringer MB, Turrisi A, Iannettoni M, Forastiere A, Strawderman M. Randomized trial of preoperative chemoradiation versus surgery alone in patients with locoregional esophageal carcinoma. J Clin Oncol 2001; 19:305–313.

31 Enzinger PC, Mayer RJ. Esophageal cancer. N Engl J Med 2003; 349:2241–2252.

32 Tachibana M, Yoshimura H, Kinugasa S, et al. Postoperative chemotherapy vs chemoradiotherapy for thoracic esophageal cancer: a prospective randomized clinical trial. Eur J Surg Oncol 2003; 29:580–587.

33 Macdonald JS, Smalley SR, Benedetti J, et al. Chemoradiotherapy after surgery compared with surgery alone for adenocarcinoma of the stomach or gastroesophageal junction. N Engl J Med 2001; 345:725–730.

34 Earlam R, Cunha-Melo JR. Oesophogeal squamous cell carcinoms: II. A critical view of radiotherapy. Br J Surg 1980; 67:457–461.

35 Earlam R. An MRC prospective randomised trial of radiotherapy versus surgery for operable squamous cell carcinoma of the oesophagus. Ann R Coll Surg Engl 1991; 73:8–12.

36 Sykes AJ, Burt PA, Slevin NJ, Stout R, Marrs JE. Radical radiotherapy for carcinoma of the oesophagus: an effective alternative to surgery. Radiother Oncol 1998; 48:15–21.

37 Okawa T, Kita M, Tanaka M, Ikeda M. Results of radiotherapy for inoperable locally advanced esophageal cancer. Int J Radiat Oncol Biol Phys 1989; 17:49–54.

38 Hyden EC, Langholz B, Tilden T, et al. External beam and intraluminal radiotherapy in the treatment of carcinoma of the esophagus. J Thorac Cardiovasc Surg 1988; 96:237–241.

39 Maingon P, d'Hombres A, Truc G, et al. High dose rate brachytherapy for superficial cancer of the esophagus. Int J Radiat Oncol Biol Phys 2000; 46:71–76.

40 Nemoto K, Matsumoto Y, Yamakawa M, et al. Treatment of superficial esophageal cancer by external radiation therapy alone: results of a multi-institutional experience. Int J Radiat Oncol Biol Phys 2000; 46:921–925.

41 Hall E. Time, Dose, and Fractionation in Radiotherapy. Radiobiology for the Radiologist, Fourth Edition. Philadelphia: JB Lippincott Company, 1994:219–221.

42 Nishimura Y, Ono K, Tsutsui K, et al. Esophageal cancer treated with radiotherapy: impact of total treatment time and fractionation. Int J Radiat Oncol Biol Phys 1994; 30:1099–1105.

43 Girinsky T, Auperin A, Marsiglia H, et al. Accelerated fractionation in esophageal cancers: a multivariate analysis on 88 patients. Int J Radiat Oncol Biol Phys 1997; 38:1013–1018.

44 Shi XH, Yao W, Liu T. Late course accelerated fractionation in radiotherapy of esophageal carcinoma. Radiother Oncol 1999; 51:21–26.

45 Herskovic A, Martz K, al-Sarraf M, et al. Combined chemotherapy and radiotherapy compared with radiotherapy alone in patients with cancer of the esophagus. N Engl J Med 1992; 326:1593–1598.

46 al-Sarraf M, Martz K, Herskovic A, et al. Progress report of combined chemoradiotherapy versus radiotherapy alone in patients with esophageal cancer: an intergroup study. J Clin Oncol 1997; 15:277–284.

47 Cooper JS, Guo MD, Herskovic A, et al. Chemoradiotherapy of locally advanced esophageal cancer: long-term follow-up of a prospective randomized trial (RTOG 85-01). Radiation Therapy Oncology Group. Jama 1999; 281:1623–1627.

48 Gaspar LE, Winter K, Kocha WI, Coia LR, Herskovic A, Graham M. A phase I/II study of external beam radiation, brachytherapy, and concurrent chemotherapy for patients with localized carcinoma of the esophagus (Radiation Therapy Oncology Group Study 9207): final report. Cancer 2000; 88:988–995.

49 Minsky BD, Pajak TF, Ginsberg RJ, et al. INT 0123 (Radiation Therapy Oncology Group 94-05) phase III trial of combined-modality therapy for esophageal cancer: high-dose versus standard-dose radiation therapy. J Clin Oncol 2002; 20:1167–1174.

50 Ilson DH, Bains M, Kelsen DP, et al. Phase I trial of escalating-dose irinotecan given weekly with cisplatin and concurrent radiotherapy in locally advanced esophageal cancer. J Clin Oncol 2003; 21:2926–2932.

51 Bedenne L MP, Bouche O, Triboulet JP, Conroy T, Pezet D. Randomized Phase III Trial in Locally Advanced Esophageal Cancer: Radiochemotherapy Followed by Surgery versus Radiochemotherapy Alone (FFCD 9102). Proc Am Soc Clin Oncol 2002; 21:130a (abstr 519).

52 Stahl M WH, Walz MK, Seeber S, Klump B, Budach W et al. Randomized Phase III Trial in Locally Advanced Squamous Cell Carcinoma (SCC) of the Esophagus: Chemoradiation with and without Surgery. Proc Am Soc Clin Oncol 2003; 22:250 (abstr 1001).

53 Kakegawa T, Yamana H, Ando N. Analysis of surgical treatment for carcinoma situated in the cervical esophagus. Surgery 1985; 97:150–157.

54 Peracchia A, Bardini R, Ruol A, et al. Surgical management of carcinoma of the hypopharynx and cervical esophagus. Hepato-gastroenterology 1990; 37:371–375.

55 Mendenhall WM, Parsons JT, Vogel SB, Cassisi NJ, Million RR. Carcinoma of the cervical esophagus treated with radiation therapy. Laryngoscope 1988; 98:769–771.

56 Iop A SM, Fongione S, Buffoli A, Terrosu C, Cedolini R. Radiochemotherapy in the Management of Locally Advanced Carcinoma of the Cervical Esophagus. Proc Am Soc Clin Oncol 2003; 22:330 (abstr 1324).

57. Mannell A, Becker PJ, Nissenbaum M. Bypass surgery for unresectable oesophageal cancer: early and late results in 124 cases. Br J Surg 1988; 75:283–286.

58. Segalin A, Little AG, Ruol A, et al. Surgical and endoscopic palliation of esophageal carcinoma. Ann Thorac Surg 1989; 48:267–271.

59. Rosenberg JC, Franklin R, Steiger Z. Squamous cell carcinoma of the thoracic esophagus: an interdisciplinary approach. Curr Probl Cancer 1981; 5:1–52.

60. Wara WM, Mauch PM, Thomas AN, Phillips TL. Palliation for carcinoma of the esophagus. Radiology 1976; 121:717–720.

61. Coia LR, Soffen EM, Schultheiss TE, Martin EE, Hanks GE. Swallowing function in patients with esophageal cancer treated with concurrent radiation and chemotherapy. Cancer 1993; 71: 281–286.

62. Sharma V, Mahantshetty U, Dinshaw KA, Deshpande R, Sharma S. Palliation of advanced/recurrent esophageal carcinoma with high-dose-rate brachytherapy. Int J Radiat Oncol Biol Phys 2002; 52:310–315.

63. Sur RK, Levin CV, Donde B, Sharma V, Miszczyk L, Nag S. Prospective randomized trial of HDR brachytherapy as a sole modality in palliation of advanced esophageal carcinoma—an International Atomic Energy Agency study. Int J Radiat Oncol Biol Phys 2002; 53:127–133.

64. Stoller JL, Brumwell ML. Palliation after operation and after radiotherapy for cancer of the esophagus. Can J Surg 1984; 27: 491–495.

65. Fidias P. Chemotherapy for Advanced Esophageal Cancer. In: UpToDate, Rose, BD (ed), UpToDate, Wellesley, MA, 2003.

66. Bleiberg H, Conroy T, Paillot B, et al. Randomised phase II study of cisplatin and 5-fluorouracil (5-FU) versus cisplatin alone in advanced squamous cell oesophageal cancer. Eur J Cancer 1997; 33:1216–1220.

67. Petrasch S, Welt A, Reinacher A, Graeven U, Konig M, Schmiegel W. Chemotherapy with cisplatin and paclitaxel in patients with locally advanced, recurrent or metastatic oesophageal cancer. Br J Cancer 1998; 78:511–514.

68. Ilson DH, Saltz L, Enzinger P, et al. Phase II trial of weekly irinotecan plus cisplatin in advanced esophageal cancer. J Clin Oncol 1999; 17:3270–3275.

69. Jatoi A. Aggressive multimodality therapy for patients with locally advanced esophageal cancer: is there a role for amifostine? Semin Oncol 2003; 30:72–75.

70. Liao Z, Milas L, Komaki R, Stevens C, Cox JD. Combination of a COX-2 inhibitor with radiotherapy or radiochemotherapy in the treatment of thoracic cancer. Am J Clin Oncol 2003; 26: S85–S91.

71. Buskens CJ, Ristimaki A, Offerhaus GJ, Richel DJ, van Lanschot JJ. Role of cyclooxygenase-2 in the development and treatment of oesophageal adenocarcinoma. Scand J Gastroenterol Suppl 2003:87–93.

72. Ilson DH, Minsky B. Irinotecan in esophageal cancer. Oncology (Huntingt) 2003; 17:32–36.

STOMACH AND SMALL BOWEL

II

9 Premalignant Lesions of the Stomach

Omid A. Shaye, MD and Andrew Ippoliti, MD

Contents

1. BACKGROUND

Dysplasia is the precursor lesion for the development of carcinoma throughout the gastrointestinal tract. Certain conditions, which may lead to the occurrence of dysplasia, are labeled precursor conditions. The most readily identified such condition is Barrett's esophagus. All esophageal adenocarcinoma follows the sequence of intestinalized Barrett's epithelium progressing to dysplasia and subsequently to adenocarcinoma with relatively measurable frequencies. Gastric dysplasia, however, is usually found in the setting of chronic atrophic gastritis. Unlike the Barrett's lesion, there are no gross endoscopic features or a demarcated anatomic location. Furthermore, patients with Barrett's esophagus are at about the same risk for progression to cancer irrespective of ethnicity, environment, and socioeconomic status. However, these are all important factors contributing to gastric cancer risk in patients with atrophic gastritis. Finally, the symptoms of gastroesophageal reflux characterize the population at risk for Barrett's, but there are no symptoms attributable to the development of chronic atrophic gastritis (CAG). This chapter reviews the premalignant gastric lesions and their management.

2. THE GASTRITIS–CANCER SEQUENCE

Based on epidemiological and pathological information, Pelayo Correa proposed a model of gastric carcinogenesis known as Correa's cascade *(1)*. He originally described the sequence as starting with chronic gastritis, which evolved to atrophy and intestinal metaplasia (IM). The metaplastic epithelium, as in Barrett's, can become dysplastic and these cells can lead to invasive malignancy. The discovery of the pathogenic role of *Helicobacter pylori* places it at the site of initiation of

From: *Endoscopic Oncology: Gastrointestinal Endoscopy and Cancer Management.* Edited by: D. O. Faigel and M. L. Kochman © Humana Press, Totowa, NJ

the sequence. In other words, *H. pylori* infection results in the chronic active gastritis that starts the process.

This model is a very useful way to approach the gastric cancer process. But the progression is not invariable. For example, chronic active gastritis may lead to duodenal ulcer, not gastric cancer. Diet, sanitary conditions, and genetics play a major role in gastric cancer development. Their impact is most likely related to the development of atrophic gastritis as well as further steps along the way. Duodenal ulcer disease arises in patients with *H. pylori* chronic active gastritis without atrophy, and a history of duodenal ulcer reduces the risk of gastric cancer. Not all atrophic gastritis is a result of *H. pylori*. The gastric body predominant, type A or autoimmune, gastritis is associated with pernicious anemia and has a risk of gastric carcinoma.

Gastric cancers are subtyped as intestinal or diffuse. The Correa model fits the intestinal type with precursor conditions of atrophic gastritis and IM. *H. pylori* infection is more frequent in patients with the intestinal type than in the general population with an odds ratio (OR) of 2.49 *(2)*. The diffuse type lacks precursor conditions, atrophic gastritis and IM are absent, but the OR for *H. pylori* infection vs the general population is 2.58, similar to the intestinal type *(2)*.

The next sections review aspects of gastritis, IM, and dysplasia as they relate to gastric cancer. But it is important to recall that these are not all inclusive in the paradigm of gastric cancer pathogenesis.

3. GASTRITIS

Probably no term in gastroenterology is so widely misused as gastritis. As an endoscopic finding it may be used to indicate redness of the mucosa, or whiteness, mucosal lesions, erosions or red dots, and the state of the stomach when yellow fluid is present. In this chapter, gastritis refers to the histological state,

Table 1
Gastritis Classification

Types	Etiology	Pathology	Acid secretion	Associated conditions
Antral	H. pylori	Chronic active inflammation of antrum with intestinal metaplasia	Increased	Duodenal ulcer
Pangastritis	H. pylori	Chronic active inflammation of antrum and body, no intestinal metaplasia	Normal	None
Multifocal atrophic gastritis	H. pylori and environmental or genetic factors	Atrophy with intestinal metaplasia in antrum and body	Decreased	Gastric ulcer or cancer
Atrophic gastritis of body	Autoimmune	Body atrophy and intestinal metaplasia, none in antrum	Absent	Pernicious anemia, gastric cancer

specifically chronic active or atrophic. The types, their features, location, and associated diseases are summarized in Table 1.

As noted earlier, the types that do not lead to atrophy may be associated with increased gastric acid secretion and duodenal ulcer. Mild IM may be present in the antrum. Consequently, the finding of IM on a gastric biopsy from the antrum is not clinically significant as regards cancer risk. H. pylori is the cause of the antral chronic active gastritis related to duodenal ulcer and, also, the pangastritis in which metaplasia is absent and acid secretion is normal. These subjects have no disease associations and are asymptomatic.

The two forms of atrophic gastritis are the conditions potentially associated with gastric cancer. Multifocal atrophic gastritis predominates in patients with intestinal-type gastric cancer. It involves the antrum and body and there are multiple foci of IM. The finding is especially common on the lesser curve near the angularis. H. pylori is an important causative factor but there are likely to be other significant cofactors such as diet and genetics. Gastric acid secretion is reduced and both gastric ulcer and gastric cancer may develop.

Body or corpus-predominant atrophic gastritis, which spares the antrum, is autoimmune in origin and is associated with antibodies to parietal cells and intrinsic factor. This results in pernicious anemia. The IM is marked. There is achlorhydria leading to hypergastrinemia. There is an association with Hashimoto's thyroiditis, insulin-dependent diabetes, and Addison's disease. There is an increased risk of cancer, 1.5–3 times the general population, but this is less than the sixfold risk of multifocal atrophic gastritis (3).

The finding of multifocal atrophic gastritis suggests that the subject may be at risk for pernicious anemia and/or gastric cancer. Thus, it is a clinically relevant finding. To best diagnose the condition, biopsies should be taken from the antrum, incisura angularis, and body (4). There is great interobserver variability among pathologists for the diagnosis of atrophic gastritis. Atrophy includes architectural distortion, loss of oxyntic glands, which are replaced by metaplastic pyloric glands (pseudopyloric metaplasia), and fibrosis. Multiple teams of

expert pathologists have been convened to create diagnostic criteria for the histopathological diagnosis. The original Sydney classification was published in 1991, updated in 1994, and there have been additional working groups since then. Thus, an accurate diagnosis requires appropriate gastric sampling and an experienced gastrointestinal pathologist.

4. DYSPLASIA

Gastric dysplasia is most often found in indistinguishable sites. In other words, the dysplastic mucosa is endoscopically no different from the surrounding mucosa. Dysplasia, manifest as an adenomatous polyp, is uncommon in the stomach. In a study of 1900 cases of early gastric cancer from Japan, 95% arose in an epithelial change within atrophic gastritis and only 3% within an adenomatous polyp (5). Most gastric polyps are non-neoplastic, the most common are hyperplastic or fundic gland. Gastric adenomas represent about 8–10% of polyps in North American series (5). These adenomas are more often flat than polypoid or sessile and arise in the setting of multifocal atrophic gastritis. Dysplasia can be found on the surface of non-neoplastic polyps, but this is rare. It is reported in about 1% of hyperplastic or fundic gland polyps. An exception are those patients with familial adenomatous polyposis (FAP). About one-fourth of fundic gland polyps in FAP can be dysplastic (5).

The prevalence of gastric dysplasia in Western countries ranges between 0.5 and 3.75% with higher rates in patients with pernicious anemia or postgastric resection, 4–40% (6). As elsewhere in the gut, dysplasia is graded as low or high. The importance of follow-up of patients with dysplasia is highlighted by the fact that 60% of cancers found after the diagnosis of dysplasia are early (6). About 15% of cases of low grade progress to high grade, and carcinoma can be diagnosed with an average follow-up of 10–30 mo. Progression from high-grade dysplasia to cancer is nearly universal, 80–85%. The diagnosis of adenocarcinoma follows the discovery of high-grade dysplasia by several weeks up to 39 mo (6). In fact, in a series of studies reviewed by Meining et al., gastric carcinoma was diagnosed in 75% of patients with high-grade dysplasia

Table 2
Helicobacter pylori **and Gastric Cancer**

Animal model—Mongolian gerbil demonstrating gastric
   carcinogensis in chronically infected animals
Increased odds ratio for gastric cancer in *H. pylori* infected subjects
   especially if cagA-positive
Development of precancerous conditions, atrophy, and intestinal
   metaplasia, after *H. pylori* infection
Regression of those lesions, to some degree, after *H. pylori* eradication

within a mean of 8 mo *(7)*. The authors indicated that the explanation for this result is likely a misdiagnosis of high-grade dysplasia rather than invasive carcinoma. In summary, the issue of dysplasia in chronic gastritis has some parallels to dysplasia in the setting of ulcerative colitis. In both cases sampling error and pathologists agreement are critical.

5. *HELICOBACTER PYLORI*

In 1994, the World Health Organization classified *H. pylori* as a human carcinogen. It is beyond the scope of this chapter to review the relevant evidence to support this finding. The evidence is summarized in Table 2. The principle issue to review here is the effect of *H. pylori* eradication on gastritis and gastric cancer risk. Because there is a long latency between the onset of *H. pylori* infection and the development of gastric cancer, prospective studies measuring the effect of eradication on development of cancer require decades of follow-up. Uemura et al. *(8)* found that there were no cancers in 253 patients treated successfully for *H. pylori* after 7.8 yr of follow-up as compared with 36 cancers in 971 patients with persistent infection *(8)*. Wong and associates studied 1630 healthy carriers of *H. pylori* after a 2-wk course of omeprazole, amoxicillin and clavulanate potassium (augmentin), and metronidazole or placebo. There was no difference found between treatment groups; 7 cancers developed in the treated group and 11 in the placebo group. However, in the subgroup without precancerous lesions at baseline endoscopy, treatment seemed to be protective. Six patients without gastric atrophy, IM, or dysplasia developed cancer. All six were in the placebo group *(9)*.

Recent studies have used surrogate end points of gastritis resolution as a sign of efficacy of *H. pylori* eradication. Sung et al. reported the effect of eradication on gastric histology after 1 yr. The degree of inflammation in both corpus and antrum decreased in the treated and the placebo groups, but there was less IM in the treated group. Neither group demonstrated a reduction in gastric atrophy *(10)*. A similar study from Mexico failed to show much change in gastric histology with eradication of *H. pylori* after 1 yr *(11)*.

A 5-yr follow-up of the patients described by Lauwers *(6)* has been reported by Lichtenstein et al. *(12)*. Cancer risk was similar, four in the treated group and six in the placebo group. The baseline histology changed in both directions: eight with IM at baseline developed cancer, in 26 the baseline IM resolved. Progression of IM, which was found in 53% of patients, was associated with persistent *H. pylori* infection, age, and some environmental factors. In summary, *H. pylori* infection is one of

several cofactors for gastric cancer. Most likely eradication, to be effective, needs to occur before the progression to extensive IM and gastric atrophy.

6. RISK FACTORS

The pathogenesis of gastric cancer is multifactorial, and numerous risk factors have been implicated with its development. Twin studies have demonstrated a relative risk of developing gastric cancer of 9.9 for monozygotic twins and 6.6 for dizygotic twins, suggesting that both environmental and genetic factors are involved in the pathogenesis of gastric cancer *(12)*. Hereditary factors have been shown to play a role in the development of gastric cancer as evidenced by clustering of this disease in families *(13)*. In addition, studies have confirmed the effect of the environment on the incidence of gastric cancer by observing distinct variations in the incidence and mortality of gastric cancer among persons of different countries, and socioeconomic groups *(14)*. Specifically, first-generation immigrants from high-risk countries have been shown to consistently have incidence rates of gastric cancer similar to that of their home country, whereas subsequent generations have risk levels approximating that of the host country *(15,16)*.

6.1. FAMILY HISTORY

A familial predisposition to gastric cancer has been demonstrated in several studies with approximately a two- to threefold increased relative risk *(17–19)*. In one large cohort study of more than 1000 patients with gastric cancer, Palli et al. found a significant association with a family history of gastric cancer in a sibling or a parent (adjusted OR, 2.6 and 1.7, respectively) after controlling for confounding risk factors. Moreover, they reported that gastric cancer risk was higher for subjects having an affected mother than an affected father (OR, 2.3 and 1.3, respectively), and also showed a further increase for subjects reporting both parents (OR, 3) or two or more siblings affected with gastric cancer (OR, 8.5) *(17)*. Others have confirmed this general increased risk but have failed to show a consistent pattern of risk with reference to the type of first-degree relationship *(20)*.

Familial clustering of gastric cancer defined by the presence of at least four cancer cases in family members has also been demonstrated in about 10% of cases *(20,21)*. Some have suggested that this familial clustering of gastric cancer corresponds, in part, to the familial clustering of *H. pylori* infection by citing studies showing higher rates of *H. pylori* infection, hypochlorhydria, and atrophic gastritis in first-degree relatives of gastric cancer patients vs healthy controls *(22)*. Despite these findings, investigators have argued that *H. pylori* infection alone cannot explain all of the family concordance of gastric cancer *(23,24)*. They maintain that *H. pylori* infection within families seems to only explain a 36% increase in family cancer rate, a smaller amount than the 100–300% increase in cancer risk that has been observed among first-degree relatives *(23)*. Some experts argue that the response to *H. pylori* infection, rather than its mere presence is important in disease outcome. They demonstrate that polymorphisms in proinflammatory cytokine genes (tumor nectosis factor-α, interleukin-10, and interleukin-1) are associated with an elevated risk for the development of precancerous conditions for gastric cancer in *H. pylori* infected patients but not in uninfected ones *(24,25)*.

FAP and hereditary nonpolyposis colorectal cancer (HNPCC) also seem to confer an increased risk of developing gastric cancer in affected patients. Patients with FAP seem to have a 10-fold increased risk of developing gastric cancer compared with the general population (26), and those with HNPCC have an about 11% likelihood of developing gastric cancer (27). As such, endoscopic screening is recommended for these populations (28,29).

6.2. DIET

Several dietary facts have been implicated as risk factors for gastric cancer. The advent of widely available refrigeration, the consequent availability of fresh foods and the decreased consumption of preserved foods seem to have contributed to the significant decline in gastric cancer incidence observed in the second half of the last century (30). In line with this trend, many studies have shown that a high intake of highly salted and preserved foods are associated with increased cancer risk (31–35). Moreover, high salt intake has been associated with increased rates of atrophic gastritis in humans and animals in the setting of *H. pylori* infection (36). Preserved meat and nitrite intake have also been linked to increased cancer risk (37), possibly owing to the formation of *N*-nitroso compounds that are known carcinogens in animal experiments (38,39).

An inverse relationship between high consumption of fresh fruits and vegetables and incidence of gastric cancer has also been demonstrated (40–42). The protective effect of fresh fruits and vegetables seems to be in part owing to increased intake of antioxidant vitamins (41,43). The possible protective micronutrients include ascorbic acid (vitamin C), α-tocopherol (vitamin E), β-carotene, and selenium (41,44). These antioxidants are believed to be free radical scavengers that reduce reactive radical-induced DNA damage (45). The evidence is strongest for ascorbic acid, with approx 50% risk reduction for gastric cancer in case–control studies (46). In addition, supplementation with ascorbic acid in a randomized controlled chemo-prevention trial in subjects with confirmed histological diagnoses of CAG or IM led to significant regression of these precancerous lesions (47). Alcohol ingestion, whereas previously thought to play a role in gastric cancer development, seems not to be an independent risk factor (48,49). Cigarette smoking, however, has been consistently found to be a risk factor for gastric cancer (48,50) and has specifically been found to contribute to the progression of precancerous lesions to gastric cancer in a high-risk population followed with serial endoscopies (49).

6.3. PERNICIOUS ANEMIA

Pernicious anemia is a disorder characterized by autoantibodies to gastric parietal cells and intrinsic factor. The resulting CAG involving the parietal cells in the fundus of the stomach leads to achlorhydria, impaired intrinsic-factor secretion, and subsequent vitamin B_{12} malabsorption. The antral mucosa, which is devoid of atrophy and achlorhydria, secretes large amounts of gastrin from antral G cells owing to the loss of negative feedback of acid (51). Although the disease is typically silent until the final stage, gastric pathology may be present many years before the development of anemia (51). Progression to an advanced stage of the disease, which is characterized by replacement of the normal parietal and zymogenic cells with those resembling IM and subsequent anemia, may take 20–30 yr (51). The significantly increased risk of progression to gastric mucosal dysplasia and even gastric carcinoma and gastric carcinoid tumors has been widely reported, particularly in populations with higher risks of gastric cancer and as such pernicious anemia is considered to be a risk factor for gastric cancer (51,52).

6.4. PARTIAL GASTRECTOMY FOR BENIGN DISEASE

Since its first description (53), numerous clinical studies have shown an increased incidence of gastric adenocarcinoma in patients who underwent stomach resection in comparison with the general population (54–56). Postgastrectomy cancers represent about 5% of all gastric cancers (57) and have been observed after Billroth I and II resections, with some reports of a higher incidence after the latter reconstruction (54,56,58). Animal studies have also shown that gastric resection promotes carcinogenesis (59). The stump carcinoma is often found to be localized at or near the surgical anastomosis, and only rarely does it reside on the intestinal side of the anastomosis (60). The increased incidence of cancer is thought to be owing to reflux of intestinal contents and bile into the gastric remnant (61). In addition, formation of *N*-nitroso carcinogens from nitrate and nitrite by gastric bacteria, which have overgrown owing to postoperative hypochlorhydia may play a role (54,59).

The development of carcinoma of the gastric remnant seems to be directly related to the postoperative time interval. Studies have consistently shown no differences between the expected and observed number of cancers occurring within 15 yr after gastric resection. However, the overwhelming majority of these studies do indicate a two- to fourfold increase in the risk of gastric cancer in patients who survived 15 or more years after gastric surgery (54–56). Moreover, an association between initial surgical indication and subsequent risk of stomach cancer has also been shown, with patients, who underwent surgery for gastric ulcer, having a twofold increased risk for stump cancer (54,56).

7. SCREENING AND SURVEILLANCE

Identification of preneoplastic conditions and early detection of gastric cancer is of great therapeutic and prognostic importance, particularly in parts of the world where gastric cancer prevalence is high. As such, mass screening of asymptomatic populations has been carried out in various endemic areas of the world with varying results. Moreover, surveillance programs in high-risk patients with preneoplastic lesions has been advocated by some. The patients targeted for screening are summarized in Table 3.

7.1. MASS POPULATION SCREENING

Mass screening programs of asymptomatic persons have been implemented in parts of the world with a high prevalence of gastric cancer with varying success (62–66). In Japan, mass screening has lead to increased detection of early gastric cancer (62), with case–control studies suggesting that detection of these more favorable lesions has resulted in up to a 50% reduction of gastric cancer mortality in the screened population (63). In a recent study, Inaba and colleagues reported a risk ratio of 0.72 of dying from gastric cancer in more than 24,000 Japanese patients

Table 3
Screening Recommendations

Positive family history
FAP/HNPCC history
Pernicious anemia
Postgastrectomy patients, after 15–20 yr
Multifocal atrophic gastritis with other associated genetic or
   environmental factors

FAP, familail adenomatous polyposis; HNPCC, hereditary nonpolyposis colon cancer.

who underwent screening endoscopy and were followed for 40 mo (64). Although this data supports the survival benefit of conducting routine endoscopic screening in high-risk populations, the cost-effectiveness of such an approach remains unknown.

However, similar mass screening programs are unlikely to be effective in Western countries, in large part owing to the significantly lower incidence of gastric cancer in this population. As such, the most recent guidelines by the American Society of Gastrointestinal Endoscopy does not support mass screening of this population group (29).

7.2. CHRONIC ATROPHIC GASTRITIS

The progression of CAG to dysplasia and even adenocarcinoma has been reported in the literature leading some to recommend endoscopic surveillance of these lesions (67,68). Although there is some controversy over the management of these lesions, the majority of experts however agree that routine endoscopic surveillance for progression to dysplasia or even gastric cancer in low-risk countries such as the United States is not cost-effective and not indicated (3,29). They cite studies showing that this progression seems to be relatively slow with a long latency period (67). Moreover, this association seems to be most pronounced in areas such as regions of South America or eastern Asia were the prevalence of gastric cancer is high. In addition, despite findings for progression of this lesion, studies have demonstrated that many patients with CAG have no progression or actually have regression on serial gastric biopsies, particularly with the eradication of H. pylori (69). A role for surveillance endoscopy has been suggested in patients with CAG and a higher risk of developing gastric carcinoma on the basis of family history, racial or ethnic origin, or emigration from an area endemic for gastric cancer (3). The frequency or cost-effectiveness of this approach is unclear.

7.3. INTESTINAL METAPLASIA

Gastric IM is considered a premalignant condition, however, controversy exists regarding whether these lesions warrant endoscopic surveillance for malignant progression. Most investigators agree that surveillance endoscopy is not indicated for IM, in general (70–72). However, some experts have suggested that a subtype of IM is more closely associated with gastric cancer and therefore argue that close endoscopic monitoring of this subtype of IM is necessary (70,73).

Other investigators maintain that IM is common in Western countries with a reported prevalence of up to one-fourth of the general population (74), and that the overall risk of malignant progression is extraordinarily low, particularly in populations with a low gastric cancer prevalence (72). Moreover, they state

that the likelihood that subsequent surveillance of individuals with IM would increase detection of curable gastric cancers in such a low-risk cancer population is extraordinarily low unless dysplasia is also present (72). Regarding subtyping IM, they refer to recent studies conducted in the United States showing no progression to gastric carcinoma in patients followed with serial endoscopy for these lesions (75,76). At the same time, they point out that routine endoscopic surveillance of IM would be problematic because this lesion is endoscopically invisible in the majority of cases and that surveillance would be difficult without the use of expensive techniques such as tissue staining (chromoendoscopy) (72,77).

Given the combination of low sensitivity and likely high cost of serial endoscopic procedures current guidelines state that endoscopic surveillance of IM is not routinely indicated (29). An endoscopic surveillance program may be considered in patients who come from a population at high risk for gastric cancer or have a positive family history of gastric malignancy, although the exact efficacy, frequency, or appropriate technique (e.g., chromoendoscopy) of a such a program is unclear (72).

7.4. DYSPLASIA

Follow-up studies have clearly established the high risk of malignant progression of gastric dysplasia (78–80). The management of dysplasia depends in large part on the severity of the lesion detected since the chronology of progression from one dysplastic grade to a higher grade or to invasive adenocarcinoma varies. High-grade dysplasia has been shown to progress to gastric carcinoma in as little as a month, suggesting concomitant invasive carcinoma, to about 39 mo with a mean between 4 and 23 mo (78). Low-grade dysplasia, however, has been found in most series to lead to gastric carcinoma on average between 10 and 30 mo but has been reported in as early as 1 mo following initial diagnosis of dysplasia, again suggesting concomitant invasive carcinoma (78). In the past, discrepancies in the diagnosis of gastric dysplasia vs carcinoma between Western and Japanese pathologists have complicated interpreting the literature and thus the management of these lesions (78,81).

With this in mind, it is critical that whenever dysplasia is diagnosed, one should get a second opinion from another pathologist, if the diagnosis was made by a pathologist who may not see many such cases (82–84). As soon as a diagnosis of dysplasia is confirmed, many experts suggest that immediate endoscopic reevaluation be undertaken to map the extent of dysplasia and to rule out concomitant gastric carcinoma (82–84). This should be done by taking biopsy specimens near any visible lesions if present, and from the rest of the stomach (e.g., eight samples equidistant from each curvature) (82).

Few experts have suggested that dysplasia of any grade should be resected citing studies showing progression to higher grade of dysplasia or even gastric carcinoma in patients even with low-grade dysplasia on initial biopsy specimens (82). On the other hand, a few have argued that careful endoscopic monitoring is sufficient for all grades of dysplasia with closer intervals for those with more advanced lesions (85). However, most investigators agree that surgical resection, whether total or subtotal, should be performed for cases in which high-grade dysplasia has been confirmed because of the intimate association of this lesion with invasive gastric adenocarcinoma *(79,83,84,86)*. As always, the age and general condition of the patient must be taken into account and in some instances a less aggressive approach may be appropriate. More recently, endoscopic mucosal resection has become a less radical alternative to gastrectomy in the management of severe dysplasia located in focally identifiable lesions *(78)*. If resection is reserved for severe grades of dysplasia, lesions of lesser severity require close endoscopic surveillance *(78,84)*. Follow-up of low-grade dysplasia has been recommended every three to 12 mo at least during the first year *(84)*. The duration of such follow-up is not clear *(78)*.

7.5. POST GASTRECTOMY

Studies have repeatedly demonstrated an increased risk of gastric stump cancer 15–20 yr following partial gastrectomy for benign conditions *(54,56,87,88)*. Although the risk is highest in countries with high gastric cancer rates, studies conducted in Western countries including the United States also demonstrate an elevated risk of gastric remnant carcinoma *(89)*. At the same time, endoscopic screening programs of this patient population have demonstrated a dramatic survival improvement when resection is performed for early-stage gastric remnant cancer *(89,90)*.

Surveillance programs of patients who have undergone partial gastrectomy for benign disease have recommended screening endoscopy starting 15–20 yr postsurgery in order to detect malignancy at an earlier stage and in turn improve prognosis *(88,89,91,92)*. A few have shown that the risk of gastric carcinoma is not significantly higher in the postgastrectomy patient as compared with the general population and have thus recommended that screening for neoplastic progression is not necessary *(93,94)*. Accounting for this discrepancy is the fact that the majority of the latter studies had a follow-up period less than 20 yr, which is often inadequate given the longer latency of malignant progression in this population. Despite the findings of a significantly elevated risk of gastric cancer, the cost-effectiveness of such surveillance has not been well established, leading to guidelines stating that such surveillance is not indicated in low-risk countries *(29)*. Yet, in populations at higher risk, screening endoscopy may be considered 15–20 yr postgastrectomy. Since early cancer in the gastric remnant may occur in the absence of a gross lesion, multiple biopsies should be obtained and a significant number of these specimens should come from the anastomotic area in which cancer is most likely to be found *(60)*. A finding of high-grade dysplasia has been shown to be a good marker for the development or the presence of malignancy and surgical resection is recommended. However, it is important that dysplasia not be confused with reactive gastritis that is common to the postoperative stomach and likely represents regenerative atypia.

7.6. PERNICIOUS ANEMIA

An excess risk of gastric carcinoma and carcinoid tumors have been reported in long-term endoscopic surveillance studies of large cohorts of patients with pernicious anemia *(51,52)*. As such, endoscopic screening protocols have been suggested for the early detection of gastric neoplasia and malignancy *(95)*. Many experts recommend that patients with pernicious anemia

should have upper endoscopy with biopsy shortly following initial diagnosis. At least six biopsies should be obtained from the fundus and body spaced equidistant along the lesser and greater curvature. In addition, four specimens should be obtained from the antrum. It is important to keep in mind that biopsies of the thinner mucosa along the lesser curvature or in the transition zones (antral-body and cardiac-body) could be misinterpreted as atrophic and therefore are not ideal in diagnosing severe fundic gland gastritis. In the majority of patients in whom dysplasia, adenomatous neoplasms, or carcinoids are not found, further endoscopic surveillance is not necessary *(29)*; except possibly for those patients with a first-degree relative with gastric cancer in which case, repeat endoscopy should be considered every 5 yr *(96)*.

REFERENCES

1. Correa P. A human model of gastric carcinogenesis. Cancer Res 1988; 48:3554–3560.
2. Sepulveda A, Graham D. Role of *Helicobacter pylori* in gastric carcinogenesis. Gastroenterol Clin North Am 2002; 31(2):517–535.
3. Faraji E, frank B. Multifocal atrophic gastritis and gastric carcinoma. Gastroenterology Clinics of North America 2002; 31(2):499–516.
4. Genta R, Rugge M. Gastric precancerous lesions: heading for an international consensus. Gut 1999; 45(Suppl I):I5–I8.
5. Haber M. Histologic precursors of gastrointestinal malignancy. Gastroenterology Clinics of North America 2002; 31(2):395–419.
6. Lauwers G. Defining the pathologic diagnosis of metaplasia, atrophy, dysplasia, and gastric adenocarcinoma. J Clin Gastroenterol 2003; 36(Suppl 1):S37–S43.
7. Meining A, Morgner A, Miehlke S, Bayerdorffer E, Stolte M. Atrophy-metaplasia-dysplasia-carcinoma sequence in the stomach: a reality or merely an hypothesis? Best Pract Res Clin Gastroenterol 2001; 15:983–998.
8. Uemura N, Okamoto S, Yamamoto S, et al. Helicobacter pylori and the development of gastric cancer. N Engl J Med 2001; 345:784–789.
9. Wong B, Lam S, Wong W, et al. *Helicobacter pylori* eradication to prevent gastric cancer in a high-risk region of China. JAMA 2004; 291:87–194.
10. Sung J, Lin S, Ching J, et al. Atrophy and intestinal metaplasia one year after cure of H. pylori infection: a prospective, randomized study. Gastroenterology 2000; 119:7–14.
11. Ley C, Mohar A, Guarner J, et al. helicobacter pylori eradication and gastric preneoplastic conditions: a randomized, double-blind, placebo-controlled trial. Cancer Epidemiol Biomark Prev 2004; 13:4–10.
12. Lichtenstein P, Holm NV, Verkasalo PK, et al. Environmental and heritable factors in the causation of cancer. N Engl J Med 2000; 343:78–85.
13. Bakir T, Can G, Siviloglu C, et al. Gastric cancer and other organ cancer history in the parents of patients with gastric cancer. Eur J Cancer Prev 2003; 12:183–189.
14. Howson CP, Hiyama T, Wynder EL. The decline of gastric cancer, epidemiology of an unplanned triumph. Epidemiol Rev 1986; 8:1–27.
15. Haenszel W, Kurihara M, Segi M, et al. Stomach cancer among Japanese in Hawaii. J Natl Cancer Inst 1972; 49:969–988.
16. Staszewski J. Migrant studies in alimentary tract cancer. Recent Results Cancer Res 1972; 39:85–97.
17. Palli D, Galli M, Caporaso NE, et al. Family history and risk of stomach cancer in Italy. Cancer Epidemiol Biomarkers 1994; 3:15–18.
18. Dhillon PK, Farrow DC, Vaughan TL, et al. Family history of cancer and risk of esophageal and gastric cancers in the United States. Int J Cancer 2001; 93:148–152.
19. Lissowska J, Groves FD, Sobin LH, et al. Family history and risk of stomach cancer in Warsaw, Poland. Eur J Cancer Prev 1999; 8:223–227.
20. La Vecchia C, Negri E, Franceschi S, et al. Family history and the risk of stomach and colorectal cancer. Cancer 1992; 70:50–55.

21. Bakir T, Can G, Siviloglu C, et al. Gastric cancer and other organ cancer history in the parents of patients with gastric cancer. Eur J Cancer Prev 2003; 12:183–189.

22. Parsonnet J. When Heredity is Infectious. Gastroenterology 2000; 118:222–224.

23. Brenner H, Bode G, Boeing H. Helicobacter pylori infection among offspring of patients with stomach cancer. Gastroenterology 2000; 118:31–35.

24. El-Omar EM, Oien K, Murray LS, et al. Increased prevalence of precancerous changes in relatives of gastric cancer patients: critical role of H. pylori. Gastroenterology. 2000; 118:22–30.

25. Machado JC, Pharoah P, Sousa S, et al. Interleukin 1B and interleukin 1RN polymorphisms are associated with increased risk of gastric carcinoma. Gastroenterology 2001; 121:823–829.

26. Zwick A, Munir M, Ryan C, et al. Gastric adenocarcinoma and dysplasia in fundic gland polyps of a patient with attenuated adenomatous polyposis. Gastroenterology 1997; 113:659–663.

27. Aarnio M, Salovaara R, Aaltonen L, et al. Features of gastric cancer in hereditary non-polyposis colorectal cancer syndrome. Int J Cancer 1997; 74:551–555.

28. Sawada T, Muto T. Familial adenomatous polyposis: Should patients undergo surveillance of the upper gastrointestinal tract? Endoscopy 1995; 27:6–11.

29. Appropriate use of gastrointestinal endoscopy. American Society for Gastrointestinal Endoscopy. Gastrointest Endosc 2000; 52: 831–837.

30. Kelley JR, Duggan JM. Gastric cancer epidemiology and risk factors. J Clin Epidemiol 2003; 56:1–9.

31. Ramon J, Serra L, Cerdo C, et al. Dietary factors and gastric cancer risk: A case control study in Spain. Cancer 1993; 71:1731–1735.

32. Ji B, Chow W, Yang G, et al. Dietary habits and stomach cancer in Shanghai, China. Int J Cancer 1998; 76:659–664.

33. Joossens JV, Hill MJ, Elliott P, et al. Dietary salt, nitrate, and stomach cancer mortality in 24 countries. Int J Epidemiol 1996; 24:494–504.

34. Hansson LE, Nyren O, Bergstrom R, et al. Diet and risk of gastric cancer. A population-based case control study in Sweden. Int J Cancer 1993; 55:181–189.

35. Lee JK, Park BJ, Yoo KY, et al. Dietary factors and stomach cancer: a case–control study in Korea. Int J Epidemiol 1995; 24:33–41.

36. Fox J, Dangler C, Taylor N, et al. High-salt intake induces gastric epithelial hyperplasia and parietal cell loss, and enhances Helicobacter pylori colonization in C57BL/6 mice. Cancer Res 1999; 59:4823–4822.

37. Buiatti E, Palli D, Decarli A, et al. A case–control study of gastric cancer and diet in Italy. II. Association with nutrients. Int J Cancer 1990; 45:896–901.

38. Correa P. Human gastric carcinogenesis: a multistep and multifactorial process. First American Cancer Society award lecture on cancer epidemiology and prevention. Cancer Res 1992; 52:6735–6740.

39. Mowat C, Carswell A, Wirz, et al. Omeprazole and dietary nitrate independently affect levels of vitamin C and nitrite in gastric juice. Gastroenterology 1999; 116:813–822.

40. You WC, Blot WJ, Chang YS, et al. Diet and high risk stomach cancer in Shandong, China. Cancer Res 1988; 48:3518–3523.

41. Steinmeitz KA, Potter JD. Vegetables, fruit and cancer prevention: a review. J Am Diet Assoc 1996; 96:1027–1039.

42. Kobayashi M, Tsubono Y, Sasazuki S, et al. Vegetables, fruit and risk of gastric cancer in Japan: a 10 year follow-up of the JPHC Study Cohort I. Int J Cancer 2002; 102:39–44.

43. Serafini M, Bellocco R, Wolk A, et al. Total antioxidant potential of fruit and vegetables and risk of gastric cancer. Gastroenterology 2002; 123:985–991.

44. Blot WJ, Li JY, Taylor PR, et al. Nutrition intervention trial in Linxian, China: supplementation with specific vitamin/mineral combinations, cancer incidence and disease-specific mortality in the general population. J Natl Cancer Inst 1993; 85:1483–1492.

45. Drake I, Davies M, Mapstone N, et al. Ascorbic acid may protect against gastric cancer by scavenging mucosal oxygen radicals. Carcinogenesis 1996; 17:559–562.

46. Neugut AI, Hayek M, Howe G. Epidemiology of gastric cancer. Semin Oncol 1996; 23:281–291.

47. Correa P, Fontham E, Bravo JC, et al. Chemoprevention of Gastric Dysplasia: Randomized trial of antioxidant supplements and anti-helicobacter pylori therapy. J Natl Cancer Inst 2000; 92:1881–1888.

48. Chow W, Swanson C, Lissowska J, et al. Risk of stomach cancer in relation to consumption of cigarettes, alcohol, tea and coffee in Warsaw, Poland. Int J Cancer 1999; 81:871–876.

49. You W, Zhang L, Gail MH, et al. Gastric dysplasia and gastric cancer: Helicobacter pylori, serum vitamin C and other risk factors. J Natl Cancer Inst 2000; 92:1607–1612.

50. Mizoue T, Tokui N, Nishisaka K, et al. Prospective study on the relation of cigarette smoking with cancer of the liver and stomach in an endemic region. Int J Epidemiol 2000; 29:232–237.

51. Toh BH, van Driel IR, Gleeson PA. Pernicious Anemia. N Eng J Med 1997; 337:1441–1448.

52. Hsing AW, Hansson LE, McLaughlin JK, et al. Pernicious anemia and subsequent cancer. A population-based cohort study. Cancer 1993; 71:745–750.

53. Balfour DC. Factors influencing the life expectancy of patients operated on for gastric surgery. Ann Surg 1922; 76:405–408.

54. Tersemette AC, Offerhaus GJ, Tersmette KW, et al. Meta-analysis of the risk of gastric stump cancer: Detection of high risk patients for stomach cancer after remote partial gastrectomy for benign conditions. Cancer Res 1990; 50:6486–6489.

55. Stalnikowicz R, Benbassat J. Risk of gastric cancer after gastric surgery for benign disorders. Arch Intern Med 1990; 150:2022–2026.

56. Tersmette AC, Goodman SN, Offerhaus GJA, et al. Multivariate analysis of the risk of stomach cancer after ulcer surgery in an Amsterdam cohort of post-gastrectomy patients. Am J Epidemiol 1991; 134:14–21.

57. Antonioli D. Gastric carcinoma and its precursors. Monogr Pathol 1990; 31:144–180.

58. Lundegardh G, Adami H-O, Helmick C, et al. Stomach cancer after partial gastrectomy for benign disease. N Engl J Med 1988; 319:195–200.

59. Sano C, Kumashiro R, Saito T, et al. Promoting effect of partial gastrectomy in carcinogenesis in the remnant stomach of rats after oral administration of N-methyl-N-nitrosoguanidine. Oncology 1984; 41:124–128.

60. Domellof L, Eriksson S, Janunger K. Carcinoma and possible precancerous changes of the gastric stump after Billroth II resection. Gastroenterology 1977; 73:462–468.

61. Kondo K. Duodenogastric reflux and gastric stump carcinoma. Gastric Cancer 2002; 5:16–22.

62. Yamakazi, H, Oshima A, Murakami R, et al. A long-term follow-up study of patients with gastric cancer detected by mass screening. Cancer 1989; 63:613–617.

63. Hisamichi S, Sugawara N, Fukao A. Effectiveness of gastric mass screening in Japan. Cancer Detect Prev 1988; 11:323–329.

64. Inaba S, Hirayama H, Nagata C, et al. Evaluation of a screening program on reduction of gastic cancer mortality in Japan: Preliminary results from a cohort study. Prev Med 1999; 29:102–106.

65. Llorens P. Gastric cancer mass survey in Chile. Sem Surg Oncol 1991; 7:339–343.

66. Pisani P, Oliver WE, Parkin DM, et al. Case–control study of gastric cancer screening in Venezuela. Br J Cancer 1994; 69:1102–1105.

67. Whiting JL, Sigurdsson A, Rowlands DC, et al. The long term results of endsocopic surveillance of premaligant gastric lesions. Gut 2002; 50:378–381.

68. Lahner E, Caruana P, D'Ambra G, et al. First endsocopic histologic follow-up in patients with body predominant atrophic gastritis: When should it be done? Gastrointestinal Endoscopy 2001; 53:443–448.

69. Dinis-Ribeiro M, Lopes C, Costa-Pereira AD, et al. A follow-up model for patients with atrophic chronic gastritis and intestinal metaplasia. J Clin Pathol 2004; 57:177–182.

70. Silva S, Filipe MI, Pinho. Variants of intestinal metaplasia in the evolution of chronic atrophic gastritis and gastric ulcer. A follow up study. Gut 1990; 31:1097–1104.

71. Sossai P, Barbazza R. Is it useful to follow-up intestinal metaplasia in the stomach? Analysis of Cost/Effectiveness. J Clin Gastroenterol 1992; 14:356–357.

72. Fennerty MB. Gastric Intestinal metaplasia on routine endoscopic biopsy. Gastroenterology 2003; 125:586–590.

73. Rokkas T, Filipe MI, Sladen GE. Detection of an increased incidence of early gastric cancer in patients with intestinal metaplasia type III who are closely followed up. Gut 1991; 32:1110–1113.

74. Petersson F, Borch K, Franzen LE. Prevalence of subtypes of intestinal metaplasia in the general population and in patients with autoimmune chronic atrophic gastritis. Scand J Gastroenterol 2002; 37:262–266.

75. El-Zimaity HMT, Ramchatesingh J, Ali Saeed M, et al. Gastric intestinal metaplasia:subtypes and natural history. J Clin Pathol 2001; 54:679–683.

76. Morales TG, Camargo E, Bhattacharyya A, et al. Long-term follow-up of intestinal metaplasia of the gastric cardia. Am J Gastroenterol 2000; 95:1677–1680.

77. Fennery MB, Sampliner RE, McGee DL, et al. Intestinal metaplasia of the stomach: identification by a selective mucosal staining technique. Gastointest Endosc 1992; 38:695–698.

78. Lauwers GY, Riddell RH. Gastric epithelial dysplasia. Gut 1999; 45:784–790.

79. Di Gregorio C, Morandi P, Fante R, et al. Gastric dysplasia. A follow-up study. Am J Gastroenterol 1993; 88:1714–1719.

80. Rugge M, Farinati F, Baffa R, et al. Gastric epithelial dysplasia in the natural history of gastric cancer: A multicenter prospective follow-up study. Gastroenterology 1994; 107:1288–1296.

81. Schlemper RJ, Riddell RH, Kato Y, ete al. The Vienna classification of gastrointestinal epithelial neoplasia. Gut 2000; 47:251–255.

82. Weinstein WM, Goldstein NL. Gastric dysplasia and its management. Gastroeneterology 1994; 107:1543–1559.

83. Farinati F, Rugge M, Di Mario F, et al. Early and advanced gastric cancer in the follow-up of moderate and severe gastric dysplasia patients. A prospective study.Endoscopy 1993; 25:261–264.

84. Fertitta AM, Comin U, Terruzzi V, et al. Clinical significance of gastric dysplasia: a multicenter follow-up study. Endoscopy 1993; 25:265–268.

85. Rugge M, Cassaro M, Di Mario, et al. The long term outcome of gastric non-invasive neoplasia. Gut 2003; 52:1111–1116.

86. Lansdown M, Quirke P, Dixon MF, et al. High grade dysplasia of the gastric mucosa: a marker for gastric carcinoma. Gut 1990; 31: 977–983.

87. Stalnikowicz R, Benbassat J. Risk of gastric cancer after gastric surgery for benign disorders. Arch Intern Med 1990; 150:2022–2026.

88. Greene FL. Gastroscopic screening of the post-gastrectomy stomach. Relationship of dysplasia to remnant cancer. Am Surg 1989; 55:12–15.

89. Greene FL. Management of gastric remnant carcinoma based on the results of a 15 year endoscopic screening program. Annals of Surgery 1996; 223:701–708.

90. Pointner R, Welscher G, Gadenstatter M, et al. Gastric remnant cancer has a better prognosis than primary gastric cancer. Arch Surg 1994; 126:615–619.

91. Lacaine F, Houry S, Huguier M. Stomach cancer after partial gastrectomy for benign ulcer disease. A critical analysis of epidemiological reports. Hepatogastroenterology 1992; 39:4–8.

92. Gannon CJ, Engbrecht B, Napolitano LM, et al. Gastric remnant carcinoma. Reevaluation of screening endoscopy. Surg Endosc 2001; 15:1488–1490.

93. Schafer LW, Larson DE, Melton LJ, et al. The risk of gastric carcinoma after surgical treatment for benign ulcer disease. A population based study in Olmsted County, Minnesota. N Engl J Med 1983; 309:1210–1213.

94. Ross AH, Smith MA, Anderson JR, et al. Late mortality after surgery for peptic ulcer. N Engl J Med 1982; 307:519–522.

95. Stockbrugger RW, Menon GG, Beilby JOW, et al. Gastroscopic screening in 80 patients with pernicious anemia. Gut 1983; 24:1141–1147.

96. Borch K. Epidemiologic, clinicopathologic and economic aspects of gastroscopic screening of patients with pernicious anemia. Scand J Gastroenterol 1986; 21:21–30.

10 Gastric Polyps

George A. Makar, MD and Gregory G. Ginsberg, MD

Contents

1. BACKGROUND

Gastric polyps are a frequent incidental finding during endoscopy that occasionally present with bleeding, obstruction, or pain. The majority are non-neoplastic. The major epithelial polyps are fundic gland, hyperplastic, and adenomatous. Sporadic fundic gland polyps (FGPs) are benign and have no malignant potential. Hyperplastic and adenomatous polyps may arise in a background of *Helicobacter pylori* infection and have malignant potential; these should be endoscopically removed. Gastric polyps can also be seen as a manifestation of polyposis syndromes most notably familial adenomatous polyposis (FAP; FGPs and to a lesser degree adenomatous), Peutz-Jegher's syndrome (harmatomas), and juvenile polyposis (hamartomas). Patients with familial polyposis may be at an increased risk of gastric cancer, particularly those with Peutz-Jegher's syndrome. Endoscopic polypectomy is safe and effective but carries a higher complication rate than polypectomy in the colon.

2. INTRODUCTION

Gastric polyps are usually found incidentally during endoscopy or gastrointestinal radiological studies performed for symptoms unrelated to gastric polyps. On occasion they might present with occult bleeding, anemia, obstruction, or abdominal pain. The majority of gastric polyps are epithelial in origin and unlike in the colon are non-neoplastic (hyperplastic and FGPs), although they may have a potential to harbor neoplastic growth (Table 1). The remainder are made up of hamartomas, carcinoids, reactive lesions (inflammatory fibroid polyps [IFP]), heterotopias, and submucosal tumors, such as leomyomas and lipomas. This chapter focuses on gastric

From: *Endoscopic Oncology: Gastrointestinal Endoscopy and Cancer Management*. Edited by: D. O. Faigel and M. L. Kochman © Humana Press, Totowa, NJ

epithelial polyps (fundic gland, hyperplastic, adenomatous) and their endoscopic management. Polyps associated with hereditary polyposis syndromes and less frequently observed gastric polyps are also discussed (Table 2).

Reported incidence in large retrospective endoscopic series is between 1 and 3% with a higher incidence in those who have had prior gastric surgery *(1–3)*. The largest endoscopic series reported on 13,000 adults undergoing endoscopy for related or unrelated gastrointestinal symptoms. Of these patients, 1.2% had gastric polyps *(2)*.

3. EPITHELIAL POLYPS

3.1. FUNDIC GLAND POLYPS

FGPs (fundic gland hyperplasia, Elster's gland cysts, and cystic hamartomatous gastric polyps) comprise up to 47% of all gastric polyps *(4)*. They are small, sessile lesions present in the cardia, fundus, and upper body of the stomach (Fig. 1). They are usually less than 5 mm in diameter but can be larger. They have a similar coloration to the background mucosa. They almost always appear on a background of healthy mucosa in *H. pylori*-negative patients. They can be single or multiple and can occur sporadically or in association with familial adenomatous polyposis. They are more common in women (2.6:1) and in patients under the age of 60 *(5)*.

Histologically they are characterized by an increase in the glandular elements of the mucosa. The glands appear dilated and tortuous with microcyst formation and are composed of parietal, chief, and occasionally mucinous cells. The pathogenesis is unknown but may be related to reversible glandular dilations caused by changes in the secretory activity of the glands.

Sporadic FGPs are becoming more frequently recognized with the routine use of high-resolution videoendoscopy. In a study by Kinoshita et al. FGPs were found in 26 of 1388 (1.9%) patients undergoing endoscopy. None of these patients

Table 1
Relative Frequency of Gastric Polypoid Lesions

Polyp	Percentage
Epithelial	>80%
Non-neoplastic	
Fundic gland	
Focal foveolar hyperplasia	
Hyperplastic	
Neoplastic	
Adenoma	
Polypoid gastric adenocarcinoma	
Heterotopias	2–3%
Pancreatic heterotopia	
Brunner's gland heterotopia	
Polypoid endocrine tumors (carcinoid)	~2%
Mesenchymal (benign and malignant)	<10%
Gastrointestinal stromal tumor	
Leiomyoma	
Lipoma, fibroma, and so on	
Others	<10%
Inflammatory fibroid	
Hamartomatous polyposis syndromes	
Mucosa-associated lymphoid tissue lymphoma	
Lymphoid follicles	
Gastritis cystica profunda	
Metastatic adenocarcinoma	
Gastritis variolifomris	

had FAP and most of these polyps were less than 2 mm and were solitary. This higher than previously reported prevalence was affirmed by Stolte et al. who re-evaluated more than 5000 gastric polyps sampled from 1969 to 1989 and found 47% were FGPs, whereas only 28.3% were hyperplastic (4). More commonly, FGPs occur in multiples rather than solitary.

FGPs were first observed and thought to be associated with FAP. FGPs are present in 40–80% (6,7) of patients with FAP and as noted earlier might be present in up to 1.9% of the general population. No differences have been detected between sporadic and FAP-associated FGPs with respect to endoscopic, morphological, or mucin histochemical features (8). Studies by Abraham reveal somatic adenomatous polyposis coli (APC) gene alterations occur much more frequently in FAP-associated FGPs than in sporadic FGPs (51 vs 8%, respectively) (9). This likely explains a low-level incidence of dysplasia noted in FAP-associated FGPs (9–11).

Sporadic FGPs are generally believed to have no malignant potential in the general population. Adenomatous changes and dysplasia have been reported in 1% of sporadic cases and 25–44% of patients with FAP (12,13). No cases of gastric adenocarcinoma have been reported in sporadic cases. However, a few published cases of patients with FAP and its attenuated form describe the development of high-grade dysplasia and gastric adenocarcinoma arising from diffuse fundic gland polyposis. These include a brother and sister with attenuated FAP who died in the fifth decade of life from metastatic gastric adenocarcinoma (14–17).

Although FGPs are generally considered themselves non-neoplastic, they can be associated with an increased rate of colorectal neoplasms. Initially described in several retro-

spective studies, this was further evaluated in a case–control study by Jung et al. Sixty-four patients with FGPs and 64 age- and sex-matched controls underwent colonoscopy. Of the 64 patients with FGPs, 8 (12.5%) had adenocarcinomas, 3 (4.7%) had high-grade intraepithelial neoplasia, and 18 (28.1%) had tubular adenomas. Only 6 (9.3%) of the control group patients had tubular adenomas and 9 (14.1%) had hyperplastic polyps on colonoscopy (18). This relationship needs to be verified by larger prospective studies. Currently, there is insufficient evidence to justify a colonoscopy in all patients with incidental FGPs.

Unlike adenomatous and hyperplastic polyps, H. pylori infection does not appear to play a role in the development of FGPs and may actually have an inhibitory effect on their development. Two series have revealed a low rate of H. pylori infection in patients with FGPs. Sakai et al. noted H. pylori infection in 3 of 84 (4%) patients with FGPs, which was significantly less than controls and in patients with hyperplastic polyps. Wu et al. found a similar rate of infection (1.9% [4/216]) in his series (12,19). There is one report of regression of multiple FGPs in two patients after H. pylori infection. FGPs recurred in one of these two patients after subsequent eradication therapy of H. pylori (20).

An association between FGPs and proton pump inhibitor (PPI) use was first reported in 1992 and later supported by retrospective reports of small numbers of patients developing FGPs while on omeprazole therapy for 1–5 yr (21,22). This relationship was further evaluated by Vieth and Stolte in 2001. In a retrospective 12-mo study, the frequency of FGPs in a 2251 patients without H. pylori infection on PPI therapy for at least 4 wk was compared with a control group of 28,096 patients who did not have H. pylori infection and were not on PPI therapy. There was no difference in frequency of FGPs between the two groups (5% in the control and 5.2% in the PPI group) suggesting that a relationship was unlikely (23).

Experienced endoscopists can recognize FGPs in the majority of cases. Weston et al. revealed a high accuracy rate of predicting FGPs based on endoscopic criteria (24). Complete excision can be achieved with single- or multiple-forceps biopsies. Electrocautery snare excision or hot biopsy forceps may be used for larger polyps but most polyps are small enough to be removed with cold biopsy forceps. In non-FAP patients with multiple typical appearing polyps, biopsy removal of several lesions may be sufficient to confirm the diagnosis without a need to remove all polyps. No further therapy or surveillance is indicated in these patients. Spontaneous regression has been reported in both FAP and sporadic FGPs (20,22,25,26).

3.2. HYPERPLASTIC POLYPS

Hyperplastic polyps comprise a majority of all gastric polyps. Initially thought to makeup 75% or more of gastric polyps (1,27), they are probably the second most common polyp after FGPs. Hyperplasiogenic, regenerative, hyeprplastic-adenomatous, adenomatous polyps, inflammatory, and benign polyps are other names in the literature used for hyperplastic polyps. They affect men and women equally and tend to develop later in life than FGPs. They are small, dome-shaped or stalked polyps with an average size of about 1 cm (range

Table 2
Characteristics of Epithelial Gastric Lesions

	Fundic gland	*Hyperplastic*	*Adenoma*
Average size	3–5 mm	10 mm	>10–20 mm
Distribution	Cardia, fundus, upper body	Throughout	Throughout (antral)
Endoscopic appearance	Small, sessile	Dome-shaped or stalked	Broad based or pedunculated
	Single or multiple	May have reddish coloration	May have irregular surface
	Normal background mucosa	May have adherent mucous or superficial erosions	Single
		Single or multiple	
Associated conditions	FAP	Type A or B gastritis	Type A or B gastritis
		Thermoablation	FAP
Risk of malignancy	Small risk in FAP	2–4%	~20–40%

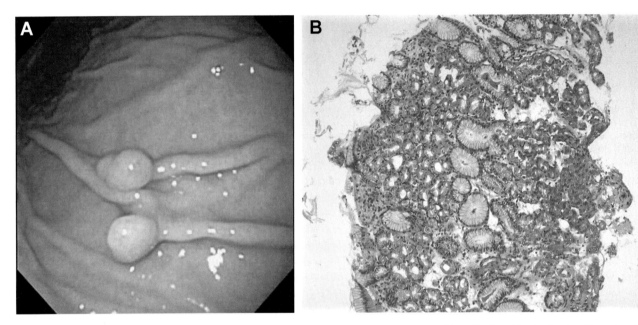

Fig. 1. **(A)** Fundic gland polyps. Two (of five) smooth sessile polyps measuring 3 mm, incidentally found in the fundus. Note the similar coloration to the background mucosa. **(B)** Gastric fundic gland polyps. Pronounced oxyntic hyperplasia with microcystic changes. (Courtesy of Emma E. Furth, MD and Zoltan Gombos, MD.)

0.1–12 cm) *(1)*. They may be single or multiple. Their coloration may be erythematous or similar to the surrounding background mucosa. They tend to be softer than other polyps with a smooth to slightly lobulated surface. The surface may be friable to palpation with adherent mucous or superficial ulceration. Unlike FGPs, they may occur anywhere in the stomach *(28)*. Large or numerous polyps may present with gastrointestinal bleeding, anemia, or intermittent gastric outlet obstruction *(29,30)* but they are usually asymptomatic (Fig. 2).

Microscopically they consist of branching, hyperplastic, and elongated gastric glands. The surface is often eroded with regenerative epithelium that can be sometimes confused with adenomatous or dysplastic changes. Regenerative epithelium is cuboidal with enlarged nuclei and distinct nucleoli associated with ulceration or granulation tissue. Although they are not inherently neoplastic, foci of dysplasia and carcinoma can occasionally develop *(28)*. A similar entity is polypoid foveolar hyperplasia which consists of a lengthening of the foveolae without the architectural changes seen in hyperplastic polyps.

Some authors consider foveolar hyperplasia to be precursor to hyperplastic polyps, whereas others consider them to be distinct entities. It is important to differentiate them from a clinical standpoint because neoplastic foci are only found in hyperplastic polyps *(27)*.

Unlike FGPs that develop on normal mucosa, hyperplastic and adenomatous polyps usually develop on a background of chronic mucosal inflammation. The pathogenesis is active regeneration in response to mucosal injury. *H. pylori* infection and chronic gastritis or intestinal metaplasia is present in most of these patients.

Treatment of the underlying inflammatory process may prevent development of new hyperplastic polyps and in some cases induce regression of current polyps. A prospective study by Ljubicic et al. evaluated the effect of *H. pylori* eradication in the setting of chronic active gastritis on the course of hyperplastic and adenomotous polyps. Among 21 patients with hyperplastic polyps, 16 were positive for *H. pylori*. Complete regression of hyperplastic polyps was observed in 7 of 16

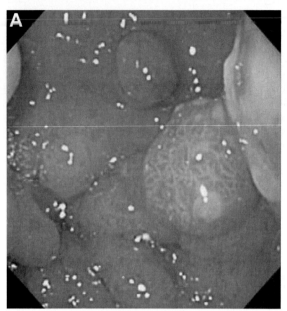
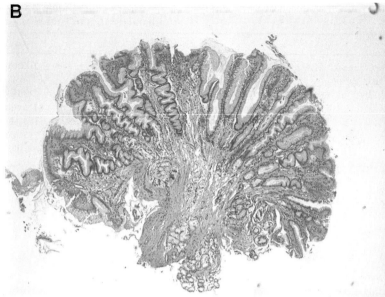

Fig. 2. (A) Numerous hyperplastic polyps in an elderly male presenting with anemia and occult gastrointestinal bleeding. (B) Gastric hyperplastic polyp, antrum. Villous surface architecture with corkscrew-like appearance. Mild amount of muscular hyperplasia is appreciated in the lamina propria. This feature is typically less pronounced that in the case of gastric Peutz-Jeghers polyp, which also shows hyperplastic features. (Courtesy of Emma E. Furth, MD and Zoltan Gombos, MD.)

(44%) patients *(31)*. A randomized controlled trial by Ohkusa et al. studied 35 patients with hyperplastic polyps at least 3 mm in size who had *H. pylori* infection. Seventeen patients received eradication therapy and 18 patients received no treatment. Follow-up endoscopy was performed 12–15 mo after therapy. The polyps disappeared in 12 of 17 treated patients (12 of 15 in whom *H. pylori* was eradicated) but in none of the control patients. It is important to note that the mean size of the polyps in this study was less than 1 cm *(32)*. The authors suggested that *H. pylori* treatment might play a role as initial therapy in patients with hyperplastic polyps and *H. pylori* infection. However, in light of the malignant potential of these polyps, others have recommended that polypectomy should still be the initial treatment *(33)*. In an effort to determine which patients were likely to respond to *H. pylori* eradication therapy, Ohkusa et al. undertook a retrospective study comparing 33 patients who had regression of hyperplastic polyps with 10 patients whose polyps did not regress after eradication therapy. The two groups were similar with respect to age, sex, co-existing diseases, and histological findings. The number and size of polyps was higher in the nonresponders, although five of these patients did have some regression in size and number of polyps. The degree of mucosal atrophy and gastrin levels were also higher in the nonresponders *(34)*.

In addition to *H. pylori* gastritis, hyperplastic polyps can develop in the setting of other causes of mucosal injury. Antral hyperplastic polyps as large as 4 cm developed in 4 of 60 patients several years after laser thermoablation therapy of gastric antral vascular ectasia. These four patients had received greater cumulative doses of thermoablation than most of the patients who did not develop polyps *(35)*. There is also a case report of a 1 cm hyperplastic polyp developing at the site of a prior resection of a gastric adenoma *(36)*. More recently, Amaro

et al. reported on the development of mostly hyperplastic polyps after solid organ transplantation in ten patients. Nine of these patients had three or more polyps, mostly in the antrum. None had adenomatous or dysplastic changes. The mechanism of this relationship is unclear and more studies would need to be performed to confirm this relationship and determine if immunosuppression plays a role in the development of these polyps *(37)*.

Hyperplastic polyps were originally believed to have no potential for malignancy but several studies have revealed a 2–4% rate of carcinoma in these lesions. Daibo et al. reviewed 477 hyperplastic polyps. Ten (2.1%) contained focal carcinomas and another 19 (4%) contained dysplastic foci. The focal carcinomas in the 10 polyps were found adjacent to dysplastic foci *(38)*. Another review of 811 benign epithelial polyps found a 2.1% (10/483) rate of focal carcinoma in hyperplastic polyps and a 7.1% of synchronous carcinoma elsewhere in the stomach. None of the 268 polypoid foveolar hyperplasia lesions contained carcinoma *(27)*. A similar rate of 3.6% (4/112) was noted in another series. The average size of these polyps was 14.5 mm. Dysplasia and intestinal metaplasia were detected in two and three of these polyps, respectively, with carcinoma arising from dysplastic regions *(39)*. In a series of 35 epithelial gastric polyps in 23 patients, 31 polyps were hyperplastic and 4 were adenomas. Six hyperplastic polyps contained focal adenomatous (dysplastic) elements. In three of these six cases focal carcinoma arose from the adenomatous portion of these polyps. All three polyps with carcinoma were less than 2 cm in size *(40)*.

3.3. ADENOMATOUS POLYPS

Gastric adenomas account for 10% or less of gastric polyps making them less common than hyperplastic or FGPs *(2,4,41–44)*. Like colonic adenomas they are neoplastic, premalignant lesions. However, gastric adenocarcinoma does not necessarily arise from adenomas. They are more likely to be

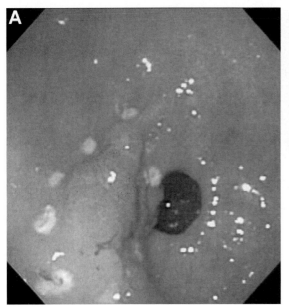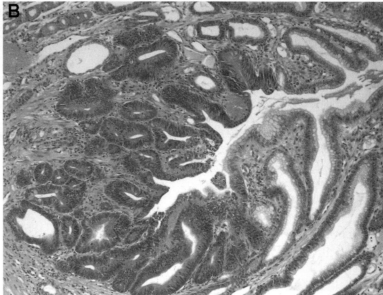

Fig. 3. **(A)** Adenomatous polyp. A single large sessile polyp is seen in the distal antrum measuring 3 cm. The perimeter of the lesion has been marked with contact thermal coagulation in advance of wide area endoscopic mucosal resection. **(B)** Gastric adenoma. Partially preserved normal epithelial lining that abruptly ends in contrast with dysplastic, hyperchromatic, and pseudostratified adenomatous epithelium. (Courtesy of Emma E. Furth, MD and Zoltan Gombos, MD.)

sessile, broad-based erythematous lesions with surface irregularities or erosions. They tend to be solitary and can be found anywhere in the stomach (Fig. 3). A majority of these polyps are at least 1 cm in size. Men and women are equally affected and mean age of onset is in the seventh or eighth decade of life *(41,42,45)*.

Histologically, they are characterized by columnar epithelium that is pseudostratified and shows elongated atypical nuclei and increased mitotic activity *(28)*. There are four types of adenomatous polyps: tubular, tubulovillous, villous (papillary), and pyloric gland adenomas. Tubular adenomas are the most common and usually present as flat or only slightly elevated polyps or even as depressed areas *(46)*. Tubulovillous adenomas are rare and tend to present as large polyps. Villous adenomas are sessile and tend to have greater potential for malignancy than the tubular form *(28)*. The epithelial lining of gastric adenomas may be of intestinal-type (containing goblet or Paneth cells) or gastric-type (lined only by gastric mucin cells). Intestinal-type adenomas occur more frequently and develop on a background of gastric atrophy and intestinal metaplasia in the surrounding mucosa. Gastric-type adenomas occur most often in the setting of FAP. They usually develop on largely bland mucosa without evidence of significant gastritis *(47)*.

After tubular adenomas, pyloric gland adenomas are the second most common type of gastric adenoma. They are made up of closely packed pyloric type glands with unique immunohistochemical staining characteristics. They tend to occur in older women and are often found in patients with autoimmune gastritis. Average size of these lesions is 17 mm at time of diagnosis. There is a 30% reported rate of conversion to adenocarcinoma which is similar to that of villous adenomas *(48)*.

It is important to identify the etiology of the underlying gastritis in these patients because the risk of developing gastric cancer is more directly related to the presence of severe long-standing gastritis and intestinal metaplasia than to the specific polyp. When *H. pylori* gastritis is present it is reasonable to attempt *H. pylori* eradication although limited data would suggest that adenomotous polyps do not regress with *H. pylori* eradication *(31)*. Therapy is also unlikely to reverse the presence of atrophic gastritis or intestinal metaplasia.

The reported incidence of carcinoma in gastric adenomas has varied from a low of 6% to a high of 75% *(1,27,43, 44,49–54)*. Risk factors for development of carcinoma include size, presence of high-grade dysplasia, and intestinal-type epithelium *(27,47,52,53,55)*. Tomasulo observed that 24% of adenomatous polyps greater than 2 cm in diameter contained carcinoma, compared with 4% of those less than 2 cm in diameter *(53)*. Other series have also reported on the development of carcinoma in adenomatous polyps less than 2 cm *(40)*. Abraham et al. reviewed 61 gastric adenomas obtained from 51 patients over a 16-yr period. There were 34 intestinal-type adenomas among 31 patients. High-grade dysplasia was present in 15 and adenocacrinoma in 8 (4 intramucosal carcinoma and 4 invasive adenocarcinoma) of the 34 polyps. All except one of these patients had evidence of intestinal metaplasia or atrophic gastritis outside of the polyp. Five of these patients had separate adenocarcinomas in the stomach. In contrast, the 25 gastric-type adenomas only contained low-grade dysplasia. None had a synchronous or metachronous gastric carcinoma and the majority had little or no inflammatory mucosal pathology in the nonpolypoid mucosa. Of the 25 polyps, 17 were from 10 patients with FAP *(47)*. These findings are consistent with the fact that patients with FAP have a higher risk of duodenal and periampullary carcinoma but not necessarily an increased risk of gastric adenocarcinoma *(56–58)*.

As with hyperplastic polyps, endoscopic resection is the initial treatment of adenomatous polyps. Again, if *H. pylori* infection is present an attempt at eradication therapy should be made, although the benefits of this intervention are uncertain. Polyps unable to be resected endoscopically or those with evidence of adenocarcinoma may require operative resection.

3.4. SYNCHRONOUS GASTRIC CARCINOMA

The incidence of extrapolypoid carcinoma is increased with adenomatous and to a lesser extent with hyperplastic polyps. This reflects the presence of chronic gastritis and intestinal metaplasia, which is the background for the development of these polyps as well as the development of adenocarcinoma. Two older studies had reported a 1.2 to 28% rate of extrapolypoid gastric cancer in the setting of hyperplastic polyps (53,59). The true incidence is probably closer to the lower end of this range.

The increased risk of extrapolypoid carcinoma with adenomatous polyps is probably a reflection of the more advanced degree of intestinal metaplasia and atrophic gastritis in these patients as compared with hyperplastic polyps. In a total of 357 Finnish subjects with gastric polyps found at endoscopy, Laxen reported synchronous or metachronous carcinoma in 38% of patients with adenomotous polyps and 4.5% of patients with hyperplastic polyps (60). Harju reported on a 14-yr follow up of 170 Japanese patients with gastric polyps and found the development of gastric cancer in 2 of 15 patients with adenomas and 3 of 142 patients with hyperplastic polyps (44). Finally, in the series by Abraham et al. 5 of 51 (9.8%) patients with gastric adenomas had synchronous carcinoma. All five adenocarcinomas were present in patients with intestinal-type adenomas (47).

4. INFLAMMATORY FIBROID POLYPS

IFPs are uncommon, accounting for 3.1% of gastric polyps in one large series (4). Seventy to 90% of IFPs are found in the stomach, most commonly in the antrum. They are found to a lesser extent in the small bowel and rarely in the esophagus and colon (61). On average, they occur more often in women than men (1.6:1), with an average age of about 64 yr at presentation. They are polypoid with a smooth surface but can have surface erosions or ulcerations. They are non-neoplastic mesenchymal tumors arising from the deep mucosa or submucosa. Histologically they are characterized by loose stroma with an eosinophilic infiltrate and an onion-skin-like arrangement of reticular fibers around blood vessels. The average size is about 1 cm but they can be much larger, up to 7 cm in one report (62,63). They are usually asymptomatic but larger lesions can present with intermittent obstruction (prepyloric) or bleeding (64,65).

IFPs are likely reactive lesions that develop in response to chronic mucosal and submucosal injury. H. pylori infection, nonsteroidal anti-inflammatory drugs gastropathy, and argon plasma coagulation therapy have been suggested as etiological factors (66,67). Although considered non-neoplastic, Mori et al. (68) noted in a series of 50 IFPs, 4 cases of adenoma or adenocarcinoma restricted to the mucosa in or adjacent to a polyp. Owing to the submucosal nature of these polyps, standard forceps biopsy is unlikely to provide adequate tissue for diagnosis (69). Endoscopic ultrasound can be used to distinguish these lesions from other submucosal abnormalities such as leiomyomas and lipomas (Fig. 4). They appear as isoechoic expansions

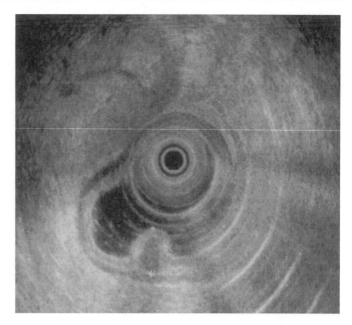

Fig. 4. IFP. EUS image (7.5 MHz) of a gastric IFP. Note the hypoechoic lesion with an indistinct border lying within the third sonographic layer. (Courtesy of Douglas O. Faigel, MD.)

of the second or third echolayer, corresponding to the deep mucosa or submucosa. They are hypoechoic and homogenous with an indistinct margin corresponding to a lack of a capsule on histology (70). Endosonographic findings are not specific for this lesion and should not be used as a substitute for histopathological diagnosis. Endoscopic resection with snare polypectomy is usually feasible as the lesion is limited to the submucosa. Endoscopic removal is curative although there is one report of recurrence after endoscopic resection (71). Patients have undergone surgical excision of these lesions because of size or atypical appearance concerning for malignancy (63,69).

5. GASTROINTESTINAL POLYPOSIS SYNDROMES

Gastrointestinal polyposis syndromes can be classified as adenomatous or hamartomatous, based on the histopathology of the predominant lesion. They are known for their association with colonic polyposis but they can also have extracolonic manifestations including gastric polyposis. The adenomatous syndromes consistent of FAP and its variants (attenuated FAP, Gardner's, and Turcot's syndrome). The most common harmatomatous syndrome is Peutz-Jeghers syndrome (PJS). The relative risk of gastric malignancy is not well defined. As such, recommendations for upper gastrointestinal surveillance are in large part based on limited evidence from case series and expert opinion.

5.1. ADENOMATOUS POLYPOSIS SYNDROMES

FAP is an autosomal dominant disorder defined by the presence of more than 100 colonic adenomas, usually thousands, and the inevitable development of colorectal cancer. The syndrome is caused by mutations of the APC gene. The phenotype of FAP and its variants is based on the specific APC gene mutation. The variants include the attenuated form (AAPC, hereditary flat adenoma syndrome), Gardner's, and Turcot's syndromes. All of these syndromes are associated with an increased rate of fundic gland and adenomatous polyposis.

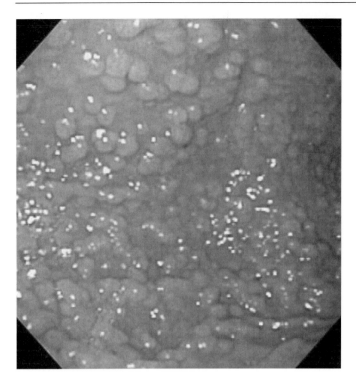

Fig. 5. FAP-associated fundic gland polyposis. No evidence of adenomatous changes were found on biopsy. (Courtesy of Michael L. Kochman, MD.)

FGPs are the most common gastric lesions in FAP. Between 26 and 84% of patients with FAP have FGPs *(6,7,72–74)*. FGPs tend to be more numerous in FAP than sporadic cases (Fig. 5). Although sporadic and FAP-associated FGPs are histologically indistinguishable, they are pathogenetically distinct. Abraham et al. reported on a series of 41 cases of FAP-associated polyps and 13 sporadic cases. Somatic *APC* gene alterations were identified in 21 of 41 (51%) FAP-associated cases but in only 1 of 13 (8%) sporadic cases *(9)*. This is consistent with the report by Bertoni et al., which revealed low-grade dysplasia in FGPs from 44% of FAP patients *(13)*. Zwick and Hofgartner reported on two siblings with attenuated FAP who died from metastatic gastric adenocarcinoma associated with fundic gland polyposis *(16,17)*.

Upper gastrointestinal tract adenomas are present in 90% or more of patients with FAP. The majority of these adenomas are duodenal or periampullary. Gastric adenomas are found in only 6–12% of Western populations *(73,74)*. These are mostly found in the antrum, although cases are reported of adenomas from the fundus or body of the stomach. Duodenal adenomas, however, are present in up to 67–92% of patients *(7,74,75)*. Offerhaus et al. calculated the relative risk of upper gastrointestinal tract cancer in patients with FAP based on the Johns Hopkins Registry. There was a relative risk of 330 for duodenal adenocarcinoma and 124 for ampullary adenocarcinoma but no significantly increased risk was found for gastric adenocarcinoma *(56)*. Although the magnitude of risk may be low, there are reports in the literature of patients with FAP developing gastric adenocarcinoma *(6,58)*. In contrast to Western populations, gastric adenomas are found in up to 50% of Japanese cases. The risk of gastric adenocarcinoma is also increased in these patients, which may be a reflection of the generally higher incidence of gastric adenocarcinoma in Japan.

Nonsteroidal anti-inflammatory drugs such as sulindac and celecoxib have had some success in decreasing the number and size of colorectal adenomas in FAP *(76–78)*. However, two small, randomized controlled trials evaluating the efficacy of sulindac have not been able to show a statistically significant reduction in the number or size of upper gastrointestinal polyps *(79,80)*. Surveillance of the upper gastrointestinal tract is focused on periampullary adenomas, because periampullary adenocarcinoma is the most common cause of death in patients with FAP who have undergone colectomy *(56,58)*. Initial endoscopy should occur close to the time of planned colectomy or early in the third decade of life with both end- and side-viewing endoscopes. Multiple biopsies should be obtained from the papilla even if the endoscopic appearance is normal as a majority of patients may harbor adenomas. When gastric polyps are seen removal by endoscopic polypectomy when feasible or at the least multiple forceps biopsy sampling should be undertaken. Any adenomatous polyps on histology should be removed on follow-up endoscopy. The frequency of surveillance endoscopy in FAP is unsettled and is dependent on the number of lesions, degrees of dysplasia and rate of growth in previously resected polyps. If no adenomas are detected it is reasonable to perform endoscopy every 3–5 yr. It may be necessary to perform surveillance endosocpy as often as every 6–12 mo in patients with dysplasia in the periampullary region *(81)*. Attenuated FAP (hereditary flat adenoma syndrome), Gardner's, and Turcot's syndromes represent variants of FAP with similar distribution of gastric polyps. Surveillance recommendations for these syndromes are the same as for patients with FAP.

5.2. HAMARTOMATOUS POLYPOSIS SYNDROMES
5.2.1. Peutz-Jeghers Syndrome

PJS is an autosomal-dominant disorder characterized by multiple hamartomatous gastrointestinal polyps and distinctive mucocutaenous pigmentation. The syndrome is caused by germline mutations of the *STK11/LKB1* gene that encodes for a serine threonine kinase, likely a tumor suppressor gene. Peutz-Jeghers polyps are composed of branching bands of smooth muscle projecting into the lamina propria. The lamina propria and surface epithelium are normal. They can range in size from 1 to 2 mm to several centimeters. These polyps can rarely occur in the absence of the syndrome.

Pigmented mucocutatenous lesions tend to develop within the first 1–2 yr of life, gradually increase in number, and then fade after puberty with the exception of those on the buccal mucosa. In contrast, gastrointestinal polyps develop during the first decade of life and become symptomatic in the second and third decades. Patients most commonly present with small bowel obstruction caused by intussception or occlusion of the lumen by a large polyp. They can also present with acute or chronic blood loss. The polyps are most frequent in the small bowel but occur in the stomach in 49% of affected patients in one series *(82)*. Carcinomas and adenomas arising from Peutz-Jeghers polyps have been described in the literature *(83–85)*. Synchronous adenomatous polyps may also develop among the hamartomatous polyps *(86)*. Patients have higher rates of both gastrointestinal and nongastrointestinal (mostly breast,

gynecological, and testicular) malignancy (87,88). In the St.
Mark's Polyposis Registry, patients with PJS had a 13-fold
relative risk of death from gastrointestinal cancer. In reviewing
the St. Marks's Polyposis Registry and the Johns Hopkins
Registry (103 patients with PJS), 24% of the gastrointestinal
malignancies were in the stomach and almost half in the small
bowel. Data supporting an increased risk of upper gastrointestinal cancer has led some experts to recommend endoscopic
surveillance every 2–5 yr, beginning at 25–30 yr of age
(83,89,90).

5.2.2. Juvenile Polyposis and Related Syndromes

Juvenile polyposis is another hamartomatous polyposis syndrome that is inherited in an autosomal-dominant fashion,
although the gene locus for this disorder has yet to be fully elucidated (91). Polyposis can be limited to the colon, limited to
the stomach or distributed throughout the gastrointestinal tract
(92,93). These polyps are characterized by abundant, loose
stroma, and elongated, rarely cystic mucinous glands covered
by normal appearing epithelium. The lamina propria is
expanded with inflammation. Unlike Peutz-Jeghers polyps,
they do not have an increased density of smooth muscle fibers
(28). They appear as smooth, firm, pedunculated lesions, and
may have a white tip. They are usually about 1 cm in diameter.
Solitary juvenile polyps may be seen in up to 2% of children
and adolescents and have no malignant potential. Hyperplastic
polyps may also be seen in familial juvenile polyposis patients.
Development of neoplasia has been documented in Peutz-Jeghers
polyps ranging from low-grade dysplasia to adenocarcinoma.

The most common presentations are anemia and protein-
losing enteropathy in the first decade of life, but these polyps
can also cause obstruction and lead to gastrointestinal malignancy (Fig. 6). Gastric cancer risk has been reported at 15–21%
(94,95). Gastric cancer has been described in patients with only
colonic polyps in addition to diffuse and gastric polyposis (94).
It is not unreasonable to perform upper endoscopy pre-operatively
in patients who are undergoing colon resection for cancer or
bleeding. One European expert panel recommends upper
gastrointestinal screening starting at age 25 with 1–2 yr intervals
contemporaneously with colorectal cancer surveillance (90).

Cowden's disease and Bannayan-Ruvalcaba-Riley syndrome
are related syndromes with autosomal-dominant inheritance
and juvenile polyposis but with a much lower risk of gastrointestinal cancer. Cowden's disease consists of multiple hamartomatous polyps of the stomach, small and large bowel, and is
related to a mutation of the PTEN tumor suppressor gene. The
extraintestinal manifestations include multiple facial trichilemmomas, breast, and thyroid cancer. There does not appear to
be an increased risk of gastrointestinal cancer in these patients
(96–99). Bannayan-Ruvalcaba-Riley syndrome consists of
hamartomatous gastrointestinal polyposis with macrocephaly,
developmental delay and pigmented spots on the penis (91).

Unlike the syndromes discussed earlier, Cronkhite-Canada
syndrome is an acquired, nonfamilial syndrome of diffuse gastrointestinal juvenile polyposis. The extraintestinal manifestations include onycholysis, alopecia and skin hyperpigmention.
Patients typically present in middle age or older (average 62 yr)
with rapid onset of progressive diarrhea, protein-losing

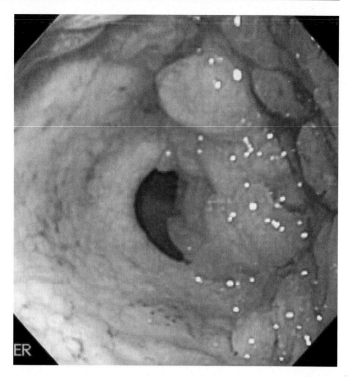

Fig. 6. Juvenile Polyposis in a young woman presenting with gastrointestinal bleeding, nausea and vomiting. The latter symptoms were
due to antral polyps prolapsing into the pylorus.

enteropathy, and associated skin changes (100). Gastric polyps
in this disorder are indistinguishable from those in juvenile polyposis (101). There have been reports of at least three patients
with gastric cancer developing in association with this syndrome, although this is probably a rare complication (102,103).

6. ENDOSCOPIC MANAGEMENT

The initial step in endoscopic evaluation and management
of gastric polyps is to determine the histology. Subepithelial
lesions can be distinguished from epithelial polyps by endoscopic and endosonographic features. The clinical setting
along with endoscopic features may suggest a diagnosis, however, polyp histology cannot be reliably assessed by endoscopic appearance alone (41,42).

Forceps biopsy sampling may not provide adequate tissue
for accurate diagnosis. Complete resection and retrieval of the
entire lesion is preferred (40,104,105). In a prospective, multicenter trial, Muehldorfer et al. reported on 222 polyps among
194 patients, excluding those with FGPs and polyposis syndromes, reviewed by the primary and a reference pathologist.
Based on primary pathologist review, there was complete
agreement in only 124 cases (55.8%) between forceps biopsy
sampling and complete polypectomy. In 77 polyps (34.7%),
there was disagreement as to the exact tissue diagnosis, the
distinction between neoplastic and non-neoplastic polyp did
not change. However, in 21 cases (9.5%) there were important
discrepancies by individual pathologists. Even after review by
the reference pathologist there were six polyps (2.7%) with
clinically significant differences including the presence of
adenocarcinoma that was not discovered with biopsy sampling

(106). Although the discrepancy rate in this study was lower than that of previous studies the evidence still supports complete removal of epithelial gastric polyps rather than forceps biopsy sampling. If the risk of polypectomy is no greater than that conveyed to the patient at the time of consent, complete excision with snare polypectomy should be performed with all tissue submitted for pathologic diagnosis. Otherwise, forceps biopsy sampling may be performed at the time of initial endoscopy with the expectation of polypectomy at a later time pending pathology results.

The risk of malignant conversion is based on polyp histology. Because they have no malignant potential, sporadic FGPs might be disregarded once a histological diagnosis by forceps biopsy has been established. Jumbo forceps or piecemeal cold biopsy resection can generally remove polyps less than 5 mm. All symptomatic polyps should be endoscopically removed when possible. All adenomatous polyps, regardless of size should be removed because of their potential for malignancy. All polyps greater than 2 cm in size should also be removed regardless of histology, as they are more likely to harbor carcinoma. The question arises with large polyps not amenable to endoscopic resection. If biopsy sampling reveals adenomatous tissue, these patients should be referred for surgical excision. If no adenomatous tissue is detected from biopsy sampling it might still be reasonable to refer for surgical excision depending on the perceived risk–benefit ratio for each patient. However, carcinoma has been documented to arise from epithelial polyps less than 2 cm in size *(39,40,53,107).* As discussed earlier forceps biopsy alone of small (<2 cm), asymptomatic hyperplastic polyps may fail to identify focal adenoma or carcinoma *(43,105–107).* Therefore total excision of these polyps, preferably by endoscopic snare resection, is recommended. Gastric polypectomy allows for definitive histological diagnosis and, in most cases, cure *(1,81,107).*

Endoscopic polypectomy is widely available and generally safe. Complications include bleeding and perforation. Bleeding associated with gastric polypectomy occurs more frequently than in colonic polypectomy. Postpolypectomy bleeding can usually be managed endoscopically *(107).* The rate of bleeding in the study by Muehldorfer was 7.2% (16/194). Hemostasis was achieved by endoscopic means in all but one patient. One patient underwent laparotomy and two patients required blood transfusions. One patient had a suspected closed perforation that was managed conservatively *(106).* As the majority of gastric polyps are benign, polypectomy is usually curative. Local recurrence is uncommon and usually attributed to incomplete polyp removal. In the series by Seifert et al., the local recurrence rate was 6.1% *(1,41,43).* At the time of polypectomy it may be reasonable to obtain random biopsies of the surrounding mucosa, especially when there is suspicion of a contributing process to polyp formation such as *H. pylori* gastritis.

6.1. MULTIPLE GASTRIC POLYPS

When multiple polyps are present, they tend to be of like histology *(41).* Hyperplastic and adenomatous polyps tend to develop on a background of chronic gastritis. Therefore, both polyps may be found together in some patients *(27,43,44,53).* Because endoscopic appearance cannot differentiate between neoplastic and non-neoplastic polyps, an attempt should be made to completely excise all polyps. When this is not feasible owing to large numbers of (nonfundic gland) polyps, the largest polyps should be removed by snare cautery and biopsy sampling of as many others as possible should be undertaken. This practice will decrease the risk of missing adenomatous or dysplastic changes. Polypectomy over several endoscopic sessions may be required to remove all significant polyps.

6.2. GASTRIC POLYPECTOMY

If gastric polypectomy is anticipated, the increased risk of bleeding and perforation should be relayed to the patient and documented on the consent form. The use of a therapeutic endoscope is preferred because it allows for more options during polyp resection and hemostasis in the setting of postpolypectomy bleeding. Intravenous glucagon administration should be considered before attempted resection to decrease the risk of polyp passage into the duodenum. Polyp removal by the Roth polyp retrieval net (Endoscopy Group Inc, Mentor, OH) prevents the accidental release of the polyp into the airway and therefore avoids the need for overtube placement. Endosonography can be useful in polyp resection. It can identify the tissue depth of the polyp to determine if endsocpic resection is feasible *(70).* It can also identify large (>2.5 mm) feeder vessels that may preclude endoscopic resection *(108).* Endoscopic hemostasis is generally effective in vessels up to 2.5 mm in diameter. Injection of 2–4 mL of 1:10,000 epinephrine into the stalk before resection may reduce the likelihood of acute postpolypectomy bleeding. Endoscopic placement of a metallic mucosal clip or injection of dehydrated alcohol into the stalk can also be used before or after polyp resection to prevent bleeding. Other creative approaches such as band ligation have been reported, although they have not been directly compared with established techniques *(109,110).* Injection with 1:10,000 epinephrine, bipolar electrocautery, mucosal clips, and argon plasma coagulation are effective in achieving endoscopic hemostasis. Rarely, patients might require interventional radiology or surgery to achieve hemostasis *(106,111).* The use of acid suppressive therapy postpolypectomy may enhance healing of ulceration at the resection site and prevent delayed bleeding. We recommend an 8-wk course of PPI therapy after polypectomy to enhance healing at the polypectomy site.

6.3. SURVEILLANCE

Appropriate surveillance recommendations require an understanding of the natural history of gastric polyps. The natural history of gastric polyps however is not as well defined as that for colonic polyps. Sporadic FGPs have no malignant potential. Their numbers may increase or decrease over time but they are likely to remain unchanged. Therefore, endoscopic surveillance is unnecessary in these patients.

Hyperplastic polyps tend to remain unchanged in size and number *(112).* In some cases they might increase or decrease in size or number and they may recur after resection *(43,112).* Changes in *H. pylori* status may affect the natural course of these lesions with some reports documenting regression or disappearance after *H. pylori* eradication *(31,32).* It is reasonable to test and treat for *H. pylori* in these patients as it may reduce the likelihood of polyp recurrence. Once these polyps are removed, a repeat endoscopy is reasonable to assess for polyp recurrence, *H. pylori* status and evidence of ongoing gastritis. Biopsy sampling of uninvolved gastric mucosa should be performed to assess for the presence of intestinal metaplasia and dysplasia. If the findings are reassuring on repeat endoscopy, continued surveillance is not necessary.

Gastic adenomas should be removed at the time of initial diagnosis. The recurrence rate for adenomas is higher than that for hyperplastic polyps at 16% in one series *(43)*. Repeat endoscopy should be performed at 1 yr to assess for polyp recurrence and survey the remaining mucosa for evidence of synchronous or metachronous adenocarcinoma. In the absence of positive findings, repeat endoscopy may be considered at 3- to 5-yr intervals *(81)*.

Several retrospective and case–control studies have documented an association between gastric polyposis and increased colorectal cancer risk *(18,26,113)*. Many of the patients in these studies had other indications for colonoscopy so it is unclear if selection bias contributed to these findings. A question for further study is whether all patients presenting with gastric polyps should undergo screening for colorectal cancer.

7. CONCLUSION

Gastric polyps are common findings at endoscopy. In the majority of cases, complete resection of gastric polyps is advocated. Adenomatous and hyperplastic gastric polyps have the potential to become malignant and management based on biopsy forceps tissue sampling alone may be inappropriate. Complete excision with snare resection should be undertaken when feasible. All FGPs do not need to be removed, once a sampling of these polyps has verified the diagnosis. FGPs in the setting of FAP may have a small risk of becoming malignant and there is evidence supporting regular surveillance. Local recurrence of gastric polyps is uncommon, especially when adequate resection margins are achieved. Endosonography may aid in diagnosis by determining the tissue layer of origin and in therapy by assessing the safety/feasibility of endoscopic resection. Endoscopic screening and surveillance for gastric polyps is appropriate in the setting of FAP and its variant syndromes. The exact interval of surveillance will depend on the numbers and types of polyps encountered on initial endoscopy. Patients with PJS and familial juvenile polyposis are also at increased risk for development of gastric cancer. They may be offered a screening endoscopy by age 30, but the optimal time of initial endoscopy and appropriate frequency of surveillance has yet to be defined.

REFERENCES

1. Ghazi A, Ferstenberg H, Shinya H. Endoscopic gastroduodenal polypectomy. Ann Surg 1984; 200:175–180.
2. Archimandritis A, Spiliadis C, Tzivras M, et al. Gastric epithelial polyps: a retrospective endoscopic study of 12974 symptomatic patients. Ital J Gastroenterol 1996; 28:387–390.
3. Dekker W. Clinical Relevance of gastric and duodenal polyps. Scand J Gastroenterol Suppl 1990; 178:7–12.
4. Stolte M, Sticht T, Eidt S, Ebert D, Finkenzeller G. Frequency, location, and age and sex distribution of various types of gastric polyp. Endoscopy 1994; 26:659–665.
5. Haruma K, Sumii K, Yoshihara M, Watanabe C, Kajiyama G, Gastric mucosa in female patients with fundic gland polyps. J Clin Gastroenterol 1991; 13:565–569.
6. Watanabe H, Enjoji M, Yao T, Ohsato K. Gastric lesions in familial adenomatosis coli: their incidence and histologic analysis. Hum Pathol 1978; 9:269–283.
7. Church JM, McGannon E, Hull-Boiner S, et al. Gastroduodenal polyps in patients with familial adenomatous polyposis. Dis Colon Rectum 1992; 35:1170–1173.
8. Odze RD, Marcial MA, Antonioli D. Gastric fundic gland polyps: a morphological study including mucin histochemistry, stereometry, and MIB-1 immunohistochemistry. Hum Pathol 1996; 27: 896–903.
9. Abraham SC, Nobukawa B, Giardiello FM, Hamilton SR, Wu TT. Fundic gland polyps in familial adenomatous polyposis: neoplasms with frequent somatic adenomatous polyposis coli gene alterations. Am J Pathol 2000; 157:747–754.
10. Abraham SC, Nobukawa B, Giardiello FM, Hamilton SR, Wu TT. Sporadic fundic gland polyps: common gastric polyps arising through activating mutations in the beta-catenin gene. Am J Pathol 2001; 158:1005–1010.
11. Abraham SC, Park SJ, Mugartegui L, Hamilton SR, Wu TT. Sporadic fundic gland polyps with epithelial dysplasia: evidence for preferential targeting for mutations in the adenomatous polyposis coli gene. Am J Pathol 2002; 161:1735–1742.
12. Wu TT, Kornacki S, Rashid A, Yardley JH, Hamilton SR. Dysplasia and dysregulation of proliferation in foveolar and surface epithelia of fundic gland polyps from patients with familial adenomatous polyposis. Am J Surg Pathol 1998; 22:293–298.
13. Bertoni G, Sassatelli R, Nigrisoli E, et al. Dysplastic changes in gastric fundic gland polyps of patients with familial adenomatous polyposis. Ital J Gastroenterol Hepatol 1999; 31:192–197.
14. Coffey RJ Jr, Knight CD Jr, van Heerden JA, Weiland LH. Gastric adenocarcinoma complicating Gardner's syndrome in a North American woman. Gastroenterology 1985; 88:1263–1266.
15. Goodman AJ, Dundas SA, Scholefield JH, Johnson BF. Gastric carcinoma and familial adenomatous polyposis (FAP). Int J Colorectal Dis 1988; 3:201–203.
16. Zwick A, Munir M, Ryan CK, et al. Gastric adenocarcinoma and dysplasia in fundic gland polyps of a patient with attenuated adenomatous polyposis coli. Gastroenterology 1997; 113:659–663.
17. Hofgartner WT, Thorp M, Ramus MW, et al. Gastric adenocarcinoma associated with fundic gland polyps in a patient with attenuated familial adenomatous polyposis. Am J Gastroenterol 1999; 94:2275–2281.
18. Jung A, Vieth M, Maier O, Stolte M. Fundic gland polyps (Elster's cysts) of the gastric mucosa. A marker for colorectal epithelial neoplasia? Pathol Res Pract 2002; 198:731–734.
19. Sakai N, Tatsuta M, Hirasawa R, et al. Low prevalence of H. pylori infection in patients with hamartomatous fundic polyps. Dig Dis Sci 1998; 43:766–772.
20. Watanabe N, Seno H, Nakajima T, et al. Regression of fundic gland polyps following acquisition of Helicobacter pylori. Gut 2002; 51:742–745.
21. el-Zimaity HM, Jackson FW, Graham DY. Fundic gland polyps developing during omeprazole therapy. Am J Gastroenterol 1997; 92:1858–1860.
22. Choudhry U, Boyce HW Jr, Coppola D. Proton pump inhibitor-associated gastric polyps: a retrospective analysis of their frequency, and endoscopic, histologic, and ultrastructural characteristics. Am J Clin Pathol 1998; 110:615–621.
23. Vieth M, Stolte M. Fundic gland polyps are not induced by proton pump inhibitor therapy. Am J Clin Pathol 2001; 116:716–20.
24. Weston BR, Helper DJ, Rex DK. Positive predictive value of endoscopic features deemed typical of gastric fundic gland polyps. J Clin Gastroenterol 2003; 36:399–402.
25. Kazantsev GB, Schwesinger WH, Heim-Hall J. Spontaneous resolution of multiple fundic gland polyps after cessation of treatment with lansoprazole and Nissen fundoplication: a case report. Gastrointest Endosc 2002; 55:600–602.

26. Eidt S, Stolte M. Gastric glandular cysts—investigations into their genesis and relationship to colorectal epithelial tumors. Z Gastroenterol 1989; 27:212–217.

27. Orlowska J, Jarosz D, Pachlewski J, Butruk E. Malignant transformation of benign epithelial gastric polyps. Am J Gastroenterol 1995; 90:2152–2159.

28. Oberhuber G Stolte M. Gastric polyps: an update of their pathology and biological significance. Virchows Arch 2000; 437: 581–590.

29. Cerwenka H, Bacher H, Mischinger HJ. Pyloric obstruction caused by prolapse of a hyperplastic gastric polyp. Hepatogastroenterology 2002; 49:958–960.

30. Gencosmanoglu R, Sen-Oran E, Kurtkaya-Yapicier O, Tozun N. Antral hyperplastic polyp causing intermittent gastric outlet obstruction: case report. BMC Gastroenterol 2003; 3:16.

31. Ljubicic N Banic M, Kujundzic M, et al. The effect of eradicating Helicobacter pylori infection on the course of adenomatous and hyperplastic gastric polyps. Eur J Gastroenterol Hepatol 1999; 11:727–730.

32. Ohkusa T, Takashimizu I, Fujiki K, et al. Disappearance of hyperplastic polyps in the stomach after eradication of Helicobacter pylori. A randomized, clinical trial. Ann Intern Med 1998; 129:712–715.

33. Metz DC. Hyperplastic gastric polyps: medical management is feasible. Am J Gastroenterol 1999; 94:1977–1978.

34. Ohkusa T, Miwa H, Hojo M, et al. Endoscopic, histological and serologic findings of gastric hyperplastic polyps after eradication of Helicobacter pylori: comparison between responder and non-responder cases. Digestion 2003; 68:57–62.

35. Geller A, Gostout CJ, Balm RK. Development of hyperplastic polyps following laser therapy for watermelon stomach. Gastrointest Endosc 1996; 43:54–56.

36. Yoshikane H, Asai T, Sakakibara A, et al. Gastric hyperplastic polyp occurring at the resection site of gastric adenoma. Endoscopy 1999; 31:563–565.

37. Amaro R, Neff GW, Karnam US, Tzakis AG, Raskin JB. Acquired hyperplastic gastric polyps in solid organ transplant patients. Am J Gastroenterol 2002; 97:2220–2224.

38. Daibo M, Itabashi M, Hirota T. Malignant transformation of gastric hyperplastic polyps. Am J Gastroenterol 1987; 82:1016–1025.

39. Zea-Iriarte WL, Sekine I, Itsuno M, et al. Carcinoma in gastric hyperplastic polyps. A phenotypic study. Dig Dis Sci 1996; 41:377–386.

40. Ginsberg GG, Al-Kawas FH, Fleischer DE, Reilly HF, Benjamin SB. Gastric polyps: relationship of size and histology to cancer risk. Am J Gastroenterol 1996 91:714–717.

41. Deppisch LM, Rona VT. Gastric epithelial polyps. A 10-year study. J Clin Gastroenterol 1989; 11:110–115.

42. Snover DC. Benign epithelial polyps of the stomach. Pathol Annu 1985; 20:303–329.

43. Seifert E, Gail K, Weismuller J. Gastric polypectomy. Long-term results (survey of 23 centres in Germany). Endoscopy 1983; 15:8–11.

44. Harju E. Gastric polyposis and malignancy. Br J Surg 1986; 73:532–533.

45. Rattan J, Arber N, Tiomny E, et al. Gastric polypoid lesions—an eight-year study. Hepatogastroenterology 1993 40:107–109.

46. Nakamura K, Sakaguchi H, Enjoji M. Depressed adenocarcinoma of the stomach. Cancer 1988; 62:2197–202.

47. Abraham SC, Montgomery EA, Singh VK, Yardley JH, Wu TT. Gastric adenomas: intestinal-type and gastric-type adenomas differ in the risk of adenocarcinoma and presence of background mucosal pathology. Am J Surg Pathol 2002; 26:1276–1285.

48. Vieth M, Kushima R, Borchard F, Stolte M. Pyloric gland adenoma: a clinico-pathological analysis of 90 cases. Virchows Arch 2003; 442(4):317–321.

49. Nakamura T, Nakano G. Histopathological classification and malignant change in gastric polyps. J Clin Pathol 1985; 38:754–764.

50. Kolodziejczyk P, Yao T, Oya M, et al. Long-term follow-up study of patients with gastric adenomas with malignant transformation. An immunohistochemical and histochemical analysis. Cancer 1994; 74:2896–2907.

51. Stolte M. Clinical consequences of the endoscopic diagnosis of gastric polyps. Endoscopy 1995; 27:32–37; discussion 59,60.

52. Park DI, Rhee PL, Kim JE, et al. Risk factors suggesting malignant transformation of gastric adenoma: univariate and multivariate analysis. Endoscopy 2001; 33:501–506.

53. Tomasulo J. Gastric polyps. Histologic types and their relationship to gastric carcinoma. Cancer 1971; 27:1346–1355.

54. Cristallini EG, Ascani S, Bolis GB. Association between histologic type of polyp and carcinoma of the stomach. Gastrointest Endosc 1992; 38:481–484.

55. Antonioli DA. Precursors of gastric carcinoma: a critical review with a brief description of early (curable) gastric cancer. Hum Path 1994 25:994–1005.

56. Offerhaus GJ, Giardiello FM, Krush AJ, et al. The risk of upper gastrointestinal cancer in familial adenomatous polyposis. Gastroenterology 1992; 102:1980–1982.

57. Marcello PW, Asbun HJ, Veidenheimer MC, et al. Gastroduodenal polyps in familial adenomatous polyposis. Surg Endosc 1996; 10:418–421.

58. Jagelman DG, DeCosse JJ, Bussey HJ. Upper gastrointestinal cancer in familial adenomatous polyposis. Lancet 1988; 1(8595): 1149–1151.

59. Yamagata S, Hisamichi S. Precancerous lesions of the stomach. World J Surg 1979; 3:671–673.

60. Laxen F. Gastric carcinoma and pernicious anemia in long-term endoscopic follow-up of subjects with gastric polyps. Scand J Gastroenterol 1984; 19:535–540.

61. Shalom A, Wasserman I, Segal M, Orda R. Inflammatory fibroid polyp and Helicobacter pylori. Aetiology or coincidence? Eur J Surg 2000; 166:54–57.

62. Stolte M, Finkenzeller G. Inflammatory fibroid polyp of the stomach. Endoscopy 1990; 22:203–207.

63. Adachi MM, Iida M, Tsuneyoshi M, Sugimachi K. Inflammatory fibroid polyp of the stomach. Report of three unusual cases. J Clin Gastroenterol 1992; 15:154–158.

64. Shigeno T, Fujimori K, Nakatsuji Y, Kaneko Y, Maejima T. Gastric inflammatory fibroid polyp manifesting massive bleeding and marked morphological changes for a short period. J Gastroenterol 2003; 38:611,612.

65. Tada S, Iida M, Yao T, et al. Endoscopic removal of inflammatory fibroid polyps of the stomach. Am J Gastroenterol 1991; 86: 1247–1250.

66. Schmeck-Lindenau HJ, Kurtz W, Heine M. Inflammatory polyps: an unreported side effect of argon plasma coagulation. Endoscopy 1998; 30:S93,S94.

67. Varis O, Laxen F, Valle J. Helicobacter pylori infection and fasting serum gastrin levels in a series of endoscopically diagnosed gastric polyps. Acta Path Micro Immunol Scand 1994; 102:759–764.

68. Mori M, Tamura S, Enjoji M, Sugimachi K. Concomitant presence of inflammatory fibroid polyp and carcinoma or adenoma in the stomach. Arch Pathol Lab Med 1988; 112:829–832.

69. Hizawa K, Iida M, Tada S, et al. Endoscopic evaluation of gastric inflammatory fibroid polyp. Surg Endosc 1995; 9:397–400.

70. Matsushita M, Hajiro K, Okazaki K, Takakuwa H. Gastric inflammatory fibroid polyps: endoscopic ultrasonographic analysis in comparison with the histology. Gastrointest Endosc 1997; 46:53–57.

71. Zinkiewicz K, Zgodzinski W, Dabrowski A, Szumilo J, Cwik G, Wallner G. Recurrent inflammatory fibroid polyp of cardia: a case report. World J Gastroenterol 2004; 10:767,768.

72. Jarvinen HJ, Sipponen P. Gastroduodenal polyps in familial adenomatous and juvenile polyposis. Endoscopy 1986; 18:230–234.

73. Jarvinen H, Nyberg M, Peltokallio P. Upper gastrointestinal tract polyps in familial adenomatosis coli. Gut 1983; 24:333–339.

74. Domizio P, Talbot IC, Spigelman AD, Williams CB, Phillips RK. Upper gastrointestinal pathology in familial adenomatous polyposis: results from a prospective study of 102 patients. J Clin Pathol 1990; 43:738–743.

75. Goedde TA, Rodriguez-Bigas MA, Herrera L, Petrelli NJ. Gastroduodenal polyps in familial adenomatous polyposis. Surg Oncol 1992; 1:357–361.

76. Giardiello FM, Offerhaus GJ, DuBois RN. The role of nonsteroidal anti-inflammatory drugs in colorectal cancer prevention. Eur J Cancer 1995; 31A:1071–1076.

77. Steinbach G, Lynch PM, Phillips RK, et al. The effect of celecoxib, a cyclooxygenase-2 inhibitor, in familial adenomatous polyposis. N Engl J Med 2000; 342:1946–1952.

78. Labayle D, Fischer D, Vielh P, et al. Sulindac causes regression of rectal polyps in familial adenomatous polyposis. Gastroenterology 1991; 101:635–639.

79. Nugent KP, Farmer KC, Spigelman AD, Williams CB, Phillips RK. Randomized controlled trial of the effect of sulindac on duodenal and rectal polyposis and cell proliferation in patients with familial adenomatous polyposis. Br J Surg 1993; 80:1618,1619.

80. Seow-Choen F, Vijayan V, Keng V. Prospective randomized study of sulindac versus calcium and calciferol for upper gastrointestinal polyps in familial adenomatous polyposis. Br J Surg 1996; 83:1763–1766.

81. Anonymous. The role of endoscopy in the surveillance of premalignant conditions of the upper gastrointestinal tract. American Society for Gastrointestinal Endoscopy. Gastrointest Endosc 1998; 48:663–668.

82. Utsunomiya J, Gocho H, Miyanaga T, Hamaguchi E, Kashimure A. Peutz-Jeghers syndrome: its natural course and management. Johns Hopkins Med J 1975; 136:71–82.

83. Konishi F, Wyse NE, Muto T, et al. Peutz-Jeghers polyposis associated with carcinoma of the digestive organs. Report of three cases and review of the literature. Dis Colon Rectum 1987; 30:790–799.

84. Perzin KH, Bridge MF. Adenomatous and carcinomatous changes in hamartomatous polyps of the small intestine (Peutz-Jeghers syndrome): report of a case and review of the literature. Cancer 1982; 49:971–983.

85. Defago MR, Higa AL, Campra JL, et al. Carcinoma in situ arising in a gastric hamartomatous polyp in a patient with Peutz-Jeghers syndrome. Endoscopy 1996; 28:267.

86. Linos DA, Dozois RR, Dahlin DC, Bartholomew LG. Does Peutz-Jeghers syndrome predispose to gastrointestinal malignancy? A later look. Arch Surg 1981; 116:1182–1184.

87. Spigelman AD, Murday V, Phillips RK. Cancer and the Peutz-Jeghers syndrome. Gut 1989; 30:1588–1590.

88. Giardiello FM, Welsh SB, Hamilton SR, et al. Increased risk of cancer in the Peutz-Jeghers syndrome. N Engl J Med 1987; 316:1511–1514.

89. Foley TR, McGarrity TJ, Abt AB. Peutz-Jeghers syndrome: a clinicopathologic survey of the "Harrisburg family" with a 49-year follow-up. Gastroenterology 1988; 95:1535–1540.

90. Dunlop MG, British Society for Gastroenterology. Association of Coloproctology for Great Britain and Ireland. Guidance on gastrointestinal surveillance for hereditary non-polyposis colorectal cancer, familial adenomatous polyposis, juvenile polyposis, and Peutz-Jeghers syndrome. Gut 2002; 51(Suppl 5):V21–V27.

91. Woodford-Richens K, Bevan S, Churchman M, et al. Analysis of genetic and phenotypic heterogeneity in juvenile polyposis. Gut 2000; 46:656–660.

92. Goodman ZD, Yardley JH, Milligan FD. Pathogenesis of colonic polyps in multiple juvenile polyposis: report of a case associated with gastric polyps and carcinoma of the rectum. Cancer 1979; 43:1906–1913.

93. Hizawa K, Iida M, Yao T, Aoyagi K, Fujishima M. Juvenile polyposis of the stomach: clinicopathological features and its malignant potential. J Clin Pathol 1997; 50:771–774.

94. Howe JR, Mitros FA, Summers RW. The risk of gastrointestinal carcinoma in familial juvenile polyposis. Ann Surg Oncol 1998:751–756.

95. Scott-Conner CE, Hausmann M., Hall TJ, Skelton DS. Anglin BL. Subramony C. Familial juvenile polyposis: patterns of recurrence and implications for surgical management. J Am Coll Surg 1995; 181:407–413.

96. Taylor AJ, Dodds WJ, Stewart ET. Alimentary tract lesions in Cowden's disease. Br J Radiol 1989; 62:890–892.

97. Marra G, Armelao F, Vecchio FM, Percesepe A, Anti M. Cowden's disease with extensive gastrointestinal polyposis. J Clin Gastroenterol 1994; 18:42–47.

98. Hizawa K, Iida M, Matsumoto T, et al. Gastrointestinal manifestations of Cowden's disease. Report of four cases. J Clin Gastroenterol 1994; 18:13–18.

99. Chilovi F, Zancanella L, Perino F, et al. Cowden's disease with gastrointestinal polyposis. Gastrointest Endosc 1990; 36:323,324.

100. Daniel ES, Ludwig SL, Lewin KJ, Ruprecht RM, Rajacich GM, Schwabe AD. The Cronkhite-Canada Syndrome. An analysis of clinical and pathologic features and therapy in 55 patients. Medicine 1982; 61:203–309.

101. Burke AP, Sobin LH. The pathology of Cronkhite-Canada polyps. A comparison to juvenile polyposis. Am J Surg Pathol 1989; 13:940–946.

102. Sagara K, Fujiyama S, Kamuro Y, Tashiro A, Sato T. Cronkhite-canada syndrome associated with gastric cancer: report of a case. Gastroenterol Jpn 1983; 18:260–266.

103. Watanabe T, Kudo M, Shirane H, et al. Cronkhite-Canada syndrome associated with triple gastric cancers: a case report. Gastrointest Endosc 1999; 50:688–691.

104. Seifert E, Elster K. Gastric polypectomy. Am J Gastroenterol 1975; 63:451–456.

105. Fabry TL, Frankel A, Waye JD. Gastric polyps. J Clin Gastroenterol 1982; 4:23–27.

106. Muehldorfer SM, Stolte M, Martus P, Hahn EG, Ell C. Multicenter Study Group "Gastric Polyps". Diagnostic accuracy of forceps biopsy versus polypectomy for gastric polyps: a prospective multicentre study. Gut 2002; 50:465–470.

107. ReMine SG, Hughes RW Jr, Weiland LH. Endoscopic gastric polypectomies. Mayo Clin Proc 1981; 56:371–375.

108. Gyrtrup HJ, Siemsen M, Vilmann P, Mogensen AM. Endoscopic ultrasonography in the evaluation of gastric polyps in juvenile polyposis. Endoscopy 1997; 29:136,137.

109. Tursi A, Brandimarte G. Endoscopic polypectomy of large pedunculated gastric polyps using a new, safe, and effective technique. Endoscopy 2002; 34:673,674.

110. Lo CC, Hsu PI, Lo GH, et al. Endoscopic banding ligation can effectively resect hyperplastic polyps of stomach. World J Gastroenterol 2003; 9:2805–2808.

111. Wahab P, Mulder CJ, den Hartog G, Thies JE. Argon plasma coagulation in flexible gastrointestinal endoscopy: pilot experiences. Endoscopy 1997; 29:176–181.

112. Kamiya T, Morishita T, Asakura H, Munakata Y, Miura S, Tsuchiya M. Histoclinical long-standing follow-up study of hyperplastic polyps of the stomach. Am J Gastroenterol 1981; 75: 275–281.

113. Cappell MS, Fiest TC. A multicenter, multiyear, case-controlled study of the risk of colonic polyps in patients with gastric polyps. Are gastric adenomas a new indication for surveillance colonoscopy? J Clin Gastroenterol 1995; 21:198–202.

11 Endoscopic Ultrasound for Staging Gastric Cancer

GREGORY OLDS, MD AND AMITABH CHAK, MD

CONTENTS

1. BACKGROUND

Although the incidence of gastric cancer is declining, it remains a leading cause of cancer-related death worldwide. Prognosis in gastric cancer is highly correlated with tumor stage. Surgical therapy remains the definitive therapy. Accurate pre-operative staging is essential, especially in patients who may be marginal surgical candidates. Accurate staging also is of particular importance in early gastric cancer in which select lesions confined to the mucosa may be treated with local endoscopic mucosal resection. Endoscopic ultrasound (EUS) currently is the most accurate test in the local–regional staging of gastric cancer. Advanced gastric cancers should be staged with a combination of EUS and computed tomography (CT). Local therapy can be appropriately applied to early gastric cancers that have no nodal involvement and are limited to the muscularis mucosa. The additional use of EUS-fine-needle aspiration (FNA) for lymph nodes distant from the primary tumor may improve staging accuracy.

2. EUS TECHNIQUE

Studies evaluating EUS staging of gastric cancers have predominantly used radial sector scanning echoendoscopes at frequencies of 7.5 and 12 MHz. A frequency of 7.5 MHz allows for a maximal depth of penetration of about 10 cm, whereas 12 MHz allows for a 3-cm maximal penetration. Although 12 MHz does not allow deep penetration, it has the advantage of providing greater resolution images that may help in evaluating more superficial, early gastric cancer lesions. Before evaluating a lesion, deaerated water is instilled into the stomach to fully cover the lesion. This provides for greater transmission of the ultrasound waves in a distended stomach, thereby enabling a larger surface

From: *Endoscopic Oncology: Gastrointestinal Endoscopy and Cancer Management.* Edited by: D. O. Faigel and M. L. Kochman © Humana Press, Totowa, NJ

of the gastric lumen to be visualized. It also allows for ultrasonographic evaluation of the lesion without direct apposition of the endoscope balloon or tip over the lesions, which could result in compression of tissue planes leading to inaccuracy in determining T category. Occasionally, it may be helpful to change the patient to a prone, supine, or even right lateral position to facilitate full immersion of the lesion. Even with change in patient position and optimal technique, the proximal lesser curve and prepyloric antrum frequently cannot be adequately visualized (1).

Ultrasonic evaluation of the normal stomach reveals five distinct layers, three hyperechoic and two hypoechoic, visible as an alternating bright–dark pattern. For practical purposes, the first two echolayers are considered to correspond histologically with the mucosa, the third with the submucosa, and the fourth with the muscularis propria and the fifth with the serosa. Gastric cancers appear as hypoechoic lesions arising in the mucosal layer that disrupt the normal layered appearance of the gastric mucosa.

3. GASTRIC CANCER STAGING

Various classification systems have been developed for the staging of gastric cancer. The two most commonly used in clinical practice include the Japanese Gastric Cancer Association system and the International Union Against Cancer/American Joint Committee on Cancer system (Tables 1 and 2) (2,3). The assessment of the extent of local tumor involvement or T category of both of these systems is essentially identical and they only vary in the method of assignment of nodal status. T1 lesions (Fig. 1) invade either the mucosa or submucosa (first three EUS layers), T2 lesions (Fig. 2) invade the muscularis propria (fourth EUS layer) or subserosa (not defined on EUS), T3 lesions (Fig. 3) penetrate the serosa (fifth EUS layer), and T4 lesions invade adjacent organs. Outcome studies have shown that stage at diagnosis correlates with survival (Table 3).

Table 1
TNM Staging Classification of Gastric Carcinoma[a]

T stage	
Tis	Carcinoma *in situ* (high-grade dysplasia without invasion of the lamina propria)
T1	Invasion of lamina propria or submucosa
T2a	Invasion of muscularis propria
T2b	Invasion of subserosa
T3	Penetration of the serosa
T4	Invasion of adjacent structures
N stage	
N0	No lymph node metastases
N1	Metastasis to 1–6 lymph nodes
N2	Metastasis to 7–15 lymph nodes
N3	Metastasis to >15 lymph nodes
M stage	
M0	No distant metastasis
M1	Distant metastasis present

[a]American Joint Committee on Cancer/International Union Against Cancer sixth edition criteria.

Table 2
Group Staging for Gastric Cancer[a]

Group stage	T stage	N stage	M stage
0	Tis	N0	M0
IA	T1	N0	M0
IB	T1	N1	M0
	T2	N0	
II	T1	N2	M0
	T2	N1	M0
	T3	N0	
IIIA	T2	N2	M0
	T3	N1	M0
	T4	N0	M0
IIIB	T3	N2	M0
IV	T4	N1–N4	M0
	T1–T3	N3	M0
	Any T	Any N	M1

[a]American Joint Committee on Cancer/International Union Against Cancer sixth edition criteria.

Studies evaluating the accuracy of EUS in the assessing the nodal status of patients of gastric cancer have almost exclusively relied on the 1987 tumor-node-metastasis (TNM) classification where the N category is determined by the distance of the involved nodes in relation to the primary gastric tumor *(4)*. Within this classification there are only three divisions: N0, N1, and N2. N1 stage (Fig. 4) is defined as nodes within 3 cm from the tumor. N2 refers to metastatic nodes greater than 3 cm from the primary tumor or nodes adjacent to the left gastric, common hepatic, splenic, or celiac artery. More recently the International Union Against Cancer/American Joint Committee on Cancer has proposed a new nodal classification with four different classifications, N0–N3, with the nodal staging based solely and incrementally on the absolute number of involved nodes from the resected specimen irrespective of the location of the nodes in relationship to the primary tumor *(3)*. Several recent studies have shown this new classification to be

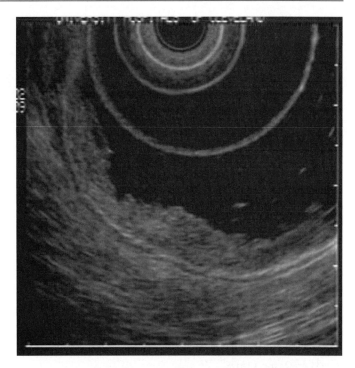

Fig. 1. Gastric cancer confined to the first three EUS layers (T1 category).

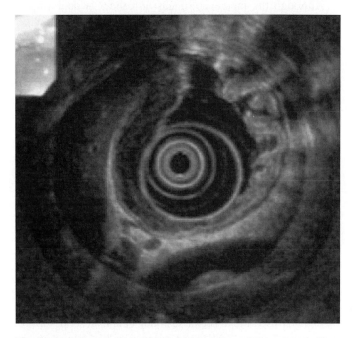

Fig. 2. Gastric cancer involving all four layers (T2 category). Note that the outer border is smooth. A small but malignant-appearing lymph node is also seen.

superior to both the 1987 TNM classification and the Japanese Gastric Cancer Association staging system *(5–9)*.

3.1. EUS STAGING

Multiple studies have evaluated the use of EUS with results of accuracy of determining the T category when staging gastric cancer varying between 70 and 92% *(1,10–22)* (*see* Table 4). Although various studies have shown somewhat disparate results, the greatest difficulty in staging gastric cancer has been

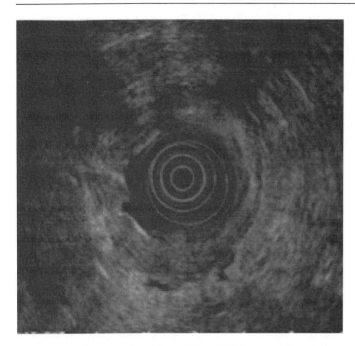

Fig. 3. A gastric cancer involving all five EUS layers with an irregular outer border (T3 category).

Table 3
Survival by Stage at Presentation

Stage	5-yr survival (%)	Presenting proportion (%)
I	50	18
II	29	16
III	13	36
IV	3	30

From ref. *23a*.

the discrimination of T2 from T3 lesions. Larger studies have consistently shown an overstaging of T2 lesions in 12–30% of tumors with an understaging rate of 4–10% (*see* Tables 5 and 6). Microscopic invasion is the most frequent cause of understaging *(17)*. Overstaging has most often been attributed to peritumor fibrosis, ulceration, and inflammation *(19,23)*. Additionally, there are several inherent anatomic features of the stomach that can lead to inaccuracy in the echoendoscopic determination of the stage of gastric cancers. The lesser curve and the posterior wall of the fundus are not covered with serosa. Therefore, in these areas, tumors with complete transmural growth are histologically classified as T2 tumors. The serosa in these cancers technically is free of invasion. Ultrasonographically, these tumors will appear as T3 lesions, potentially leading to overstaging *(14)*. T2 lesions may also be overstaged in areas of the stomach where there is attachment of the gastrocolic ligament, gastrohepatic ligament, and omentrum major and minor. In these areas, there is fatty tissue between the muscularis propia and serosa. Therefore, lesions invading into fatty tissue may appear ultrasonographically consistent with T3 lesions when in fact they are histologically T2 *(16)*.

The overall accuracy of determining N category for EUS in gastric cancer has ranged from 65 to 90%, predominantly based on the 1987 TNM classification (Table 7). Within these studies, various criteria have been used to characterize nodes as malignant. The majority of studies have classified nodes that are hypoechoic and sharply demarcated as being indicative of malignant nodes (Figs. 2 and 4), irrespective of lymph node size *(1,11,14–17,21)*. In addition to these characteristics, round configuration was also occasionally used as an additional criterion to suggest malignancy *(1,21)*. A few studies have used absolute node size to characterize malignant nodes, with 8–10 mm used as the cutoff point, irrespective of the sonographic features of the visualized nodes *(18,19,22)*.

EUS has limited usefulness in the detection of metastatic disease. Ascites can frequently be detected during echoendoscopic evaluation in the staging of gastric cancer. Chen et al. *(24)* retrospectively reviewed 57 consecutive gastric cancer patients who underwent subsequent surgery. Twenty patients (39%) had ascites detected by echoendoscopic evaluation. Although the presence of ascites was correlated with depth of tumor invasion and lymph node metastasis, it did not correlate with peritoneal carcinomatosis found upon surgery. Chu et al. *(25)* prospectively evaluated 402 consecutive patients with gastric cancer with a 12.5 MHz catheter probe ultrasound with particular attention to the presence of ascites. Compared with the findings at laparoscopy or laparotomy, EUS was 60.7% sensitive and 99.4% specific for detecting ascites. Peritoneal metastasis was noted in 63.9% of patients with ascites detected by EUS. This correlation was highly statistically significant. Of patients without ascites detected on EUS, 11.3% had peritoneal metastasis. These results suggest that although EUS is very specific for diagnosing ascites, the presence of ascites itself does not necessarily indicate the presence of peritoneal metastasis, as nearly 40% of these patients will be free of peritoneal disease at laparoscopy.

The majority of studies evaluating the accuracy of EUS for the staging of gastric cancer have not blinded the endoscopist to the patient's clinical history including previous radiographic and endoscopic evaluation. This has raised the concern of whether the true accuracy of EUS has been inflated by additional information gained from the clinical history. In one study, videotaped examinations of 33 patients who had undergone EUS for the evaluation of gastric cancer were blindly reviewed and these results were compared to the initial non-blinded EUS assessment obtained during the routine clinical evaluation *(26)*. The authors found that the non-blinded initial routine evaluation yielded an overall accuracy of 66.7% for determining T category, which fell to 45.5% under blinded evaluation. The same authors subsequently performed a similar study of videotaped endoscopic ultrasonographic examinations in 55 patients with gastric cancer to assess interobserver variability between five blinded experienced examiners in determining T and N category accuracy *(27)*. κ-values for assessing T1, T2, T3, and T4 lesions were 0.47, 0.38, 0.39, and 0.34, respectively, consistent with a substantial degree of interobserver variability. Interobserver variability for determining N category fared worse with a κ-value of 0.46, 0.34, and 0.29 for N0, N1, and N2 tumors, respectively.

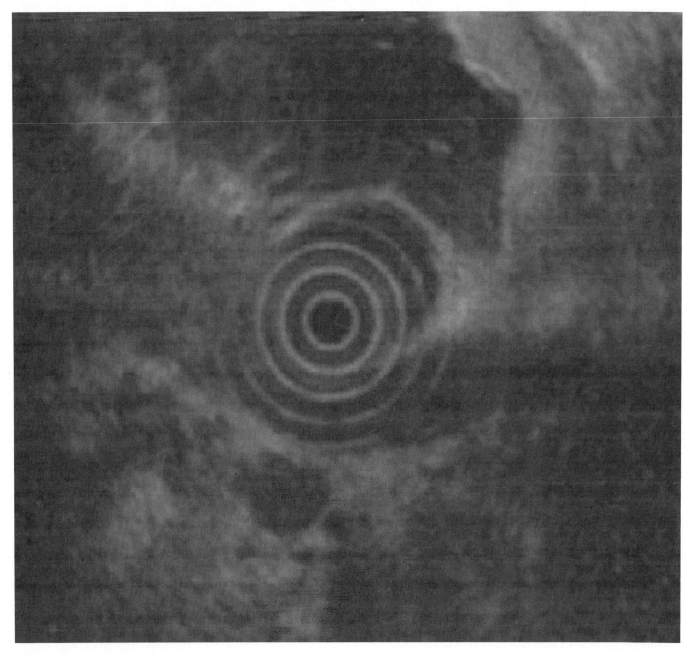

Fig. 4. A gastric cancer involving all five EUS layers with irregular border and an involved hypoechoic rounded enlarged lymph node (T3N1).

3.2. COMPARISON OF CT AND EUS

Several studies have compared CT scan directly with EUS for the staging of gastric cancer (Table 8). The greatest limitation of CT is its limited ability to accurately determine the T category of lesions with several studies showing less than 50% accuracy *(13,16,18)*. Ziegler et al. *(16)* reported that CT scan failed to detect 6 T1 lesions and overstaged 12 T1 lesions out of a total of 22 patients with T1 tumors. CT also tends to over-stage T2 lesions as T3 lesion. EUS has also consistently shown superior ability to determine the N category when compared with CT. However, many of these studies were conducted using older CT technology, potentially biasing these studies in favor of EUS. Habermann et al. *(22)* recently compared new-generation helical CT to EUS for the staging of gastric cancer in 51 patients. In order to enhance accuracy, CT scan was also performed after having the patent drink 500–800 mL of tap water to fully distend the stomach. The authors were able to demonstrate a T category accuracy of 76% compared with 86% for EUS, a difference that was not statistically significant. The N category accuracy of CT scan in this study was also higher than previous comparative studies with 70% accuracy. An advantage of CT compared with EUS is a greater ability to detect distant metastatic disease. Therefore, currently CT and EUS are considered complementary in the staging of gastric cancer.

3.3. EUS IN EARLY GASTRIC CANCER

The subset of T1 gastric lesions confined to the mucosa or submucosa has traditionally been referred to as early gastric cancer. T1 lesions confined only to the mucosa are candidates for curative endoscopic mucosal resection, whereas those that invade the submucosa usually require surgical resection owing

Table 4
EUS Studies Evaluating Accuracy in Determining T Category When Staging Gastric Cancer (1,10–22)

Author	Year	MHz	Patients	Type	T category accuracy (%)
Murata	1988	7.5–10	146	R	79
Tio	1989	7.5–12	72	P	81
Akahoshi	1991	7.5–12	74	R	81
Botet	1991	7.5–12	50	R	92
Caletti	1993	7.5–12	35	P	91
Dittler	1993	7.5–12	254	R	83
Grimm	1993	7.5	147	P	78
Ziegler	1993	7.5–12	108	P	86
Massari	1996	7.5–12	65	P	89
Perng	1996	7.5–12	69	P	71
Wang	1998	7.5–12	119	P	70
Tseng	2000	7.5–12	74	R	85
Willis	2000	7.5–12	116	R	78
Habermann	2004	7.5–12	51	P	86

R, retrospective study; P, prospective study.

Table 5
Accuracy of EUS in Respect to Individual T Category in the Assessment of Gastric Cancer Stage (1,10–22)

Author	MHz	Patients	T1	T2	T3	T4
Murata	7.5–10	146	93	50	41	–
Tio	7.5–12	72	77	93	81	88
Akahoshi	7.5–12	74	93	57	100	60
Botet	7.5–12	50	92% T1+T2		97	86
Caletti	7.5–12	35	83	100	86	100
Dittler	7.5–12	254	81	71	87	79
Grimm	7.5	147	74	73	85	85
Ziegler	7.5–12	108	91	81	84	94
Massari	7.5–12	65	100	86	85.7	88.8
Perng	7.5–12	69	58	63	79	83
Wang	7.5–12	119	68	67	81	53
Tseng	7.5–12	74	100	74	87	86
Willis	7.5–12	116	80	63	95	83
Habermann	7.5–12	51	–	90	79	100

Table 6
Overstaging and Understaging Rate (%) of EUS With Respect to Determining T Category (1,10–12,14–22)

Author		T1 over	T2 under	T2 over	T3 under	T3 over	T4 under
Murata	146	4	36	14	7	0	–
Tio	72	23	0	7	9	9	13
Akahoshi	74	7.5	33	10	0	0	40
Caletti	35	17	0	0	14	0	0
Dittler	254	19	2	27	7	5	21
Grimm	147	26	4	23	9	6	15
Ziegler	108	9	67	13	11	5	0
Massari	65	0	14	0	5	10	11
Perng	69	57	50	14	22	17	11
Wang	119	33	10	23	7	10	47
Tseng	74	0	9	17	0	13	14
Willis	116	21	9	30	5	0	17
Habermann	51	–	0	10	21	0	0

Over, overstaging; under, understaging.

Table 7
EUS Studies Evaluating Accuracy of Determining N Category When Staging Gastric Cancer (1,11,13–22)

Author	Year	MHz	No.	N	N0	N1	N2
Tio	1989	7.5–12	72	68	50	62	90
Botet	1991	7.5–12	50	78	91	68	82
Caletti	1993	7.5–12	35	69	–	–	–
Dittler	1993	7.5–12	254	66	93	65	52
Grimm	1993	7.5	148	83	79	46	91
Ziegler	1993	7.5–12	108	74	71	74	100
Massari	1996	7.5–12	56	68	58	65	73
Perng	1996	7.5–12	69	65	75	53	60
Wang	1998	7.5–12	119	68	73	69	52
Willis	2000	7.5–12	116	77	82	75	64
Habermann	2004	7.5–12	51	90	100	83	84

Table 8
Comparitive Studies of CT vs EUS in the Staging of Gastric Cancer (13,16,18,22)

Author	Year	No.	Type	EUS T stage	EUS N stage	CT T stage	CT N stage
Botet	1991	33	R	92	78	42	48
Ziegler	1993	108	P	86	74	43	51
Perng	1996	69	P	71	65	42	49
Habermann	2004	51	P	86	90	76	70

to an approx 20% rate of lymph node metastasis (28). Therefore, with these lesions, it is imperative that an accurate assessment be available, before a decision about definitive therapy. The majority of studies evaluating dedicated 7.5 and 12 MHz radial endoscopes have not attempted to subclassify T1 lesions into mucosal vs submucosal involvement.

High-frequency ultrasound catheter probes that can be inserted through the accessory channel of a standard upper endoscope have been evaluated in the assessment of early gastric cancer. The higher frequency of these probes, in the range of 15–20 MHz, allows for greater resolution imaging, which can potentially discriminate muscosal from submucosal invasion. Smaller lesions may also be more easily targeted by these "mini" probes, because they allow for the lesion to be targeted under direct endoscopic visualization. Occasionally, with higher frequency ultrasound probes a nine-layered bright–dark alternating pattern will be visualized instead of the usual five. The first three layers roughly correspond to the mucosa, the fourth with the subserosa, the six through eighth with the muscularis propria, and the ninth with the subserosa and serosa (29).

Several studies have evaluated these high-frequency ultrasound catheters in the evaluation of early gastric cancer. Overall accuracy has ranged from 65 to 72% (23,29–31) (Table 9). High-frequency catheter probe ultrasound has a tendency to overstage T1 mucosal lesions as T1 submucosal lesions with an overstaging rate that has varied from 29-46%. Fortunately, T1 submucosal understaging is less frequent with a rate that has ranged from 6 to 48%, with four of five studies reporting an understage rate of less than 17% (Table 10).

Table 9
Accuracy of High-Frequency Catheter Probe Ultrasounds in Determining T Category When Staging Early Gastric Cancer (23,29–32)

Author	Type	MHz	No.	Overall accuracy	T1m	T1sm	T2	T3
Yanai 1996	linear	20	47	72	69	96	–	–
Yanai 1997	linear/ radial	20	108	65	68	44	25 for T2+T3	
Akahoshi 1998	radial	15	78	67	70	46	71	–
Okamura 1999	radial	20	46	72	76	77	33	–
Yanai 1999	radial	20	52	71	64	88	50	

All accuracies reported as percent.

Table 10
Over- and Understaging Rate of High-Frequency Catheter Probe Ultrasound in Determining T Category When Staging Early Gastric Cancer (23,29–32)

Author	Type	MHz	No.	Overall	T1m overstage	T1sm understage	T1sm overstage
Yanai 1996	linear	20	47	72	29	13	0
Yanai 1997	linear/ radial	20	108	65	32	48	8
Akahoshi 1998	radial	15	78	67	30	15	15
Okamura 1999	radial	20	46	71.7	24	17	0
Yanai 1999	radial	20	52	71	36	6	6

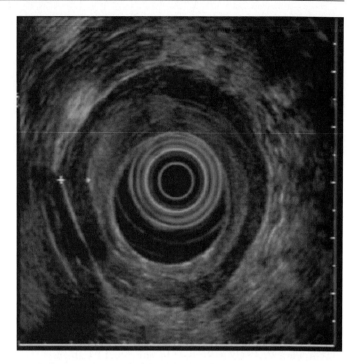

Fig. 5. Typical thickening of the fourth EUS layer seen in linitis plastica.

An inherent disadvantage of high-frequency probes is a limited depth of penetration. Studies evaluating high-frequency ultrasound have shown that accuracy decreases as the size of the tumor increases and these probes should be reserved for tumors less than 2 cm in size. Okumura et al. *(31)* reported that the accuracy of a 20 MHz was 85.7% for lesions less than 20 mm but that this accuracy fell to 50% for lesions greater than 20 mm. Attenuation of the ultrasound by gastric folds or protruding lesions can lead to a suboptimal evaluation. One study using a 15 MHz linear catheter probe reported the muscularis propria was only visualized in 34% of examinations *(30)*.

The lack of sufficient depth of penetration of high-frequency ultrasound probes limits the sensitivity in detecting lymph node metastasis. Studies evaluating lymph node metastasis in 15–20 MHz have shown sensitivity of only 17–33% in the detection of regional lymph nodes *(30,31,33)*.

A few studies have evaluated lower frequency catheter probe ultrasound in the routine evaluation of gastric cancer. These probes that have a frequency in the range of standard echoendoscopes (12.5 MHz) have the advantage that they can be used to evaluate stenotic areas not traversable by a dedicated echoendoscope and that they can potentially be used on demand through the accessory channel of a standard upper endoscope. These lower frequency probes also provide deeper penetration and therefore unlike higher frequency miniprobes can be used to assess lymph node status. Hunerbein et al. evaluated 30 patients with gastric cancer with a 12.5 MHz catheter probe ultrasound. Overall accuracy was 82% for determining T category and 80% for N category *(34)*. Chu et al. reported that of 402 consecutive patients with gastric cancer, 12% could not be traversed with a standard endoscope. Using a 12.5 MHz catheter probe ultrasound all the patients could be sufficiently evaluated *(25)*.

4. GASTRIC CANCER AND EUS-GUIDED FNA

There is limited literature concerning the use of FNA as an adjunct to standard gastric cancer endoscopic evaluation. The potential role for EUS-FNA in the evaluation of gastric cancer includes sampling of enlarged lymph nodes, particularly lymph nodes that would confirm metastatic disease, and also sampling of ascitic or pleural fluid and FNA of liver lesions. Mortensen et al. reported with EUS-FNA, they were able to confirm metastatic disease in eight gastric cancer patients with enlarged mediastinal (*n* = 3) or para-aortic (*n* = 5) lymph nodes *(35)*. Chang et al. *(36)* reported diagnosing malignant ascites and malignant pleural effusion with EUS-FNA in one gastric cancer patient and malignant pleural effusion in another gastric cancer patient. In the first patient, neither the effusion nor the ascites were noted on prior CT scan. EUS-guided FNA of suspected liver metastases in patients with gastric cancer has also been described, although data are currently limited in this regard *(37)*.

5. EUS IN THE EVALUATION OF LINITIS PLASTICA

Limited data exist regarding the features of EUS in the evaluation of linitis plastica or scirrhous type of gastric cancer. A few small retrospective studies describe the EUS characteristics of linitis plastica as a subset of patients undergoing evaluation of large gastric folds (39–41). The five-layer structure is usually preserved in linitis plastic, as opposed to gastric lymphoma in which the five-layer structure is frequently destroyed. In the majority of cases of linitis plastica, thickening of the fourth layer (Fig. 5) is noted with occasionally thickening of the second and third layers. Thickening of the fourth layer is rarely if ever seen in benign conditions and thickening of this layer in the setting of large gastric folds should raise the concern of gastric carcinoma or gastric lymphoma. Fujishima et al. (42) compared 16 patients with scirrhous gastric cancer and 7 patients with hypertrophic gastritis to 16 control patients. Patients with scirrhous gastric cancer were noted to have preservation of the five-layer structure with irregular hypoechoic thickening of the third and fourth layers. The thickness of the third and fourth layers was sixfold and threefold that of controls. In patients with hypertrophic gastritis, only the mucosal layer was noted to be thickened. Saito et al. reviewed the role EUS in determining T category accuracy in 34 patients with scirrhous gastric cancer. In this study, the deepest layer showing thickening or irregularity was interpreted as the endoscopic T category of the tumor. Overall accuracy for determining T category was 88%. Accuracy of lymph node involvement was not reported.

REFERENCES

1. Caletti G, Ferrari A, Brocchi E, Barbara L. Accuracy of endoscopic ultrasonography in the diagnosis and staging of gastric cancer and lymphoma. Surgery 1993; 113:14–27.
2. Nishi M, Omori Y, Miwa K, Japanese classification of gastric carcinoma. Japanese Research Society for Gastric Cancer. 1st edn. Tokyo: Kanehara & Co., 1995.
3. Hermanek P, Sobin LH, editors. UICC TNM classification of malignant tumors. 4th edition. Berlin: Springer; 1987.
4. Sobin LH, Wittekin CH. TNM classification of malignant tumors. International Union Against Cancer. 5th edn. New York:John Wiley & Sons; 1997.
5. Katai H, Yoshimura K, Maruyama K, Sasako M, Sano T. Evaluation of the New International Union Against Cancer TNM staging for gastric carcinoma. Cancer 2000; 88:1796–1800.
6. Hayashi H, Ochiai T, Suzuki T, et al. Superiority of a new UICC-TNM staging system for gastric carcinoma. Surgery 2000; 127:129–135.
7. Roder JD, Bottcher K, Busch R, Wittekind C, Hermanek P, Siewert JR. Classification of regional lymph node metastasis from gastric carcinoma. German Gastric Cancer Study Group. Cancer 1998; 82:621–631.
8. Yoo CH, Noh SH, Kim YI, Min JS. Comparison of prognostic significance of nodal staging between old (4th edition) and new (5th edition) UICC TNM classification for gastric carcinoma. International Union Against Cancer. World J Surg 1999; 23:492–497; discussion 497–498.
9. Hermanek P, Altendorf-Hofmann A, Mansmann U, Dworak O, Wittekind C, Hohenberger W. Improvements in staging of gastric carcinoma from using the new edition of TNM classification. Eur J Surg Oncol 1998; 24:536–541.
10. Murata Y, Suzuki S, Hashimoto H. Endoscopic ultrasonography of the upper gastrointestinal tract. Surg Endosc 1988; 2:180–183.
11. Tio TL, Schouwink MH, Cikot RJ, Tytgat GN. Preoperative TNM classification of gastric carcinoma by endosonography in comparison with the pathological TNM system: a prospective study of 72 cases. Hepatogastroenterology 1989; 36:51–56.
12. Akahoshi K, Misawa T, Fujishima H, Chijiiwa Y, Maruoka A, Ohkubo A, Nawata H. Preoperative evaluation of gastric cancer by endoscopic ultrasound. Gut 1991; 32:479–482.
13. Botet JF, Lightdale CJ, Zauber AG, Gerdes H, Winawer SJ, Urmacher C, Brennan MF. Preoperative staging of gastric cancer: comparison of endoscopic US and dynamic CT. Radiology 1991; 181:426–432.
14. Dittler HJ, Siewert JR. Role of endoscopic ultrasonography in gastric carcinoma. Endoscopy 1993; 25:162–166.
15. Grimm H, Binmoeller KF, Hamper K, Koch J, Henne-Bruns D, Soehendra N. Endosonography for preoperative locoregional staging of esophageal and gastric cancer. Endoscopy 1993; 25:224–230.
16. Ziegler K, Sanft C, Zimmer T, et al. Comparison of computed tomography, endosonography, and intraoperative assessment in TN staging of gastric carcinoma. Gut 1993; 34:604–610.
17. Massari M, Cioffi U, De Simone M, et al. Endoscopic ultrasonography for preoperative staging of gastric carcinoma. Hepatogastroenterology 1996; 43:542–546.
18. Perng DS, Jan CM, Wang WM, et al. Computed tomography, endoscopic ultrasonography and intraoperative assessment in TN staging of gastric carcinoma. J Formos Med Assoc 1996; 95:378–385.
19. Wang JY, Hsieh JS, Huang YS, Huang CJ, Hou MF, Huang TJ. Endoscopic ultrasonography for preoperative locoregional staging and assessment of resectability in gastric cancer. Clin Imaging 1998; 22:355–359.
20. Tseng LJ, Mo LR, Tio TL, et al. Video-endoscopic ultrasonography in staging gastric carcinoma. Hepatogastroenterology 2000; 47: 897–900.
21. Willis S, Truong S, Gribnitz S, Fass J, Schumpelick V. Endoscopic ultrasonography in the preoperative staging of gastric cancer:accuracy and impact on surgical therapy. Surg Endosc 2000;14: 951–954.
22. Habermann CR, Weiss F, Riecken R, et al. Preoperative staging of gastric adenocarcinoma: comparison of helical CT and endoscopic US. Radiology 2004; 230:465–471.
23. Yanai H, Matsumoto Y, Harada T, et al. Endoscopic ultrasonography and endoscopy for staging depth of invasion in early gastric cancer: a pilot study. Gastrointest Endosc 1997; 46:212–216.
23a. Waneb HJ, Kennedy BJ, Chmiel J, Steele G Jr, Winchester D, Osteen R. Cancer of the stomach. A patient care study by the American College of Surgeons. Ann Surg 1993; 218:583–592.
24. Chen CH, Yang CC, Yeh YH. Preoperative staging of gastric cancer by endoscopic ultrasound: the prognostic usefulness of ascites detected by endoscopic ultrasound. J Clin Gastroenteroln 2002; 35:321–327.
25. Chu KM, Kwok KF, Law S, Wong KH. A prospective evaluation of catheter probe EUS for the detection of ascites in patients with gastric carcinoma. Gastrointest Endosc 2004; 59:471–474.
26. Meining A, Dittler HJ, Wolf A, et al. You get what you expect? A critical appraisal of imaging methodology in endosonographic cancer staging. Gut 2002; 50:599–603.
27. Meining A, Rosch T, Wolf A, et al. High interobserver variability in endosonographic staging of upper gastrointestinal cancers. Z Gastroenterol 2003; 41:391–394.
28. Ichikura T, Uefuji K, Tomimatsu S, Okusa Y, Yahara T, Tamakuma S. Surgical strategy for patients with gastric carcinoma with submucosal invasion. A multivariate analysis. Cancer 1995; 76: 935–940.
29. Akahoshi K, Chijiwa Y, Hamada S, et al. Pretreatment staging of endoscopically early gastric cancer with a 15 MHz ultrasound catheter probe. Gastrointest Endosc 1998; 48:470–476.
30. Yanai H, Tada M, Karita M, Okita K. Diagnostic utility of 20-megahertz linear endoscopic ultrasonography in early gastric cancer. Gastrointest Endosc 1996; 44:29–33.
31. Okamura S, Tsutsui A, Muguruma N, et al. The utility and limitations of an ultrasonic miniprobe in the staging of gastric cancer. J Med Invest 1999; 46:49–53.
32. Yanai H, Noguchi T, Mizumachi S, et al. A blind comparison of the effectiveness of endoscopic ultrasonography and endoscopy in staging early gastric cancer. Gut 1999; 44:361–365.

33. Akahoshi K, Chijiiwa Y, Sasaki I, et al. Pre-operative TN staging of gastric cancer using a 15 MHz ultrasound miniprobe. Br J Radiol 1997; 70:703–707.

34. Hunerbein M, Ghadimi BM, Haensch W, Schlag PM. Transendoscopic ultrasound of esophageal and gastric cancer using miniaturized ultrasound catheter probes. Gastrointest Endosc 1998; 48:371–375.

35. Mortensen MB, Pless T, Durup J, Ainsworth AP, Plagborg GJ, Hovendal C. Clinical impact of endoscopic ultrasound-guided fine needle aspiration biopsy in patients with upper gastrointestinal tract malignancies. A prospective study. Endoscopy 2001; 33:478–483.

36. Chang KJ, Albers CG, Nguyen P. Endoscopic ultrasound-guided fine needle aspiration of pleural and ascetic fluid. Am J Gastroenterol 1995; 90(1):148–150.

37. tenBerge J, Hoffman BJ, Hawes RH, et al. EUS-guided fine needle aspiration of the liver: indications, yield, and safety based on an international survey of 167 cases. Gastrointest Endosc 2002; 55:859–862

38. Chen TK, Wu CH, Lee CL, Lai YC, Yang SS. Endoscopic ultrasonography in the differential diagnosis of giant gastric folds. J Formos Med Assocm1999; 98:261–264.

39. Caletti G, Fusaroli P, Bocus P. Endoscopic ultrasonography in large gastric folds. Endoscopy 1998; 30 Suppl 1:A72–A75.

40. Mendis RE, Gerdes H, Lightdale CJ, Botet JF. Large gastric folds: a diagnostic approach using endoscopic ultrasonography. Gastrointest Endosc 1994; 40:437–441.

41. Songur Y, Okai T, Watanabe H, Motoo Y, Sawabu N. Endosonographic evaluation of giant gastric folds. Gastrointest Endosc 1995; 41:468–474.

42. Fujishima H, Misawa T, Chijiwa Y, Maruoka A, Akahoshi K, Nawata H. Scirrhous carcinoma of the stomach versus hypertrophic gastritis: findings at endoscopic US. Radiology 1991; 181:197–200.

43. Saito N, Takeshita K, Habu H, Endo M. The use of endoscopic ultrasound in determining the depth of cancer invasion in patients with gastric cancer. Surg Endosc 1991; 5:14–19.

15 Carcinoid Tumors

WILLSCOTT E. NAUGLER, MD AND GORDON C. HUNT, MD

CONTENTS

1. BACKGROUND

Carcinoid tumors are of neuroendocrine origin, and can produce bioactive peptides or amines that rarely produce clinical symptoms. These tumors are slow growing, and infrequently produce the so-called carcinoid syndrome, cardinal features of which are flushing and diarrhea. About two-thirds of carcinoid tumors are found in the gastrointestinal (GI) tract, one-fourth in the bronchopulmonary tree, and the remainder in the urogenital tract. Presentation, behavior, and malignant potential of carcinoid tumors are determined by the site at which they originate. Resection of the tumor is the only curative option, but advances in the understanding of the biology of carcinoids have produced therapies that can effectively treat symptoms caused by these tumors.

2. INTRODUCTION

Carcinoid tumors arise from neuroendocrine cells usually located within the gut or tracheobronchial tree. A confusing array of names has been applied to the carcinoid cell of origin, including chromaffin, enterochromaffin, enterochromaffin-like (ECL), Kulchitsky, and enteroendocrine. It was once thought that these cells originated in neural-crest tissue, but it now appears that these cells develop within the gut (or other organs) (1), and perform various neuroendocrine functions, which may differ according to the anatomical site.

Lubarsch first described the pathological entity of carcinoid in 1888 (2) after finding multiple ileal tumors in two autopsied patients. In 1907, Oberndorfer offered the name "karzinoide" to describe an ileal tumor morphologically distinct and much less clinically aggressive than the typical intestinal adenocarcinoma (3). Masson argued in 1928 that carcinoids should be considered endocrine tumors because the tumor cells displayed amine precursor uptake and decarboxylation (4). The name amine precursor uptake and decarboxylation, previously thought to adequately characterize such cells, has fallen into disfavor as many of the secretory products are now known to be peptides, rather than bioactive amines.

The presence of serotonin in carcinoid tumors was first described in 1953 (5), and elevated levels of the serotonin metabolite 5-hydroxyindoleacetic acid (5-HIAA) were initially found in the urine of patients with the carcinoid syndrome in 1955 (6). Gastric carcinoids are present in 9% of patients with multiple endocrine neoplasia (MEN), and often in patients with the Zollinger-Ellison (ZE) syndrome.

Recognition that this tumor causes a syndrome of flushing and diarrhea has fascinated physicians for years, although such presentations are rare. Most carcinoid tumors are discovered incidentally at surgery or endoscopy, or on work-up of vague symptoms such as weight loss, abdominal pain, or occasionally anemia or pellagra. Because of its relatively slow growth, the carcinoid tumor can present clinicians with challenges unusual for malignant neoplasms. Managing carcinoid syndrome, pellagra, valvular disease, or bowel obstruction in patients who have metastatic disease can be clinically difficult.

From: *Endoscopic Oncology: Gastrointestinal Endoscopy and Cancer Management*. Edited by: D. O. Faigel and M. L. Kochman © Humana Press, Totowa, NJ

3. CLINICAL PRESENTATION

Carcinoid tumor presentation depends largely on the anatomical site in which the neoplasm originates. Bronchopulmonary carcinoids frequently manifest with cough, hemoptysis, or recurrent respiratory infections (7). Gastric carcinoids can produce abdominal pain or rarely GI bleeding, whereas small intestine tumors may present with signs and symptoms of obstruction owing to the desmoplastic reaction caused by carcinoid tumors (8). Colonic tumors are usually right-sided, and present with obstructive symptoms or manifestations of disseminated disease. Rectal carcinoids are nearly always found incidentally on routine rectal examination, or on endoscopic exam for unrelated reasons. Rarely, rectal pain or bleeding will result in a diagnosis of a carcinoid tumor.

Many studies have found that about half of patients (40–60%) diagnosed with carcinoid tumors are asymptomatic (9,10). Indeed, studies have noted that more than half of carcinoids were unsuspected before autopsy (9,11). In the epidemiological study of carcinoid tumors by Modlin et al., an increasing incidence of these tumors (with the notable exception of appendicial carcinoids) is evident in the past decade. However, this may be because of an increase in the availability and use of diagnostic tools, especially endoscopy (12).

Infrequently, the initial manifestation of a malignant carcinoid is the carcinoid syndrome, or a variant. This classical syndrome is rare, complicating approx 5–10% of all carcinoid tumors. Most tumors that cause the carcinoid syndrome arise from the small intestine. Gastric carcinoids may rarely produce an atypical carcinoid syndrome. Less often, syndromes are produced from other biologically active substances secreted by carcinoids (e.g., 1% of Cushing's syndrome are a result of adrenal corticotropic hormone production by a carcinoid) (13,14).

4. EPIDEMIOLOGY

The largest epidemiological study of carcinoids to date is that of Modlin et al., which compiled data from three National Cancer Institute registries including 13,715 patients with carcinoid tumors (12). Carcinoids are rare, consisting of 0.45% of all malignancies, with an incidence rate of about 2–4 per 100,000 people in the United States (12,15). Incidence rates are similar in European countries and Japan, although autopsy rates can be much higher (9,11,16–19).

In the Modlin et al. study, 66.9% of carcinoids originated in the GI tract (Fig. 1A), 24.5% in the bronchopulmonary tree, and the remainder being found mostly in the urogenital tract. Women comprised 55% of all carcinoids, including most of the gastric, colon, appendix, and gallbladder cases. Males predominated with esophageal location. Black patients had a higher frequency of rectal carcinoids but a lower frequency of tracheobronchial carcinoids when compared with white patients. Differing incidences of site-specific carcinoids in various populations are detailed in Table 1 (12).

Modlin et al. analysis of more than 13,000 carcinoids illustrates some interesting trends. From 1950 to 1999, there has been an increase (>fivefold) in the proportion of gastric malignancies that are carcinoids, and a decrease (from 77 to 15%) in the portion of appendiceal malignancies that are carcinoids. Carcinoids persist at a stable 44% of all cancers in the small intestine. Reasons for theses trends are not clear.

The most recent tumor registry (Surveillance, Epidemiology, and End-Results [SEER] Program) reveals 22.4% of patients with a carcinoid tumor had another, noncarcinoid neoplasm (12). Indeed, there has been prior speculation that patients with carcinoids were more likely to develop other tumors, which is supported by the SEER data. Reasons for such associations are unclear, but a hypothesis is that carcinoid tumors produce local growth factors, which stimulate cellular proliferation, and potential malignant degeneration (20). Alternatively, there may be a genetic predisposition to cancer development, which could explain the increased risk of non-carcinoid tumors in carcinoid patients.

5. PATHOLOGY

Grossly, carcinoid tumors are usually well-circumscribed submucosal lesions, and are tan-yellow on cut surface owing to their high fat content (see Fig. 1B). With typical H&E staining, the tumors reveal monotonous sheets of uniform cells with few mitotic figures (see Fig. 1C,D) (21). Immunohistochemical staining has demonstrated that carcinoids make numerous secretory products, including serotonin, histamine, dopamine, corticotropin, substance P, neurotensin, kallekrein, gastrin, insulin, and even prostaglandins (21,22). Although these tumors may stain for secretory products, they usually do not produce a significant amount of these products to cause a clinical syndrome. However, immunohistochemical staining may be helpful in the diagnosis of carcinoid tumors. Common markers include chromogranin, synaptophysin, neuron specific enolase, endocrine granule constituent, gremileus silver stain and specific acetylcholine esterase (23). On electron microscopy, membrane bound secretory vesicles are visible in carcinoid tumors, as are synaptic vesicles, affirming the neuroendocrine function of the cells (22,24).

In 1963, Williams and Sanders grouped carcinoid tumors into divisions based on the embryological site of origin, corresponding to the foregut, midgut, and hindgut (25). Foregut tumors (esophageal, gastric, pancreatic, duodenal) arise in the distribution of the celiac artery, midgut (jejunum, ileum, appendix, ascending colon) from the superior mesenteric artery, and hindgut (colon and rectum) from the inferior mesenteric artery. The classification system was based largely on silver staining characteristics (argyrophilic, argentaffin, and nonreactive) and propensity for metastatic disease.

Cells from which carcinoid tumors arise synthesize peptides and bioamine products, indicating neuroendocrine function. A characteristic of these bioamine cells is the ability to take up silver. Depending on the endogenous reducing power of the cells, they are termed "argentaffin" (able to reduce silver) and "argyrophilic" (unable to reduce silver). Traditional teaching is that foregut tumors are usually argyrophilic, midgut tumors are more often argentaffin, and hindgut tumors are argyrophilic or nonreactive to silver staining (26).

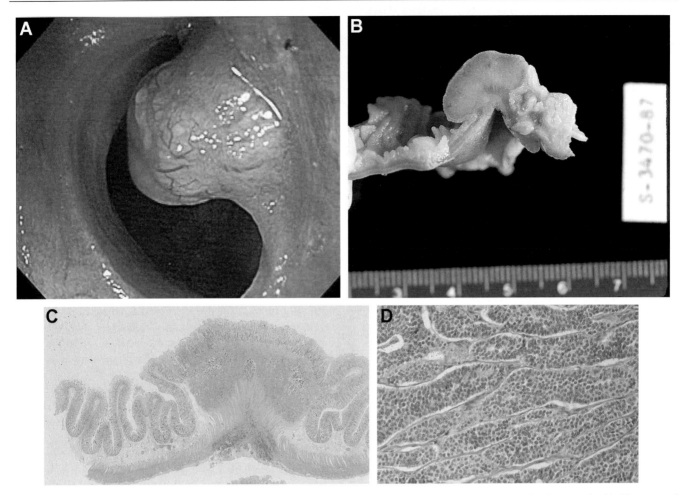

Fig. 1. (**A**) Endoscopic view of submucosal tumor in the terminal ileum seen on colonoscopy. The tumor proved to be a carcinoid. (Courtesy of Dr. Jaime Chen, GI fellow, UCSD.) (**B**) Gross specimen of resected ileal carcinoid. (Courtesy of Dr. Katsumi Miyai, Professor of Pathology, UCSD.) (**C**) Higher magnification of the ileal carcinoid. (Courtesy of Dr. Katsumi Miyai, Professor of Pathology, UCSD.) (**D**) H&E stain of the ileal carcinoid, demonstrating monotonous sheets of round cells, characteristic of neuroendocrine tumors. (Courtesy of Dr. Katsumi Miyai, Professor of Pathology, UCSD.)

With more sophisticated methods for differentiating these heterogeneous tumors available, it is clear that silver staining characteristics do not always correlate with clinical behavior, site of origin, or secretory products *(27)*. Aggressive clinical behavior occurs in tumors possessing nuclear atypia, increased mitoses or areas of necrosis *(21)*. However, categorizing carcinoid tumors by malignant potential has proven to be difficult. The terms "anaplastic" and "atypical" have been used synonymously for those tumors with the worrisome features listed earlier.

A widely accepted classification system simply denotes carcinoids as well or poorly differentiated neuroendocrine tumors *(24)*. Many authors accept this classification system, arguing that the best prognostic information is determined by the site of origin, state of differentiation, and size of the cancer. Although often cited, the terms *foregut*, *midgut*, and *hindgut* are less precise than naming the specific site of origin. Because of the great variability of these tumors, this chapter details carcinoids by the organ of origin despite popular use of the embryological divisions.

6. CHARACTERISTICS OF CARCINOIDS BY SITE OF ORIGIN

6.1. ESOPHAGUS

Carcinoids in the esophagus rarely occur. A review in 1997 found only 14 cases reported in the literature, although the SEER database (1973–1999) reported 6 cases *(12,28)*. Esophageal carcinoids have been found predominantly in men, usually in the lower esophagus, and may present with dysphagia and weight loss. Most have been treated with surgical resection, with a few anecdotal cases of radiotherapy. There are too few cases to make generalizations about esophageal carcinoids, but when staged like other esophageal cancers, it is apparent that stages I and II have better clinical prognosis than stages III and IV *(28)*.

6.2. STOMACH

The stomach is the most common location of foregut enteric carcinoids. The incidence of carcinoids as a proportion of gastric malignancies has increased over the past several decades for unclear reasons *(15)*. It is clear that the low acid state (as in atrophic gastritis) is associated with the

Table 1
Distribution of Carcinoid Tumors by Site

Site	Percentage of all carcinoids
Bronchopulmonary	25–28
Digestive system	70–74
Esophagus	<1
Stomach	4
Liver/biliary	<1
Pancreas	<1
Small intestine	25
Duodenum	3
Jejunum	2
Ileum	14
Meckel's	<1
NOS	6
Large intestine	36
Cecum/appendix	12
Rectum	10–17
Digestive system NOS	4
Other[a]	5

NOS, not otherwise specified.

[a]Other includes ovaries, testes, and other neuroendocrine sites, including the thymus.

Table 2
Characteristics of Gastric Carcinoids by Type

	Type 1	Type 2	Type 3
Location	Fundus	Fundus	Fundus or Antrum
Size	<2cm	<2cm	2–5 cm
Number	Usually multicentric	Often multicentric	Solitary
Total (%)	69–75%	5–8%	20–23%
Potential for metastases	RarelyLow	Higher	
Plasma gastrin level	High	High	Normal
Gastric acid output	Absent	High	Low or normal
Presumed cell of origin	ECL-cell	ECL-cell	ECL-cell

Type 1 are associated with chronic atrophic gastritis type A.
Type 2 are associated with MEN type 1 and ZE syndrome.
Type 3 are sporadic.

development of gastric carcinoids *(29)*. The hypergastrinemia consequent to the low acid state induces proliferation of the ECL cell, and promotes initiation of neoplastic transformation. Supporting this theory, ECL hyperplasia has been shown to occur adjacent to gastric carcinoids *(30)*. Although induction of hypergastrinemia in rats with proton pump inhibitors has led to the development of gastric carcinoids *(31)*, there is no evidence that such agents have led to gastric carcinoids in humans *(32)*.

A recent review of 562 gastric carcinoids collected from 1973 to 1999 revealed that these tumors comprise nearly 2% of gastric malignancies and 9% of enteric carcinoids. There appears to be a 2:1 female-to-male predominance, the average age at diagnosis is 63 yr, and the 5-yr survival rate for all patients with gastric carcinoids is 63% *(29)*.

Three categories of gastric carcinoid have been described, each with different presentations and prognoses *(see* Table 2) *(33,34)*. Approximately 75% of gastric carcinoids are type 1, and are associated with chronic atrophic gastritis type A. More than half of type 1 gastric carcinoids present with pernicious anemia *(35–37)*. These tumors tend to be multicentric, occurring primarily in the fundus, and may be found incidentally at endoscopy. Type 1 gastric carcinoids are usually slow growing and rarely metastasize. Tumors less than 1 cm are almost always benign, and endoscopic submucosal–mucosal resection (ESMR) has been used successfully to manage these tumors *(38)*. Antrectomy to reduce the hypergastrinemic state has been reported in cases of multifocal disease, but long-term benefits of this approach are uncertain given the benign nature of the disease *(33,39)*.

Type 2 gastric carcinoids arise in the context of MEN type 1 or ZE syndrome, and are associated with hypergastrinemia and high gastric acid output. Like type 1 gastric carcinoids, type 2 carcinoids are often multicentric, usually less than 2 cm, and clinically indolent at the time of diagnosis. Type 2 gastric carcinoids metastasize at a slightly higher rate than type 1. The tumor suppressor MEN 1 locus may be involved in the pathogenesis of these carcinoids *(40)*, which consists of 5–8% of gastric carcinoids.

Sporadic gastric carcinoids, type 3, make up nearly 25% of these tumors in the stomach, and are not associated with hypergastrinemia but rather a normal gastric acid output *(34)*. This type is the most aggressive of the gastric carcinoids, often presenting with relatively large masses and hepatic or regional lymph node metastases *(33,39)*. Type 3 tumors more often produce the carcinoid syndrome, perhaps related to their ability to metastasize.

Overlap between the three types occurs, but in general a hypergastrinemic state portends a more favorable prognosis. The overall 5-yr survival rates for patients with gastric carcinoids (of any type) is 67%, falling to 21% when there is metastatic disease at the time of presentation *(29)*.

6.3. PANCREAS

Because the pancreas produces other neuroendocrine tumors (gastrinomas, insulinomas, etc.), distinguishing between carcinoids can be difficult. When pancreatic carcinoids are defined as neuroendocrine tumors that produce serotonin, they comprise only 29 cases in a review of the literature from 1966 to 1995 *(41)*. Compared with other enteric carcinoids, those originating in the pancreas are more often metastatic at presentation (76%), and have a poor 5-yr survival rate (34%) *(15)*. However, pancreatic carcinoids do compare favorably with the 0.5% 5-yr survival rate seen in adenocarcinoma at this location *(42)*. Less than 1% of GI carcinoids occur in the pancreas *(12)*.

6.4. LIVER AND GALLBLADDER

A review of the literature in 2003 by Knox et al. found less than 50 cases of primary hepatic carcinoid *(43)*. Out of the 13,715 carcinoids compiled by Modlin et al., only 25 cases were primary gallbladder carcinoid *(12)*. Primary hepatic carcinoid tumors appear to be amenable to surgical resection, and have been reported to be relatively slow growing. High (68%) 10-yr survival rates have been cited *(43)*, although others have reported much lower rates *(12)*. Neither chemotherapy, radiotherapy, or embolization seemed to provide a survival benefit *(43)*. Carcinoids of the extrahepatic bile ducts have been reported, but are exceedingly rare *(44)*.

6.5. DUODENUM AND AMPULLA OF VATER

Duodenal carcinoids make up 2.6% of all carcinoids *(12)*, but have different characteristics than carcinoids elsewhere in the small intestine. Typically staining argyrophilic as opposed to argentaffin as seen in most other small bowel locations, duodenal carcinoids also produce gastrin rather than serotonin. Despite histochemical evidence of gastrin production in nearly half of duodenal carcinoids, the carcinoid syndrome is unusual and associated ZE syndrome is also rare *(45,46)*. In Burke et al.'s study of 99 duodenal tumors, 5 cases of ZE were found, and 21% had metastatic disease *(46)*. Immunohistochemical identification of somatostatin did not correlate with symptoms suggestive of the somatostatin syndrome (diabetes mellitus, cholelithiasis, and diarrhea).

Ampullary carcinoids are rare. As expected, these tumors frequently present with jaundice *(22)*. Interestingly, approx 25% of periampullary carcinoids are associated with neurofibromatosis type 1 (von Recklinghausen's disease) and express somatostatin *(45,47)*.

The limited data on duodenal or ampullary tumors has made it difficult to outline optimal management. Surgical resection has been the mainstay for therapy. For many tumors, especially duodenal carcinoids less than 2 cm, endoscopic resection has been used and may be a reasonable approach *(38,48–50)*.

6.6. SMALL INTESTINE

Malignant carcinoid tumors of the small intestine make up only about 1–2% of malignancies in the GI tract *(51,52)*. Carcinoids are the second most common malignant tumor of the small bowel (behind adenocarcinoma), accounting for 26–38% of cancers. Small bowel carcinoids account for about one-third of all enteric carcinoids *(12,52)*. Most of these occur in the ileum, are often multifocal and are frequently found within 60 cm of the ileocecal valve *(12)*. An unusual feature of the small intestinal carcinoid is that it often produces a dramatic fibrotic (desmoplastic) reaction in the surrounding mesentery, which can lead to intermittent bowel obstruction, abdominal pain, intussusception, and even mesenteric ischemia *(53)*. As with other tumors of the GI tract, bleeding may be the initial presentation of ileal or jejunal carcinoids.

Although the small bowel produces tumors that give rise to the carcinoid syndrome more than any other location, the syndrome complicates only 5–7% of small intestinal carcinoids *(9,54)*. Serotonin production is frequent in small intestinal carcinoids, but hepatic metabolism prevents systemic circulation of secreted bioactive products. Thus, the carcinoid syndrome usually represents hepatic or retroperitoneal metastatic disease and is therefore a grim prognostic sign.

Compared with carcinoids arising from other sites, the size of small intestinal tumors is a less reliable indicator of metastatic spread. Up to 18% of small intestinal carcinoids less than 2 cm have hepatic metastases *(55)*, a far greater percentage than those seen in other regions of the GI tract. Almost half of small intestinal carcinoid tumors larger than 2 cm have spread to the liver.

Surgical resection is the treatment of choice for small bowel carcinoids *(1,21,22)*. These tumors often present late with a mesenteric desmoplastic reaction and bulky lymphadenopathy, often making surgery a challenge. With small presenting tumors, surgical resection is straightforward with the goal of complete cure. With regional or distant spread, surgical debulking may provide significant palliation given the debilitating symptoms of intestinal obstruction or of the carcinoid syndrome *(56,57)*.

Carcinoids are rarely found in Meckel's diverticula. Less than 150 cases have been reported in the literature, and they have often been found incidentally at surgery (i.e., at laparoscopic cholecystectomy) *(58)*. On pathological and immunohistochemical analysis, these tumors appear to be most closely related to carcinoids of the small intestine *(59)*.

6.7. APPENDIX

Appendiceal carcinoids complicate less than 1% of appendectomies *(60)*, but are among the most frequently occurring tumors at this site. Carcinoid tumors comprise one-third to one-half of all tumors in the appendix *(15,60,61)*. The relative frequency of appendiceal carcinoids as a proportion of all carcinoids has decreased over the past five decades. It has been suggested that this is a result of a decreasing number of appendectomies over the past 20 yr, many of which had incidental carcinoids diagnosed at the time of appendectomy *(15)*. Tumors arising in this location have the best prognosis of all carcinoids, with a 5-yr survival rate exceeding 80%.

Like other carcinoids, those in the appendix exhibit more malignant behavior as the size increases. Most appendiceal tumors are less than 1 cm, and it has been reported that metastatic disease does not occur in tumors smaller than 2 cm *(62)*. Tumors larger than 2 cm have a significant risk of metastasizing, and this risk increases further for tumors larger than 3 cm. Varying opinions exist as to the optimal treatment of appendiceal carcinoids measuring between 1 and 2 cm. Many authors agree that simple appendectomy is a reasonable approach for tumors less than 2 cm, reserving right hemicolectomy for more extensive disease *(60,62)*.

6.8. COLON

Although carcinoids make up less than 1% of colon malignancies *(15)*, their presentation is similar to that of adenocarcinoma. Average age at diagnosis is 65 yr *(15)*. The most common site in the colon (aside from the appendix) is the cecum, where one-third of colon carcinoids are found *(29)*. It is unclear from the available data if some of those reported in the cecum were actually extensions from the appendix. Carcinoids in the extra-appendiceal colon may present with pain, anorexia, and weight loss *(63)*; less than 5% produce the carcinoid syndrome *(63,64)*. Tumors in the colon generally have a poor prognosis, with nodal or metastatic disease present at diagnosis in 55–85% of patients, *(12)* and 5-yr survival rates of 20–41% *(29,65–67)*. Adenocarcinomas of the colon have a 5-yr survival rate of 60% for all patients *(12)*. It has been proposed that the poor survival rate for colonic carcinoids could be skewed by misdiagnosing poorly differentiated adenocarcinomas as carcinoids *(68)*.

The average size of nonappendiceal colon carcinoids is 5 cm *(64,69)*. Some experts recommend endoscopic resection if the tumors are small (<2 cm) *(1,67)*, but most require local resection or colectomy *(21)*.

6.9. RECTUM

Carcinoids in the rectum might be found on investigation for rectal bleeding, pain, or change in stool caliber. Many are found incidentally at endoscopy performed for other reasons *(70,71)*. These tumors usually appear as submucosal nodules, and almost never produce the carcinoid syndrome, despite their direct access to the systemic circulation *(72)*. As in other carcinoids, malignant behavior in rectal carcinoids is related to the size of the tumor at presentation. Approximately two-thirds of such tumors are less than 1 cm, of which less than 5% have metastasized. Incidence of extra-rectal disease increases with size, with metastatic disease present in the majority of cases of tumors larger than 2 cm *(73)*. Endoscopic ultrasound is helpful in determining the depth of the tumor invasion (i.e., wall layer of the rectum), whether it has invaded blood vessels, and if there is local nodal disease *(74)*.

Given that most rectal carcinoids are less than 1 cm and the risk for metastatic disease is low, these lesions are usually treated with local excision surgically or endoscopically. Treatment of lesions larger than 1 cm is controversial. Some authors advocate low anterior or abdominoperineal resection for tumors larger than 2 cm, but others have argued that for these tumors the prognosis is poor and surgery does not alter the outcome *(75,76)*. Rectal carcinoids in the 1–2 cm range can sometimes be excised endoscopically, or with local surgical excision. Given the conflicting data regarding tumors larger than 1 cm, an individualized approach is recommended, taking into account patient preference, comorbid state, and so on *(21,22)*.

6.10. BRONCHOPULMONARY TREE

Approximately 28% of all carcinoids appear in the bronchi or lungs. They generally are slow growing and have a much better prognosis than other cancers arising in the lung *(12)*. Carcinoids are not associated with smoking. Histological features such as nuclear atypia and high mitotic rates signify more aggressive tumors with resultant lower survival rates *(77)*. These tumors rarely produce the carcinoid syndrome (<5% of patients), and other endocrine neoplastic syndromes such as Cushing's syndrome or acromegaly *(13,78,79)*. Surgical resection is the treatment of choice for bronchopulmonary carcinoids.

6.11. METASTATIC DISEASE

Metastatic spread of carcinoid tumors has been reported in an autopsy series *(11)* to occur in 29% of patients, with the majority of the metastases coming from small intestinal tumors (61%). Other series report that carcinoids that metastasize most frequently are located in the ileum, cecum, and colon *(66,80)*. Lymph nodes are the most frequent site of carcinoid metastases (89%), followed by liver (44%), lung (13%), and peritoneum (13%). Metastatic disease is more likely to produce a paraneoplastic endocrine syndrome and has a worse prognosis than localized disease, with a 5-yr survival rate of 39% *(34)*.

7. CARCINOID SYNDROME

As detailed earlier, the carcinoid syndrome is an infrequent manifestation of carcinoid tumors, and usually indicates systemic disease. Since its initial description in the early 1950s *(81,82)*, the rare constellations of flushing, diarrhea, telangiectasias, heart disease, and occasionally pellagra, have fascinated physicians. Because carcinoid tumors have been found to secrete many different bioactive amines, peptides, and prostaglandins *(8,83–85)*, different combinations of symptoms are possible. Most divide these manifestations into "typical" and "atypical" carcinoid syndromes.

The typical carcinoid syndrome complicates 5–7% of small bowel tumors, and occurs when venous drainage bypasses the liver (hepatic or retroperitoneal metastases). Of all presentations of carcinoid syndrome, 75–80% are from small bowel tumors, 1% are from appendiceal carcinoids, and rectal (hindgut) tumors virtually never produce a carcinoid syndrome *(86)*. The remaining cases of the carcinoid syndrome are produced by gastric or bronchial tumors, and often produce different bioactive secretions that lead to different symptoms (atypical).

The most prominent and distinctive features of the typical carcinoid syndrome are flushing and diarrhea, which occur in 30–94% and 38–86% of patients, respectively *(87–90)*. Flushing episodes have an abrupt onset, and are characterized by the appearance of a red to purple violaceous rash on the neck, face, and sometimes upper chest. The episodes usually last 20–30 s, although the duration may increase as the disease progresses. A burning sensation accompanies the rash, and hypotension or bronchoconstriction might develop. Flushing episodes do not correlate with elevated plasma levels of serotonin, but with its metabolite, 5-HIAA, which will be elevated in the urine. Elevated levels of urinary 5-HIAA may distinguish the flushing of carcinoid syndrome from other causes of flushing. The tachykinins (especially substance P) have been implicated as the secreted culprits that cause flushing, but the precise etiology of flushing in the carcinoid syndrome is not completely understood. Somatostatin analogs help to relieve the symptoms of flushing, whereas serotonin antagonists do not *(91–93)*.

Serotonin, however, plays a major causal role in the diarrhea of carcinoid syndrome. Intestinal ischemia, kinking of the bowel from mesenteric fibrosis and altered colonic transit may also contribute *(94,95)*. In 85–90% of cases, diarrhea presents in conjunction with the episodic flushing of the typical carcinoid syndrome, although both symptoms rarely occur simultaneously *(86)*. The diarrhea is secretory in nature, and may present with up to 30 bowel movements per day, which are watery and nonbloody. Serotonin antagonists such as methysergide and ondansetron have been shown to relieve the symptoms of diarrhea in the carcinoid syndrome, thus strongly suggesting that this substance is implicated in the pathogenesis of the symptom *(96)*.

A small number of patients will have dyspnea from bronchoconstriction, often during a flushing episode. It is important to recognize this symptom as originating from the carcinoid syndrome, as treatment of such wheezing with β-adrenergic agonists can trigger significant vasodilation and hypotension. Anti-cholinergic agents such as ipratroprium bromide are useful in such cases.

In homeostatic conditions, 99% of dietary tryptophan is converted to nicotinic acid, and less than 1% is made into 5-hydroxytryptophan (5-HTP), the precursor to serotonin. Carcinoid tumors may shunt the majority of tryptophan into the 5-HTP and serotonin pathway, which can deplete nicotinic acid stores and result in deficiency *(1,83,97,98)*. Pellagra, the resultant syndrome, may manifest with dermatitis (rough scaly skin, glossitis, angular stomatitis), diarrhea, and dementia.

Cardiac valvular lesions occur in a moderate number of patients with the carcinoid syndrome (45–75%) *(99–103)*. Lesions typically occur on the tricuspid valve, but are common on the pulmonary valve as well. The pathogenesis of these lesions is unknown, but is hypothesized to be related to excess circulating serotonin. Fibrous plaques may cause both stenosis and insufficiency of the involved valves, and right-heart failure can ensue. Valve replacement has been undertaken in such patients, but the peri-operative mortality is high. Rarely, left-sided heart disease will present with signs/symptoms of heart failure, usually because there is a bronchial carcinoid secreting substances directly into the systemic circulation.

Bronchopulmonary and gastric carcinoids rarely produce a so-called atypical variant of the carcinoid syndrome. These tumors generally lack the enzyme to convert 5-HTP to serotonin; plasma levels of 5-HTP are elevated and serotonin levels are normal in these patients *(22)*. Atypical carcinoid syndromes from bronchopulmonary tumors manifest with flushing that is marked and much longer than that of the typical syndrome. Neuropsychiatric symptoms such as disorientation and anxiety may accompany these episodes *(53)*.

Gastric tumors may produce an atypical carcinoid syndrome manifested by a blotchy erythematous rash that is sharply demarcated with central clearing, and is intensely pruritic. This variant is thought to be mediated by histamine production by the tumor *(104)*, and can be ameliorated by histamine antagonists.

The aptly named carcinoid crisis presents with flushing, profound hypotension (sometimes hypertension), and occasionally, bronchospasm or tachyarrhythmias *(105)*. Stressors such as anesthetic induction for surgery or surgical manipulation of the tumor usually precipitate this phenomenon, which is believed to be mediated by a massive release of vasoactive amines by the tumor. The hypotension is difficult to treat because it is resistant to sympathomimetic agents. These agents may actually induce more release of vasoactive substances from the tumor *(89)*. A recommended therapy for the hypotension of carcinoid crisis is the combination of fluid administration in conjunction with an infusion of octreotide, which often corrects the hypotensive episode in 10 min *(89,106)*.

8. DIAGNOSIS

Identification of primary tumors usually relies on endoscopy, GI contrast studies (small bowel follow-through or enteroclysis), or CT scan. More sophisticated imaging modalities (such as scintigraphy) may be employed when these diagnostic modalities fail to identify a lesion or when there is other evidence of the carcinoid syndrome. Incidental carcinoids (especially in the stomach, appendix, and rectum) may be discovered on investigation of unrelated matters. Ultimately, a biopsy of the tumor showing typical pathological features is diagnostic.

A 24-h urine collection for 5-HIAA has a specificity of 88% for carcinoid tumors *(107)*, and is the usual test to obtain when metastatic carcinoid is suspected. Of the other potential peptides and markers, chromogranin levels have been most studied. Chromogranin levels are sensitive but nonspecific for diagnosis of carcinoids, as they are elevated in other types of neuroendocrine tumors *(108)*.

If suspected, metastatic disease should be ruled out before curative resection is undertaken. Assessment for hepatic metastases with biochemical means is unreliable *(21)* because levels of transaminases and alkaline phosphatase can be normal in the face of extensive involvement of the liver. When metastatic disease is suspected (elevated urinary levels of 5-HIAA or presence of the carcinoid syndrome), a CT of the abdomen with and without contrast is appropriate to assess for liver lesions.

Most carcinoid tumors express somatostatin receptors. This feature has stimulated the development of nuclear medicine scans that aid in the diagnostic work-up of metastatic (and occasionally local) carcinoid disease. An [111]Indium-labeled somatostatin analog (pentetreotide) has been used with success to identify and localize carcinoid tumors, with a sensitivity of 80–90% *(109)*. Scintigraphy with this modality detects lesions that conventional imaging (CT and MRI) fails to capture *(110,111)*, but is most often used in concert with CT and MRI *(112–116)*.

Positron emission tomography (PET) scanning takes advantage of differing metabolic activity of tumor cells as compared to normal tissue, and may be used to assess for metastatic carcinoid disease. Labeling with 5-HTP has been used to detect carcinoids with this technology *(117,118)*. Sensitivity and specificity of PET have yet to exceed that of conventional imaging. The availability and expanding experience with PET scans may make this modality useful in the future, but further supporting data are required *(108)*.

9. TREATMENT

The only potentially curative therapy for carcinoid tumors is resection of the primary tumor. Surgery is appropriate for local resection of tumors smaller than 2 cm, and radical surgical approaches may be indicated for tumors larger than 2 cm. Endoscopic resection of tumors in the stomach and rectum is becoming more feasible as technology and experience increase, especially in cases in which the tumor is less than 1 cm. Small tumors can be amenable to endoscopic resection by a variety of methods.

The mainstay of treatment for metastatic carcinoids is somatostatin analogs. Somatostatin inhibits the release of bioactive peptides and amines, and can be cytostatic to tumor cells *(119,120)*. A somatostatin analog, octreotide, is administered subcutaneously every 6–12 h, and causes dramatic decreases in flushing and diarrhea in patients with the carcinoid syndrome *(108)*. Lantreotide is another somatostatin analog, and requires dosing every 10–14 d (not available in the United States). Depot octreotide is given once a month once a steady state is reached *(90)*.

In addition to symptomatic relief, somatostatin analogs may result in shrinkage of tumor mass. Several studies examining this theory have been undertaken *(121–127)*. Biochemical responses (decrease in urinary 5-HIAA levels) range from 27 to 72%, but objective tumor shrinkage in these studies has been less than 10%. Stabilization of disease progression *(124)* now seems a more reasonable endpoint with currently available somatostatin analogs. These medications are generally well tolerated, but observation for several unique side effects (cholelithiasis, arrhythmias) is warranted.

Treatment of symptomatic carcinoid tumors with interferons was initially proposed in 1983 *(128)*. Since that time, additional trials have examined the use of human leukocyte interferon, interferon-α and -γ *(125,129–138)*. These studies report modest biochemical response (about 40%) and minimal tumor response (12%) for the interferons *(108)*. Three studies addressed the utility of combining octreotide and interferon alpha, and report good biochemical responses (72–77%) but no tumor regression *(126,139)*.

Single-agent chemotherapy for carcinoid tumors has been evaluated and is not effective. As well, several multiagent regimens have been investigated and have minimal response rates. Many authors believe that systemic chemotherapy for carcinoid tumors should be reserved for patients with metastatic disease who are symptomatic and unresponsive to other therapies *(1,21,22,108)*. Chemotherapy in combination with interferon has proved to be disappointing as well *(125,140)*.

Vascular occlusion has been used to treat carcinoid tumors metastatic to the liver, taking advantage of tumor dependence on the hepatic artery. Various vascular occluding agents have been employed, with success reported in select patient populations. Small trials using intra-arterial chemotherapy in addition to embolization have been undertaken, but no significant improvement has been found *(141–149)*. Intra-arterial chemoembolization has been employed successfully in relieving symptoms from the carcinoid syndrome, although responses in tumor size are minimal *(150)*.

The role of radiotherapy in the treatment of disseminated carcinoid disease is palliation. External beam radiation has been most useful in treating symptomatic disease that involves the bone or central nervous system *(151)*.

Surgical resection of hepatic metastases is a reasonable option when the liver is the only site of spread (which is often the case). One series reported hepatic resection results of neuroendocrine tumors in 74 patients, of whom 50 had carcinoid tumors *(152)*. Relapse was common, but the overall 4-yr survival rate exceeded 70%. A small number of patients have received orthotopic liver transplants for metastatic disease to the liver, but there is not enough experience with this approach to recommend it.

Most patients with metastatic carcinoid tumors live for some time after diagnosis, given the slow-growing nature of the tumor (Table 3). Physicians are often left with palliative treatment of symptoms, and should do so in these challenging cases. Conservative treatment of symptoms with agents such as loperamide for mild diarrhea, nicotinic acid to prevent pellagra, bronchodilators for bronchospasm, and controlling symptoms of heart failure when valvular problems occur, are an integral part of supporting patients with this illness.

Table 3
5-Yr Survival Rates for Carcinoid Tumors by Site

Site	5-yr survival rates (%)
All carcinoids	65–67
Bronchopulmonary	70–74
Digestive system	63–68
Stomach	63
Liver	18
Biliary	60
Pancreas	38
Small intestine	61
Colon (not rectum or appendix)	61
Appendix	71
Rectum	88

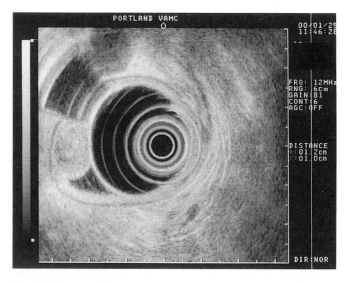

Fig. 2. EUS image of a gastric carcinoid. (Courtesy of Raquel Davila, MD, Oregon Health & Science University.)

10. ROLE OF ENDOSCOPY

As previously mentioned, carcinoid tumors of the stomach, duodenum, rectum, colon, appendix, and terminal ileum may be found incidentally when other conditions are being investigated via endoscopy. Infrequently, a carcinoid tumor will produce symptoms such as abdominal or rectal pain, blood per rectum, bowel obstruction, or mass felt on rectal exam, necessitating a diagnostic endoscopy. Simple biopsy of a luminal mass may be adequate to diagnose a carcinoid tumor. However, the submucosal location of most tumors sometimes results in nondiagnostic biopsies. In these cases, endoscopic ultrasound (EUS) may provide images of the internal structure of the GI wall, determine the depth of mucosal carcinoid tumors *(153)* as well as provide fine-needle aspiration or ESMR to obtain diagnostic tissue (Fig. 2). One group has advocated endoscopic resection of gastric carcinoids less than 2 cm if EUS can confirm that the tumor is confined to the submucosa without local adenopathy *(154)*.

Modified techniques of ESMR include cap-assisted endoscopic mucosal resection (EMRC) and endoscopic mucosal resection with ligation (EMRL) *(155)*. EMRC requires a specialized transparent plastic cap to be placed on the end of a standard or therapeutic endoscope. After submucosal injection to raise the tumor, a crescent-shaped snare is advanced into a groove on the inner cap while briefly suctioning normal mucosa to seal the cap outlet. Next, the lesion is sucked into the cap and the snare is closed around the lesion. Blended electrosurgical current is applied to resect the lesion, followed by aspiration of the specimen into the plastic cap for removal (156). EMRL uses a standard endoscopic variceal ligation device that is fitted onto a single-channel endoscope. After marking the periphery of the lesion, about 5–10 mL of submucosal injectant is applied. The submucosal nodule is suctioned into a ligator device and a ligating band is deployed. The snare is placed below the band, blended electrosurgical current is applied, and deep vertical resection margins are achieved (157).

In addition to ESMR, other diagnostic methods utilized for submucosal carcinoids include snare polypectomy with and without saline injection, strip biopsy, aspiration lumpectomy, and Nd:Yag laser ablation (48–50,158–161). Snare polypectomy without saline injection, known as "inject and cut technique," may not provide adequate resection margins; lifting the lesion with submucosal injection of saline solution or by aspiration and banding followed by snare resection as described above, are more effective techniques (162). Strip biopsy technique with hypertonic saline and epinephrine injection has been advocated for duodenal carcinoids located in the submucosal layer, but there may be a risk of perforation (48). This risk is perceived to be owing to inadvertent entrapment of the muscularis propria layer during the snare technique. To perform strip biopsy (also referred to as "inject, lift, and cut technique"), a two-channel endoscope is required. A needle is stabbed into the submucosal space to lift the tumor, which is then grasped with a snare and pulled up through the snare with a wide-mouthed forceps. Electrosurgical blended current is applied to remove the submucosal tumor (48). Given the various methods of endoscopic mucosal resection the method chosen should be that with which the endoscopist is most experienced.

It is important to determine the completeness of resection after ESMR or after other modified techniques. In cases of positive margins after attempted endoscopic resection, followup endoscopy is recommended (155). However, interval guidelines may vary from several weeks to several months. Repeat ESMR, endoscopic thermal/laser therapy such as argon plasma coagulation, or surgery have all been advocated when residual recurrent lesions are found (155). Maeda et al. report that 24–42% of rectal tumors less than 2 cm have incomplete resections or unclear margins when treated endoscopically, and thus recommend minimally invasive surgical resection (163). Another study with a follow up of 29–237 mo found no evidence of recurrent local or metastatic disease in 18 of 22 patients with rectal carcinoids less than 10 mm treated with endoscopic resection (164).

When conventional diagnostic tests as outlined above are unsatisfactory, capsule endoscopy holds promise in improving the diagnosis of deep small bowel pathology (165). It is a relatively new, painless adjunctive method of imaging the entire small bowel with good to excellent visualization. In one study,

wireless capsule endoscopy had a similar diagnostic yield to small bowel enteroclysis for 22 patients with suspected small bowel pathology (166). Capsule endoscopy has also been used to diagnose metastatic carcinoid tumor of unknown primary, when the primary tumor lies in the small bowel (167). These studies comprehensively demonstrate that capsule endoscopy may be a valuable tool for diagnosing primary small intestine tumors, but due to their small sample sizes, further studies regarding efficacy are warranted.

No studies have proven the utility of screening or of surveillance of populations for carcinoid tumors. Bresky et al. biannually surveilled 128 patients with pernicious anemia for the development of gastric neoplasms, finding only two carcinoids in the course of the study (168). They concluded that such surveillance with esophagogastroduodenoscopy was not warranted. Given that carcinoid tumors are rare, screening cannot be recommended. Though there is little supporting evidence, it might be reasonable to follow patients with locally resected carcinoids to determine if there is recurrence, which may be amenable to further local therapy.

11. PROGNOSIS

The prognosis for carcinoid tumors is good when compared with many other neoplasms, notably adenocarcinoma. The 5-yr survival rates from the past decade (see Table 3) are encouraging. As with most malignancies, survival decreases significantly as disease progresses from local to regional to distant. Key to treatment of these usually indolent tumors is early resection, and effective palliation when there is extensive disease.

REFERENCES

1. Caplin ME, et al. Carcinoid tumour. Lancet 1998; 352(9130): 799–805.
2. Lubarsch O. Ueber den primaren Krebs des Ileum, nebst Bemerkungen uber das gleichzeitige Vorkommen von Krebs und Tuberkolose. Virchows Arch 1888; 111:280–317.
3. Oberndorfer S. Karzinoide tumoren des dunndarms. Frank Z Pathol 1907; 1:425–429.
4. Masson P. Carcinoids (argentaffin-cell tumors) and nerve hyperplasia of appendicular mucosa. Am J Pathol 1928; 4:181–212.
5. Lembech F. 5-hydroxytryptamine in carcinoid tumor. Nature 1953; 172:p. 910–911.
6. Page I, Corcoran A, Vollenfrend S. Argentaffinoma as an endocrine tumor. Lancet 1955; 1:198,199.
7. Todd TR, et al. Bronchial carcinoid tumors: twenty years' experience. J Thor Cardiovasc Surg 1980; 79(4):532–536.
8. Neary PC, et al. Carcinoid disease: review of the literature. Dis Colon Rectum 1997; 40(3):349–362.
9. Moertel C, et al. Life history of the carcinoid tumor of the small intestine. Cancer 1961; 14:901–912.
10. Eller R, Frazee R, Roberts J. Gastrointestinal carcinoid tumors. Am Surgeon 1991; 57:434–437.
11. Berge T, Linell F. Carcinoid tumours. Frequency in a defined population during a 12-year period. Acta Pathol et Microbiol Scand—Section A Pathol 1976; 84(4):322–330.
12. Modlin IM, Lye KD, Kidd M. A 5-decade analysis of 13,715 carcinoid tumors. Cancer 2003; 97(4):934–959.
13. Limper AH, et al. The Cushing syndrome induced by bronchial carcinoid tumors. Ann Int Med 1992; 117(3):209–214.
14. Wajchenberg BL, et al. Ectopic ACTH syndrome. (erratum appears in J Steroid Biochem Mol Biol 1995 Sep;54(5–6):287). J Steroid Biochem Mol Biol 1995; 53(1–6):139–151.

15. Modlin IM, Sandor A. An analysis of 8305 cases of carcinoid tumors. Cancer 1997; 79(4):813–829.

16. Woods HF Bax ND, Ainsworth I. Abdominal carcinoid tumours in Sheffield. Digestion 1990; 45(Suppl 1):17–22.

17. Newton JN, et al. The epidemiology of carcinoid tumours in England and Scotland. Br J Cancer 1994; 70(5):939–942.

18. Lu Cortez L, et al. (Carcinoid tumor. An analysis of 131 cases). Revista Clinica Espanola 1994; 194(4):291–293.

19. Soga J. Carcinoids of the rectum an evaluation of 1271 reported cases Surgery Today 1997; 27(2):112–119.

20. Waldum HL, Haugen OA, Brenna E. Do neuroendocrine cells particularly the D-cellplay a role in the development of gastric stump cancerCancer Detection & Prevention 1994; 18(6):431–46.

21. Kulke MH, Mayer RJ. Carcinoid tumors. N Eng J of Med 1999; 340(11):858–868.

22. Anthony T, Kim L. Gastrointestinal Carcinoid Tumors and the Carcinoid Syndromein Sleisenger & Fordtran's Gastrointestinal and Liver Disease Feldman M Friedman LS, Sleisenger MH. eds. Saunders: Philadelphia; 2002; 2151–2168.

23. Vyberg M, et al. Immunohistochemical identification of neuron-specific enolasesynaptophysinchromogranin and endocrine granule constituent in neuroendocrine tumours. Acta Histochemica—Supplement B 1990; 38:179–181.

24. Capella C, et al. Revised classification of neuroendocrine tumors of the lungpancreas and gut. Digestion. 1994; 55(Suppl 3):11–23.

25. Williams E, Sanders M. The classification of carcinoid tumors. Lancet 1963; 1:238,239.

26. Soga J, Tazawa K. Pathologic analysis of carcinoids. Histologic reevaluation of 62 cases. Cancer 1971; 28(4):990–998.

27. Yang K, et al. The neuroendocrine products of intestinal carcinoids. An immunoperoxidase study of 35 carcinoid tumors stained for serotonin and eight polypeptide hormones. Cancer 1983; 51(10): 1918–1926.

28. Lindberg GM, et al. Atypical carcinoid of the esophagus: a case report and review of the literature. Cancer 1997; 79(8): 1476–1481.

29. Modlin IM, Lye KD, Kidd M. A 50-year analysis of 562 gastric carcinoids: small tumor or larger problem Am J Gastroenterol 2004; 99(1):23–32.

30. Rindi G, et al. Gastric carcinoids and neuroendocrine carcinomas, pathogenesis, pathology and behavior. World J Surg 1996; 20(2): 168–172.

31. Havu N. Enterochromaffin-like cell carcinoids of gastric mucosa in rats after life-long inhibition of gastric secretion. Digestion 1986; 35(Suppl 1):42–55.

32. Klinkenberg-Knol EC, et al. Long-term treatment with omeprazole for refractory reflux esophagitisefficacy and safety (see comment) Ann Intern Med 1994; 121(3):161–167.

33. Bordi C. Endocrine tumours of the stomach. Pathol Res Pract 1995; 191(4):373–380.

34. Modlin IM, Lye KD, Kidd M. Carcinoid tumors of the stomach. Surg Oncol 2003; 12(2):153–172.

35. Rindi G, et al. Three subtypes of gastric argyrophil carcinoid and the gastric neuroendocrine carcinomaa clinicopathologic study (see comment) Gastroenterology 1993; 104(4):994–1006.

36. Gough DB, et al. Diverse clinical and pathologic features of gastric carcinoid and the relevance of hypergastrinemia. World J Surg 1994; 18(4):473–479 discussion 479, 480.

37. Moses RE, et al. The syndrome of type A chronic atrophic gastritis pernicious anemia and multiple gastric carcinoids. J Clin Gastroenterol 1986; 8(1):61–65.

38. Hunt GC, Smith PP, Faigel DO. Yield of tissue sampling for submucosal lesions evaluated by EUS. Gastrointestinal Endosc 2003; 57(1):68–72.

39. Gilligan CJ, et al., Gastric carcinoid tumors: the biology and therapy of an enigmatic and controversial lesion. Am J Gastroenterol 1995; 90(3):338–352.

40. Debelenko LV, et al. The multiple endocrine neoplasia type I gene locus is involved in the pathogenesis of type II gastric carcinoids. Gastroenterology 1997; 113(3):773–781.

41. Maurer CA, et al. Carcinoid of the pancreas: clinical characteristics and morphological features. Eur J Cancer 1996; 32A(7):1109–1116.

42. Gudjonsson B., Carcinoma of the pancreas: critical analysis of costs, results of resectionsand the need for standardized reporting (see comment) J Am College Surgeons 1995; 181(6):483–503.

43. Knox CD, et al. Long-term survival after resection for primary hepatic carcinoid tumor(see comment) Ann Surgical Oncol 2003; 10(10):1171–1175.

44. Podnos YD, et al. Carcinoid tumors of the common bile duct: report of two cases. Surg Today 2003; 33(7):553–535.

45. Makhlouf HR, Burke AP, Sobin LH. Carcinoid tumors of the ampulla of Vater: a comparison with duodenal carcinoid tumors. Cancer 1999; 85(6):1241–1249.

46. Burke AP, et al. Carcinoid tumors of the duodenum. A clinicopathologic study of 99 cases. Arch Pathol Lab Med 1990; 114(7):700–704.

47. Klein A, Clemens J, Cameron J. Periampullary neoplasms in von Recklinghausen's disease. Surgery 1989; 106(5):815–819.

48. Yoshikane H, et al. Endoscopic resection of small duodenal carcinoid tumors with strip biopsy technique. Gastrointestinal Endoscopy 1998; 47(6):466–470.

49. Yamamoto C, et al. Carcinoid tumors of the duodenum: report of three cases treated by endoscopic resection. Endoscopy 1997; 29(3):218–221.

50. Nishimori I, et al. Endosonography-guided endoscopic resection of duodenal carcinoid tumor. Endoscopy. 1997; 29(3):214–217.

51. Barclay TH, Schapira DV. Malignant tumors of the small intestine. Cancer 1983; 51(5):878–881.

52. North JH, Pack MS. Malignant tumors of the small intestine: a review of 144 cases. Am Surgeon 2000; 66(1):46–51.

53. Eckhauser FE, et al. Mesenteric angiopathy, intestinal gangrene, and midgut carcinoids. Surgery 1981; 90(4):720–728.

54. Burke AP, et al. Carcinoids of the jejunum and ileum: an immunohistochemical and clinicopathologic study of 167 cases. Cancer 1997; 79(6):1086–1093.

55. Loftus JP, van Heerden JA. Surgical management of gastrointestinal carcinoid tumors. Advances in Surg 1995; 28:317–336.

56. Wangberg B, et al. Survival of patients with disseminated midgut carcinoid tumors after aggressive tumor reduction. World J Surg 1996; 20(7):p. 892–899; discussion 899.

57. Makridis C, et al. Progression of metastases and symptom improvement from laparotomy in midgut carcinoid tumors. World Surg. 1996; 20(7):900–906; discussion 907.

58. Anderson DJ. Carcinoid tumor in Meckel's diverticulum: laparoscopic treatment and review of the literature. J Am Osteopathic Assoc 2000; 100(7):432–434.

59. Moyana TN. Carcinoid tumors arising from Meckel's diverticulum. A clinical, morphologic, and immunohistochemical study. Am J Clin Pathol. 1989; 91(1):52–56.

60. Goede AC, Caplin ME, Winslet MC. Carcinoid tumour of the appendix. Br J Surg. 2003; 90(11):1317–1322.

61. McCusker ME, et al. Primary malignant neoplasms of the appendix: a population-based study from the surveillance, epidemiology and end-results program, 1973-1998. Cancer 2002; 94(12):3307–3312.

62. Moertel CG, et al. Carcinoid tumor of the appendix: treatment and prognosis. N Engl J Med 1987; 317(27):1699–1701.

63. Rosenberg JM. Welch JP. Carcinoid tumors of the colon. A study of 72 patients. Am J Surg 1985; 149(6):775–779.

64. Berardi RS. Carcinoid tumors of the colon (exclusive of the rectum): review of the literature. Dis Colon Rectum 1972;15(5):383–391.

65. Saha S, et al. Carcinoid tumors of the gastrointestinal tract: a 44-year experience. Southern Med J. 1989; 82(12):1501–1505.

66. Olney JR, et al. Carcinoid tumors of the gastrointestinal tract. Am Surgeon 1985; 51(1):37–41.

67. Ballantyne GH, et al. Incidence and mortality of carcinoids of the colon. Data from the Connecticut Tumor Registry. Cancer 1992; 69(10):2400–2405.

68. Thomas RM, Sobin LH. Gastrointestinal cancer. Cancer 1995; 75 (1 Suppl):154–170.

69. Spread C, et al. Colon carcinoid tumors. A population-based study. Dis Colon Rectum 1994; 37(5):482–491.

70. Schindl M, et al. Stage-dependent therapy of rectal carcinoid tumors. World J Surg. 1998; 22(6):628–633; discussion 634.

71. Jetmore AB, et al. Rectal carcinoids: the most frequent carcinoid tumor. Dis Colon & Rectum 1992; 35(8): 717–725.

72. Mani S, et al. Carcinoids of the rectum. J Am College Surgeons. 1994; 179(2):231–248.

73. Naunheim KS, et al. Rectal carcinoid tumors—treatment and prognosis. Surgery. 1983; 94(4):670–676.

74. Yoshida M, et al. Endoscopic assessment of invasion of colorectal tumors with a new high-frequency ultrasound probe. Gastrointestinal Endoscopy. 1995; 41(6):587–592.

75. Sauven P, et al. Anorectal carcinoid tumors. Is aggressive surgery warranted? (see comment). Ann Surg 1990; 211(1):67–71.

76. Koura AN, et al. Carcinoid tumors of the rectum:effect of size, histopathology, and surgical treatment on metastasis free survival. Cancer. 1997; 79(7):1294–1298.

77. Mc Mullan DM, Wood DE. Pulmonary carcinoid tumors. Sem Thor Cardiovasc Surg 2003; 15(3):289–300.

78. Carroll DG, et al. Resolution of acromegaly after removal of a bronchial carcinoid shown to secrete growth hormone releasing factor. Austr N Zeal J Med1987; 17(1):63–67.

79. Chughtai TS, et al. Bronchial carcinoid—twenty years' experience defines a selective surgical approach. Surgery 1997; 122(4):801–808.

80. Marshall JB, Bodnarchuk G. Carcinoid tumors of the gut. Our experience over three decades and review of the lite J Clin Gastroenterol. 1993; 16(2):123–129.

81. Rosenbaum FD, Claudon D. Essential telangiectasia, pulmonic and tricuspid stenosis, and neoplastic liver disease: A possible new clinical syndrome. J Lab Clin Med 1953; 42:941.

82. Thorson A, Bjork G, Bjorkman G. Malignant carcinoid of the small intestine with metastasis to the liver, valvular disease of the right heart (pulmonary stenosis and tricuspid regurgitation without septal defect), peripheral vasomotor symptoms, bronchoconstriction and an unusual type of cyanosis. Am Heart J 1954; 47:794.

83. Creutzfeldt W. Historical background and natural history of carcinoids. Digestion 1994; 55(Suppl 3):3–10.

84. Kloppel G, Heitz PU. Classification of normal and neoplastic neuroendocrine cells. Ann NY Acad Sci 1994; 733:19–23.

85. Wilander E. Diagnostic pathology of gastrointestinal and pancreatic neuroendocrine tumours. Acta Oncologica. 1989; 28(3):363–369.

86. Feldman JM. Carcinoid tumors and the carcinoid syndrome. Curr Problems Surg 1989; 26(12):835–885.

87. Creutzfeldt W. Carcinoid tumors: development of our knowledge. World J Surg. 1996; 20(2):126–131.

88. Bax ND, et al. Clinical manifestations of carcinoid disease. World J Surg 1996; 20(2):142–146.

89. Vaughan DJ, Brunner MD, Anesthesia for patients with carcinoid syndrome. Inter Anesthesiol Clinics 1997; 35(4):129–142.

90. Rubin J, et al. Octreotide acetate long-acting formulation versus open-label subcutaneous octreotide acetate in malignant carcinoid syndrome. J Clinical Oncol 1999; 17(2):600–606.

91. Creutzfeldt W, Stockmann F. Carcinoids and carcinoid syndrome. Am J Med 1987; 82(5B):4–16.

92. Richter G, et al. Serotonin release into blood after food and pentagastrin. Studies in healthy subjects and in patients with metastatic carcinoid tumors. Gastroenterol 1986; 91(3):612–618.

93. Lucas KJ, Feldman JM. Flushing in the carcinoid syndrome and plasma kallikrein. Cancer 1986; 58(10):2290–2293.

94. Saslow SB, et al. Octreotide inhibition of flushing and colonic motor dysfunction in carcinoid syndrome. Am J Gastroenterol 1997; 92(12):2250–2256.

95. von der Ohe MR, et al. Motor dysfunction of the small bowel and colon in patients with the carcinoid syndrome and diarrhea. (erratum appears in N Engl J Med 1993 Nov 18;329(21):1592). New Engl J Med. 1993; 329(15):1073–1078.

96. Ahlman H, et al. The pentagastrin test in the diagnosis of the carcinoid syndrome. J Cardiovascular Pharmacol. 1985; 7(Suppl 7): S86—S88.

97. Moertel CG. Karnofsky memorial lecture. An odyssey in the land of small tumors. J Clin Oncol 1987; 5(10):1502–1522.

98. Sin LL, Chapman W, Moore MJ. Use of the somatostatin analogue octreotide acetate in the treatment of encephalopathy associated with carcinoid tumor. Case report. Am J Clinical Oncol 1997; 20(6):558–561.

99. Pellikka PA, et al. Carcinoid heart disease. Clinical and echocardiographic spectrum in 74 patients. Circulation 1993; 87(4):1188–1196.

100. Lundin L, et al. Transoesophageal echocardiography improves the diagnostic value of cardiac ultrasound in patients with carcinoid heart disease. Br Heart J 1990; 64(3):190–194.

101. Howard RJ, et al. Carcinoid heart disease: diagnosis by two-dimensional echocardiography. Circulation 1982; 66(5):1059–1065.

102. Lundin L, et al. Carcinoid heart disease: relationship of circulating vasoactive substances to ultrasound-detectable cardiac abnormalities. Circulation 1988; 77(2):264–269.

103. Moyssakis IE, et al. Incidence and evolution of carcinoid syndrome in the heart. J Heart Valve Dis 1997; 6(6):625–630.

104. Roberts LJ, 2nd, Marney SR, Jr, Oates JA. Blockade of the flush associated with metastatic gastric carcinoid by combined histamine H1 and H2 receptor antagonists. Evidence for an important role of H2 receptors in human vasculature. N Engl J Med 1979; 300(5):236–238.

105. Basson MD, et al. Biology and management of the midgut carcinoid. Am J Surg 1993; 165(2):288–297.

106. Veall GR, et al. Review of the anaesthetic management of 21 patients undergoing laparotomy for carcinoid syndrome. (see comment) Br J Anaesthesia 1994; 72(3):335–341.

107. Tormey WP, Fitz Gerald RJ. The clinical and laboratory correlates of an increased urinary 5-hydroxyindoleacetic acid. Postgraduate Mel Jl. 1995; 71(839):542–545.

108. Schnirer II, Yao JC, Ajani JA. Carcinoid—a comprehensive review. Acta Oncologica. 2003; 42(7):672–692.

109. Krenning EP, et al. Radiotherapy with a radiolabeled somatostatin analogue (111In-DTPA-D-Phe1)-octreotide. A case history. Ann NY Acad Sci 1994; 733:496–506.

110. Westlin JE, et al. Somatostatin rec eptor scintigraphy of carcinoid tumours using the (111In-DTPA-D-Phe1)-octreotide. Acta Oncologica. 1993; 32(7–8):783–786.

111. Shi W, et al. Localization of neuroendocrine tumours with (111In) DTPA-octreotide scintigraphy (Octreoscan): a comparative study with CT and MR imaging. Qjm 1998; 91(4): 295–301.

112. Anthony LB, et al. Somatostatin receptor imaging: predictive and prognostic considerations. Digestion 1996; 57(Suppl 1):50–53.

113. Krenning EP, et al. Somatostatin receptor: scintigraphy and radionuclide therapy. Digestion. 1996; 57(Suppl 1):57–61.

114. Kwekkeboom DJ, Krenning EP. Somatostatin receptor scintigraphy in patients with carcinoid tumors. World J Surg 1996; 20(2): 157–161.

115. Ahlman H, et al. Somatostatin receptors on neuroendocrine tumors—a way to intraoperative diagnosis and localization. Yale J BioMed 1994; 67(3–4):215–221.

116. Lobrano MB, et al. Metastatic carcinoid tumor imaged with CT and a radiolabeled somatostatin analog: a case report. Am J Gastroenterol 1997; 92(3): 513–515.

117. Eriksson B, et al. Positron emission tomography (PET) in neuroendocrine gastrointestinal tumors. Acta Oncologica. 1993;32(2): 189–196.

118. Eriksson B, et al. The role of PET in localization of neuroendocrine and adrenocortical tumors. Ann NY Acad Sci 2002; 970:159–169.

119. Lamberts SW, et al. Long-term treatment of acromegaly with the somatostatin analogue SMS 201-995. New Engl J Med. 1985; 313(25):1576–1580.

120. Schally AV. Oncological applications of somatostatin analogues. (erratum appears in Cancer Res 1989 Mar 15;49(6):1618). Can Res 1988; 48(24 Pt 1):6977–6985.

121. Kvols LK, et al. Treatment of the malignant carcinoid syndrome. Evaluation of a long-acting somatostatin analogue. New Engl J Med 1986; 315(11):663–666.

122. Oberg K Norheim I. Theodorsson E. Treatment of malignant midgut carcinoid tumours with a long-acting somatostatin analogue octreotide. Acta Oncologica. 1991; 30(4):503–507.

123. Tomassetti P, Migliori M, Gullo L. Slow-release lanreotide treatment in endocrine gastrointestinal tumors. Am J Gastroenterol 1998; 93(9):1468–1471.

124. Saltz L, et al. Octreotide as an antineoplastic agent in the treatment of functional and nonfunctional neuroendocrine tumors. Cancer. 1993; 72(1):244–248.

125. Janson ET, et al. Treatment with alpha-interferon versus alpha-interferon in combination with streptozocin and doxorubicin in patients with malignant carcinoid tumors: a randomized trial. Ann Oncol 1992; 3(8):635–638.

126. Janson ET, Oberg K. Long-term management of the carcinoid syndrome. Treatment with octreotide alone and in combination with alpha-interferon. Acta Oncologica. 1993; 32(2):225–229.

127. Arnold R, et al. Somatostatin analogue octreotide and inhibition of tumour growth in metastatic endocrine gastroenteropancreatic tumours. Gut. 1996; 38(3):430–438.

128. Oberg K, Funa K, Alm G. Effects of leukocyte interferon on clinical symptoms and hormone levels in patients with mid-gut carcinoid tumors and carcinoid syndrome. New Engl J Med 1983; 309(3):129–133.

129. Creutzfeldt W, et al. Treatment of gastrointestinal endocrine tumours with interferon-alpha and octreotide. Acta Oncologica 1991; 30(4):529–535.

130. Hanssen LE, et al. Treatment of malignant metastatic midgut carcinoid tumours with recombinant human alpha2b interferon with or without prior hepatic artery embolization. Scandinavian J. Gastroenterol. 1989; 24(7):787–795.

131. Moertel CGJ, Kvols LK. Therapy of metastatic carcinoid tumor and the malignant carcinoid syndrome with recombinant leukocyte A interferon. J Clin Oncol 1989; 7(7):865–868.

132. Oberg K, et al. Treatment of malignant carcinoid tumors with recombinant interferon alfa-2b: development of neutralizing interferon antibodies and possible loss of antitumor activity. J National Cancer Institute 1989; 81(7):531–535.

133. Oberg K, Eriksson B. The role of interferons in the management of carcinoid tumours. Bri J Haematol 1991; 79(Suppl 1):74–77.

134. Schober C, et al. Antitumour effect and symptomatic control with interferon alpha 2b in patients with endocrine active tumours. Euro J Cancer.,1992; 28A(10):1664–1666.

135. Joensuu H, Kumpulainen E, Grohn P. Treatment of metastatic carcinoid tumour with recombinant interferon alfa. Eur J Cancer 1992; 28A(10):1650–1653.

136. Bajetta E, et al. Treatment of metastatic carcinoids and other neuroendocrine tumors with recombinant interferon-alpha-2a. A study by the Italian Trials in Med Oncol Group. Cancer 1993;72(10):3099–3105.

137. Di Bartolomeo M, et al.Treatment of carcinoid syndrome with recombinant interferon alpha-2a(erratum appears in Acta Oncol 1993;32(5):592). Acta Oncologica 1993; 32(2):235–238.

138. Jacobsen MB, et al. Interferon-alpha 2b, with or without prior hepatic artery embolization: clinical response and survival in midgut carcinoid patients. The Norwegian carcinoid study. Scand J Gastroenterol 1995; 30(8):789–796.

139. Frank M, et al. Combination therapy with octreotide and alpha-interferon: effect on tumor growth in metastatic endocrine gastroenteropancreatic tumors. Am J Gastroenterol 1999;94(5):1381–1387.

140. Saltz L, et al. A phase II trial of alpha-interferon and 5-fluorouracil in patients with advanced carcinoid and islet cell tumors. Cancer 1994; 74(3):958–961.

141. Nobin A, Mansson B, Lunderquist A. Evaluation of temporary liver dearterialization and embolization in patients with metastatic carcinoid tumour. Acta Oncologica 1989; 28(3):419–424.

142. Carrasco CH, et al. The carcinoid syndrome: palliation by hepatic artery embolization. AJR. Am J Roentgenol 1986;147(1):149–154.

143. Eriksson BK, et al. Liver embolizations of patients with malignant neuroendocrine gastrointestinal tumors. Cancer 1998;83(11):2293–2301.

144. Ruszniewski P, et al. Hepatic arterial chemoembolization in patients with liver metastases of endocrine tumors. A prospective phase II study in 24 patients. Cancer 1993; 71(8):2624–2630.

145. Therasse E, et al. Transcatheter chemoembolization of progressive carcinoid liver metastasis. Radiology 1993; 189(2):541–547.

146. Perry LJ, et al. Hepatic arterial chemoembolization for metastatic neuroendocrine tumors. Surgery 1994; 116(6):1111–1116; discussion 1116–1117.

147. Drougas JG, et al. Hepatic artery chemoembolization for management of patients with advanced metastatic carcinoid tumors. Am J Surg 1998; 175(5):408–412.

148. Diamandidou E, et al. Two-phase study of hepatic artery vascular occlusion with microencapsulated cisplatin in patients with liver metastases from neuroendocrine tumors. AJR. Am J Roentgenol 1998; 170(2):339–344.

149. Kim YH, et al. Selective hepatic arterial chemoembolization for liver metastases in patients with carcinoid tumor or islet cell carcinoma. Cancer Investigation 1999; 17(7):474–478.

150. Gates J, et al. Chemoembolization of hepatic neoplasms: safety, complications, and when to worry. Radiographics 1999;19(2):399–414.

151. Schupak, KD. Wallner KE. The role of radiation therapy in the treatment of locally unresectable or metastatic carcinoid tumors. Inter J Radiation Oncol Biol Physics 1991; 20(3):489–495.

152. Que FG, et al. Hepatic resection for metastatic neuroendocrine carcinomas. Am J Surg 1995; 169(1):36–42; discussion 42, 43.

153. Inai M, et al. Endosonographic characterization of duodenal elevated lesions. Gastrointest Endosc1996; 44(6):714–719.

154. Chak A. EUS in submucosal tumors. Gastrointestinal Endoscopy 2002; 56(4 Suppl):S43–S48.

155. Soetikno RM, et al. Endoscopic mucosal resection. Gastrointest Endosc 2003; 57(4):567–579.

156. Inoue H, et al. Endoscopic mucosal resection with a cap-fitted panendoscope for esophagus, stomach, and colon mucosal lesions. Gastrointest Endosc 1993; 39(1):58–62.

157. Suzuki Y, et al. Treatment of gastric tumors by endoscopic mucosal resection with a ligating device. Gastrointest Endosc1999; 49(2): 192–199.

158. Rau BK, Harikrishnan KM. KrishnaS.Endoscopic laser ablation of duodenal carcinoids: a new treatment modality. J Clin Laser MedSurg 1995; 13(1):37–38.

159. Berkelhammer C, et al. "Band-snare" resection of small rectal carcinoid tumors. Gastrointestinal Endoscopy 1999; 50(4):582–585.

160. Lachter J, Chemtob J. EUS may have limited impact on the endoscopic management of gastric carcinoids. Inter J Gastrointestinal Cancer 2002; 31(1–3):181–183.

161. Ichikawa J, et al. Endoscopic mucosal resection in the management of gastric carcinoid tumors. Endoscopy 2003; 35(3):203–206.

162. Ono A, et al. Endoscopic submucosal resection of rectal carcinoid tumors with a ligation device. Gastrointest Endosc 2003; 57(4): 583–587.

163. Maeda K, et al. Minimally invasive surgery for carcinoid tumors in the rectum. Biomed Pharmacotherapy 2002; 56 (Suppl 1):222s–226s.

164. Higaki S, et al. Effectiveness of local endoscopic resection of rectal carcinoid tumors. Endoscopy 1997; 29(3):171–175.

165. de Mascarenhas-Saraiva MN, da Silva Araujo Lopes LM. Small-bowel tumors diagnosed by wireless capsule endoscopy: report of five cases. Endoscopy 2003; 35(10):865–868.

166. Voderholzer WA, et al. Diagnostic yield of wireless capsule enteroscopy in comparison with computed tomography enteroclysis. Endoscopy 2003; 35(12):1009–1014.

167. Coates SW Jr, DeMarco DC. Metastatic carcinoid tumor discovered by capsule endoscopy and not detected by esophagogastroduodenoscopy. Dig Dis Sci 2004; 49(4):639–641.

168. Bresky G, et al. Endoscopic findings in a biennial follow-up program in patients with pernicious anemia. Hepatogastroenterology 1999; 50(54):2264–2266.

16 Medical and Surgical Therapy for Gastric Cancer

DIANE HERSHOCK, MD, PhD

CONTENTS

1. BACKGROUND

Gastric cancer remains among the 10 most common cancers in the world with variations in incidence and survival based on geographic sites. Gastric cancer is the second most common tumor worldwide with 60% of cases in developing countries (1). It appears that, worldwide, gastric cancer is second only to lung cancer with a reported 798,300 new cases in 1990 and is more common than, breast and colorectal cancer outside of the United States. The highest incidences are in Japanese men; rates are also increased in eastern Europe, South America, and eastern Asia, but lower in the United States, North Africa, and Australia (1). In contrast, esophageal cancer is relatively rare, being the seventh leading cause of death in men in the United States (2). Survival is poor, being only 37% for stage II, 11–18% for stage III, and 5% for stage IV. The effectiveness of surgery, chemotherapy, radiation therapy or the combination of the above modalities has been investigated for decades with varied results.

2. INCIDENCE/EPIDEMIOLOGY

The patterns of occurrence of gastric cancer has changed over the years with population migration. Although it remains the second most common tumor in the world, the incidence of gastric cancer declined dramatically since 1930 in the developed countries, particularily the United States (3). This decline may be attributed to reclassification of adenocarcinomas of the gastric cardia and the lower third of the esophagus as gastro-esophageal junction (GEJ) cancers because both behave in a similar biological and clinical fashion. Additionally, there has been a decline in the well-differentiated adenocarcinomas of the fundus and antrum (4).

3. PATHOGENESIS AND ETIOLOGY

The pathogenesis of gastric cancer has not been well established. It has been postulated that p53 mutations, the adenomatous polyposis coli (APC) gene, K-ras alterations, loss of heterozygosity of the deleted-in-colorectal-cancer (DCC) gene and translocated promoter region-MET rearrangement may play a role in gastric cancer development (5–7). It is unclear, as in colon cancer, whether there is a sequenced order of progression from an adenoma. However, it has been suggested by one study that translocated promoter region-MET activation may play an early role in gastric cancer development; K-ras may predict further progression (7,8). Variations in p53 mutations may explain differences in Asian and European cases (9). G:C → A:T transitions are seen more commonly in Europeans whereas A:T → G:C transitions/transversions are seen in Asians (9). Food associations and other risk factors may also be more closely linked to p53 differences in the pathogenesis of Western vs Asian gastric cancers (10). Microsatellite instability and LOH are purported to cause progression of gastric cancers (11–14).

Familial aggregates of gastric cancer have also been observed and may account for a substantial number of cases. Carriers of mismatch repair gene mutations, such as hMSH2, responsible for hereditary non-polyposis colorectal carcinoma syndrome, have a significant risk (approx 19 times) of developing gastric cancer as well (15–17). Microsatellite instability and LOH may be due to other genes responsible for DNA replication fidelity (18,19). Additionally, those with familial adenomatous polyposis are at increased risk of gastric cancer as well,

From: *Endoscopic Oncology: Gastrointestinal Endoscopy and Cancer Management*. Edited by: D. O. Faigel and M. L. Kochman © Humana Press, Totowa, NJ

although secondary to mutations at exon 10–15H *(20)*. Those with Li-Fraumeni syndrome (germline mutation of the *p53* gene) infrequently develop gastric cancer suggesting that risk may not be increased by a *p53* mutation *(21–23)*.

4. CLASSIFICATION/PROGNOSTIC INDICATORS

Suspected causative agents in gastric cancer include dietary factors such as poor nutrition, salted and smoked foods, alcohol, decreased intake of fruits/vegetables, and nitrates *(24,25)*. Lifestyle issues such as smoking and low socioeconomic status have been noted. Vitamins E, C, β-carotene, selenium, and other micronutrients have been reported to be protective but data are relatively inconsistent *(26,27)*.

GEJ appear to differ significantly in their etiology as compared with gastric cancers. GEJ tumors arise from gastroesophageal reflux resulting in esophagitis, gastric metaplasia, and Barrett's esophagitis. It appears also that obese people are at increased risk of GEJ cancers *(28)*. It may be related to increased intra-abdominal pressure from an increased body mass index resulting in hiatal hernia formation and gastroesophageal reflux. Tobacco, alcohol, and low socioeconomic status are also risk factors for GEJ tumors *(67,68)*.

Helicobacter pylori has been investigated as an etiological agent in non-GEJ gastric cancer. *Helicobacter* has been listed as a known carcinogen and has been postulated initially as inducing an inflammatory response that leads to the release of proinflammatory cytokines, many of which cause a reactive oxygen species, leading to oxidative stress and a milieu conducive to carcinogen development *(31–33)*. Controversy remains, however, and it may be the cytotoxin, CagA, causing an increased risk. Those individuals positive for both CagA and *Helicobacter* appear to have an increased risk of developing gastric cancer *(34–36)*.

Histologically, gastric cancers are classified as intestinal or diffuse. Diffuse gastric cancers consist of small cells, which grow diffusely into the surrounding gastric tissue; intestinal type is more glandular in appearance and forms more well-defined tumors. Linitis plastica is an antomical–pathological entity due to diffuse infiltration by the small, diffuse type of cancer cells resulting in a stomach that appears rigid and tubular like a "leather bottle." The diffuse type appears to have an overall worse prognosis even after tumor-metastasis-node staging is considered. World Health Organization classifies gastric cancer cells histologically into mucinous, tubular, signet ring, and papillary *(37)*. Diffuse-type cancer cells typically have a signet ring morphology.

Immunohistochemical and molecular prognostic indicators are now coming into investigation. To date, *p53* has been evaluated to the greatest extent. An inverse relationship between *p53* protein overexpression and survival has been reported, but studies have been limited by a lack of multivariate analyses considering other factors, and incomplete inclusion of all patient *(38–40)*. Serum antibodies to p53 were measured in 501 patients with gastric cancer and were associated with a poor prognosis, lymph node metastasis and poorly differentiated nuclear grade *(41)*. Other prognostic markers include Bcl-2, c-met, c-erb, vascular endothelial growth factor, urokinase plasminogen activator, DNA ploidy, CD-44 expression and nm23 *(42–50)*. Large trials investigating their utility in predicting outcome have not been done.

In general, gastric cancers have a poor outcome and thus prognosis. The overall survival rate particularly in the United States has been reported at 37, 18, 11, and 5% for stages II, IIIA, IIIB, and IV diseases *(51)*. The survival rates are thought to be so poor in this country owing to late detection. However, rates are similar in Europe. In Japan, stage IA and IB cancers are more frequently found owing to earlier detection programs and thus the 5-yr survival is reported at 75% *(52,53)*.

Until the last decade, the management of gastric cancer for curative intent was with surgery; chemotherapy, and radiotherapy were generally used for palliation. With newer chemotherapy and radiotherapy techniques, multimodality approaches are now coming into existence, with newer data suggesting curative benefit.

5. SURGICAL MANAGEMENT

Surgery has been the mainstay of treatment of gastric cancers for curative intent for the past century. Debate now exists as to the optimum surgical technique in terms of total vs subtotal gastrectomy, the extensive lymph node dissections done by Japanese surgeons and approaches to early gastric cancers.

Two randomized trials in western Europe were designed to address the question of total vs subtotal gastrectomy. The French Association for Surgical Research randomized 169 patients with adenocarcinoma to total or subtotal gastrectomy *(54)*. The 5-yr survival in either group was the same at 48% with a higher surgical mortality in the subtotal group. A second study conducted by the Italian Gastrointestinal Tumour Study Group randomized 624 patients with gastric cancer in the distal half of the stomach to subtotal or total gastrectomy *(55)*. Again, 5-yr survival rates were similar at 65 and 62%, respectively, but those with subtotal gastrectomy and lymphadenectomy of compartments one and two had a better quality of life and nutritional status.

Lymph node metastasis clearly affects prognosis in gastric cancer. The issue of performing extensive lymph node dissection when performing a gastrectomy has been debated over the past 30 yr *(56–59)*. Removal of the perigastric lymph nodes only is called D1 resection. D2 lymphadenectomy adds removal of the lymphatic chains along the celiac axis, the common hepatic and splenic artery and at the hilus of the spleen. The Japanese Society for Research in Gastric Cancer attempted to standardize this procedure by classifying 16 lymph node stations or four levels. The D2 procedure is done to achieve accurate staging and regional lymph node disease control. It is safe if done by a skilled surgeon, avoids pancreatic and splenic resections and benefits a group with occult disease in D2 nodes.

Studies have differed as to the benefits of more extensive lymphadenectomy. Eight prospective randomized trials demonstrated a significant survival advantage for D2 over D1 resections especially in patients with stage II or IIIA disease. A small trial from South Africa looked at 43 patients who were randomized to D1 or D2 resections showed no survival advantage in the D2 arm with increased surgical morbidity and prolonged hospital courses *(60)*. Another trial from Hong Kong in which 55 patients either underwent subtotal gastrectomy or more extensive resections showed an overall survival advantage in the more limited surgery group with increased surgical morbidity and mortality in those receiving the more extensive resctions *(61)*. Two major randomized trials from the United Kingdom and Dutch Gastric Cancer Group have been reported *(62–65)*; 711 and 400 patients, respectively either underwent D1 or D2 resections. Again, the complication rates were higher in the D2 resection, even in the Dutch trial in which supervision in the operating room by Japanese surgeons was made available. Neither trial showed a survival advantage with D2 resection although the 5-yr survival rate was slightly better in the Dutch study, which was attributed to a lower number of patients with T4 disease. The morbidity associated with D2 resections is postulated owing to lesions to the pancreatic tail or because the pancreas needs to be resected to achieve complete removal of the lymph nodes at the splenic hilus. Splenectomy was also included in the D2 resection and it is also thought that T-cell immunosuppression from splenectomy may contribute to surgical mortality. It is now recommended that splenectomy is an adverse prognostic factor and should only be performed in locally advanced tumors in the upper third of the stomach, greater curvature, gastric cardia, or macroscopic disease to the splenic hilum *(66)*.

In Japan, early gastric cancer represents 50% of newly diagnosed cases. The 10-yr survival in Japan is between 80 and 95% *(67)*. Submucosal invasion has been noted in 20% of cases, which can be associated with lymph node involvement, thus suggesting a poorer prognosis *(68–70)*. Thus, detection of early lymph node involvement is controversial and an ongoing debate in terms of accuracy of staging endoscopy/endoscopic ultrasound *(71–73)*. It has been suggested that size and submucosal invasion should determine the extent of surgical resection *(74,75)*.

Surgery remains an integral part of curative management of resectable gastric cancer. Debate continues as to the extent of resection. Adding other effective modalities of treatment may be important, particularly in the adjuvant setting. The next sections review the current literature on chemotherapy and radiation.

6. MEDICAL THERAPY OF GASTRIC CANCER

6.1. SYSTEMIC CHEMOTHERAPY

In order to understand the current literature in the neoadjuvant and adjuvant settings, a review of chemotherapy agents in the metastatic disease will be discussed. As with many cancers, gastric cancer was thought to be relatively insensitive to chemotherapy. Most agents used in gastric cancer did not induce a complete response, responses in general were poor, and time to progression was short. Table 1 shows a list of single-agent drugs with activity in gastric cancer.

The standard first-line salvage regimen through the 1980s was 5-fluorouracil (5FU), adriamycin, and mitomycin C (FAM) with an initial reported response rate of 50% *(77)*. This combination, though, was subsequently evaluated by multiple other investigators with less-convincing response rates *(78–81)*. Randomized trials subsequently followed, the largest from the

Table 1
Single-Agent Chemotherapeutic Agents for Gastric Cancer

Drug	Patients studied (first line/second line)	Responses (%)
5-Fluorouracil	392	21
Mitomycin C	211	30
Cisplatin	14/115	36/20
Etoposide	14	21
Doxorubicin	124/78	17/17
Methotrexate	28	11
Carboplatin	29	7
BCNU	55	20

From ref. *76*.

European Organization for Research and Treatment of Cancer (EORTC). Response rates were reported at 9% with a median survival of 6.5 mo *(82)*. In the United States, 252 patients were evaluated comparing 5FU to FAM as well as other combinations such as lomustine (CCNU) with FAM, and low-dose cisplatin with 5-FU and adriamycin *(83)*. None of these combination agents had any advantage.

Attempts to evaluate more aggressive multiple drug combinations was then pursued. FAMTX, or the addition of high-dose methotrexate to the standard FAM with leucovorin rescue (LV), was compared with FAM alone *(82,84,85)* FAM again demonstrated a 9% response compared to 42% with FAMTX; additionally, a median survival of 29 vs 42 wk with FAMTX was reported. Thus, FAMTX became the standard of care in metastatic gastric cancer.

Cisplatin (CDDP) in single-agent trials had only mediocre response rates. Synergy was known to exist between 5FU and cisplatin and thus trials were designed to exploit this. Regimens such as FUP (5FU/CDDP), FLP (5FU/LV/CDDP), PELF (CDDP/Epirubicin/LV/5FU), and ELF (Etoposide/LV/5FU) had responses ranging from 37 to 72% with duration of response reported between 4 and 7 mo (Table 2) *(86–91)*.

Phase III trials compared the previous regimens to each other. FAM vs 5FU vs FUP, which is 5FU/CDDP suggested responses of 25, 51, and 26% in 166 patients with measurable disease *(93)*. Time to progression was 21 wk in the FUP arm compared with 12 wk for either 5FU or FAM; however, no statistical significance was found. FAM was compared with PELF with PELF nonstatistically superior in terms of median time to progression *(91)*. FAMTX was compared with etoposide, adriamycin, and CDDP (EAP) but suspended owing to unacceptable toxicities *(92)*. The EORTC did a multicenter trial comparing FAMTX, FUP, and ELF with responses of 12, 20, and 9% with median survivals of 6.7–7.2 mo *(94)*.

Continuous infusion 5FU was investigated based on new knowledge of the pharmacokinetics of the drug and method of administration. Bolus 5FU appears to favor binding of the drug into RNA leading to disruption of maturation of nuclear RNA. Infusional 5FU on the other hand favors inhibition of thymidylate synthetase after its conversion to 5-fluoro-2′-deoxy-5′ monophosphate and thus DNA synthesis. Based on data derived from colon cancer, response rates with the infusional form were noted to be 32 vs 7% for the bolus arm with no

Table 2
Combination Chemotherapy for Gastric Cancer

Combination	Patients	Response rate (RR%)	Survival (mo)
FAMTX	317	25	6–10 (84,85,92)
FUP/FLP	226	44	8–11 (89,93)
PELF	85	43	8 (91)
ELF	63	49	7–11 (88)

FAMTX, 5-fluorouracil (5FU), adriamycin, mitomycin C, methotrexate; FUP/FLP, 5FU, cisplatin/5FU, leucovorin, cisplatin; PELF, cisplatin/epirubicin/leucovorin/5FU; ELF, Etoposide/LV/5FU.

survival advantage to either arm (95). This led to the evolution of 5FU continuous infusion with epirubicin and CDDP (ECF) with responses of 71% (96–98). Responses of ECF compared to FAMTX were 45 vs 21% with a superior median time to progression of 7.4 vs 3.4 mo and a significant survival advantage (8.9 vs 5.7 mo) (99).

Many of the above regimens have been given on the every 3–4 wk cycling owing to various toxicities. High-dose weekly regimens have been investigated such as epirubicin, CDDP, 5FU, and LV (EPFL) with 62% response rates but unacceptable neutropenia (100). Another study looked at an additional drug, etoposide with the EPFL regimen with responses of 71% but again with considerable toxicity (101).

Other active agents have now been looked at in the past 5–10 yr, including the taxanes paclitaxel or docetaxel as well as irinotecan (CPT11) as single agents and in combination. Other newer agents include Oxaliplatin and Xeloda or oral 5FU.

Paclitaxel or Taxol™ is an antimitotic agent that binds microtubules, which promotes microtubular assembly and stabilizes microtubules (102). Taxol as a single agent in gastric cancer has reported response rates of 5–17% as well as 20% (103–105). Taxol in combination with 5FU or CDDP or both have reported responses of 32–64% with time to progression of 4–8 mo and overall median survival from 6 to 11 mo (106–109). Paclitaxel with CDDP and etoposide was evaluated in 25 chemotherapy-naïve patients with locally advanced, unresectable, or metastatic gastric and esophageal cancer with a high response rate; both adenocarcinoma and squamous cell were included and thus differences may have been owing to histology as well as the inclusion of locally advanced but non-metastatic patients (110).

Docetaxel or Taxotere™ is reported to be twice as potent as paclitaxel inhibiting microtubule depolymerization. Using docetaxel as a single agent, three phase II trials report responses ranging from 17 to 24% in gastric cancer (111–113). Phase I studies combining CDDP with docetaxel revealed dose-limiting myelosuppression (114). Lower doses appeared tolerable and the Europeans reported combinations of CDDP with docetaxel as well as continuous infusion 5FU with docetaxel and CDDP (115,116). The first study evaluated 47 patients with every 3 wk CDDP at 75 mg/m² and docetaxel at 85 mg/m². Responses were reported at 56% with median time to progression of 6.6 mo and overall survival of 9 mo. Toxicity profile was acceptable. The second trial involving this regimen with continuous infusion 5FU was then pursued. Fifty percent of patients (52 patients) responded with an overall survival of 9.3 mo. Further

investigations and randomized studies are underway in the first-line metastatic setting.

In those patients in which docetaxel was used as second-line therapy, studies have demonstrated 20% responses as a single agent and 21% responses in combination with epirubicin (117,118).

Irinotecan or CPT11 is a DNA topoisomerase I inhibitor converted to its active metabolite SN38 by hepatic carboxyesterase. It has been shown to have first-line activity as a single agent of 18–23% (119,120). Studies incorporating CDDP have been done in both gastric and esophageal cancer with reported responses of 42–58% in chemotherapy-naïve patients.

Oxaliplatin is a third-generation cisplatin analog with a 1,2-diaminocyclohexane carrier ligand. It forms diaminocyclo-hexane-platinum adducts with DNA. It appears to have activity in tumors marginally sensitive to other platinum agents and is neither nephrotoxic or ototoxic. Its main side effect is cold neuropathy, which can be exacerbated by cold exposure. Oxaliplatin has been demonstrated to have additive or synergistic activity with 5FU, especially in 5FU resistant as well as CDDP resistant tumor cell lines (124). A recent phase II study in which bolus 5FU at 400 mg/m² with oxaliplatin at 85 mg/m² followed by infusional 5FU over 48 h reported response rates of 26% with median time to progression of 4.3 mo (125). Toxicity profiles were tolerable. Thus, this is yet another chemotherapeutic agent that has promise.

Matrix metalloproteinases agents are zinc-containing enzymes responsible for degradation of various proteins in the extracellular matrix. These may be important in invasion and metastatic spread of tumors. A study done in patients with gastric cancer who failed other chemotherapies looked at oral Marimastat for 18 mo; median survival was more than 5 mo (126). Many other agents are currently under investigation.

In conclusion, the ECF regimen is standard in Europe and is being investigated in the United States because data suggests superiority to FAMTX, hitherto the standard regimen for metastatic disease. Other agents such as taxanes, CPT11, and Oxaliplatin are encouraging in phase II trials and warrant further investigation.

6.2. ADJUVANT CHEMOTHERAPY

It is well known that despite complete resections for curative intent, patients can subsequently present with local disease, peritoneal carcinomatosis, or distant metastases. Over the years, various neoadjuvant and adjuvant strategies have been investigated with the intent of treating microscopic residual disease post-surgery. Meta-analysis have suggested benefit to adjuvant chemotherapy but more recently, the Intergroup 0116 Study reported information with improved disease-free and overall survival with combination chemoradiotherapy, which will be discussed in detail subsequently (127).

Initial adjuvant chemotherapy trials revealed less than encouraging data. The Gastrointestinal Tumor Study Group published a positive trial looking at methyl-CCNU with 5FU (128). The median survival was reported at 33 mo in those who did not receive postoperative chemotherapy; the median survival in the chemotherapy arm was more than 4 yr. Unfortunately, these results were not confirmed in a larger trial setting. Mitomycin C was used by the Japanese Surgical Adjuvant Chemotherapy Group with various dosing schedules; all trials but one were negative (129).

Multiple adjuvant trials have been conducted in Japan; unfortunately, few had surgery alone as a control arm and many of these trials merely compared chemotherapy regimens. Several studies in the United States and Europe looked at regimens such as FAM and compared soft surgery alone as the control; most were negative trials with sufficient numbers of patients enrolled.

Several meta-analyses have attempted to prove or disprove the use of adjuvant chemotherapy by creating larger sample sizes. One study published by the Dutch, based on 14 randomized trials including 2096 patients, did not suggest a survival advantage from adjuvant chemotherapy (130). Another meta-analysis in 1999 analyzed 13 trials demonstrating a small but significant survival benefit for patients receiving postoperative chemotherapy (131). There was an absolute risk reduction from 65 to 61% in relapse-free survival after postoperative chemotherapy. A third meta-analysis based on 20 trials was published by the Gruppo Italiano per lo Studio dei Carcinomi dell'Apparato Digerente. Patients received either 5FU alone or in combination with adriamycin-based chemotherapy with a reduced risk of death of 18% in the chemotherapy arm (132). This translated to an overall absolute risk reduction of about 4% in 5-yr survival.

Thus, from the earlier trials and published meta-analyses, many negative trials appear to exist in the adjuvant setting, none of which were powered to show a 5-yr survival advantage. The few positive trials published were too small in sample size to suggest validity. The effectiveness of adjuvant chemotherapy alone remains controversial at best; if a benefit exists in terms of survival, it needs to be evaluated in terms of acceptable toxicity and quality of life.

6.3. RADIOTHERAPY

The rationale for adjuvant radiation therapy is similar to chemotherapy; it is used to decrease the locoregional relapse rate observed after surgery. Based on tissue tolerance/toxicity to the local area such as spinal cord, pancreas, small bowel, liver, kidneys, the dose of external beam is limited to 45 Gy (133,134).

Many of the radiation studies published were retrospective in nature, and many had methodical issues making evaluation and interpretation difficult. Issues include underpowered studies, variations in doses of radiation, no control arm (no treatment), or inadequate randomization if done. Only one study using chemotherapy in one arm, radiation in another arm and surgery alone suggested a benefit from radiation (135). In general, none of the studies suggested a true survival benefit to radiation alone in the adjuvant setting.

Intra-operative radiation therapy (IORT) is another modality in which a single dose of radiation is given directly into the operative field at the time of surgery. The initial theory is based on immediate local treatment of any residual microscopic disease, which may remain in the operative bed, sparing normal tissue from field effects. There are technical difficulties associated with this type of treatment in that radiation equipment must be available in the sterile arena of the operative suite, which is not necessarily practical.

The Japanese have conducted several nonrandomized trials of IORT in which single doses of 30–35 Gy were given to the local area, particularly lymph nodes less than 3 cm; if no nodes were noted, 28 Gy was given to the operative bed alone (136,137). Further data suggested that doses of 30–40 Gy decreased primary tumor size but was insufficient to eradicate all disease (138). Many of the above studies were feasibility studies; little has been determined regarding improvement in overall survival. Patterns of local recurrence after this type of radiation were assessed and felt to be of little to no benefit if surgical margins were positive (139).

Two comparative trials evaluating IORT have been published with varied results. One study conducted at the National Cancer Institute (NCI) compared IORT (20 Gy) to a control group consisting of surgery alone in stages I/II disease or surgery followed by postoperative external beam radiation (50 Gy) in those with stages III/IV disease (140). Forty-one patients were evaluable; locoregional failure occurred in 44% of IORT patients and 92% of surgery alone patients ($p < 0.001$). No difference in median survival was documented. The second study reviewed 211 patients with no comment on staging or type of surgical resection performed; patients were randomized at the time of the procedure (141). This report suggested a significant survival benefit but again, major flaws appear to exist based on the information published.

Based on local and regional recurrence rates at the tumor bed, the anastomosis site, or regional lymph nodes 40–65% of the time in those undergoing surgery for curative resection and the unsatisfying data from adjuvant chemotherapy and radiation trials alone, the SWOG/ECOG/RTOG/CALGB/NCCTG cooperative groups designed the landmark Intergroup 0116 trial (127). This study demonstrated that adjuvant chemoradiotherapy after surgical resection of high-risk localized gastric cancer resulted in an improved relapse-free survival from 31 to 48% at 3 yr. Overall survival at 3 yr was 52 vs 41% ($p = 0.005$). The treatment arm consisted of the Mayo Clinic method of administration of one cycle of 5FU/LV (425 mg/m^2 + 20 mg/m^2 LV daily times 5 d) followed 1 mo later by combined 5FU/LV days 1–4 as above with 180 cGy/d of external beam radiation and the same chemotherapy again in the last week of radiation for 3 d. The total fraction of radiation was 4500 Gy. Two subsequent cycles of adjuvant chemotherapy alone at the above doses were given thereafter. There was a 44% relative improvement in relapse-free survival and a 28% relative improvement in survival with median survival of 42 and 27 mo, respectively. Radiotherapy techniques were closely monitored owing to variations in target volume. Flaws in this study included the initial requirement that all patients have D2 resections; 54% of the patients ultimately only received a D1 resection, which is less than standard. Thus, the issue of benefit from chemoradiation might have been because of inadequate surgery.

6.4. NEOADJUVANT CHEMOTHERAPY

The rationale for preoperative neoadjuvant chemotherapy is based on treating an intact vascular tumor with no reason for treatment induced resistance for a better response rate de novo. There have always been arguments that responses are improved with the fibrotic remodeling of the tumor bed following surgical removal. Additionally, surgery may be less invasive if an adequate response occurs prior to that procedure and thus issues of organ preservation are considered.

There have been extensive debates in the literature as to the utility of neoadjuvant chemotherapy in the treatment of any cancer. In locoregionally advanced rectal cancers, neoadjuvant radiotherapy has been considered superior to surgery alone or followed by adjuvant radiotherapy in terms of risk of locoregioanl relapse *(142,143)*. Neoadjuvant chemotherapy is also used in inflammatory breast cancer as well as osteosarcoma *(144,145)*.

There are several issues as to the use of neoadjuvant chemotherapy in gastric cancer. The decision for adjuvant treatment is often made based on the final pathological diagnosis and features postoperatively; the decision to perform or not a pre-operative intervention relies on clinical staging, which is not as accurately known without the benefit of surgery. The primary tumor extension is not necessarily obvious on routine CT scans or MRIs and the invaded lymph nodes might not be detectable on conventional scans. Endoscopic ultrasonography is the only option for estimating the T and N stage with a known diagnostic accuracy of 70% *(146)*. Peritoneal carcinomatosis is also difficult to determine without surgical exploration and thus many trials investigating neoadjuvant therapy have suggested laparoscopic staging.

Few randomized studies have been done comparing neoadjuvant chemotherapy followed by surgery vs surgery alone. One study looked at 107 patients after receiving two to three cycles of CDDP/VP16/5FU with surgery vs surgery alone *(147)*. A higher curative resection rate was noted in the investigative arm, with evidence of downstaging after chemotherapy. As with many studies, though, no survival advantage was reported. Another randomized trial looked at two to four cycles of FAMTX/surgery vs surgery alone *(148)*. Fifty-nine patients were studied and the study was ultimately suspended owing to toxicity and poor accrual.

Two randomized trials with neoadjuvant radiation have been published as well. Three hundred seventeen patients with adnenocarcinoma of the cardia were randomized to radiation therapy/surgery vs surgery alone *(149)* and 40 Gy were administered as 2 Gy/d; surgery was done 2–4 wk later. The reported 5-yr survival was 30 vs 20% in the radiation therapy/ surgery arm vs surgery. Issues with this study include inadequate staging and the variation in the radiation fields. Another randomized study investigated radiation therapy/surgery, radiation therapy/local hyperthermia followed by surgery vs surgery alone *(150)*. Again 20 Gy were given. The 5-yr survival rates were 45, 52, and 30%, respectively.

The MRC Adjuvant Gastric Infusional Chemotherapy (MAGIC) trial, a United Kingdom-driven trial, is investigating the role of pre- and postoperative epirubicin, CDDP, and 5FU chemotherapy in combination with surgery compared with surgery alone; results are pending. The EORTC is comparing neoadjuvant systemic therapy with surgery vs surgery alone using weekly CDDP and high-dose 5FU/LV. The French have a similar trial to the EORTC using infusional 5FU/CDDP every 3–4 wk. Taxotere with 5FU/CDDP is currently in trial in Italy with four neoadjuvant cycles followed by surgery.

7. MULTIMODALITY THERAPY

The treatment of gastric cancer with potential curative resection has become a question of multidisciplinary management. The roles of surgery, radiation, and chemotherapy and their sequence in treatment is still evolving. New treatment regimens based on novel cytotoxic agents such as docetaxel, paclitaxel, irinotecan, and biological agents such as epidermal growth factor receptor inhibitors and antiangiogenesis might find a role in the management of gastric cancer, either in the neoadjuvant, adjuvant, or combined modality setting. The limited benefit from adjuvant therapy in many trials to date might be owing to residual tumor burden after sugery, delay in the administration of chemotherapy, insufficient activity of current chemotherapy, inadequate sample sizes of treatable patients, or the need for better local therapies with combination radiation/chemotherapy. Optimal surgical intervention needs to be better defined as well. Thus, much work remains in determining the best strategies for the treatment of gastric cancer.

REFERENCES

1. Parkin DM. Epidemiology of cancer global patterns and trends. Toxicol Lett 1998; 102,103:227–234.
2. Ilson DH. Oesophageal cancer: new developments in systemic therapy. Cancer Treatment Rev 2003; 29:525–532.
3. Howson CP, Hiyama T, Wynder EL. The decline in gastric cancer epidemiology of an unplanned triumph. Epidemiol Rev 1986; 8:1–27.
4. Correa P. The epidemiology of gastric cancer. World J Surg 1991; 15:228–234.
5. Dijkhuizen SM, et al. Multiple hyperplastic polyps in the stomach: evidence for clonality and neoplastic potential. Gastroenterology 1997; 112:561,562.
6. Shiao YH, et al. Implications of p53 mutation spectrum for cancer etiology in gastric cancers of various histologic types from a high-risk area of central Italy. Carcinogenesis 1998; 10:2145–2149.
7. Correa P, Shiao YH. Phenotypic and genotypic events in gastric carcinogenesis. Cancer Res 1994; 54:1941s–1943s.
8. Gong C, et al. KRAS mutations predict progression of preneoplastic gastric lesions. Cancer Epidemiol Biomarkers Prev 1999; 8:167–171.
9. Hongyo T, et al. Mutations of the K-ras and p53 genes in gastric adenocarcinomas from a high-incidence region around Florence, Italy. Cancer Res 1995; 55:2665–2672.
10. Fedriga R, et al. Relation between food habits and p53 mutational spectrum in gastric cancer patients. Int J Oncol 2000; 17:127–133.
11. Strickler JG, et al. P53 mutations and microsatellite instability in sporadic gastric cancer: when guardians fail. Cancer Res 1994; 54:4750–4755.
12. Chong JM, et al. Microsatelllite instability in the progression of gastric carcinoma. Cancer Res 1994; 54:4595–4597.
13. Kobayashi K, et al. Genetic instability in intestinal metaplasia is a frequent event leading to well-differentiated early adenocarcinoma of the stomach. Eur J Cancer 2000; 36:1113–1119.
14. Palli D, et al. Red meat, family history, and increased risk of gastric cancer with microsatellite instability. Cancer Res 2001; 61:5415–5419.
15. Lin KM, et al. Cumulative incidence of colorectal and extracolonic cancers in MLH1 and MSH2 mutation carriers of hereditary non-polyposis colorectal cancer. J Gastrointest Surg 1998; 2:67–71.
16. Vasen HF, et al. Cancer risk in families with hereditary nonpolyposis colorectal cancer diagnosed by mutation analysis. Gastroenterology 1996; 110:1020–1027.
17. Akiyama Y, et al. Frequent microsatellite instabilities and analyses of the related genes in familial gastric cancers. Jpn J Cancer Res 1996; 87:595–601.
18. Yanagisawa Y, et al. Methylation of the hMLH1 promoter in familial gastric cancer with microsatelllite instability. Int J Cancer 2000; 85:50–53.

19. Keller G, et al. Microsatellite instability and loss of heterozygosity in gastric carcinoma in comparison to family history. Am J Pathol 1998; 152:1281–1289.

20. Enomoto M, et al. The relationship between frequencies of extracolonic manifestations and the position of APC germline mutation in patients with familial adenomatous polyposis. Jpn J Clin Oncol 2000; 30:82–88.

21. Shinmura K, et al. Familial gastric cancer: clinicopathological characteristics, RER phenotype and germline p53 and E-cadherin mutaiton. Carcinogenesis 199; 20:1127–1131.

22. Varley JM, et al. An extended li-Fraumeni kindred with gastric carcinoma and a codon 175 mutation in PT53. J Med Genet 1995; 32:942–945.

23. Sugano K, et al. Germline p53 mutaiton in a case of Li-Fraumeni syndrome presenting as gastric cancer. Jpn J Clin Oncol 1999; 29:513–516.

24. Neugut AI, Hayek M, Howe G. Epidemiology of gastric cancer. Semin Oncol 1996; 23:281–291.

25. Chyou PH, et al. A case-cohort study of diet and stomach cancer. Cancer Res 1990; 50:7501–7504.

26. Blot WJ, et al. Nutrition intervention trials in Linxian, China: supplementation with specific vitamin/mineral combinations, cancer incidence, and disease-specific mortality in the general population. J Natl Cancer Institute 1993; 85:1483–1492.

27. Benner SE, Hong Wk. Clinical chemoprevention: developing a cancer prevention strategy. J Natl Cancer Inst 1993; 85:1446–1447.

28. Chow WH, et al. Body mass index and risk of adenocarcinomas of the esophagus and gastric cardia. J Natl Cancer Inst 1998; 90:150–155.

29. Gammon MD, et al. Tobacco, alcohol, and socioeconomic status and adenocarcinomas of the esophagus and gastric cardia. J Natl Cancer Inst 1997; 89:1277–1284.

30. Zhang ZF, Kurtz RC, Marshall JR. Cigarette smoking and esophageal and gastric cardia adenocarcinoma. J Natl Cancer Inst 1997; 89:1247–1249.

31. Ernst P. Review article: the role of inflammation in the pathogenesis of gastric cancer. Aliment Pharmacol Ther 1999; 13:13–18.

32. Graham DY. Helicobacter pyylori infection in the pathogenesis of duodenal ulcer and gastric cancer: a model. Gastroenterolgy 1997; 113:1983–1991.

33. Danesh J. Helicobacter pylori and gastric cancer: time for megatrials? Br J Cancer 1999; 80:927–929.

34. Parsonnet J, et al. Risk for gastric cancer in people with CagA positive or CagA negative *Helicobacter pylori* infeciton. Gut 1997; 40:297–301.

35. Blaser MJ, et al. Infection with Helicobacter pylori strains possessing cagA is associated with an increased risk of developing adenocarcinoma of the stomach. Cancer Res 1995; 55:2111–2115.

36. Deguchi R, et al. Association between CagA + Helicobacter pylori infection and p53, bax and transforming growth factor-beta-RII gene mutations in gastric cancer patients. Int J Cancer 2001; 91:481–485.

37. Oota K, Sobin LH. Histological typing of gastric and oesophageal tumors in international histological classification of tumors, WHO, Editor. 1977, WHO: Geneva.

38. Maehara Y, et al. Prognostic value of p53 expression for patients with gastric cancer-a multivariate analysis. Br J Cancer 1999; 79:1255–1261.

39. Fonseca L, et al. P53 detection as a prognostic factor in early gastric cancer. Oncology 1994; 51:485–490.

40. Aizawa K, et al. Apoptosis and bcl-2 expression in gastric cartcinomas: correlation with clnicopathological variables, p53 expression, cell proliferation and prognosis. Int J Oncol 1999; 14:85–91.

41. Wu CW, et al. Serum anti-p53 antibodies in gastric adenocarcinoma patients are associated with poor prognosis lymph node metastatsis and poorly differentiated nuclear grade. Br J Cancer 1999; 79:1255–1261.

42. Maeda K, et al. Expression of p53 and vascular endothelial growth factor associated with tumor angiogenesis and prognosis in gastric cancer. Oncology 1998; 55:594–599.

43. Martin HM, et al. P53 expression and prognosis in gastric carcinoma. Int J Cancer 1992; 50:859–862.

44. Polkowski W, et al. Prognostic value of Lauren classification and c-erbB-2 oncogene overexpression in adenocarcinoma of the esophagus and gastroesophageal junction. Ann Surg Oncol 1999; 6:290–297.

45. Nakajtma M, et al. The prognostic significance of amplification and overexpression of c-met and c-erb B-2 in human gastric carcinomas. Cancer 1000; 85:1894–1902.

46. Heiss MM, et al. Tumor-associated proteolysis and prognosis: new functional risk factors in gastric cancer defined by the urokinase-type plasminogen activator system. J Clin Oncol 1995; 13:2084–2093.

47. Heiss MM, et al. Individual development and uPA-receptor expression of disseminated tumour cells in bone marrow: a reference to early systemic disease in solid cancer. Nat Med 1995; 1:1035–1039.

48. Yonemura Y, et al. Prediction of lymph node metastasis and prognosis from the assay of the expresion of porliferating cell nuclear antigen and DNA ploidy in gastric cancer. Oncology 1994; 51:251–257.

49. Muller W, et al. Expression and prognostic value of the CD44 splicing variants v5 and v6 in gastric cancer. J Pathol 1997; 183:222–227.

50. Yoo CH, et al. Prognostic significance of CD44 and nm23 expression in patients with stage Ii and stage IIIA gastric carcinoma. J Surg Oncol 1999; 71:22–28.

51. Hundahl SA, et al. The National Cancer Data Base report on gastric carcinoma. Cancer 1997; 80:2233–2241.

52. Nakamura K, et al. Pathology and prognosis of gastric carcinoma. Findings in 10000 patientes who underwent primary gastrectomy. Cancer 1992; 70:1030–1037.

53. Fuchs CS, Mayer RJ. Gastric carcinoma. New Engl J Med 1995; 333:32–41.

54. Gouzi JL, et al. Total versus subtotal gastrectomy for adenocarcinoma of the gastric antrum. A French prosepctive controlled study. Ann Surg 1989; 209:162–166.

55. Italian Gastrointestinal Tumor Study Group, Bozzetti F, et al. Subtotal versus total gastrectomy for gastric cancer five-year survival rates in a multicenter randomized Italian trial. Ann Surg 1000; 230:170–178.

56. Roukos DH, Kappas AM, Encke A. Extensive lymph-node dissection in gastric cancer is it of therapeutic value. Cancer Treat Rev 1996; 22:247–252.

57. Roukos DH. Extended lymphadenectomy in gastric cancer when, for whom and why. Ann R Colll Surg Engl 1998; 80:16–24.

58. Jessup JM. Is bigger better. J Clin Oncol 1995; 13:5–7.

59. Lawrence W, Jr, Horsley JS. Extended lymph node dissections for gastric cancer-is more better? (editorial). J Surg Oncol 1996; 61:85–89.

60. Dent DM, Madden MV, Price SK. Randomized comparison of R1 and R2 gastrectomy for gastric carcinoma. Br J Surg 1988; 75:110–112.

61. Robertson CS, et al. A prospective randomized trial comparing P1 subtotal gastrectomy with R3 total gastrectomy for antral cancer (see comments). Ann Surg 1994; 220:176–182.

62. Dutch Gastric Cancer Group, Bonenekamp JJ, et al. Extended lymph-node dissection for gastric cancer. New Engl J Med 1999; 340:908–914.

63. Bonenkamp JJ, et al. Randomised comparison of morbidity after D1 and D2 dissection for gastric cancer in 996 Dutch patients. Lancet 1995; 345:745–748.

64. Surgical Cooperative Group, Cushieri A, et al. Patient survival after D1 and D2 resections for gastric cancer: long-term results of the MRC randomized surgical trial. Br J Cancer 1999; 79:1522–1530.

65. The Surgical Cooperative Group, Cuchieri A, et al. Post-operative morbidity and mortality after D1 and D2 resections for gastric cancer preliminary results of the RMC randomised controlled surgical trial. Lancet 1996; 347:995–999.

66. Maruyama K, et al. Pancreas-preserving total gastrectomy for proximal gastric cancer. World J Surg 1995; 19:532–536.

67. Jentschura D, et al. Surgery for early gastric cancer, a European one-center experience. World J Surg 1997; 21:845–848.

68. Iriyama K, et al. Is extensive lymphadenectomy necessary for surgical treatment of intramucosal carcinoma of the stomach. Arch Surg 1989; 124:309–311.

69. Hanazaki K, et al. Clinicopathologic features of submucosal carcinoma of the stomach. J Clin Gastroenterol 1997; 24:150–155.

70. Hanazaki K, et al. Surgical outcome in early gastric cancer with lymph node metastasis. Hepatogastroenterology 1997; 44:907–911.

71. Yanai H, et al. Diagnostic utility of 20-megahertz linear endoscopic ultrasonography in early gastric cancer. Gastrointest Endosc 1996; 44:29–33.

72. Akahoshi K, et al. Pre-operative TN staging of gastric cancer using a 15 MHz ultrasound miniprobe. Br J Radiol 1997; 70:703–707.

73. Akahoshi K, et al. Endoscopic ultrasonography: a promising method for assessing the prospects of endoscopic mucosal resection in early gastric cancer. Endoscopy 1997; 29:614–619.

74. Takeshita K, et al. Rational lymphadenectomy for early gastric cancer with submucosal invasion: a clinicopathological study. Surg Today 1998; 28:580–586.

75. Sano T, Kobori O, Muto T. Lymph node metastatsis from early gastric cancer: endoscopic resection of tumour. Br J Surg 1992; 79:241–244.

76. Roth AD. Curative treatment of gastric cancer: towards a multidisciplinary approach? Critical Rev in Oncology Hematology. 2003; 46:59–100.

77. Macdonald JS, et al. 5-fluorouracil, adriamycin and mitomycin-C (FAM) combination chemotherapy in the treatment of advanced gastric cancer. Cancer 1979; 44:42–47.

78. Cunningham D, et al. Advanced gastric cancer experience in Scotland using 5-fluorouracil adriamycin and mitomycin-C. Br J Surg 1984; 71:673–676.

79. Haim N, et al. Treatment of advanced gastric carcinoma with 5-fluorouracil adriamycin and mitomycin C (FAM). Cancer Chemother Pharmacol 1982; 8:277–280.

80. Haim N, et al. Further studies on the treatment of advanced gastric cancer by 5-fluorouracil, Adriamycin (doxorubicin) and mitomycin C (modified FAM). Cancer 1984; 54:1999–2002.

81. Macdonald JS, Gohmann JJ. Chemotherapy of advanced gastric cancer: present status, future prospects. Semin Oncol 1988; 15:42–49.

82. Wils JA, et al. Sequential high-dose methotrexate and fluorouracil combined with doxorubicin-A step ahead in the treatment of advanced gastric cancer. A trial of the Euopean Organization for Research and Treatment of Cancer Gastrointestinal Tract Cooperative Group. J Clin Oncol 1991; 9:827–831.

83. North Central Cancer Treatment Group, Cullinan SA, et al. Controlled evaluation of three drug combination regimens versus fluorouracil alone for the therapy of advanced gastric cancer. J Clin Oncol 1994; 12:412–416.

84. Wils J, et al. An EORTC Gastrointestinal Group evaluation of the combination of sequential methotrexate and 5-fluorouracil, combined with adriamycin in advanced measurable gastric cancer. J Clin Oncol 1986; 4:1799–1803.

85. Murad Am, et al. Modified therapy with 5-fluorouracil, doxorubicin and methotrexate in advanced gastric cancer. Cancer 1993; 72: 37–41.

86. Leichman L, Berry BT. Cisplatin therapy for adenocarcinoma fo the stomach. Semin Oncol 1991; 18 (Suppl 3):25–33.

87. Wilke H, et al/ Preoperative chmeotherapy in locally advanced and nonresectable gastric cancer: a phase II study with etoposide, doxorubicin and cisplatin. J Clin Oncol 1989; 7:1318–1326.

`88. Wilke H, et al. Etoposide, folinic acid and 5-fluorouracil in carboplatin-pretreated patients with advanced gastric cancer. Cancer Chemother Pharmacol 1991; 29:83–84.

89. Ychou M, et al. A phase II study of 5-fluorouracil, leucovorin and cisplaitn (FLP) for metastatic gastric cancer. Eur J Cancer 1996; 32A:1933–1937.

90. Preusser P, Wilke H, Achterrath W. Phase II study with the combination etoposide, doxorubicin and cisplatin in advanced measurable gastric carcinoma. J Clin Oncol 1989; 7:1310–1317.

91. Cocconi G, et al. Fluorouracil, doxorubicin and mitomycin combination versus PELF chemotherapy in advanced gastric cancer: a prospective randomized trial of the Italian Oncology Group for Clinical Research. J Clin Oncol 1994; 12:2687–2693.

92. Kim NK, et al. A phase III randomized study of 5-fluorouracil and cisplatin versus 5-fluorouracil, doxorubicin and motomycin C versus 5-fluorouracil alone in the treatment of advanced gastric cancer. Cancer 1993; 71:3813–3818.

93. Kelsen D, et al. FAMTX versus etoposide, doxorubicin and cisplatin: a random assignment trial in gastric cancer. J Clin Oncol 1992; 10:541–548.

94. Vanhoefer U, et al. Final results of a randomized phsae III trial of sequential high-dose methotrexate, fluorouracil and doxorubicin versus etoposide, leuocovorin and fluorouracil versus infusional fluorouracil and cisplatin in advanced gastric cancer: a trial of the European Organization for Research and Treatment of Cancer Gastrointestinal Tract Cacner Cooperative Group. J Clin Oncol 2000; 11:301–306.

95. Lokich JJ, et al. A prospective randomized comparison of continuous infusion fluorouracil with a conventional bolus schedule in metastatic colorectal carinaoma: a Mid-Atlantic Oncology Program Study. J Clin Oncol 1989; 7:425–432.

96. Findlay M, et al. A phase II study in advanced gastroesophageal cancer using epirubicin and cisplatinin combination with continuous infusion 5-fluorouracil (ECF). Ann Oncol 1994; 5:609–6616.

97. Bamias A, et al. Epirubicin, cisplatin, and protracted venous infusion of 5-fluorouracil for esophagogastric adenocarcinoma: response, toxicity, quality oflife and survival. Cancer 1996; 77:1978–1985.

98. Zaniboni A, et al. Epirubicin, cisplatin and continuous infusion 5-fluorouracil is an active and safe regimen for patients with advanced gastric cancer. An Italian Group for the Study of Digestive Tract Cancer (GISCAD) report. Cancer 1995; 76:1694–1699.

99. Webb A, et al. Randomized trial comparing epirubicin, cisplatin, and fluorouracil versus fluorouracil, doxorubicin and methotrexate in advanced esophagogastric cancer. J Clin Oncol 1997; 15:261–267.

100. Cascinu S, et al. Intensive weekly chemotherapy for advanced gastric cancer using fluorouracil, cisplatin, epi-doxorubicin, 6S-leucovorin, glutathione and filgrastim: A report from the Italian Group for the Study of Digestive Tract Cancer. J Clin Oncol 1997; 15:3313–3319.

101. Chi KH, et al. Weekly etoposide, epirubicin, cisplatin 5-fluorouracil and leucovorin: an effective chemotherapy in advanced gastric cancer. Br J Cancer 1998; 77:1984–1988.

102. Schiff PB, Horwitz SB. Taol assembles tubulin in the absence of exogenous guanosine 5´triphosphate or microtubule-associated proteins. Biochemistry 1981; 20:3247–3252.

103. Einzig AI, et al. Phase II trial of Taxol in patients with adenocarcinoma of the upper gastrointestintal tract (UGIT). The Eastern Cooperative Oncology group (ECOG) results. Invest New Drugs 1995; 13:223–227.

104. Ajani JA, et al. Phase II study of Taxol in patients with advanced gastric carcinoma. Cancer J Sci Am 1998; 4:269–275.

105. Ohtsu A, et al. An early phase II study of a 3 h infusion of paclitaxel for advanced gastric cancer. Am J Clin Oncol 1998; 21:416–419.

106. Cascinu S, et al. A phase I study of paclitaxel and 5-fluorouracil in advanced gastric cancer. Eur J Cancer 1997; 33:1699–1702.

107. Bokemeyer C, et al. A phase II trial of paclitaxel and weekly 24 h infusion of 5-fluorouracil/folinic acid in patients with advanced gastric cancer. Anticancer Drugs 1997; 8:396–399.

108. Chun H, et al. Chemotherapy (CT) with cisplatin, fluorouracil (FU) and paclitaxel for adenocarcinoma (AC) of the stomach and gastroesophageal junction (GEJ). ASCO Proc 1999; 18:280a.

109. Kim YH, et al. Paclitaxel, 5-fluorouracil and cisplatin combination chemotherapy for the treatment of advanced gastric carcinoma. Cancer 1999; 85:295–301.

110. Lokich JJ, et al. Combined paclitaxel, cisplatin and etoposide for patients with previously untreated esophageal and gastroesophageal carcinomas. Cancer 1999; 85:2347–2351.

111. Einzig AI, et al. Phase II trial of docetaxel (Taxotere) in patients with adenocarcinoma of tehupper gastrointestinal tract previously untreated with cytotoxic chemotherapy: the Eastern Cooperative Oncology Group (ECOG) results of protocol E1293. Med Oncol 1996; 13:87–93.

112. EORTC Early Clinical Trials Group, Sulkes A, et al. Docetaxel (Taxotere) in advanced gastric cancer, results of a Phase II clinical trial. Br J Cancer 1994; 70:380–383.

113. Mai M, et al. A late phase II clinical study of RP56976 (docetaxel) in patients with advanced or recurrent gastric cancer; a cooperative study group grial (group B). Gan To Kagaku Ryoho 1999; 26:487–496.

114. Verweij J, Clavel M, Chevalier B. Paclitaxel(Taxol) and docetaxel (Taxotere): not simply two of a kind. Ann Oncol 1994;5:495–505.

115. Roth AD, et al. Docetaxel (taxotere)-cisplatin (TC): an effective drug combination in gastric carcinoma. Swiss Group for Clinical Cancer Research (SAKK) and the European Institute of Oncology (EIO). Ann Oncol 2000; 11:301–306.

116. Roth AD, et al. 5FU as protracted continuous IV infusion (5Fupiv) can be added to full dose taxotere-cisplatin (TC) in advanced gastric carcinoma (AGO). Eur J Cancer 1999; 35:S130–S139.

117. Vanhoefer U, et al. Phase II study of docetaxel as second line chemotherapy (CT) in metastatic gastric cancer. ASCO Proc 1999; 18:303a.

118. Andre T, et al. Docetaxel-epirubicine as second-line treatment for patients with advanced gastric cancer. ASCO Proc 1999; 18:277a.

119. CPT-11 Gastrointestinal Cancer Study Group, Futatsuki K, et al. Late phase II study of irinotecan hydrochloride (CPT-11) in advanced gastric cancer. Gan To Kagaku Ryoho 1994; 21:1033–1038.

120. Kohne CH, et al. Final results of a phase II trial of CPT-1 in patients with advanced gastric cancer. ASCO Proc 1999; 18:258a.

121. Shirao K, et al. Phase I-II study of irinotecan hydrochloride combined with cisplatin in patients with advanced gastric cancer. J Clin Oncol 1997; 15:921–927.

122. Boku N, et al. Phase II study of a combination of irinotecan and cisplatin against metastatic gastric cancer. J Clin Oncol 1999; 17:319–323.

123. Ajani JA, et al. Irinotecan plus cisplatin in advanced gastric or gastroesophageal junction carcinoma. Oncology 2001; 15:52–54.

124. Raymond E, Chaney SG, Taamma A, et al. Oxaliplatin: a review of preclinical and clinical studies. Ann Oncol 1998; 9:1053–1071.

125. Kim DY, Kim JH, Lee SH, et al. Phase II study of oxaliplatin, 5-fluorouracil and leucovorin in previously platinum-treated patients with advanced gastric cancer. Ann Oncol 2003; 14:383–387.

126. Murray GI, et al. Matrix metalloproteinases and their inhibitors in gastric cancer. Gut 1998; 43:791–797.

127. Macdonald JS, Smalley SR, Benedetti J, et al. Chemoradiotherapy after surgery compared with surgery alone for adenocarcinoma of the stomach or gastroesophageal junction. N Engl J Med 2001; 345:725–730.

128. The Gastrointestinal Tumor Study Group. Controlled trial of adjuvant chemotherapy following curative resection for gastric cancer. Cancer 1982; 49:1116–1122.

129. Imanaga H, Nakazato H. Results of surgery for gastric cancer and effect of adjuvant mitomycin C on cancer recurrence. World J Surg 1977; 2:213–221.

130. Hermans J, et al. Adjuvant therapy after curative resection for gastric caner: meta-analysis of randomized trials. J Clin Oncol 1993; 11:1441–1447.

131. Pignon JP, Ducreux M, Rougier P. Meta-analysis of adjuvant chemotherapy in gastric cancer: a critical reappraisal. J Clin Oncol 1994; 12:877–878.

132. Mari E, et al. Efficacy of adjuvant chemotherapy after curative resection for gastric cancer: a meta-analysis of published randomised trials. A study of the GISCAD (Gruppo Italiano per lo Studio dei Carcinomi dell' Apparato Digerente). Ann Oncol 2000; 11:837–843.

133. Minsky BD. The role of radiation therapy in gastric cancer. Semin Oncol 1996; 23:390–396.

134. Budach VG. The role of radiation therapy in the management of gastric cancer. Ann Oncol 1994; 5:37–48.

135. Hallissey MT, et al. The second British Stomach Cancer Group trial of adjuvant radiotherapy or chemotherapy in resectable gastric cancer: a 5 year follow-up. Lancet 1994; 343:1309–1312.

136. Abe M, et al. Clinical experiences with intraoperative radiotherapy of locally advanced cancers. Cancer 1980; 45:40–48.

137. Abe M, et al. Japan gastric trials in intraoperative radiation therapy. Int J Radiat Oncol Biol Phys 1988; 15:1431–1433.

138. Abe M, et al. Intraoperative radiotherapy of gastric cancer. Cancer 1974; 34:2034–2041.

139. Pelton JJ, et al. The influence of surgical margins on advanced cancer treated with intraoperative radiation therapy (IORT) and surgical resection. J Surg Oncol 1993; 53:30–35.

140. Sindelar WF, et al. Randomized trial of intraoperative radiotherapy in carcinoma of the stomach. Am J Surg 1993; 165:178–186.

141. Abe M, et al. Intraoperative radiotherapy in carcinoma of the stomach and pancreas. World J Surg 1987; 11:459–464.

142. Frykholm GJ, Glimelius B, Pahlman L. Preoperative or postoperative irradiation in adenocarcinoma of the rectum: final treatment results of a randomized trial and an evaluation of late secondary effects. Dis Colon Rectum 1993; 36:564–572.

143. Swedish Rectal Cancer Trial. Improved survival with preoperative radiotherapy in resectable rectal cancer. New Engl J Med 1997; 336:980–987.

144. Singletary Se. Current treatment options for inflammatory breast cancer. Ann Surg Oncol 1999; 6:228–229.

145. Provisor AJ, et al. Treatment of nonmetastatic osteosarcoma of the extremity with preoperative and postoperative chemotherapy: a report from the Children's Cancer Group. J Clin Oncol 1997; 15:76–84.

146. Martinez-Monge R, et al. Patterns of failure and long-term results in high-risk resected gastric cancer treated with post-operative radiotherapy with or without intraoperative electron boost. J Surg Oncol 1997; 66:24–29.

147. Kang YK, et al. A phase III randomized comparison of neoadjuvant chemotherapy followed by surgery versus surgery for locally advanced stomach cancer. ASCO Proc 1996; 15:210–215.

148. The Dutch Gastric Cancer Group (DGCD), Songun I, et al. Chemotherapy for operable gastric cancer: results of the Dutch randomised FAMTX trial. Eur J Cancer 1999; 35:558–562.

149. Zhang ZX, et al. Randomized clinical trial on the combination of preoperative irradiation and surgery in the treatment of adenocarcinoma of gastric cardia (AGC): Report on 370 patients. Int J Radiat Oncol Biol Phys 1998; 42:929–934.

150. Shchepotin IB, et al. Intensive preoperative radiotherapy with local hyperthermia for the treatment of gastric carcinoma. Surg Oncol 1994; 3:37–44.

COLON III

17 Colorectal Cancer Screening

Jason A. Dominitz, md, mhs and William M. Grady, md

Contents

1. BACKGROUND

Colorectal cancer (CRC) remains the second leading cause of cancer death in the United States *(1)*. It is estimated that approx 148,610 will be diagnosed with CRC and 55,170 will die from it in 2006 *(1)*. However, mortality from CRC has been declining over the past 20 yr, felt largely to be due to earlier detection. The average lifetime risk is 6%, with men and women almost equally affected. Most cases are sporadic, apparently resulting from a combination of environmental and genetic factors (Fig. 1), although there are many known risk factors (Table 1). Screening for CRC has been advocated on the grounds that CRC is a major public health problem, it is preventable through removal of precursor lesions, it is curable if detected early (Fig. 2), and screening tests have been proven to impact disease outcomes. In fact, some screening strategies have been proven to reduce cancer mortality and many strategies are cost-effective *(2,3)*. Unfortunately, CRC screening is underutilized because of a variety of barriers to screening.

We now have a wide assortment of screening modalities to offer our patients, each with its own strengths and limitations. It is important to keep in mind that screening should be viewed as a program that occurs over time, not as an individual test administered at one point in time. Therefore, there are costs associated with the original screening test, as well as with the evaluation of positive tests, surveillance, complications, and the cost of cancers not avoided. This chapter focuses on screening for CRC among average-risk individuals, and follows the algorithm proposed by the Multisociety Task Force (Fig. 3) *(4)*. Readers can find additional information on screening and surveillance of individuals at increased risk (e.g., prior personal history of adenomatous polyps, CRC, or inflammatory bowel disease, and family history of colonic neoplasia) covered in Chapters 18 and 19 of this text, as well as in published guidelines *(4)*. Patients with signs or symptoms of CRC should undergo an appropriate diagnostic evaluation.

2. WHEN TO START AND WHEN TO STOP SCREENING

Based on data indicating a rapid rise in the incidence of CRC around age 50 (Fig. 4), screening for CRC should begin at age 50 for average-risk individuals. Those believed to be at increased risk (e.g., first-degree relative with CRC before 60 yr of age) should begin screening at an earlier age.

Although there are no clear guidelines for when to stop screening, one general principal is that screening should cease when the patient is unlikely to benefit from further screening. From a population perspective, the impact of CRC on life expectancy is rather minimal beyond age 80 *(5)* (Fig. 5). Therefore, it is reasonable to discontinue screening of individuals whose age or comorbidity limits their life expectancy.

3. SCREENING TESTS

3.1. DIGITAL RECTAL EXAM

Although there is no direct evidence of the effectiveness of digital rectal examination (DRE) and only 5–10% of all cancers could be detected by DRE *(6)*, its use is generally part of other screening tests (i.e., sigmoidoscopy, colonoscopy, and barium enema). Moreover, DRE is usually performed as part of a routine physical exam in patients of appropriate age for CRC screening (i.e., prostate evaluation in men, pelvic examination in women). Therefore, the additional effort required on the part of providers and patients is minimal, and DRE can be included as an adjunctive screening method in a CRC screening program.

From: *Endoscopic Oncology: Gastrointestinal Endoscopy and Cancer Management*. Edited by: D. O. Faigel and M. L. Kochman © Humana Press, Totowa, NJ

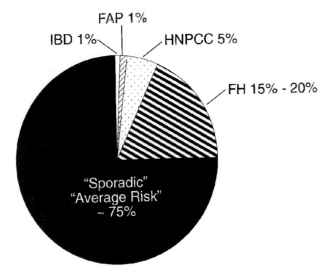

Fig. 1. Factors associated with annual new cases of CRC. Sporadic, men and women age 50 and older with no special risk factors. FH, positive family history; FAP, familial adenomatous polyposis; HNPCC, hereditary nonpolyposis colorectal cancer; IBD, inflammatory bowel disease. (Reprinted with permission from ref. *91*.)

Table 1
Risk Factors for Colorectal Cancer

Inflammatory bowel disease
   Chronic ulcerative colitis
   Crohn's colitis
Adenomatous polyposis
   Familial polyposis
   MYH-associated polyposis
Turcot's syndrome
Oldfield's syndrome
Juvenile polyposis
Hereditary nonpolyposis colorectal cancer
Family history
   Colorectal adenomas younger than 60 yr
   Colorectal cancer
Past history
   Colorectal adenomas
   Colorectal cancer
   Breast, ovarian, and uterine cancer

Adapted from ref. *85.*

3.2. FECAL OCCULT BLOOD TESTS
3.2.1. Guaiac-Based Stool Tests

The American College of Physicians has published comprehensive guidelines for fecal occult blood testing (FOBT) and interpretation with review of the data *(7,8)*. FOBT has been estimated to detect around 90% of cancers with repeated testing over several years *(9)*. However, a one-time FOBT (three samples) has an estimated sensitivity for advanced neoplasia of only 23.9% *(10)*. FOBT is most commonly performed using a guaiac-based test for peroxidase activity. Therefore, it is important that patients avoid other substances with peroxidase or pseudoperoxidase activity, such as rare red meat and some fruits and vegetables (e.g., turnips and horseradish). False-positive results can also occur as a result of other sources of gastrointestinal bleeding (e.g., hemorrhoids, peptic ulcer, and gum disease). False-negatives can result from tumors,

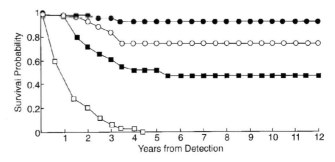

Fig. 2. Correlation of survival with stage of CRC. Stage I (63); s, stage II (49); j, stage III (55); h, stage IV (32). (Reprinted with permission from ref. *92*.)

which do not bleed at the time the stool is sampled, or from vitamin C use, which can interfere with the test reaction. Rehydration of the stool specimen with a drop of water has been demonstrated to increase the sensitivity at the expense of decreased specificity. The positive predictive value for cancer is 10–17% without rehydration, and 2–6% with rehydration. Despite the apparent simplicity of the test, improper test interpretation can be a significant problem *(11)*.

FOBT is the only screening modality that has been proven to reduce mortality from CRC in randomized controlled trials (Table 2) *(9,12–14)*. FOBT has also been demonstrated to reduce CRC incidence *(15)*. In the Minnesota Colorectal Cancer Control Trial, 46,551 people without symptoms of CRC were randomized to undergo either annual FOBT, biennial FOBT, or usual care *(9)*. For most of the trial, FOBT was performed with rehydrated slides. Colonoscopy was recommended for those with a positive FOBT. Over 13 yr of follow-up, the annually screened group evidenced a 33% reduction in CRC mortality (*see* Fig. 6). There was no significant reduction in mortality with biennial screening during 13 yr of follow-up, although after 18 yr, CRC mortality was reduced by 21% *(16)*. Of note, 38% of the annually screened subjects and 28% of the biennial group underwent colonoscopy at some point during the initial 13-yr study. Also of interest, patients in the annual FOBT group completed 75% of the screening offered and 90% completed at least one screening.

In a second randomized controlled trial, conducted in the Nottingham, England area, more than 150,000 patients aged between 45 and 74 were randomly offered FOBT without hydration biennially or received usual care *(12)*. Again, colonoscopy was recommended for those with a positive FOBT. After a mean of 7.8 yr of follow-up, CRC mortality was reduced by 15% in the screened group (odds ratio [OR] 0.85, 95% confidence interval [CI] 0.74–0.98). Compliance with at least one FOBT was 59.6%. A similar study conducted of nearly 62,000 Danes aged 45–75 found an 18% reduction in CRC mortality 10 yr after the study began (OR 0.82, 95% CI 0.68–0.99) *(13)*. In this study, 67% of the screening group completed the first screening round and more than 90% of those accepted repeated screening. Based on the above studies, annual FOBT appears to be more effective than biennial screening. Complications of FOBT testing include the negative effects patients endure as a result of false-positive test results,

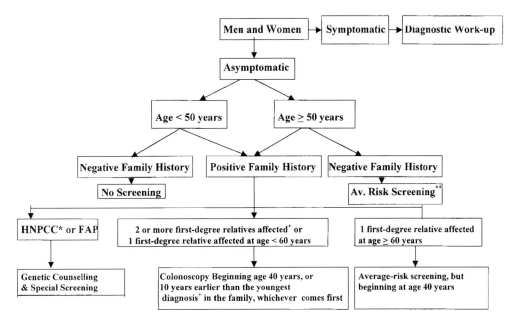

Fig. 3. Algorithm for colorectal cancer screening. +, either colorectal cancer or adenomatous polyp; *, hereditary nonpolyposis colorectal cancer; **, *see* text. FAP, familial adenomatous polyposis. (Reprinted with permission from ref. *4*.)

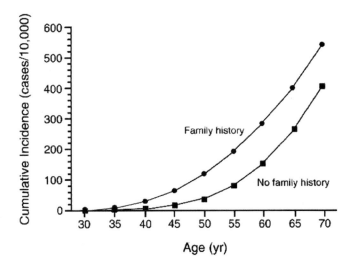

Fig. 4. Cumulative incidence of colorectal cancer according to age and the presence or absence of a family history of the disease. (Reprinted with permission from ref. *93*.)

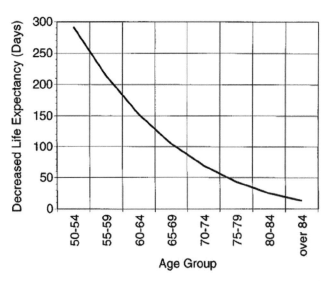

Fig. 5. The impact of colorectal cancer on life expectancy. The *x*-axis depicts age in 5-yr groups; the *y*-axis indicates the decrease in life expectancy in days owing to colorectal cancer. (Reprinted with permission from ref. *5*.)

the danger of misleading reassurance in those with false-negative results, and complications related to the diagnostic evaluation of positive FOBT results.

3.2.2. Immunochemical-Based Stool Testing

Given concerns about the need for dietary restriction and detection of clinically insignificant bleeding from the upper gut with the guaiac-based FOBT, immunochemical tests for human hemoglobin have been developed. Immunochemical tests have performed well compared to guaiac-based tests in clinical studies, but commercially available tests have not been studied in large populations of average-risk individuals in order to clearly demonstrate their accuracy *(17)*. Although immunochemical tests may be easier to interpret than guaiac-based tests, the processing of the available immunochemical tests must occur in a central lab. Also, the cost of immunochemical

tests is considerably higher than guaiac-based tests (e.g., $28 for InSure™ *[18]* compared to typically less than $4 for guaiac-based tests *[19]*). As noted by Levin et al. *(20)*, these tests have not found wide usage for technical and commercial reasons. As a result, some immunochemical tests (e.g., FlexSureOBT™ and HemeSelect™) are no longer on the market. Our experience with immunochemical tests failed to show any clear benefit with respect to patient compliance and overall rate of positive results when compared with a guaiac-based test *(21)*.

3.2.3. Fecal DNA-Based Molecular Marker Assays

Genetic and epigenetic alterations of DNA are a fundamental aspect of virtually all cancers, including CRC (Fig. 7). Consequently, testing of stool samples for altered DNA has been

Table 2
Evidence of the Effectiveness of Fecal Occult Blood Testing

	Minn (9)	*Minn (16)*	*UK (12)*	*Denmark (13)*	*France (14)*
Frequency of testing	Annual	Biennial	Biennial	Biennial	Biennial
Duration (yr)	13	18	8	10	11
Slide rehydration	Yes	Yes	No	No	No
Colonoscopy performed (%)	38	>28	5	4	4
Colorectal cancer mortality reduction (%)	33	21	15	18	16

proposed as a potential screening test for colon cancer. In 1992, Sidransky et al. *(22)* demonstrated the feasibility of this approach by detecting mutant *KRAS2* DNA in stool samples from people with colon cancer. Since that time, a number of other investigators have demonstrated that other DNA alterations, including *APC* mutations, *TP53* mutations, and microsatellite unstable DNA (i.e., *BAT26* alterations), can be detected in fecal DNA and can serve as molecular markers for colon adenomas and colon cancer *(23–26)*. Furthermore, with the recent demonstration of the common occurrence of aberrantly methylated genes in colon adenomas and cancer and the development of a technique called methylation-specific polymerase chain reaction (PCR), considerable interest in the use of aberrantly methylated genes as serum or stool-based molecular marker assays for colon cancer has developed *(27,28)*. As proof of principle, methylated *SFRP2*, the gene for secretory frizzled related protein 2, has been shown to be a potential stool-based molecular marker for colon cancer *(29)*.

DNA-based markers are a promising class of potential early detection markers because DNA is stable in the stool, is shed continuously, and can be detected in minute amounts through the use of PCR-based technologies *(30)*. However, a substantial technical limitation to the use of DNA alterations as markers for colon cancer is the lack of a single alteration that can serve as a marker for all colon cancers. For example, *APC* mutations, which are believed to be the most common mutation in colon cancer, can be found in at most 70% of colon cancers using conventional mutation detection techniques *(31)*. In fact, it is now well appreciated that colon cancers are genetically heterogeneous, which has led to the belief that assay panels that include tests that detect a variety of gene alterations will be needed to generate a clinically useful test *(25)*. One of these assay panels is commercially available and marketed under the name PreGen-Plus (EXACT Sciences and LabCorp). This assay is a stool-based panel of 23 assays that targets known point mutations in *APC, KRAS2, TP53, BAT26* and also tests for long fragments of DNA, which has been called the DNA Integrity Assay (DIA®). Of note, the mechanism responsible for the long fragments of DNA found in individuals with colon neoplasms is not known but may be DNA from nonapoptotic cells. Data using this assay panel from a small pilot study of symptomatic patients undergoing colonoscopy (*N* = 61) found that the sensitivity for cancer was 91% (95% CI, 71–99%), the sensitivity for large adenomas was 82% (95% CI, 48–98%), and the specificity for adenomas or cancer was 93% (95% CI, 76–99%) *(25)*. Exclusion of *KRAS2* mutations in the assay panel increased the specificity to 100% (95% CI, 88–100%)

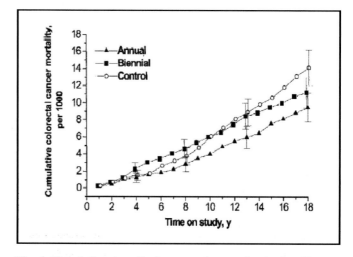

Fig. 6. Cumulative mortality by years since randomization (time on study) for each randomization group (annual, biennial, and control), with bars at 4, 8, 13, and 18 yr representing 95% confidence intervals. Early in the study, cumulative colorectal cancer mortality was greater in the biennial group than in the control group. The trend was reversed by the 11th year of follow-up and resulted in a 21% reduction by year 18. (Reprinted with permission from ref. *16*.)

with a fall in sensitivity for adenomas to 73% (95% CI, 39–94%). In this highly selected sample, the positive predictive value was 100%, with a negative predictive value of 85%. In this study, Hemoccult performed poorly at detecting adenomas (0/11 detected). Other studies of fecal-based DNA markers have demonstrated similar levels of specificity and sensitivity for colon cancer and colon adenomas. For example, Traverso et al. demonstrated that an assay that detects *APC* mutations in DNA extracted from stool had a sensitivity of 57% (95% CI, 41–71%) for colon cancer or colon adenomas more than 1 cm in size and a specificity of 100% (95% CI, 88–100%) *(23)*. Imperiale et al. demonstrated in a large prospective study of people undergoing colonoscopy for colon cancer screening that the PreGen Plus assay could detect individuals with CRC (sensitivity 51.6%) and advanced adenomas (sensitivity 18.2%) with 95% specificity. Thus, these studies have demonstrated the feasibility of an approach using molecular markers for the early detection or prevention of colon cancer; however, their performance as screening assays in this large cross-sectional study demonstrated that the sensitivity of these assays using current technological approaches is not ideal because the sensitivity is less than that of other available CRC screening methods. Thus, studies are ongoing using

Chromosome Unstable (CIN) Pathway

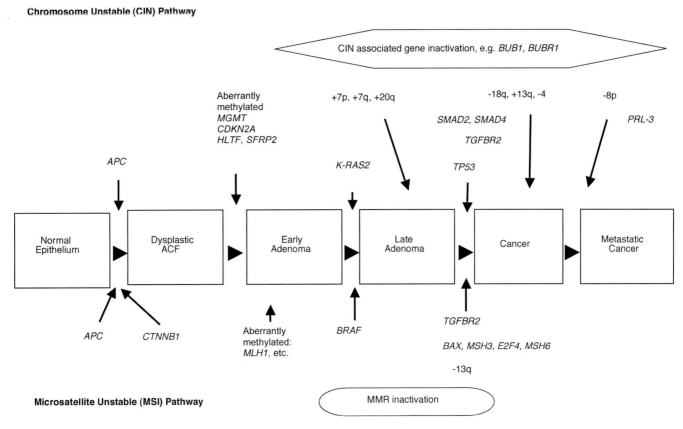

Fig. 7. Schematic representation of the adenoma–carcinoma progression sequence that highlights histological stages that are believed to represent critical steps in the evolution of normal colon epithelial cells to adenocarcinomas cells. Genetic and epigenetic events that have been identified at these different histological steps are shown above and below the histological representations of the steps. Colon cancers are believed to be heterogeneous in regards to the genetic and epigenetic events they acquire during this progression sequence, and this figure is not intended to imply that all colon cancers will have all of the alterations listed. In addition, there are at least two different types of colon cancers that can be defined by the type of genomic DNA instability they display, and these have been called chromosome unstable (CIN) tumors and microsatellite unstable (MSI) tumors. The genetic and epigenetic alterations observed in these two types of colon cancers vary as shown above.

second-generation molecular marker assays to improve on the performance of the first-generation assay panels. It is widely believed that the performance of the molecular marker assays will improve substantially with advances in sample collection methods, choice of targets for the assays, and target detection technology *(32)*.

The potential advantages and disadvantages of stool-based DNA mutation testing have been discussed in some detail by Levin et al. *(20)* and are summarized below. These advantages include the following: (1) a high specificity for neoplasia, because the mutation assays developed to date do not appear to generate false-positive results from other causes of gastro-intestinal bleeding as occurs with fecal occult blood; (2) a theoretical ability to detect cancers proximal to the colon (e.g., aerodigestive cancers); (3) the noninvasive nature of the assay, which requires no preparation; and (4) the potential for high accuracy for the early detection of colon cancer. However, as noted earlier, there are still major limitations currently to the application of these assays as colon cancer screening tests, including the lack of data of the performance characteristics of most of these assays when run on screening populations, the need for test refinement to improve sensitivity without sacrificing specificity, the high cost (currently >$600 per test), and

finally concerns about adherence because an entire bowel movement must be expeditiously delivered to the laboratory to perform the assays. In addition, these tests can theoretically identify clinical and pre-clinical disease because they detect DNA alterations that may precede the onset of histologically evident disease, which raises issues about how these "false-positive" results will be evaluated. It is not clear what should be done if the test is positive but the colonoscopic exam does not reveal any adenomas or cancer, especially in light of the fact that at least some of these assays can detect aerodigestive tract cancers. Thus, molecular marker assays for colon cancer show considerable promise to be inexpensive and accurate noninvasive screening tests, however, their performance as colon cancer screening assays in comparison to other currently available screening tests remains to be determined.

3.3. FLEXIBLE SIGMOIDOSCOPY

The advantages of sigmoidoscopy over FOBT include direct visualization of the bowel lumen and the ability to biopsy lesions at the time of the procedure, thereby increasing the sensitivity and specificity for detecting cancer within the limits of the length of the scope. Moreover, there may be an indirect benefit of screening with sigmoidoscopy through two mechanisms. First, removal of small polyps during sigmoidoscopy may prevent progression of these polyps to future CRC. Second, adenomas found during sigmoidoscopy often prompt full colonoscopy with subsequent detection of premalignant or malignant lesions in the portion of the colon not seen with the sigmoidoscope. It is estimated that approximately half of all polyps and cancers are within reach of a standard 60-cm flexible sigmoidoscope. Several studies have evaluated the proportion of patients with advanced proximal neoplasia according to the findings in the distal colon (Table 3). There is still controversy as to the necessity for full colonoscopy if only one or two small adenomas are detected and removed at sigmoidoscopy (33). The prevalence of proximal advanced neoplasia in patients without distal adenomas is under 5%.

To date, no randomized controlled trials have been completed that evaluate the effectiveness of screening sigmoidoscopy, although studies are underway (34). Nonetheless, there is good evidence of the effectiveness from four case–control studies (35–38) (Table 4). Selby et al. (36) performed a case–control study of the effect of rigid sigmoidoscopy on CRC mortality using enrollees of Kaiser Permanente of Northern California (261 cases and 868 controls). They found a 59% reduction in CRC mortality for those cancers within reach of the sigmoidoscope (OR 0.41, 95% CI 0.25–0.69). Importantly, they found no benefit of sigmoidoscopy with respect to mortality from cancers beyond the reach of the sigmoidoscope (OR 0.96, 95% CI 0.61–1.50). This internal control helps to adjust for potential unmeasured differences between the cases and controls with respect to other cancer risk factors.

The correct interval at which to screen with sigmoidoscopy is unknown. From the study by Selby et al., it appears as though the benefit of screening persists for as much as 10 yr. The Muller and Sonnenberg study suggests that the benefit persists for at least 6 yr (35). A repeat colonoscopy 5 yr after a negative colonoscopy will infrequently identify advanced neoplasia (39), although the quality of the preparation and completeness of the exam may be less for sigmoidoscopy than for colonoscopy. The current recommendation is to offer flexible sigmoidoscopy (FS) every 5 yr. The decision to perform colonoscopy after a small polyp is found on sigmoidoscopy is controversial.

3.4. FS COMBINED WITH FOBT

The rationale behind combining FOBT and sigmoidoscopy stems from a belief that each test offers some benefit to counter the limitations of the other. Although sigmoidoscopy fails to screen above the reach of the sigmoidoscope, FOBT can detect proximal lesions that bleed. Although FOBT fails to detect many nonbleeding cancers, sigmoidoscopy directly visualizes the bowel and offers the possibility of reducing cancer incidence through polyp removal. In fact, in the Nottingham trial of FOBT, two-thirds of the cancers missed by FOBT were in the rectosigmoid region (40). There has been one controlled trial of more than 12,000 people in the Sloan-Kettering Institute and Strang Clinic in New York, which compared annual rigid sigmoidoscopy to annual rigid sigmoidoscopy with FOBT (41). CRC mortality was reduced by 43% in the group receiving combination screening after 5–11 yr of follow-up. In addition, this study demonstrated a shift toward earlier stage

of cancer diagnosis in the combination group (70 vs 48%). In an ongoing randomized trial of sigmoidoscopy with or without FOBT, there is no evidence from their preliminary report that FOBT adds to the proportion of patients found to have high-risk neoplasia compared with sigmoidoscopy alone (42). A recommendation of the Multisociety Task Force is to offer screening including both FOBT and sigmoidoscopy (as described in the earlier recommendations for the individual tests) together, although FOBT should be done first (as a positive test will result in a colonoscopy and obviate the need for sigmoidoscopy) (4).

3.5. BARIUM ENEMA

Barium enemas can be used to visualize the entire colon in most patients. An air-contrast, or double-contrast barium enema (DCBE) is better at identifying small mucosal lesions than a single-contrast study. The performance characteristics of DCBE are difficult to determine precisely owing to methodological problems in the available studies. However, it is estimated that the sensitivity of DCBE is 53% for polyps 6–10 mm in size and 48% for polyps larger than 1 cm (43). False-negative tests result from inadequate visualization of the bowel or improper interpretation. False-positive tests result from adherent stool and other non-neoplastic mucosal lesions. One case–control study suggested there might be some association with reduced CRC mortality, although the confidence interval was wide (44). There are no controlled trials that show that barium enema is effective in reducing adverse health outcomes related to CRC. Therefore, any recommendation for screening with barium enema is based on indirect evidence stemming from the ability of barium enema to detect colonic neoplasms. Furthermore, there are no studies that help us to determine the appropriate frequency of screening with DCBE. Complications relating to barium enema include perforation (estimated 1/25,000), radiation exposure (300–500 mrem) and minor complications directly attributable to the test, as well as complications from colonoscopy resulting from positive screening tests.

The Multisociety Task Force clinical guidelines recommend that DCBE be offered every 5 yr (4). This recommendation is based on evidence that screening DCBE is better at detecting cancers and large polyps than FOBT and is probably safer than sigmoidoscopy or colonoscopy. DCBE is less sensitive to small polyps than endoscopy, can result in false-positives that require colonoscopic evaluation, and involves patient discomfort and inconvenience. Although adding FS will increase the sensitivity, the clinical benefit of such an approach for colon cancer screening has not been demonstrated and may not justify the additional effort.

3.6. COLONOSCOPY

Colonoscopy is attractive for CRC screening for several reasons. First, unlike sigmoidoscopy, colonoscopy offers the ability to visualize the entire colon in most patients. Second, it allows for one to both detect, biopsy, and/or remove mucosal lesions in one setting. Moreover, colonoscopy does not rely on polyps or cancers to bleed in order for them to be detected. Finally, as colonoscopy is the final common pathway for the evaluation of positive screening tests (e.g., FOBT, barium enema), it is reasonable to attribute much of the benefits of

Table 3
Rate of Advanced Proximal Neoplasm[a] According to Colorectal Findings in the Distal Colon

| Reference | Normal | Hyperplastic polyp | Findings in the distal colon (%) (no./total) | | Advanced neoplasm |
			Tubular adenoma <1 cm	Multiple tubular adenomas <1 cm[b]	
10	2.7 (48/1765)	2.8 (13/464)	6.4 (35/543)	9.1 (4/44)	11.7 (32/274)
86	Not reported	Not reported	0.8 (1/124)	Not reported	11.8 (12/102)
87	Not reported	Not reported	6.9 (13/189)[c]	Not reported	28.6 (4/14)
88	Not reported	Not reported	2.9 (15/521)	2.4 (2/85)	5.9 (27/460)
89	Not reported	Not reported	1.6 (3/90)	10.4 (5/48)	7.4 (5/63)
90	5.3 (29/544)	Not reported	5.0 (22/444)	6.3 (20/319)	8.8 (147/1665)
45	1.5 (23/1564)	4.0 (8/201)	7.1 (12/168)	Not reported	11.5 (7/61)[d]

Modified from ref. *33*.
[a]Defined as invasive cancer of adenoma 1 cm or larger in diameter or with villous features or high-grade dysplasia.
[b]Defined as three of more adenomas.
[c]Includes adenomas with villous features.
[d]Does not include adenomas 1 cm or larger.

Table 4
Case–Control Studies of Mortality Reduction Associated With Sigmoidoscopy Screening

Study characteristics	Selby et al. (36)	Newcomb et al. (37)	Muller and Sonnenberg (35)
No. of cases of colorectal cancer	261	66	4411
Type of sigmoidoscope	Rigid	Rigid and flexible	Rigid and flexible
Odds ratio (95% CI) for colorectal cancer death	0.41 (0.25–0.69)	0.21 (0.08–0.52)	0.41 (0.33–0.5)
Interval of apparent protective effect (yr)	9–10	Not specified	5

Modified from ref. *33*. CI, confidence interval.

other screening strategies to the colonoscopy itself. Two large, cross-sectional screening colonoscopy studies have been published showing that approximately half of those patients with advanced proximal neoplasia have no distal adenomas *(45,46)*. The sensitivity and specificity of colonoscopy are difficult to measure, because colonoscopy is often considered to be the gold standard. Tandem colonoscopy studies have shown that 0–6% of large polyps (≥1 cm) are missed and up to 27% of smaller lesions are missed *(47,48)*. In the Office of Technology Assessment study of the cost-effectiveness of CRC screening, the sensitivity of colonoscopy for polyps and cancer was estimated at 90% *(49)*. Given that lesions can be biopsied at the time of colonoscopy, the specificity is near 100%.

There are no controlled studies that directly assess the effectiveness of screening colonoscopy in reducing CRC mortality. There are case–control studies, which demonstrate that colonoscopy with or without polypectomy decreases the incidence of CRC *(50)*. The National Polyp Study found that colonoscopy with polypectomy reduces the incidence of CRC *(51)* (Fig. 8). Similar results were seen in a cohort study from Italy *(52)*. Moreover, a randomized, controlled study of sigmoidoscopy with follow-up colonoscopy did show a significant reduction in CRC incidence in screened subjects *(53)*. It is not known how often screening colonoscopy should be performed. However, given that polyps usually require many years to progress to CRC, the high accuracy of colonoscopy for detecting advanced neoplasia *(47)*, and the evidence of protection from cancer mortality for many years following

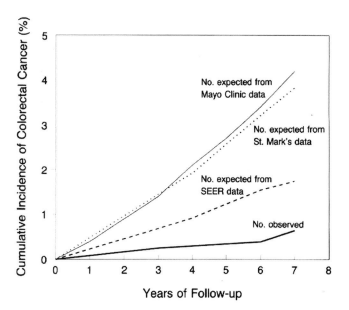

Fig. 8. Observed and expected CRC incidence in National Polyp Study cohort after colonoscopic polypectomy. (Reprinted with permission ref. *51*.)

proctosigmoidoscopy, recent data on the low yield of colonoscopy 5 yr after a negative colonoscopy support the recommendation for screening colonoscopy every 10 yr in the absence of neoplasia.

However, there are several problems with colonoscopy as a screening test. First, its performance is operator-dependent, with the endoscopist's experience playing a role in how often an adequate exam is obtained. It is estimated that the cecum can be reached in 98.6% of screening colonoscopies *(54)*. Colonoscopy performed by nongastroenterologists, however, has been shown to be less sensitive for detecting cancer than colonoscopy by gastroenterologists *(55)*. Therefore, screening colonoscopy should only be performed by well-trained providers. Second, patient discomfort or embarrassment may limit acceptance, although the use of conscious sedation during most colonoscopies can alleviate most patient discomfort. In fact, many patients prefer colonoscopy to barium enema *(56)*. Third, colonoscopy is the most expensive screening test under consideration when viewed from the perspective of cost per test. However, inclusion of downstream costs in the analysis alters this assessment. Finally, colonoscopy can result in complications such as perforation, bleeding, infection, and reactions to medications used for conscious sedation *(57)*. Commonly used estimates of the risk of perforation and bleeding are probably overstated, as these data often include patients undergoing therapeutic procedures, patients with comorbidity which would usually exclude screening, or they include complications during early experience with colonoscopy. In the Minnesota Colon Cancer Control Study, 12,246 colonoscopies were performed at the university hospital, resulting in 4 perforations (all requiring surgery) and 11 serious bleeding episodes (3 requiring surgery) *(9)*. There were no perforations among more than 5000 patients in the two large screening colonoscopy studies *(45,46)*.

3.7. COMPUTED TOMOGRAPHIC COLONOGRAPHY

Computed tomographic colonography (CTC) is performed using a spiral CT scan. Magnetic resonance imaging techniques are also under development. Computer software generates a virtual image of the bowel lumen, allowing one to perform a "fly-through" examination of the bowel looking for polyps and cancer. This non-invasive technique for total colonic evaluation is rapidly evolving. If CTC can accurately distinguish patients with polyps or cancer from those without, then the cost and risks of colonoscopy can be limited to those most likely to benefit and overall screening rates may improve.

Unfortunately, there is considerable variability in the reported sensitivity and specificity of CTC, with most studies reporting results that indicate further improvements are needed before widespread clinical application *(58–60)*. There is one study that stands out for its impressive results *(61)*. In this study, Pickhardt et al. performed CTC followed by colonoscopy in 1233 subjects. Unlike other studies, these investigators employed software techniques to electronically "cleanse" the bowel mucosa and utilized primary three-dimensional reconstruction for review of the images. Although they demonstrated that CTC sensitivity was similar to optical colonoscopy (88.7 vs 92.3% for polyps >5 mm), their results have yet to be reproduced. Other investigators have reported markedly lower sensitivities, although differences in technique, hardware, and radiologist training may contribute to these differences.

For example, the study reported by Cotton et al. *(58)* utilized widely available CT technology, whereas the Pickhardt study used only more state-of-the-art four- or eight-section CT scanners. Interestingly, subsequent three-dimensional imaging in the Cotton study did not dramatically improve the test characteristics. Radiologist experience may play a role, because the Cotton study required 10 prior CTC cases and the Pickhardt study required 25 prior CTC cases. The previously documented very poor interobserver variation of CTC interpretation among experienced radiologists raises concerns about the performance of CTC in routine clinical practice *(60)*. Further studies are needed to confirm the findings of Pickhardt et al. before CTC is endorsed as a screening test for CRC. Clearly, the technique is still evolving and the role of CTC in clinical care is yet to be fully defined.

4. COST-EFFECTIVENESS OF SCREENING

It is critical to understand that the cost of screening for CRC entails more than just the cost of the initial screening test. Other costs include those associated with the evaluation of true- and false-positive results, costs of complications, and costs of cancer care. Some costs are very difficult to measure and are usually not included in cost-effectiveness models. These include the costs of time lost from work and early mortality with loss of income for the patient's family.

There have been several formal analyses of the cost-effectiveness of CRC screening *(3,49,62,63)*. In Lieberman's model of the cost-effectiveness of preventing death from CRC, several key points were highlighted *(63)*. Although FOBT achieves reduction in CRC mortality through detection of early stage cancer, it prevents the fewest cancers when compared with other screening modalities. One-time colonoscopy achieves the greatest reduction in CRC and mortality from CRC. The model assumed that 100% of patients with a positive FOBT would undergo colonoscopy. This assumption is unlikely to be met in clinical practice, as the Minnesota Colon Cancer Control Study only had 81% compliance with follow-up colonoscopy. Importantly, the cost of cancer care is a key variable in the cost-effectiveness analysis, for when the cost of cancer care exceeds $45,000, the cost per death prevented is similar for FOBT, FS/FOBT, and colonoscopy. Failure to screen will result in additional costs to provide care for the cancers, which could have been prevented. As the cost of cancer care rises, therefore, screening becomes increasingly cost-effective, and potentially cost-saving. When the cost of colonoscopy falls below $750, then one-time colonoscopy is more cost-effective than the other strategies studied. Finally, compliance is a key factor in determining the relative cost-effectiveness of the screening strategies. When compliance is 100% for all strategies, FOBT ($225,000 per death prevented) appears much more cost-effective than colonoscopy ($274,000 per death prevented). However, when compliance falls to 50% for all tests, FOBT ($331,000 per death prevented) is negligibly more cost-effective than colonoscopy ($337,000 per death prevented). Because FOBT requires annual testing, whereas colonoscopy is modeled as a one-time procedure, one could speculate that compliance may actually be higher for colonoscopy. Clearly, compliance is critical to any discussion of cost-effectiveness. A program of FOBT testing would

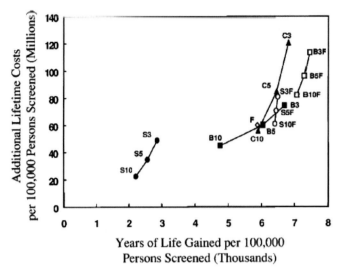

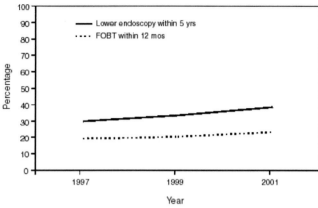

* 1997 and 1999 surveys did not include responses within 10 years.
† Age-adusted to the 2001 BRFSS population.

Fig. 9. Effects and costs of CRC screening. S, sigmoidoscopy; B, DCBE; C, colonoscopy; F, annual fecal occult blood test (FOBT). The number next to the letter indicates screening interval in years. For example, S5F is sigmoidoscopy every 5 yr combined with annual FOBT. (Reprinted with permission from ref. *49*.)

Fig. 10. Percentage of people aged 50 yr or older who reported receiving a fecal occult blood test (FOBT) within 12 mo preceding survey and/or lower endoscopy within 5 yr* preceding survey, by test type and year—Behavioral Risk Factor Surveillance System (BRFSS), United States, 1997–2001.† (Reprinted with permission from ref. *67*.)

require 80% compliance to achieve the same mortality reduction seen when screening colonoscopy is performed with 50% compliance. Unfortunately, we lack good data on reasonable compliance rates for colonoscopy. Although there is some evidence of poor participation in screening colonoscopy studies *(64)*, participation may be dramatically improved if physicians, professional organizations and third-party payers strongly recommend and support screening colonoscopy.

The model performed by the Office of Technology Assessment of the Unites States Congress *(49)* studied the cost-effectiveness of FOBT, FS, DCBE and colonoscopy, both individually and in combination, for patients aged 50–85 yr (Fig. 9). Although it accounted for years of life lost as a result of detection and treatment of cancer, it did not account for imperfect compliance. The most striking finding of this study is that all strategies cost less than $20,000 per year of life saved. This is well within the commonly accepted range (<$40,000) of cost-effectiveness for US health care (dialysis costs approximately $35,000 per year of life saved).

5. COMPLIANCE

Compliance with screening for CRC in the United States and Canada has been disappointingly low *(65–67)*. The Centers for Disease Control conducts a state-based, random-digit-dialed telephone survey of the civilian US population on a biennial basis *(67)*. In 2001, 87,729 persons aged 50 yr or older responded. An estimated 44.6% had ever had FOBT, with 23.5% indicating they had FOBT in the past 12 mo. Overall, 47.3% had ever had lower endoscopy and 43.4% had lower endoscopy within 10 yr. An estimated 53.1% had FOBT in the past 12 mo and/or lower endoscopy in the past 10 yr. Comparison to similar surveys conducted in 1997 and 1999 indicates a trend toward increasing participation (Fig. 10). Recent data from Ontario suggests that screening participation is much lower in Canada *(65)*. In this study of nearly 1 million individuals aged 50–59 yr without

prior evidence of screening in administrative databases, less than 20.5% were screened during 6 yr of follow-up.

There is marked variation in screening participation rates in studies of CRC screening. Much of this variation in compliance is explained by study design, with studies of high-risk subjects and volunteers generally finding higher compliance than mass screening studies. One British study has found that refusal to undergo screening may be related to fear of further tests and surgery, feeling well, and unpleasantness of the screening procedure *(68)*. Myers et al. *(69)* have found that prior exposure to health education interventions is associated with increased compliance with screening. Thus, compliance may be associated with positive attitudes toward screening and a willingness to risk the complications of the screening test in return for the assurance that is obtained for a negative test. Unwillingness to undergo screening may represent perceived lack of vulnerability to CRC, fear of discomfort or discovery of illness, or possibly belief that finding cancer will not impact on treatment and survival. Weller et al. *(70)* in an Australian population-based study, found that although awareness of FOBT is high, only 15% of subjects over age 40 had been tested. Moreover, only 28% stated that they intend to be tested. Many patients denied susceptibility to CRC, had knowledge deficits related to treatment success, or felt uncomfortable about taking the test. Kelly and Shank have shown that perceptions of discomfort with screening and perception of how well the physician explained the importance of the test are significant predictors of adherence to a screening program *(71)*.

Although many of these factors are inherent to the patient, there are a number of system level barriers to CRC screening. Although many professional societies have long endorsed CRC screening *(72)*, screening guidelines from national task forces (e.g., US Preventive Services Task Force and Canadian Task Force on Preventive Health Care) have only endorsed many screening modalities relatively recently *(2,73,74)*. As a result, physicians and other health care providers may not yet be convinced of the

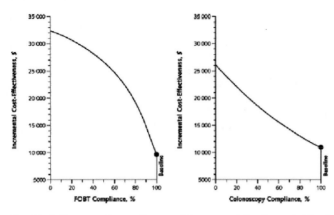

Fig. 11. Influence of compliance with repeated fecal occult blood testing (FOBT) once per year (left) and repeated colonoscopy (right) once per decade on the incremental cost-effectiveness ratio compared with no screening. (Reprinted with permission from ref. *94*.)

benefits of screening. In addition, there are financial barriers to screening, especially because many insurance companies do not fully cover CRC screening. Nevertheless, screening participation is highest among those with health insurance, as well as those with higher education and recent routine doctors visits *(75)*. Although a CRC screening benefit was introduced for Medicare beneficiaries in 1998, early data suggests that this has not yet had measurable impact on test utilization *(76)*.

Compliance with screening colonoscopy requires further study. When medical personnel and their spouses were invited to undergo a free screening colonoscopy, less than 15% accepted *(64)*. Adherence to recommended follow-up colonoscopy after polypectomy was 80% in the National Polyp Study *(77)*. However, there is much interest in the idea of a one-time screening colonoscopy *(78)*. This strategy may achieve a significant reduction in CRC mortality without requiring longitudinal compliance, one of the most difficult problems with CRC screening. This is especially important as the cost-effectiveness of screening is reduced as compliance falls (Fig. 11).

6. PATIENT PREFERENCES FOR CRC SCREENING

A variety of studies have assessed patient preferences for CRC screening. It is difficult to generalize findings from these studies, as the most defensible conclusion is that there is considerable variability in patient attitudes toward these screening modalities. In a survey of outpatients, Leard et al. *(79)* found that colonoscopic screening was preferred to sigmoidoscopy or barium enema. In a hospital-based randomized trial of screening sigmoidoscopy vs screening colonoscopy, patients found the preparation for sigmoidoscopy easier *(80)*. However, colonoscopy was less uncomfortable and less embarrassing than sigmoidoscopy, likely resulting from use of sedation with colonoscopy. In their study, colonoscopy was as acceptable to patients and only 20% more expensive. Patients clearly express anxiety and fear regarding endoscopy. McCarthy and Moskowitz found that although many patients undergoing screening sigmoidoscopy experienced pain and embarrassment, they reported significantly less pain and embarrassment than they had expected *(81)*. In a study of veterans with and without CRC *(82)*, substantial variation in attitudes toward screening

sigmoidoscopy and colonoscopy was demonstrated. Drossman et al. *(83)* have shown that younger patients, women, and patients without prior personal experience with endoscopic procedures were more likely to express concerns relating to endoscopy, including finding out what is wrong, experiencing pain, and finding cancer. These concerns may result in failure of the patient to undergo screening. Recent studies of CT colonography have assessed patient preferences for standard colonoscopy vs CT colonography. Unfortunately, there is no consistent pattern to the results, likely resulting from variation in how the subjects are queried about their preferences. One study has directly assessed preferences through the offering of either CT colonography or colonoscopy to 451 Australians in a community-based study. Of these, only 62 people chose to undergo screening, with 61% choosing colonoscopy and 39% choosing CT colonography ($p = 0.075$) *(84)*.

Therefore, decisions regarding recommendations for CRC screening must take into account the variability in patient preferences. Ideally, patients should be offered a menu of test options from which to choose the test that best suits their preference. Although not all tests may be available in a given situation, patients should understand the advantages and limitations of each test in order to make an informed decision.

7. SUMMARY

CRC is a significant health care problem for which screening has been shown to be effective in improving health related outcomes related to this cancer, as well as to be cost-effective. Unfortunately, participation rates in screening programs have been disappointingly low. Given the availability of several good screening tests, it is incumbent on providers to educate their patients about the benefits of screening, and the test options. Efforts to remove barriers to screening should be supported.

REFERENCES

1. American Cancer Society. Cancer Facts and Figures, 2006. Atlanta: American Cancer Society; 2006.
2. Pignone M, Rich M, Teutsch SM, Berg AO, Lohr KN. Screening for colorectal cancer in adults at average risk: a summary of the evidence for the U.S. Preventive Services Task Force. Ann Intern Med 2002; 137(2):132–141.
3. Frazier AL, Colditz GA, Fuchs CS, Kuntz KM. Cost-effectiveness of screening for colorectal cancer in the general population. JAMA 2000; 284(15):1954–1961.
4. Winawer S, Fletcher R, Rex D, et al. Colorectal cancer screening and surveillance: clinical guidelines and rationale-Update based on new evidence. Gastroenterology 2003; 124(2):544–560.
5. Inadomi JM, Sonnenberg A. The impact of colorectal cancer screening on life expectancy. Gastrointest Endosc 2000; 51(5):517–523.
6. Winawer SJ. Surveillance overview. In: Cohen AM, Winawer SJ, eds. Cancer of the colon, rectum, and anus. New York: McGraw-Hill; 1995:265.
7. Anonymous. Suggested technique for fecal occult blood testing and interpretation in colorectal cancer screening. American College of Physicians. Ann Intern Med 1997; 126(10):808–810.
8. Ransohoff DF, Lang CA. Screening for colorectal cancer with the fecal occult blood test: a background paper. American College of Physicians. Ann Intern Med 15 1997; 126(10):811–822.
9. Mandel JS, Bond JH, Church TR, et al. Reducing mortality from colorectal cancer by screening for fecal occult blood. Minnesota Colon Cancer Control Study. N Engl J Med 1993; 328(19):1365–1371.

10. Lieberman DA, Weiss DG. One-time screening for colorectal cancer with combined fecal occult-blood testing and examination of the distal colon. N Engl J Med 2001; 345(8):555–560.

11. Selinger RR, Norman S, Dominitz JA. Failure of health care professionals to interpret fecal occult blood tests accurately. Am J Med 2003; 114(1):64–67.

12. Hardcastle JD, Chamberlain JO, Robinson MH, et al. Randomised controlled trial of faecal-occult-blood screening for colorectal cancer. Lancet 1996; 348(9040):1472–1477.

13. Kronborg O, Fenger C, Olsen J, Jorgensen OD, Sondergaard O. Randomised study of screening for colorectal cancer with faecal-occult-blood test. Lancet 1996; 348(9040):1467–1471.

14. Faivre J, Dancourt V, Lejeune C, et al. Reduction in colorectal cancer mortality by fecal occult blood screening in a French controlled study. Gastroenterology 2004; 126(7):1674–1680.

15. Mandel JS, Church TR, Bond JH, et al. The effect of fecal occult-blood screening on the incidence of colorectal cancer. N Engl J Med 2000; 343(22):1603–1607.

16. Mandel JS, Church TR, Ederer F, Bond JH. Colorectal cancer mortality: effectiveness of biennial screening for fecal occult blood. J Natl Cancer Inst 1999; 91(5):434–437.

17. Young GP, St John DJ, Winawer SJ, Rozen P. Choice of fecal occult blood tests for colorectal cancer screening: recommendations based on performance characteristics in population studies: a WHO (World Health Organization) and OMED (World Organization for Digestive Endoscopy) report. Am J Gastroenterol 2002; 97(10):2499–2507.

18. InSure™. How much does the InSure™ FOBT cost? Available at: http://www.insurefobt.com/faq01.html#option03. Accessed March 25, 2003.

19. Allison JE, Tekawa IS, Ransom LJ, Adrain AL. A comparison of fecal occult-blood tests for colorectal-cancer screening. N Engl J Med 1996; 334(3):155–159.

20. Levin B, Brooks D, Smith RA, Stone A. Emerging technologies in screening for colorectal cancer: CT colonography, immunochemical fecal occult blood tests, and stool screening using molecular markers. CA Cancer J Clin 2003; 53(1):44–55.

21. Ko CW, Dominitz JA, Nguyen TD. Fecal occult blood testing in a general medical clinic: comparison between guaiac-based and immunochemical-based tests. Am J Med 2003; 115(2):111–114.

22. Sidransky D, Tokino T, Hamilton SR, et al. Identification of ras oncogene mutations in the stool of patients with curable colorectal tumors. Science 1992; 256(5053):102–105.

23. Traverso G, Shuber A, Levin B, et al. Detection of APC mutations in fecal DNA from patients with colorectal tumors. N Engl J Med 2002; 346(5):311–320.

24. Traverso G, Shuber A, Olsson L, et al. Detection of proximal colorectal cancers through analysis of faecal DNA. Lancet 2002; 359(9304):403–404.

25. Ahlquist DA, Skoletsky JE, Boynton KA, et al. Colorectal cancer screening by detection of altered human DNA in stool: feasibility of a multitarget assay panel. Gastroenterology 2000; 119(5):1219–1227.

26. Dong SM, Traverso G, Johnson C, et al. Detecting colorectal cancer in stool with the use of multiple genetic targets. J Natl Cancer Inst 2001; 93(11):858–865.

27. Laird PW. The power and the promise of DNA methylation markers. Nat Rev Cancer 2003; 3(4):253–266.

28. Herman JG, Graff JR, Myohanen S, Nelkin BD, Baylin SB. Methylation-specific PCR: a novel PCR assay for methylation status of CpG islands. Proc Natl Acad Sci USA 1996; 93(18):9821–9826.

29. Muller HM, Oberwalder M, Fiegl H, et al. Methylation changes in faecal DNA: a marker for colorectal cancer screening? Lancet 2004; 363(9417):1283–1285.

30. Ahlquist DA, Shuber AP. Stool screening for colorectal cancer: evolution from occult blood to molecular markers. Clin Chim Acta 2002; 315(1–2):157–168.

31. Grady WM, Markowitz SD. Genetic and epigenetic alterations in colon cancer. Annu Rev Genomics Hum Genet 2002; 3:101–128.

32. Imperiale TF, Ransohoff DF, Itzkowitz SH, Turnbull BA, Ross ME. Fecal DNA versus fecal occult blood for colorectal-cancer screening in an average-risk population. N Engl J Med 2004; 351(26):2704–2714.

33. Walsh JM, Terdiman JP. Colorectal cancer screening: scientific review. JAMA 2003; 289(10):1288–1296.

34. Single flexible sigmoidoscopy screening to prevent colorectal cancer: baseline findings of a UK multicentre randomised trial. Lancet 2002; 359(9314):1291–1300.

35. Muller AD, Sonnenberg A. Protection by endoscopy against death from colorectal cancer. A case–control study among veterans. Arch Intern Med 1995; 155(16):1741–1748.

36. Selby JV, Friedman GD, Quesenberry CP, Jr., Weiss NS. A case–control study of screening sigmoidoscopy and mortality from colorectal cancer. N Engl J Med 1992; 326(10):653–657.

37. Newcomb PA, Norfleet RG, Storer BE, Surawicz TS, Marcus PM. Screening sigmoidoscopy and colorectal cancer mortality. J Natl Cancer Inst 1992; 84(20):1572–1575.

38. Kavanagh AM, Giovannucci EL, Fuchs CS, Colditz GA. Screening endoscopy and risk of colorectal cancer in United States men. Cancer Causes Control 1998; 9(4):455–462.

39. Rex DK, Cummings OW, Helper DJ, et al. 5-year incidence of adenomas after negative colonoscopy in asymptomatic average-risk persons (see comment). Gastroenterology. 1996; 111(5):1178–1181.

40. Hardcastle JD, Thomas WM, Chamberlain J, et al. Randomised, controlled trial of faecal occult blood screening for colorectal cancer. Results for first 107,349 subjects. Lancet. May 27 1989; 1(8648):1160–1164.

41. Winawer SJ, Flehinger BJ, Schottenfeld D, Miller DG. Screening for colorectal cancer with fecal occult blood testing and sigmoidoscopy. J Natl Cancer Inst 1993; 85(16):1311–1318.

42. Gondal G, Grotmol T, Hofstad B, Bretthauer M, Eide TJ, Hoff G. The Norwegian Colorectal Cancer Prevention (NORCCAP) screening study: baseline findings and implementations for clinical work-up in age groups 50–64 years. Scand J Gastroenterol 2003; 38(6):635–642.

43. Winawer SJ, Stewart ET, Zauber AG, et al. A comparison of colonoscopy and double-contrast barium enema for surveillance after polypectomy. National Polyp Study Work Group (see comments). N Engl J Med 2000; 342(24):1766–1772.

44. Scheitel SM, Ahlquist DA, Wollan PC, Hagen PT, Silverstein MD. Colorectal cancer screening: a community case–control study of proctosigmoidoscopy, barium enema radiography, and fecal occult blood test efficacy. Mayo Clinic Proc 1999; 74(12):1207–1213.

45. Imperiale TF, Wagner DR, Lin CY, Larkin GN, Rogge JD, Ransohoff DF. Risk of advanced proximal neoplasms in asymptomatic adults according to the distal colorectal findings. N Engl J Med 2000; 343(3):169–174.

46. Lieberman DA, Weiss DG, Bond JH, Ahnen DJ, Garewal H, Chejfec G. Use of colonoscopy to screen asymptomatic adults for colorectal cancer. Veterans Affairs Cooperative Study Group 380. N Engl J Med 2000; 343(3):162–168.

47. Rex DK, Cutler CS, Lemmel GT, et al. Colonoscopic miss rates of adenomas determined by back-to-back colonoscopies (see comments). Gastroenterology 1997; 112(1):24–28.

48. Hixson LJ, Fennerty MB, Sampliner RE, McGee D, Garewal H. Prospective study of the frequency and size distribution of polyps missed by colonoscopy. J Natl Cancer Inst 1990; 82(22):1769–1772.

49. Wagner JL, Tunis S, Brown ML, Ching A, Almeida R. Cost-effectiveness of colorectal cancer screening in average-risk adults. In: Young G, Levin B, eds. Prevention and early detection of colorectal cancer. London: Saunders; 1996.

50. Muller AD, Sonnenberg A. Prevention of colorectal cancer by flexible endoscopy and polypectomy. A case–control study of 32,702 veterans. Ann Intern Med 1995; 123(12):904–910.

51. Winawer SJ, Zauber AG, Ho MN, et al. Prevention of colorectal cancer by colonoscopic polypectomy. The National Polyp Study Workgroup. N Engl J Med. Dec 30 1993; 329(27):1977–1981.

52. Citarda F, Tomaselli G, Capocaccia R, Barcherini S, Crespi M. Efficacy in standard clinical practice of colonoscopic polypectomy in reducing colorectal cancer incidence. Gut 2001; 48(6):812–815.

53. Thiis-Evensen E, Hoff GS, Sauar J, Langmark F, Majak BM, Vatn MH. Population-based surveillance by colonoscopy: effect on the

incidence of colorectal cancer. Telemark Polyp Study I. Scand J Gastroenterol 1999; 34(4):414–420.

54. Rex DK, Lehman GA, Hawes RH, Ulbright TM, Smith JJ. Screening colonoscopy in asymptomatic average-risk persons with negative fecal occult blood tests (*see* comments). Gastroenterology 1991; 100(1):64–67.

55. Haseman JH, Lemmel GT, Rahmani EY, Rex DK. Failure of colonoscopy to detect colorectal cancer: evaluation of 47 cases in 20 hospitals (*see* comments). Gastrointestinal Endoscopy 1997; 45(6):451–455.

56. Van Ness MM, Chobanian SJ, Winters C, Jr., Diehl AM, Esposito RL, Cattau EL, Jr. A study of patient acceptance of double-contrast barium enema and colonoscopy. Which procedure is preferred by patients? Arch Intern Med 1987; 147(12):2175–2176.

57. Dominitz JA, Eisen GM, Baron TH, et al. Complications of colonoscopy. Gastrointest Endosc 2003; 57(4):441–445.

58. Cotton PB, Durkalski VL, Pineau BC, et al. Computed tomographic colonography (virtual colonoscopy): a multicenter comparison with standard colonoscopy for detection of colorectal neoplasia. JAMA 2004; 291(14):1713–1719.

59. Rockey DC, Paulson E, Niedzwiecki D, et al. Analysis of air contrast barium enema, computed tomographic colonography, and colonoscopy, prospective comparision. Lancet 2005; 365(9456):305–311.

60. Johnson CD, Harmsen WS, Wilson LA, et al. Prospective blinded evaluation of computed tomographic colonography for screen detection of colorectal polyps. Gastroenterology 2003; 125(2): 311–319.

61. Pickhardt PJ, Choi JR, Hwang I, et al. Computed tomographic virtual colonoscopy to screen for colorectal neoplasia in asymptomatic adults. N Engl J Med 2003; 349(23):2191–2200.

62. Song K, Fendrick AM, Ladabaum U. Fecal DNA testing compared with conventional colorectal cancer screening methods: a decision analysis. Gastroenterology 2004; 126(5):1270–1279.

63. Lieberman DA. Cost-effectiveness model for colon cancer screening. Gastroenterology 1995; 109(6):1781–1790.

64. Rex DK, Lehman GA, Ulbright TM, et al. Colonic neoplasia in asymptomatic persons with negative fecal occult blood tests: influence of age, gender, and family history (*see* comments). Am J Gastroenterol 1993; 88(6):825–831.

65. Rabeneck L, Paszat LF. A population-based estimate of the extent of colorectal cancer screening in Ontario. Am J Gastroenterol 2004; 99(6):1141–1144.

66. Breen N, Wagener DK, Brown ML, Davis WW, Ballard-Barbash R. Progress in cancer screening over a decade: results of cancer screening from the 1987, 1992, and 1998 National Health Interview Surveys. J Natl Cancer Inst 21 2001; 93(22):1704–1713.

67. Colorectal cancer test use among persons aged > or = 50 years — United States, 2001. MMWR Morb Mortal Wkly Rep 2003; 52(10): 193–196.

68. Hynam KA, Hart AR, Gay SP, Inglis A, Wicks AC, Mayberry JF. Screening for colorectal cancer: reasons for refusal of faecal occult blood testing in a general practice in England. J Epidemiol Community Health 1995; 49(1):84–86.

69. Myers RE, Ross E, Jepson C, et al. Modeling adherence to colorectal cancer screening. Prev Med 1994; 23(2):142–151.

70. Weller DP, Owen N, Hiller JE, Willson K, Wilson D. Colorectal cancer and its prevention: prevalence of beliefs, attitudes, intentions and behaviour. Aust J Public Health 1995; 19(1):19–23.

71. Kelly RB, Shank JC. Adherence to screening flexible sigmoidoscopy in asymptomatic patients. Med Care 1992; 30(11):1029–1042.

72. Smith RA, Cokkinides V, Eyre HJ. American Cancer Society guidelines for the early detection of cancer, 2004. CA Cancer J Clin 2004; 54(1):41–52.

73. Screening for colorectal cancer: recommendation and rationale. Ann Intern Med 2002; 137(2):129–131.

74. Colorectal cancer screening. Recommendation statement from the Canadian Task Force on Preventive Health Care. CMAJ 2001; 165(2):206–208.

75. Ioannou GN, Chapko MK, Dominitz JA. Predictors of colorectal cancer screening participation in the United States. Am J Gastroenterol 2003; 98(9):2082–2091.

76. Ko CW, Kreuter W, Baldwin LM. Effect of Medicare coverage on use of invasive colorectal cancer screening tests. Arch Intern Med 2002; 162(22):2581–2586.

77. Winawer SJ, Zauber AG, O'Brien MJ, et al. Randomized comparison of surveillance intervals after colonoscopic removal of newly diagnosed adenomatous polyps. The National Polyp Study Workgroup. N Engl J Med 1993; 328(13):901–906.

78. Lieberman D. Endoscopic colon screening: is less more? Gastroenterology 1996; 111(5):1385–1387.

79. Leard LE, Savides TJ, Ganiats TG. Patient preferences for colorectal cancer screening. J Fam Pract 1997; 45(3):211–218.

80. Elwood JM, Ali G, Schlup MM, et al. Flexible sigmoidoscopy or colonoscopy for colorectal screening: a randomized trial of performance and acceptability. Cancer Detect Prev 1995; 19(4):337–347.

81. McCarthy BD, Moskowitz MA. Screening flexible sigmoidoscopy: patient attitudes and compliance. J Gen Intern Med 1993; 8(3):120–125.

82. Dominitz JA, Provenzale D. Patient preferences and quality of life associated with colorectal cancer screening. Am J Gastroenterol 1997; 92(12):2171–2178.

83. Drossman DA, Brandt LJ, Sears C, Li Z, Nat J, Bozymski EM. A preliminary study of patients' concerns related to GI endoscopy. Am J Gastroenterol 1996; 91(2):287–291.

84. Scott RG, Edwards JT, Fritschi L, Foster NM, Mendelson RM, Forbes GM. Community-based screening by colonoscopy or computed tomographic colonography in asymptomatic average-risk subjects. Am J Gastroenterol 2004; 99(6):1145–1151.

85. Winawer SJ, Fletcher RH, Miller L, et al. Colorectal cancer screening: clinical guidelines and rationale (*see* comments) (published errata appear in Gastroenterology 1997; 112(3):1060 and 1998; 114(3):625). Gastroenterology 1997; 112(2):594–642.

86. Zarchy TM, Ershoff D. Do characteristics of adenomas on flexible sigmoidoscopy predict advanced lesions on baseline colonoscopy? Gastroenterology 1994; 106(6):1501–1504.

87. Read TE, Read JD, Butterly LF. Importance of adenomas 5 mm or less in diameter that are detected by sigmoidoscopy. N Engl J Med 1997; 336(1):8–12.

88. Schoen RE, Corle D, Cranston L, et al. Is colonoscopy needed for the nonadvanced adenoma found on sigmoidoscopy? The Polyp Prevention Trial. Gastroenterology 1998; 115(3):533–541.

89. Wallace MB, Kemp JA, Trnka YM, Donovan JM, Farraye FA. Is colonoscopy indicated for small adenomas found by screening flexible sigmoidoscopy? Ann Intern Med 1998; 129(4):273–278.

90. Levin TR, Palitz A, Grossman S, et al. Predicting advanced proximal colonic neoplasia with screening sigmoidoscopy. JAMA 1999; 281(17):1611–1617.

91. Winawer SJ, Schottenfeld D, Flehinger BJ. Colorectal cancer screening. J Natl Cancer Inst 1991; 83:243–253.

92. Winawer SJ, Enker WE, Levin B. Colorectal cancer. In: Winawer SJ, ed. Management of gastrointestinal diseases. New York: Gower Medical, 1992.

93. Fuchs CS, Giovannucci EL, Colditz GA, Hunter DJ, Speizer FE, Willett WC: A prospective study of family history and the risk of colorectal cancer. N Engl J Med 1994; 331(25): 1669–1674.

94. Sonnenberg A, Delcò F, Inadomi JM. Cost-effectiveness of colonoscopy in screening for colorectal cancer. Ann Intern Med 2000; 133:573–584.

18 Polyposis and Familial Cancer Syndromes

FERNANDO S. VELAYOS, MD, MADHULIKA G. VARMA, MD,
AND JONATHAN P. TERDIMAN, MD

CONTENTS

1. INTRODUCTION

Colorectal cancer (CRC) is the second leading cause of cancer death in the United States. Each year approx 130,000 Americans are diagnosed with the disease and 50,000 will die of it (1). The cumulative lifetime risks of CRC and mortality from CRC are approx 3–6% and 2%, respectively. The majority of CRCs occur in individuals over 60 yr old, whom have no previous personal or family history of the disease. The major risk factors for these sporadic cases are advancing age and environmental exposures, most importantly diet. Approximately 20–25% of CRCs are in younger individuals or in those with a personal or family history of cancer, suggesting a heritable susceptibility (2).

The genetic predisposition to CRC falls into two major groups, common familial CRC (15–20% of CRC) and hereditary CRC (5% of CRC) (Fig. 1) (3). In common familial CRC, first-degree relatives of persons with CRC or adenomatous polyps have an approximately twofold risk of developing CRC, and the risk increases with the number of relatives affected and the earlier the age of onset in the family (4). Increased risk for CRC in common familial CRC is conveyed by the inheritance of one or more, of the likely many, low penetrance susceptibility alleles, most of which have yet to be identified (5). Carriage of these susceptibility alleles increases the risk of acquiring CRC, but by no means is the development of CRC certain. In fact, in the large majority of allele carriers, CRC does not occur.

From: *Endoscopic Oncology: Gastrointestinal Endoscopy and Cancer Management.* Edited by: D. O. Faigel and M. L. Kochman © Humana Press, Totowa, NJ

More than 5% of CRCs are hereditary in etiology, meaning that they are caused by carriage of a highly penetrant, dominantly inherited, susceptibility allele. Hereditary CRC is conventionally divided between the polyposis syndromes and hereditary nonpolyposis colorectal cancer (HNPCC) (Table 1) (3). The polyposis syndromes are defined by the presence of multiple polyps in the gut lumen, and have conventionally been categorized by polyp histology. The most common and important of the polyposis syndromes is familial adenomatous polyposis (FAP). FAP carries a life-time risk of CRC approaching 100% if the colon is not removed (6). The other major category of hereditary polyposes is the hamartomatous polyposis syndromes, most importantly Peutz-Jeghers syndrome (PJS), hereditary juvenile polyposis, and Cowden syndrome. There are a number of other very rare hereditary polyposis syndromes, as well as several nonhereditary polyposis syndromes that may or might not confer an increased risk for CRC.

Much more common than any of the polyposis syndromes is HNPCC. At least 2–3% of all CRC is secondary to HNPCC (7,8). In HNPCC, the lifetime risk of CRC approaches 70–80%, but not as a consequence of an increased number of colorectal adenomas (6).

The primary importance of familial and hereditary colorectal cancer is the increased risk of CRC, and often, other cancers, for individuals with these conditions. Failure to recognize common familial CRC, or more importantly, one of the hereditary syndromes, will lead to inadequate cancer screening and surveillance in individuals at risk, with subsequent premature loss of life. Recently, the elucidation of the genes responsible for many of these syndromes has revolutionized the care of at-risk individuals and families. Genetic testing has the potential to greatly improve the efficiency and reduce the costs and morbidity of cancer screening and surveillance. Genetic testing is now commercially available and is often offered to individuals and families with, or suspected of having, FAP or HNPCC *(9,10)*. Genetic testing will most likely affect the management of individuals at risk for common familial CRC as well. However, genetic testing raises a number of vexing clinical, ethical, legal, and psychosocial questions.

This chapter discusses the clinical features, genetics, diagnosis, and management of common familial and hereditary CRC, specifically the polyposis syndromes and HNPCC.

2. POLYPOSIS SYNDROMES

2.1. FAMILIAL ADENOMATOUS POLYPOSIS

2.1.1. Clinical Features: Intestinal

FAP is an autosomal-dominant disorder that affects about one in 10,000–15,000 individuals and accounts for probably less than 0.1% of CRCs *(11)*. In classic FAP, affected individuals develop hundreds to thousands of colonic adenomas by the mid to late teens, with more than 95% of affected individuals demonstrating polyposis by age 35. CRC is inevitable in untreated patients, with the majority of cancers appearing by age 40 and more than 90% by age 45 *(12,13)*. Variants of FAP are now recognized in which polyps are greatly reduced in number, are predominantly or exclusively located in the right colon, and occur approximately a decade later than in classic FAP. This latter condition has been termed attenuated adenomatous polyposis coli (AAPC) or attenuated FAP *(14,15)*.

In addition to colonic polyps, up to 90% of individuals with FAP will develop small bowel adenomas, most commonly at or near the ampulla of Vater *(16–19)*. These lesions are usually multiple and sessile, often forming carpet-like lesions. Because the ampulla of Vater is almost invariably involved, to assess the full extent of duodenal polyposis, duodenoscopy, in addition to routine upper endoscopy, is required *(20)*. The lifetime risk for small bowel carcinoma is approx 5%, and duodenal cancer is the leading cause of cancer death in FAP patients that have undergone a colectomy *(13,21–23)*.

Most FAP patients also will develop gastric polyposis. Gastric polyps are usually of the fundic gland histological type, but adenomas rarely do occur *(19)*. Gastric carcinoma risk is not much increased in Western families, but is reported to be increased three- to fourfold in Japanese and Korean families with FAP. Overall the lifetime risk of gastric cancer in individuals with FAP has been reported at 0.5% *(19)*.

2.2. CLINICAL FEATURES: EXTRAINTESTINAL

Approximately two-thirds of FAP patients will have congenital hypertrophy of the retinal pigment epithelium (CHRPE). Although CHRPE does not affect vision or have any malignant potential, it is important as an early marker to identify susceptible individuals, as it can be detected at birth. In CHRPE-positive families nearly all individuals with FAP in the family will have CHRPE. Thus, an examination of the fundus can identify susceptible family members at a young age *(24)*.

Other benign extraintestinal manifestations of FAP include dental abnormalities, osteomas, lipomas, epidermoid cysts, and

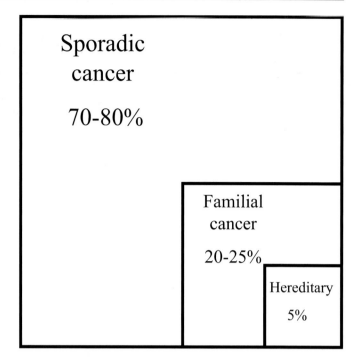

Fig. 1. Frequency of sporadic, familial, and hereditary colorectal cancer.

desmoid tumors *(12,17)*. Desmoids develop in about 9–17% of individuals with FAP. Approximately half are intra-abdominal and involve the small bowel and its mesentery. The rest occur in the abdominal wall or other extraabdominal sites such as the neck, thigh, breast, axilla, or back *(17,25–27)*. Although desmoids are not malignant, they may cause considerable morbidity and mortality by local invasion. Surgical treatment of intraabdominal desmoids is associated with high morbidity and mortality and therefore is reserved for those who have severe symptoms *(25,28)*. FAP in conjunction with soft tissue tumors, osteomas, and dental abnormalities is often referred to as the Gardner syndrome.

FAP is associated with increased risk for extraintestinal cancers, including hepatoblastoma in young children, medulloblastoma, papillary carcinoma of the thyroid, and pancreatic cancer *(12,29,30)*. The association of FAP and central nervous systems tumors, primarily medulloblastoma, has been termed Turcot syndrome *(31,32)*.

2.3. GENETICS

The great majority of cases of FAP are caused by a germline mutation of the tumor suppressor *APC* gene located on chromosome 5q21 *(33–35)*. Individuals with FAP only have one functional copy of *APC* per cell, and mutation or loss of this functional copy can initiate the pathway of colonic neoplasia *(36–42)*. The specific location of a germline mutation in *APC* may determine in part the disease phenotype *(43–55)*. Such genotype–phenotype correlation will prove useful in increasing the accuracy and effectiveness of screening, surveillance, and treatment *(56–58)*.

Recently, a small number cases of FAP have been attributed to inherited defects of the base excision repair gene *MYH* *(59,60)*. *MYH* is responsible for repair of G:C to T:A mutations that occur as a consequence of oxidative DNA

Table 1
Classification of Hereditary Colorectal Cancer Syndromes

Polyposis syndromes (<1% of all colorectal cancers)
Adenomatous polyposis syndromes
    Familial adenomatous polyposis
        Gardner syndrome
        Turcot syndrome
        Attenuated adenomatous polyposis coli
Hamartomatous polyposis syndromes
    Peutz-Jeghers syndrome
    Juvenile polyposis
        Hereditary mixed polyposis syndrome
    Cowden syndrome
        Bannayan-Riley-Ruvalcaba syndrome
        Ruvulcaba-Myhre syndrome
        Bannayan-Zonana syndrome
        Soto syndrome
        Lhermitte-Duclos disease
    Gorlin syndrome
Hereditary nonpolyposis colorectal cancer (3–5% of all
    colorectal cancers)
    Lynch syndrome
    Muir-Torre syndrome
    Turcot syndrome

damage *(59)*. Germline *MYH* mutations must be biallelic to cause polyposis, so in this circumstance the adenomatous polyposis is the consequence of recessive rather than dominant inheritance as it is with germline *APC* mutations. Mutations in *MYH* may account for some of the cases of FAP that occur without a family history that had previously been felt to be secondary to spontaneous germline mutations of *APC (61)*.

2.4. DIAGNOSIS

Genetic testing for FAP is commercially available and discussion of the option is the standard of care for families suspected of having the syndrome *(9,10)*. Testing starts with a family member suspected of having FAP based on clinical presentation. If the disease causing mutation can be identified, nonaffected family members can then be tested to determine if they carry the mutation. Family members proven not to have inherited the family mutation may then be spared burdensome screening and surveillance.

2.5. SURVEILLANCE AND TREATMENT

Because CRC occurs in nearly 100% of untreated patients with FAP, the goals of management include early identification of at-risk family members, endoscopic surveillance of colonic polyps in the premalignant stage, and definitive surgical treatment to eradicate the progression of colorectal polyposis to cancer. Colonic and extracolonic screening and surveillance recommendations for FAP are summarized in Table 2 *(3,62)*.

Endoscopic surveillance will reduce rates of CRC and mortality in FAP patients *(63)*. Individuals at risk for FAP should undergo annual flexible sigmoidoscopy beginning at age 10–12 yr. Once adenomas have been identified, yearly colonoscopy is required. Colectomy should be undertaken once any of the polyps is 5 mm or larger or if any polyp biopsies

demonstrate villous features or high-grade dysplasia. In families with suspected AAPC, surveillance should be undertaken with complete colonoscopy, rather than sigmoidoscopy because of the proximal location of the polyps. Owing to the later onset of polyposis in these families, some experts recommend that surveillance can sometimes be safely deferred until approximately age 20. However, in the author's opinion, delaying the onset of surveillance in AAPC families can be problematic because of the potential for phenotypic variability in such families.

Surveillance for upper tract adenomas is indicated in patients with FAP as well *(20)*. Upper gastrointestinal (GI) endoscopy and duodenoscopy, with biopsy of the ampulla of Vater, should be initiated once colonic adenomas have been identified, and no later than age 25 *(62)*. Multiple random biopsies taken from duodenal folds have been recommended if polyps are not visible *(64)*. Enteroscopy and/or enteroclysis also are advocated by some experts to exclude small bowel adenomas distal to the duodenum. However, significant lesions in the middle or distal small bowel are rare. The upper GI surveillance interval remains empirical, but generally screening should be undertaken every 1–3 yr depending on the Spigelman stage, a measure of the burden of duodenal polyposis *(65)*. Once detected, upper tract adenomas can be removed or ablated by a variety of methods, though there are no data to show that this will improve long-term outcomes *(66–68)*. If invasive cancer or high-risk adenomas are encountered (Spigelman stage IV), then operative resection is indicated *(69)*.

After colectomy, ongoing surveillance is required. If the rectum is retained, endoscopic examination should be performed approximately every 6–12 mo to remove or ablate any adenomas found. The risk of rectal cancer is individuals with FAP with an ileorectal anastomosis (IRA) exceeds 10%, and more than 20% of patients that undergo a colectomy with IRA will ultimately require completion proctectomy *(70)*. Even after ileal pouch-anal anastomosis, a substantial risk of the development of pouch adenomas exists, although the risk of developing invasive cancer appears to be low *(71,72)*. Therefore, endoscopic examination of the ileal pouch is recommended every 1 to 2 yr.

In addition to endoscopic screening, cancer prevention efforts in FAP may be augmented by chemoprevention with use of non-steroidal anti-inflammatory drugs (NSAIDs) or cyclooxygenase 2 (COX-2) selective inhibitors. Both the NSAIDs, sulindac, and the COX-2 inhibitor, celecoxib, have been demonstrated to reduce the size and number of adenomas in individuals with FAP *(73,74)*. Unfortunately, in a recent study, use of sulindac did not prevent the development of adenomas *(75)*, but sulindac, celecoxib, and like drugs, may slow polyp progression *(76)*. Recent data tempers enthusiasm for the use of COX-2 inhibitors and other classes owing to the concern over long-term side-effects. They are unlikely to obviate the need for surgery in patients, but might serve to delay the timing or prevent the need for a second operation in those with retained rectums *(77)*. The exact role of these medications in the management of FAP remains to be elucidated.

Table 2

Options for Cancer Prevention in FAP for Known or Suspected Gene Mutation Carriers

Primary recommendations

- Annual flexible sigmoidoscopy beginning by age 10–12 yr
- Annual colonoscopy, beginning by age 20 yr, when attenuated FAP suspected
- Prophylactic colectomy in teen years or when polyps detected at colonoscopy
- Endoscopic surveillance every 4–6 mo after IRA and annually after ileoanal anastomosis
- Upper endoscopy, including duodenoscopy, every 6 mo to 3 yr starting by age 20–25 yr

Secondary recommendations

- Annual thyroid exam beginning by age 10–12 yr
- Annual palpation of liver during first decade of life (consider annual hepatic ultrasound and measure of α-fetoprotein)
- Consider serial MRI of brain in families with Turcot syndrome
- Consider serial MRCP or endoscopic ultrasound in families with multiple pancreatic cancers
- Consider use of sulindac or celecoxib chemoprevention in individuals with colorectal adenomas

3. HEREDITARY HAMARTOMATOUS POLYP SYNDROMES

3.1. PEUTZ-JEGHERS SYNDROME

3.1.1. Clinical Features

PJS is a rare, autosomal-dominant cancer predisposition syndrome occurring in approx 1 in 200,000 births *(12)*. It is characterized by the presence of numerous hamartomatous polyps in the GI tract *(78)*. The classic mucocutaneous melanin pigment spots occur on the lips and buccal mucosa, but can also be found on other areas of the skin, such as the dorsal and volar aspects of the hands and feet *(79)*. PJS occurs among all races and skin types. Pigment spots can be identified in 95% of PJS patients, often from birth or early infancy. However, the spots can fade with age, and therefore the absence of typical pigmentation does not exclude the diagnosis. No malignant potential has been ascribed to the hyperpigmentation of PJS.

The predominant clinical feature of PJS is the presence of numerous GI hamartomatous polyps. The polyps have a distinctive histology with an arborizing pattern of smooth muscle in the lamina propria that distinguishes them from the hamartomas seen in juvenile polyposis or Cowden syndrome *(80)*. The polyps can be pedunculated or sessile, and they range in size from several millimeters to giant polyps, 3–4 cm in size. The polyps occur throughout the GI tract, from esophagus to rectum. Polyps are seen in the stomach in approx 40% of cases, in the small bowel in 80%, especially the jejunum, and in the colon and rectum in 40% *(79,80)*. The polyps occur at a young age, and the typical age of diagnosis of PJS secondary to polyp complications is in the mid-20s. One-third of PJS patients will experience polyp-related symptoms by age 10, and 50–60% will have symptoms before the age of 20 yr *(81)*. The major complications related to PJS polyps are recurrent GI bleeding and obstruction, often secondary to intussusception. More than 40–50% of PJS patients will require operation for polyp-related bowel obstruction at some point in time *(79,82)*.

Although the typical PJS polyp is benign and without dysplasia, there is no doubt that PJS is associated with very high rates of intestinal and extraintestinal cancer *(83,84)*. The majority of PJS-related deaths after age 30 are secondary to malignancy, and the lifetime risk of cancer in PJS approaches 90% *(84)*. Intestinal cancers may be secondary to the malignant degeneration of the hamartomatous polyps, and foci of dysplasia can sometimes be found in large PJS polyps *(85)*. The majority of intestinal cancers are adenocarcinomas, although an increased risk for malignant GI stromal tumors, such as leiomyosarcoma, exists as well. Extraintestinal cancers are very common, and in fact, are more common than intestinal cancers. The most common extraintestinal cancer is cancer of the pancreas. Increased risk for cancer of the breast, ovary, lung, cervix, uterus, and testes has been documented, as well as others (Table 3) *(79,84)*. In addition, PJS is associated with an increased frequency of unusual neoplastic and non-neoplastic tumors of the genital tract *(12)*.

3.1.2. Genetics

PJS is caused by a germline mutation in the tumor-suppressor *STK11* gene (also called *LKB1*) located on 19p *(86,87)*. Mutations in *STK11* can be documented in about one-half of PJS families. Other PJS families may be the consequence of germline mutations in other genes, possibly one or more of those in the *STK11* molecular pathway *(88)*. As with FAP testing, if a pathogenic gene alteration can be detected in an affected family member, nonaffected family members can then be tested with essentially 100% accuracy.

3.1.3. Surveillance and Treatment

Though the lifetime risk of cancer in PJS is extremely high, the ability to reduce cancer incidence and cancer-related mortality in PJS patients through intensive surveillance remains unproved. Surveillance guidelines remain empirical and have not been formally adopted by any of the major professional organizations (Table 4) *(62,79,89)*. However, most experts recommend surveillance and they further recommend that any intestinal polyps encountered, especially those greater than 1–1.5 cm in size be removed, even if that requires exploratory laparotomy and intraoperative endoscopy *(90)*.

3.2. JUVENILE POLYPOSIS

3.2.1. Clinical Features

Juvenile polyps are common, occurring in about 2% of children. Typically, juvenile polyposis is defined as the presence of 10 or more juvenile polyps. Approximately one-third of cases of juvenile polyposis have a hereditary etiology, whereas the remainder are sporadic. Hereditary juvenile polyposis is rare, occurring in roughly 1 in 100,000 individuals *(89)*. Histologically, juvenile polyps are hamartomas with a characteristic hyperplastic

Table 3
Cancer Risk in Peutz-Jeghers Syndrome

Cancer site	Approximate lifetime risk (%)
All cancers	93
Gastrointestinal Cancers	
Colorectal	39
Pancreas	36
Stomach	29
Small bowel	13
Esophagus	0.5
Nongastrointestinal cancers	
Breast	54
Ovary	21
Lung	15
Cervix	10
Uterus	9
Testes	9

Table 4
Cancer Prevention Options in Peutz-Jeghers Syndrome

- Upper endoscopy every 2 yr starting age 10–15 yr
- Enteroscopy/small bowel X-ray (small bowel follow through or enteroclysis) every 2 yr starting age 10–15 yr
- Colonoscopy every 3 yr starting age 15–20 yr
- Removal of all polyps found >1–1.5 cm (either by endoscopy methods or at laparotomy with intra-operative endoscopy)
- Endoscopic ultrasound or MRCP every 1–2 yr starting at age 30 yr
- Annual breast exam and mammography starting age 25 yr
- Annual pelvic exam, pap smear, transvaginal ultrasound, and CA-125 levels starting at age 20–25 yr
- Annual testicular exam starting at age 10, with testicular ultrasound for onset of feminizing features

appearance of the surface epithelium, expansion of the lamina propria and frequent cyst formation with mucus engorgement. The characteristic cystically dilated glands have led these polyps also to be termed juvenile retention polyps *(91)*. The polyps can range in size from several millimeters to several centimeters, and they might be sessile or pedunculated, more often the latter. Juvenile polyps are most commonly found in the colon and rectum, but in hereditary juvenile polyposis, the polyps can be found throughout the GI tract *(92)*. In contrast to individuals with sporadic juvenile polyps, those with hereditary juvenile polyposis will continue to form polyps throughout their lifetime.

The primary clinical manifestation of juvenile polyposis is colorectal bleeding. The blood loss might be occult, with subsequent development of iron deficiency anemia, or overt GI bleeding may occur *(89)*. Bleeding from juvenile polyps is one the leading causes of lower GI hemorrhage among children.

As with the other hereditary hamartomatous polyp syndromes, juvenile polyposis is associated with an increased risk for CRC *(93,94)*. CRC occurs at a young age, often in the mid-30s *(92,93)*. Cancer will arise from a juvenile polyp that has developed dysplastic/adenomatous features, and therefore, increased cancer risk can extend to other segments of the bowel involved with polyps. Individuals with many polyps with mixed histological features of juvenile polyps and adenomas are

termed as having hereditary mixed polyposis syndrome. However, CRC can occur in individuals with no prior evidence of dysplastic polyps *(89)*. Increased cancer risk is not seen among individuals with sporadic juvenile polyps. The exact magnitude of the risk in hereditary juvenile polyposis remains uncertain, but may approach that seen in FAP *(95)*. It is not clear if there is an increased risk of extraintestinal cancer, such as pancreatic cancer.

3.2.2. Genetics

Hereditary juvenile polyposis is an autosomal-dominant disorder, and disease causing germline mutations can be found in about 50% of patients. The majority of mutations are found in *SMAD4*, located on 18q, and commercial genetic testing is available *(92,96–98)*. *SMAD4* is a tumor suppressor gene of importance in the development of sporadic pancreatic and CRC, among others *(99)*. Some juvenile polyposis families are found to have disease-causing mutations in the *PTEN* gene *(100)*, or in the bone morphogenetic protein receptor 1A *(BMPR1A)* gene *(101)*. *BMPR1A* is a serine-threonine kinase type receptor belonging to the superfamily of *TGF*-β receptors involved in growth inhibitory signaling.

3.2.3. Surveillance and Treatment

No formal screening or surveillance recommendations exist for hereditary juvenile polyposis. In asymptomatic children from families with the syndrome, complete colonoscopy should commence in the early teen years and should be repeated every 1–3 yr depending on the size and number of polyps found *(62,89)*. Polyps found should be removed. In hereditary juvenile polyposis, as with all the hereditary polyposis syndromes, polyps will continue to recur throughout the patient's lifetime, and intensive surveillance should continue until age 70 *(62)*. If the number of polyps is great, especially if polyps with dysplastic features are encountered, colectomy is indicated. At the time that colonic polyps are detected, upper endoscopy and small bowel contrast X-rays should be performed to look for extra-colonic polyps. If none are found, repeat upper GI screening exams may be performed approximately every 1–3 yr *(62,89)*.

3.3. COWDEN SYNDROME

3.3.1. Clinical Features

Cowden syndrome, also termed the gingival multiple hamartoma syndrome, is a rare autosomal-dominant syndrome (1 in 200,000 individuals) characterized by skin lesions, intestinal hamartomas, and an increased risk of cancer *(12)*. The characteristic mucocutaneous lesions are found in about 85% of affected patients and include facial trichilemmomas, acral keratoses, café au lait spots, and verrucous papules of the oral mucosa, gingiva, and tongue. Subcutaneous lipomas and fibromas are common, as are benign thyroid nodules, uterine leiomyomas, and fibrocystic disease of the breast.

Sixty percent of Cowden patients develop hamartomatous polyps of the GI tract *(89,102)*. The GI polyps most often resemble juvenile polyps, but other benign GI tract polyps can occur as well, including lipomas, ganglioneuromas, inflammatory polyps, and lymphoid hyperplasia *(91)*. Juvenile type polyps that contain some neural elements are particularly characteristic of the syndrome.

The syndrome is often associated with congenital abnormalities (50% of the time) that include craniomegaly and mental retardation. Families with macrocephaly, lipomas, and pigmentation of the glans penis belong to the Bannayan-Ruvalcaba-Riley syndrome (syndrome variations have been termed Soto syndrome, Ruvalcaba-Myhre syndrome and Bannyan-Zonana syndrome), although those with glial mass in the cerebellum leading to altered gait and seizures belong to the sub-syndrome called Lhermitte-Duclos disease *(12)*.

Cowden syndrome is a cancer-susceptibile syndrome, and cancer is the primary source of morbidity and mortality among affected individuals. The lifetime incidence of breast cancer among women with Cowden syndrome is 25–50%, and the cancer often is bilateral and with an early age of onset (median age 41 yr) *(12)*. Individuals with Cowden syndrome also have a lifetime risk of follicular carcinoma of the thyroid that approaches 10%. Although many affected individuals have GI tract hamartomas, an excess of GI cancer risk has not been clearly described *(89,102)*. There is probably a modest increased risk for CRC among individuals with colorectal hamartomas. Increased risk other cancers also likely is present, including skin, ovary, uterus, lung, and kidney.

3.3.2. Genetics

Cowden syndrome, and its associated sub-syndromes, are caused by a germline mutation in the tumor suppressor gene *PTEN* on 10q *(103,104)*. *PTEN* mutation testing is commercially available, and mutations can be detected in about 90% of affected individuals *(12)*. Principles of clinical genetic testing would mirror those in FAP, PJS, and hereditary juvenile polyposis.

3.3.3. Surveillance and Treatment

The major cancer morbidity from Cowden syndrome is secondary to breast cancer. Breast cancer surveillance should commence at age 20 yr (monthly self-exam and yearly physician exam and mammography *[12]*). Annual thyroid exams are recommended to start in the teens. No guidelines regarding GI screening or surveillance have been established *(102)*. On diagnosis, it makes sense to perform upper and lower GI endoscopy to look for GI polyps. Among individuals with GI polyps, regular surveillance and polypectomy is likely wise. Those without polyps initially might undergo screening colonoscopy starting at age 40, with repeat exams every 3–5 yr.

3.4. GORLIN SYNDROME

Gorlin syndrome is a rare autosomal-dominant inherited condition (1 in 55,000 people) characterized by multiple basal cell nevi and carcinomas *(12)*. The condition is also called the basal cell nevus syndrome and accounts for about 0.5% of persons with basal cell carcinoma. The carcinomas often first occur before 30 yr of age, with 90% of affected individuals with cancer by age 40 yr. Other features of the syndrome include odontogenic or polyostotic bone cysts, facial congenital defects including macrocephaly, cleft lip or palate, congenital skeletal abnormalities of the ribs, and/or spine, ectopic calcification of the falx cerebri, cardiac or ovarian fibromas, medulloblastoma, and characteristic pits of the skin of the palms and soles (three or more pits). Rarely, GI hamartomas occur *(12,102)*. The syndrome is caused by a germline mutation in the *PTC* gene on 9q *(12)*. Spontaneous germline mutations of *PTC* are the cause of Gorlin syndrome in more than 50% of cases.

4. HEREDITARY NEURAL POLYPOSIS SYNDROMES

4.1. NEUROFIBROMATOSIS TYPE 1

Neurofibromatosis type (NF) 1, also called von Recklinghausen disease, is defined by the presence of café-au-lait spots (five or more > 0.5 cm), multiple cutaneous or subcutaneous neurofibromas, multiple axillary or inguinal freckles, bilateral optic nerve gliomas, multiple hamartomas of the iris, and congenital abnormalities of the long bones (bowing or thinning of the cortex) *(12,102)*. Seizures are reported in 3–5% of affected individuals, and learning disabilities in 25–40%. This condition is caused by the autosomal-dominant inheritance of a mutated *NF1* gene located on 17q *(12)*. Approximately 25% of patients with *NF1* have intestinal polypoid neurofibromas or ganglioneuromas *(102)*. The polyps are most commonly found in the small bowel, but can occur in the stomach and colon as well. In most cases, the polyps are clinically silent, but can rarely cause abdominal pain or hemorrhage.

4.2. MULTIPLE ENDOCRINE NEOPLASIA TYPE 2

Multiple endocrine neoplasia type (MEN) 2 is characterized by the presence of medullary carcinoma of the thyroid, pheochromocytoma, parathyroid hyperplasia or adenomas, marfanoid habitus, and ganglioneuromas of the GI tract *(12)*. The ganglioneuromas occur in nearly all patients with MEN2B, and they occur throughout the GI tract, but are most common in the colon and rectum *(102)*. The polyps are often clinically silent. However, generalized dysmotility of the GI tract is often associated with the disease, and may be in part secondary to the intestinal ganglioneuromas. MEN2 is caused by a germline mutation in the *RET* proto-oncogene *(12)*. The condition is transmitted in autosomal dominant fashion, though about 50% of cases are secondary to a spontaneous, new germline mutation.

5. SPORADIC (NONHEREDITARY) POLYPOSIS SYNDROMES

5.1. HYPERPLASTIC POLYPOSIS

Hyperplastic polyposis is defined as the presence of 10 or more typical colorectal hyperplastic polyps. Most cases of hyperplastic polyposis involve the occurrence of diminutive (one to several millimeters) polyps located in the rectum and left colon. This phenomenon likely is sporadic in etiology and not associated with an increased risk for CRC. Rarely, patients may have tens to hundreds of diminutive hyperplastic polyps throughout the colon, simulating FAP *(105,106)*. Whether or not cancer risk is increased in these patients is unclear. Very rarely, patients with hyperplastic polyposis have giant (up to 2–3 cm) polyps, often found in the proximal colon *(105–107)*. In this circumstance, an increased risk for CRC is likely *(105,106,108)*, although the magnitude of the risk remains uncertain. Some experts recommend polypectomy for these large hyperplastic polyps and increased colonic surveillance in these patients *(105)*. However, the risks and benefits of this approach are unknown and such recommendations remain controversial. If the hyperplastic polyps have a mixed hyperplastic/adenomatous histology, the polyps are properly classified as being serrated adenomas. When serrated polyposis is present, the increased risk for CRC is clear, and the polyps must be removed, if possible by endoscopy, or if necessary, by colectomy.

5.2. CRONKHITE-CANADA SYNDROME

Cronkhite-Canada syndrome is a rare acquired condition, with an average age of onset during the sixth to seventh decade of life (105,109). The syndrome has a worldwide distribution, and has no known cause. It is more common in men (60%) than women, and is characterized by the onset of generalized GI polyposis, with esophageal sparing, in association with cutaneous hyperpigmentation, hair loss, nail atrophy, and hypogeusia (105). The polyps are sessile and innumerable, and they range in size from several millimeters to several centimeters. On histological examination the polyps resemble juvenile polyps, although dysplastic changes do rarely occur (110).

Cronkhite-Canada syndrome has an acute onset and is progressive, although symptomatic remission does occur in a minority of cases (102,105,111). The primary clinical manifestations are that of progressive diarrhea, often with significant malabsorption and protein-losing enteropathy (105). Malnutrition is common, and the condition can be fatal. For those with a more protracted course of illness, the lifetime incidence of CRC exceeds 10% (112,113). The primary therapy is supportive care (102). Patients often require nutritional support and may require total parenteral nutrition to prevent severe dehydration and malnutrition (114). If a particular segment of the GI tract is heavily involved with polyps, then operative resection might be helpful (105). Other interventions that have been tried with uncertain efficacy include administration of corticosteroids and antibiotics (114).

5.3. INFLAMMATORY POLYPOSIS

Inflammatory polyps, often called pseudopolyps, can occur during the healing phase of any inflammatory injury to the GI tract. Inflammatory polyps are most commonly seen in individuals with ulcerative colitis or Crohn's disease affecting the colon (115). They can also occur during the healing phase of other colitides, such as ischemic colitis (105). The polyps have a characteristic filiform appearance and on histological examination the polyps represent tissues with inflammatory elements that persist during healing (116). Inflammatory polyps may be few in number, or they may be innumerable, and their size ranges from several millimeters to several centimeters (105). The polyps have no malignant potential themselves, though they are often associated with longstanding chronic colitis and its attendant risk of colitis-related dysplasia and cancer. Inflammatory polyposis is an acquired condition. However, a case of familial inflammatory intestinal polyposis has been described and termed Devon polyposis (102).

5.4. LIPOMATOUS POLYPOSIS

Intestinal lipomas are benign tumors consisting of collections of adipose tissue in the submucosa. Solitary lipomas are common in the intestine, most often occurring in the vicinity, or involving the ileocecal valve. Diffuse lipomatous polyposis is an extremely rare condition (105,117). The polyps may occur in the small bowel, large bowel, or both. There is an association of diffuse intestinal lipomatous polyposis and lipomatosis or hypertrophy of the appendices epiploicae of the colon (118). Diffuse lipomatous polyposis is usually asymptomatic, but patients may present with GI bleeding, diarrhea, intussusception, or obstruction (105,119).

5.5. NODULAR LYMPHOID HYPERPLASIA

Nodular lymphoid hyperplasia refers to a condition in which numerous lymphoid nodules are found in the small intestine, large intestine, or both (120). Histologically, the nodules are enlarged lymphoid clusters with germinal centers in the lamina propria or submucosa (120). Lymphoid hyperplasia occurs most frequently in individuals with immune deficiencies such as common variable immune deficiency (CVID) or the AIDS (105,121). Nodular lymphoid hyperplasia can also occur in individuals without immune system dysfunction, and might be identified at as many as 3% of autopsies (105). In most cases, nodular lymphoid hyperplasia is asymptomatic, but it can be associated with diarrhea and malabsorption (105,122).

5.6. LYMPHOMATOUS POLYPOSIS

Multiple lymphomatous polyposis (MLP) is a rare manifestation of intestinal lymphoma. MLP is a non-Hodgkin B-cell lymphoma that appears to be the GI counterpart of mantle cell lymphoma, and extra-intestinal lymphoma is often present (102,105). Multiple nodular/polypoid lesion of the GI tract also may be seen in Mediterranean-type lymphoma. Mediterranean-type lymphoma of the gut begins as an intense proliferation of plasma cells in the lamina propria, with eventual malignant transformation (102). This lymphoma is almost always associated with production of an abnormal IgA paraprotein (102).

6. HEREDITARY NONPOLYPOSIS CANCERS

6.1. HEREDITARY NONPOLYPOSIS CRC
6.1.1. Clinical Features

HNPCC, like FAP is an autosomal-dominant disorder characterized by the occurrence of multiple CRCs in a family. HNPCC is also called the Lynch syndrome after Henry Lynch, MD (123), a pioneer in the field of familial cancer, who has devoted much of his career to the description of the syndrome and the care of affected families. HNPCC accounts for about 1–5% of all CRC cases (7,8,124–127). The number of polyps appears not much greater than in the general population, but the polyps are far more likely to be flat, to have villous features or high-grade dysplasia, and more importantly, to grow rapidly and progress to invasive cancer (123,128–132).

Individuals with HNPCC have a lifetime risk of CRC of about 80% (133–136). The mean age of onset of CRC in HNPCC is approx 45, but may appear in the teens (123,128). Compared with sporadic cases, synchronous, and metachronous CRC is more common in HNPCC. HNPCC cancers are also more commonly on the right side of the colon, more poorly differentiated, and have other unusual histological characteristics, most importantly, the presence of tumor-infiltrating lymphocytes (137–139). Nonetheless, several studies have found that survival is better than in sporadic cancer when matched for stage (140–144).

Table 5
Lifetime Risk for Cancer Among HNPCC Gene Carriers

Cancer type	Lifetime risk (%)
Colorectal	70–80
Endometrial	20–60
Ovarian	10–12
Gastric	5–13
Renal pelvis/ureter/kidney	4–10
Biliary tract/gallbladder/pancreas	2–18
Small bowel	1–4
CNS (usually glioblastoma)	1–4

The risk for other cancers in HNPCC is greatly increased. Individuals with HNPCC, are at an increased risk of endometrial, gastric, ovarian, small bowel, transitional cell (renal pelvis, ureter), sebaceous, central nervous system, and possibly other cancers (Table 5) *(133,134,136,145)*. When HNPCC was first described in the 1920s, gastric cancer was the primary malignancy. The decreasing frequency of gastric cancers and increasing frequency of CRCs in HNPCC kindred has mirrored this change in the general population in Western Europe and the United States *(128,146)*. Gastric cancer is still an important part of HNPCC in regions in which that cancer is endemic, such as Korea *(147,148)*. The occurrence of sebaceous adenomas, carcinomas, and keratoacanthomas in conjunction with HNPCC-related visceral malignancies define the Muir-Torre syndrome, a variant of HNPCC *(149,150)*. Some cases of Turcot syndrome are also variants of HNPCC, with glioblastoma as the associated central nervous system cancer *(31,32)*.

6.1.2. Diagnostic Criteria

Obtaining a personal and family cancer history from all patients is critical, and a high index of suspicion needs to be maintained if individuals with HNPCC are to be detected. Many diagnostic criteria have been proposed for HNPCC, the best known of which are the Amsterdam criteria *(151)*. The criteria were designed specifically to facilitate research on HNPCC before the mutations responsible for the syndrome had been identified *(152–155)*. A number of other less stringent diagnostic criteria and guidelines for HNPCC have been promulgated, including the Amsterdam II criteria and the recently revised Bethesda guidelines (Table 6) *(156–158)*. At the heart of all of these criteria are certain basic features that are typical of HNPCC: early age of onset of CRC or endometrial cancer (<50 yr of age), multiple family member with colorectal, endometrial or another HNPCC-related cancer, and multiple HNPCC-related cancers in the same individual. If one or more of these features is identified, the diagnosis of HNPCC should be considered. It should be pointed out, however, that the personal and family cancer history need not be very striking in cases of HNPCC detected in the general population, so vigilance is required.

6.1.3. Genetics

The genetic basis of HNPCC is a germline mutation in one of a set of genes responsible for DNA mismatch repair (MMR), and the syndrome might be best termed the hereditary deficient MMR syndrome *(159)*. The growing number of MMR genes include *MSH2, MLH1, PMS1, PMS2, MSH3, MSH6,* and others *(160–165)*. More than 90% of the identified mutations are in

two genes, *MSH2* and *MLH1*, located on chromosome 2p and 3p, respectively *(166)*. More than 5–10% of HNPCC families, often with some atypical or attenuated features, will be accounted for by a germline mutation in *MSH6 (165,167–172)*. Persons with HNPCC have a non-functioning copy of the gene in the germline, usually through an inherited, or occasionally spontaneous, germline mutation. When the remaining working copy of the gene is inactivated by mutation, loss or other mechanisms, the cell loses the ability to repair the inevitable mismatches of DNA basepairs during DNA replication, as well as short insertion and deletion loops *(173,174)*.

Particularly vulnerable to mutation during replication are microsatellites, or DNA regions distributed throughout the genome in which nucleotide bases are repeated several or many times. More than 90% of CRCs in HNPCC demonstrate multiple change-of-length mutations of these microsatellites, termed microsatellite instability (MSI) *(175–177)*. MSI is classified as being absent, low, or high depending on the frequency of microsatellite mutation. The instability of HNPCC tumors is almost always high frequency *(178,179)*. A simple laboratory assay can detect the presence or absence and degree of MSI in tumor tissue using a standard set of microsatellite markers. In addition, tumors that have lost the function of one of the MMR genes show negative staining for the protein product of that gene by immunohistochemistry. Staining tumors for *MSH2* or *MLH1* also may aide in the diagnosis of HNPCC *(180–183)*.

As with *APC*, the specific mutations in the MMR genes (genotype) correlates with the observed phenotype. For example, extra-colonic tumors are more common with *MSH2* mutation than *MLH1* mutation. Families with an *MSH6* mutation tend to have a more attenuated phenotype (later age of onset and lower percentage of gene carriers developing cancer) and an abundance of endometrial cancers when compared with *MSH2* or *MLH1* gene carrying families *(136,184–186)*. As in FAP, a better understanding of genotype–phenotype correlation will lead to improved HNPCC screening, surveillance, and treatment.

Genetic testing for HNPCC, as well as tumor analysis for microsatellite instability and MMR protein immunostaining, is commercially available. Molecular diagnostics for HNPCC is now recommended *(9)*, and in the correct circumstances, can greatly facilitate the care of individuals and families suspected of having the syndrome *(187)*.

6.1.4. Surveillance and Treatment

Recommendations for surveillance in individuals with known or suspected HNPCC are summarized in Table 7. Colonoscopy is recommended every 1–3 yr staring at age 20, or at least 10 yr before the earliest age of cancer in the family *(188)*. Some experts have recommended more frequent surveillance *(62,189)*, for example, that the surveillance frequency be increased to yearly starting at age 40 yr *(190)*. Complete colonoscopy is essential because the preponderance of right-sided tumors in HNPCC. Colonoscopy needs to be repeated frequently because of accelerated rate at which adenomas transform into invasive cancer in HNPCC. Individuals that undergo regular total colonic surveillance have a markedly lower incidence of CRC, CRC-related mortality and all cause mortality, than those not

Table 6
Clinical Criteria for HNPCC

Name	Criteria
Amsterdam	There should be at least three relatives with CRC; all the following criteria should be present • One should be the first-degree relative of the other two • At least two successive generations should be affected • At least one CRC should be diagnosed before age 50 • Familial adenomatous polyposis should be excluded
Amsterdam II	There should be at least three relatives with an HNPCC-associated cancer (CRC, cancer of the endometrium, small bowel, ureter, or renal pelvis); all the following criteria should be present. • One should be the first-degree relative of the other two • At least two successive generations should be affected • At least one CRC should be diagnosed before age 50 • Familial adenomatous polyposis should be excluded
Bethesda 1997	• Individuals with cancer in families that meet the Amsterdam criteria. (*Note*: Three affected relatives with histologically verified CRC with one of them a first-degree relative of the other two and two affected generations and one member diagnosed with colorectal cancer before age 50; FAP should be excluded.) • Individuals with two HNPCC-related cancers, including synchronous and metachronous CRC or associated extracolonic cancers. (*Note*: Endometrial, ovarian, gastric, hepatobiliary or small bowel cancer or transitional cell carcinoma of the renal pelvis or ureter.) • Individuals with CRC and a first-degree relative with CRC and/or HNPCC-related extracolonic cancer and/or a colorectal adenoma; one of the cancers diagnosed at age less than 45 yr, and the adenoma diagnosed at age less than 40 yr. • Individuals with CRC or endometrial cancer diagnosed at age less than 45 yr. • Individuals with right-sided CRC with an undifferentiated pattern (solid/cribiform) on histopathology diagnosed at age less than 45 yr. (*Note*: Solid/cribiform defined as poorly differentiated or undifferentiated carcinoma composed of irregular, solid sheets of large eosinophilic cells, and containing small gland-like spaces.) • Individuals with signet-ring-cell-type CRC diagnosed at age less than 45 yr. (*Note*: Made up of 50% signet-ring cells.) • Individuals with adenomas diagnosed at age less than 40 yr.
Bethesda (Revised 2004)	• CRC diagnosed in a patient less than 50 yr of age. • Presence of synchronous, metachronous CRC, or other HNPCC associated tumor, regardless of age. (*Note*: Stomach, ovarian, pancreas, ureter and renal pelvis, biliary tract, and brain, sebaceous gland adenomas and keratocanthomas, and small bowel.) • CRC with MSI-high histology diagnosed in a patient less than 60 yr of age. (*Note*: Tumor infiltrating lymphocytes, Crohn's like lymphocytic reaction, mucinous/signet ring differentiation, or medullary growth pattern.) • CRC diagnosed in at least one first-degree relative with an HNPCC-related tumor diagnosed under age 50 yr. • CRC diagnosed in two or more first- or second-degree relatives with HNPCC-related tumors, regardless of age.

CRC, colorectal cancer; HNPCC, hereditary nonpolyposis colorectal cancer; MSI, microsatellite instability.

undergoing regular surveillance *(191)*, and surveillance is cost-effective *(192,193)*.

In addition to CRC surveillance, surveillance for endometrial cancer is recommended for individuals at-risk for HNPCC *(188)*. There is no consensus on the optimal method of surveillance, but choices include yearly endometrial biopsy or yearly transvaginal ultrasound, which also serves as a surveillance test for ovarian cancer, especially if coupled with regular (every 6–12 mo) determination of CA-125 levels. Surveillance for other HNPCC-related cancers is not recommended generally. However, recommendations should be tailored to the tumors appearing in the family being treated. For example, genitourinary cancers may be screened by periodic urine, cytology, and gastric cancer by upper GI endoscopy. The need for and efficacy of surveillance for extracolonic cancer in HNPCC remains unproved *(194,195)*.

Many experts advocate total abdominal colectomy with IRA at the time of the initial cancer resection because of the high rate of metachronous tumors *(62,196)*. However, what appears to be most important is adequate postoperative surveillance, rather than the extent of the initial resection *(193)*. Unless patients are diagnosed with synchronous cancers, or they cannot be relied on to follow-up for colonoscopic surveillance, a partial colectomy can be offered. As with FAP, the rate of rectal cancer in HNPCC can exceed 10% over an extended follow-up period, so ongoing surveillance is essential, even if an IRA is performed *(197)*. When adenomas are encountered during surveillance colonoscopy, they are removed endoscopically using standard techniques, and in general, colonoscopic surveillance is continued. However, HNPCC-related polyps are often sessile, so adequate endoscopic resection can be difficult to perform. If there is any doubt, one should proceed with operative resection. Because of the high risk of endometrial and ovarian cancer, some experts have advocated prophylactic hysterectomy and oophorectomy for women beyond the age of child bearing, especially if they are undergoing a colonic resection for CRC. A recent panel of experts, however, found insufficient evidence to recommend for or against prophylactic hysterectomy and oophorectomy *(188)*.

Table 7
Options for Cancer Prevention in HNPCC for Known or Suspected Gene Mutation Carriers

Primary recommendations

- Colonoscopy every 1–2 yr beginning at age 20–25 (or 10 yr before the earliest diagnosis of colorectal cancer in the family, whichever comes first) until age 40 and then annual colonoscopy
- Annual transvaginal ultrasound with color Doppler and/or endometrial aspirate beginning at age 25–35

Secondary recommendations

- Consider total abdominal colectomy with IRA at diagnosis of colorectal cancer
- Consider prophylactic hysterectomy and oophorectomy in known gene carriers at time of colonic operation, or after child bearing complete
- Consider annual measure of CA-125 level
- Consider serial upper endoscopy among families with gastric cancer
- Consider annual urine cytology among families with urinary tract cancers

Table 8
Risk for CRC Based on Family History

Family history	Lifetime risk for CRC (%)
No family history	3–6
One first-degree relative with CRC	Two- to threefold increased risk
One first-degree relative with CRC < age 50	Three- to fivefold increased risk
Two first-degree relatives with CRC	Three- to fivefold increased risk
One second- or third-degree relative with CRC	1.5-fold increased risk
Two second- or third-degree relative with CRC	Two- to threefold increased risk
One first-degree relative with adenoma	1.5–2-fold increased risk

CRC, colorectal cancer.

6.2. COMMON FAMILIAL CRC
6.2.1. Clinical Features

FAP and HNPCC confer the highest risks of colon cancer; however, account for no more than 5% of all CRCs. Nevertheless, familial history is an important risk factor the development of CRC, suggesting a critical hereditary component in more than 25% of cases *(3,198)*. The magnitude of the risk depends on the number of first-degree relatives affected and the age at diagnosis (Table 8) *(4)*. Individuals with a single first-degree relative with CRC have a risk about 2.25 times that in the general population. Individuals with more than one first-degree relatives with CRC have a risk about 4.25 times that in the general population, and individuals with a relative diagnosed with CRC before the age of 45 have a risk about four times higher than the general population *(4)*. Individuals with a first-degree relative with colorectal adenoma also have a risk of colon cancer about twice that in the general population *(199)*. Colon cancer in a second- or third-degree relative increases colon cancer risk, but only about 50% above average risk *(190)*. Importantly, individuals with a first-degree relative with a family history of colon cancer have a colon cancer risk at age 40, which is similar to the general population risk at age 50 (Fig. 2) *(190,200)*. Although family history of CRC increases an individual's risk for the disease, especially at a younger age than seen in pure sporadic cancer, there is no convincing evidence yet that the clinical presentation of these common familial CRCs differ in important ways from sporadic CRC with respect to features such as tumor location or aggressiveness.

6.2.2. Genetics

The gene alterations responsible for common familial CRC are being discovered in increasingly greater numbers, although for the most part these cancer susceptibility alleles remain unknown *(2,5)*. Kindred studies suggest that these genes are dominantly inherited, but unlike in true hereditary CRC, the altered genes that cause familial CRC are generally low penetrance *(201)*. Thus, inheriting a disease susceptibility gene increases one's risk for CRC, but by no means guarantees that the disease will occur. Candidate susceptibility alleles are many and include minor mutations in the same genes that cause hereditary CRC. An example of this is the *I1307K* allele of *APC* found in Ashkenazi Jews *(202)*. Inheritance of this unstable *APC* allele increases the chance of developing CRC by approx 1.5- to 2-fold, rather than the near 100% risk of CRC that occurs in classic FAP *(203)*.

6.2.3. Surveillance and Treatment

Several different screening recommendations for individuals with familial risk have been published. A recent task force, comprising several different professional organizations, recommended that CRC screening in individuals with a family history of CRC be the same as the screening recommended for the general public, but that this screening start at age 40 yr *(190)*. The American College of Gastroenterology recommends that individuals with a strong family history of colon cancer should undergo screening colonoscopy starting at age 40, or 10 yr younger than the age at diagnosis of the youngest affected relative. They then recommend that colonoscopy be repeated at 3- to 5-yr intervals *(204)*. The US Preventive Services Task Force does not address familial risk outside of the hereditary syndromes *(205)*. Treatment of colon and rectal cancer in this setting involves partial colectomy with close surveillance of the residual colon and rectum thereafter.

7. GENETIC TESTING FOR HEREDITARY CRC
7.1. AVAILABLE TESTS

Genetic tests are commercially available for FAP, HNPCC (*MSH2* and *MLH1*), and the *I1307K APC* allele. Testing for PJS, juvenile polyposis, and Cowden syndrome also is becom-

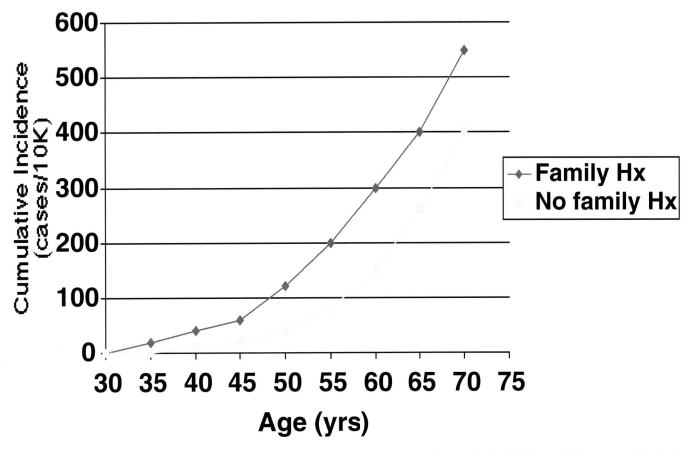

Fig. 2. Cumulative incidence of colorectal cancer according to age and the presence or absence of a family history of the disease. (Reprinted with permission from ref. *200*.)

ing available through commercial laboratories *(206–208)*. Genetic testing for common familial CRC will certainly become common in the near future. The germline genetic tests typically are performed on DNA extracted from white blood cells obtained from a blood sample. The laboratories that provide these tests, the tests themselves, and their costs are constantly changing. An online reference for genetic testing laboratories and location of genetics professionals can be found at www.geneclinics.org.

7.2. GENETIC COUNSELING AND INFORMED CONSENT

Before genetic testing for hereditary CRC, genetic counseling and informed consent are essential *(209)*. Genetic counseling for hereditary cancer is best performed by trained genetic counselors in conjunction with physicians who are experts on the disease, such as a gastroenterologist, oncologist, or surgeon *(206)*. The role of the counselor can be filled by other trained professionals, such as nurses or physicians with a special interest and expertise in hereditary cancer. Cancer genetic counseling may involve several family members, some of whom might have had cancer, and others who have not and it often involves multiple visits *(206,210)*.

7.3. INDICATIONS AND STRATEGY FOR GENETIC TESTING IN HEREDITARY CRC

The American Society of Clinical Oncology (ASCO) recommends that cancer predisposition testing be offered only when

(1) the person has a strong family history of cancer or very early age of onset of disease, (2) the test can be adequately interpreted, and (3) the results will influence the medical management of the patient or family member *(211)*. ASCO recognizes three general categories of indications for genetic testing. In the first category testing may already be considered part of the standard care, in the second category the value of testing is presumed, but not clearly established, and in the third category the benefit of testing is not yet established. There is no doubt that intensive cancer screening among individuals at risk for FAP and HNPCC will save lives and has been found to be cost-effective *(63,191–193)*. Detection of FAP and HNPCC gene carriers is beneficial because it will improve the efficiency of cancer prevention in families with these conditions by allowing those who do not carry the predisposition allele to avoid costly and burdensome screening tests, and has also been found to be cost-effective *(10,187,212)*. Therefore, genetic testing for FAP and HNPCC falls under the first ASCO category and is now the standard of care for families suspected of having these syndromes *(9,10,206,208)*. Genetic testing for other rare polyposis syndromes, and for the gene alterations that cause common familial CRC is becoming commercially available, but the benefits of such testing are not yet clearly established *(62)*.

7.3.1. Familial Adenomatous Polyposis

Testing for FAP mutations is a standard part of the care of affected individuals and families *(9,213)*. The indications and strat-

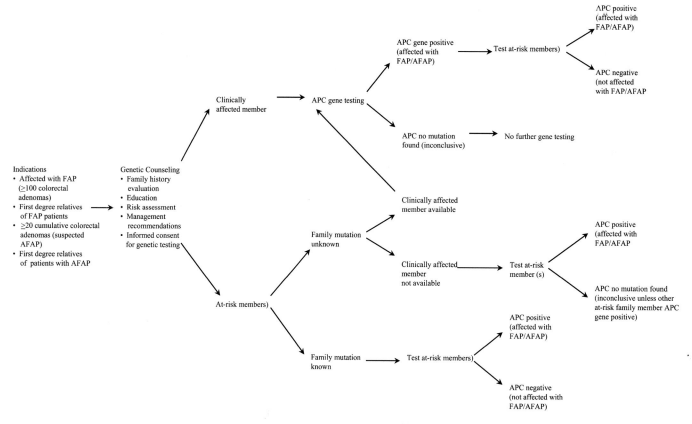

Fig. 3. FAP gene testing recommendations and strategy. (Adapted from ref. *217*.)

Table 9
Appropriate Interpretation of Genetic Test Results

Proband result	Family member result	Interpretation
Positive	Positive	Positive
Positive	Negative	Negative
Negative	Do not test	Not informative[a]
Ambiguous	Do not test	Not informative[a]

[a]Must assume that family member carries the deleterious gene given the inability to prove otherwise because of the negative test in the proband. Proceed with cancer screening appropriate for a gene carrier in the family member.

egy for FAP testing are summarized in Fig. 3. Genetic testing of an FAP family should start with an affected family member. If a mutation is found, then at-risk members of the family can proceed to testing. If the mutation is not found in an affected person, it does not mean that FAP is not present, but that the test is non-informative (Table 9) *(214)*. Because up to one-third of individuals with FAP have a spontaneous germline *APC* mutation, testing should not be limited to members of classic FAP kindred. Individuals with the FAP phenotype, but without a family history, are also eligible for testing. Because minors can develop polyposis and therefore require cancer screening, predisposition testing of minors is appropriate, although this is best deferred until early adolescence *(208,215)*. Ophthalmological exams of families with CHRPE can be used as a surrogate for genetic testing, but the validity of this approach to FAP screening has not been conclusively demonstrated. It may be difficult to determine whether an individual has

Table 10
Likelihood of Detecting a Germline *MSH2* or *MLH1* Mutation Depending on Family History and Tumor MSI Status

Clinical criteria met	Likelihood of detecting a mutation (%)
Amsterdam criteria met	40–70
Amsterdam criteria met and MSI-H tumor	80
Near Amsterdam criteria met	20–50
Near Amsterdam and MSI-H tumor	50–60
Bethesda guidelines met	30
Bethesda guidelines met and MSI-H tumor	50
Early onset CRC w/o family history	0–30
Early onset CRC and MSI-H tumor	30
Sporadic CRC	<1
Sporadic CRC with MSI-H tumor	10

the FAP phenotype and therefore merits testing, especially if the diagnosis of attenuated FAP is being considered. A finding of multiple polyps in an individual over age 45–50, especially in the absence of a family history, is far more likely to be part of the spectrum of sporadic colonic neoplasms rather than FAP, but this remains an area of controversy. Some experts would test patients with 20 or more cumulative colorectal adenomas *(3,10)*.

7.3.2. Hereditary Nonpolyposis CRC

As with FAP, genetic testing is a standard part of the care of individuals and families at risk for HNPCC *(9,213)*. However, determining when genetic testing is indicated for HNPCC is a far more difficult problem than in FAP, because individuals

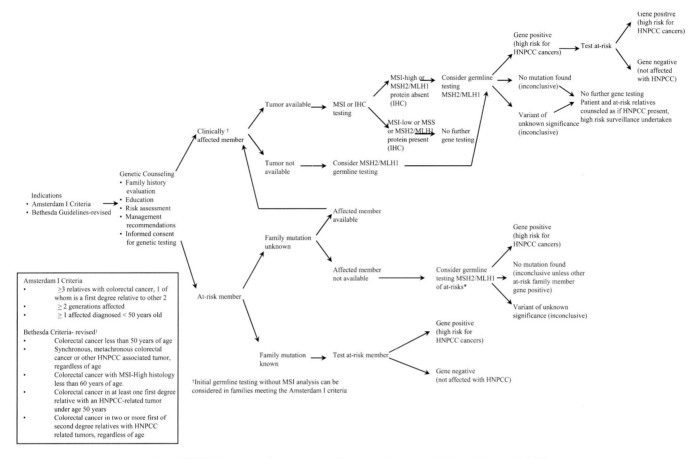

Fig. 4. HNPCC gene testing recommendations and strategy. (Adapted from ref. *217*.)

with HNPCC do not have a unique phenotype to help establish the clinical diagnosis. Some investigators have suggested direct germline *MSH2* and *MLH1* testing of CRC patients that meet appropriate and fairly stringent clinical criteria, such as Amsterdam, Amsterdam II, or the first three Bethesda guidelines *(152,153)*. The likelihood of detecting a germline *MSH2* or *MLH1* mutation based on clinical criteria met is summarized in Table 10. Other investigators have suggested that tumor MSI testing or MSH2/MLH1 protein immunohistochemistry should be performed first, and that germline testing be reserved for those found to have MSI-H tumors or those with loss of MMR protein expression *(155,157,183,216)*. The decision to perform tumor MSI or immunohistochemistry testing is again based on clinical criteria, although often less stringent criteria than used to decide for germline testing, such as revised Bethesda guidelines *(158)*. The likelihood of detecting a germline mutation following a positive tumor MSI test also is summarized in Table 10.

Once a germline mutation is detected in the affected proband, germline testing can then be carried out in other family members. In this situation, if family members are found not to carry the family mutation, their result is considered a true negative, and there risk for cancer is that of the general population. As with FAP, if a mutation is not detected in a family suspected of having HNPCC, the test result is not informative. Failure to detect a mutation in a family without a known mutation does not mean that the family does not have HNPCC

(Table 9). The indications and strategy for HNPCC gene testing are summarized in Fig. 4 *(9)*.

8. CONCLUSIONS

Heredity plays an important causative role in a large percentage of CRCs. Clinical recognition of the hereditary polyposis syndromes, HNPCC, and common familial CRC, is essential because screening, surveillance and treatment among affected individuals, and their family members differs from that recommended to the general population. More intensive cancer screening and surveillance is required if premature death is to be avoided. Genetic testing is commercially available for most of the hereditary CRC syndromes, and can greatly facilitate the management of patients if properly undertaken.

REFERENCES

1. Greenlee RT, Hill-Harmon MB, Murray T, Thun M. Cancer statistics, 2001. California Cancer J Clin 2001; 51:15–36.
2. Calvert PM, Frucht H. The genetics of colorectal cancer. Ann Intern Med 2002; 137:603–612.
3. Burt RW. Colon cancer screening. Gastroenterol 2000; 119:837–853.
4. Johns LE, Houlston RS. A systematic review and meta-analysis of familial colorectal cancer risk. Am J Gastroenterol 2001; 96: 2992–3003.
5. Houlston RS, Tomlinson IP. Polymorphisms and colorectaltumor risk Gastroenterology 2001; 121:282–301.
6. Terdiman JP, Conrad PG, Sleisenger MH. Genetic testing in hereditary colorectal cancer indications and procedures. Am J Gastroenterol 1999; 94:2344–2356.

7. Samowitz WS, Curtin KI, Ju Robertson H, Schaffer MA, Nichols DM, Gruenthal K, Leppert MF, Slattery ML. The colon cancer burden of genetically-defined hereditary nonpolyposis colon cancer. Gastroenterology 2001.

8. Salovaara R, Loukola A, Kristo P, et al. Population-based molecular detection of hereditary nonpolyposis colorectal cancer. J Clin Oncol 2000; 18:2193–2200.

9. American Gastroenterological Association Medical Position Statement Hereditary colorectal cancer and genetic testing. Gastroenterology 2001; 121:195–197.

10. Giardiello FM, Brensinger JD, Petersen GMAG. A technical review on hereditary colorectal cancer and genetic testing. Gastroenterology 2001; 121:198–213.

11. Bisgaard ML, Fenger K, Bulow S, Niebuhr E, Mohr J. Familial adenomatous polyposis (FAP) frequency penetrance and mutation-rate. Hum Mutat 1994; 3:121–125.

12. Lindor NM, Greene MH. The concise handbook of family cancer syndromes. Mayo Familial Cancer Program. J Natl Cancer Inst 1998; 90:1039–1071.

13. Galle TS, Juel K, Bulow S. Causes of death in familial adenomatous polyposis Scand J Gastroenterol 1999; 34:808–812.

14. Spirio L, Olschwang S, Groden J, et al. Alleles of the APC gene an attenuated form of familial polyposis Cell 1993; 75:951–957

15. Lynch HT, Smyrk T, McGinn T, Lanspa S, Cavalieri J, Lynch J, Slominski-Castor S, Cayouette MC, Priluck I, Luce MC. Attenuated familial adenomatous polyposis (AFAP). A phenotypically and genotypically distinctive variant of FAP Cancer, 1995; 76:2427–2433

16. Church JM, McGannon E, Hull-Boiner S Sivak V, VanStolk R, Jagelman DG, Fazio VW, Oakley JR, Lavery IC, Milsom JW. Gastroduodenal polyps in patients with familial adenomatous polyposis. Dis Colon Rectum 1992; 35:1170–1173.

17. Campbell WJ, Spence RA, Parks TG. Familial adenomatous polyposis Br J Surg 1994; 81:1722–1733.

18. Offerhaus GJ, Giardiello FM, Krush AJ, Booker SV, Tersmette AC, Kelley NC, Hamilton SR. The risk of upper gastrointestinal cancer in familial adenomatous polyposis (see comments). Gastroenterology 1992; 102:1980–1982.

19. Wallace MH, Phillips RK. Upper gastrointestinal disease in patients with familial adenomatous polyposis. Br J Surg 1998; 85:742–750.

20. Saurin JC, Chayvialle JA, Ponchon T. Management of duodenal adenomas in familial adenomatous polyposis. Endoscopy 1999; 31:472–478.

21. Belchetz LA, Berk T, Bapat BV, Cohen Z, Gallinger S. Changing causes of mortality in patients with familial adenomatous polyposis. Dis Colon Rectum 1996; 39:384–387.

22. Bjork J, Akerbrant Hiselius L, Bergman A, Engwall Y, Wahlstrom J, Martinsson T, Nordling M, Hultcrantz RP. Periampullary adenomas and the adenocarcinomas in familial adenomatous polyposis cumulative risks and APC gene mutations. Gastroenterology 2001; 121:1127–1135.

23. Kadmon M, Tandara A, Herfath C. Duodenal adenomatosis in familial adenomatous polyposis coli A review of the literature and results from the Heidelberg Polyposis Register. Int J Colorectal Dis 2001; 16:63–75.

24. Ruhswurm I, Zehetmayer M, Dejaco C, Wolf B, Karner-Hanusch J. Ophthalmic and genetic screening in pedigrees with familial adenomatous polyposis Am J Ophthalmol 1998; 125:680–686.

25. Clark SK, Johnson Smith TG, Katz DE, Reznek RHRKP. Identification and progression of a desmoid precursor lesion in patient with familial adenomatous polyposis. Br J Surg 1998; 85:970–973.

26. Church JM, McGannon E. Prior pregnancy ameliorates the course of intra-abdominal desmoid tumors in patients with familial adenomatous polyposis. Dis Colon Rectum 2000; 43:445–450.

27. Soravia C, Berk T, McLeod RS, Cohen Z. Desmoid disease in patients with familial adenomatous polyposis. Dis Colon Rectum 2000; 43:363–369.

28. Rodriguez-Bigas MA, Mahoney MC, Karakousis CP, Petrelli NJ. Desmoid tumors in patients with familial adenomatous polyposis. Cancer 1994; 74:1270–1274.

29. Giardiello FM, Offerhaus GJA, Lee DH, et al. Increased risk of thyroid and pancreatic carcinoma in familial adenomatous polyposis. Gut 1993; 34:1394–1396.

30. Cetta F, Montalto G, Gori M, Curia MC, Cama A, Olschwang S. Germline mutations of the APC gene in patients with familial adenomatous polyposis-associated thyroid carcinoma results for a European cooperative study. J Clin Endocrinol Metab 2000; 85:286–292.

31. Hamilton SR, Liu B, Parsons RE, et al. The molecular basis of Turcot's syndrome (see comments). N Engl J Med 1995; 332:839–847.

32. Paraf F, Jothy S, Van Meir EG. Brain tumor-polyposis syndrome two genetic diseases J Clin Oncol 1997; 15:2744–2758.

33. Kinzler KW, Nilbert MC, Su LK, et al. Identification of FAP locus-genes from chromosome 5q21 Science, 1991; 253:661–665.

34. Groden J, Thliveris A, Samowitz W, et al. Identification and characterization of the familial adenomatous polyposis coli gene. Cell 1991; 66:589–600.

35. Miyoshi Y, Ando H, Nagase H, et al. Germ-line mutations of the APC gene in 53 familial adenomatous polyposis patients. Proc Natl Acad Sci USA 1992; 89:4452–4456.

36. Polakis P. The adenomatous polyposis coli (APC) tumors uppress or Biochim Biophys Acta 1997; 1332:F127–147.

37. Dihlmann S, Gebert J, Siermann A, Herfath C, von Knebel Doeberitz MD. Ominant negative effect to the APC1309 mutation a possible explanation for genotype-phenotype correlations in familial adenomatous polyposis. Cancer Res 1999; 59:1857–1860.

38. Bullions LC, Levine AJ. The role of beta-catenin in cell adhesion signal transduction and cancer Curr Opin Oncol 1998; 10:81–87.

39. Behrens J, Jerchow BA, Wurtele M, et al. Functional interaction of an axin homolog conductin with beta-catenin APC and GSK3 beta. Science 1998; 280:596–599.

40. Kishida S, Yamamoto H, Ikeda S, et al. Axina negative regulator of the wnt signaling pathway directly interacts with adenomatous polyposis coli and regulates the stabilization of beta-catenin. J Bio Chem 1998; 273:10,823–10,826.

41. He TC, Sparks AB, Rago C, et al. Identification of c-MYC as a target of the APC pathway (see comments). Science 1998; 281:1509–1512.

42. Tetsu O, McCormick F. Beta-catenin regulates expression of cyclin D1 in coloncarcinoma cells. Nature 1999; 398:422–426.

43. Wallis YL, Morton DGCMM, Macdonald F. Molecular analysis of the APC gene in 205 families extended genotype-phenotype correlations in FAP and evidence for the role of AP C aminoacid changes in colorectal cancer predisposition. J Med Genet 1999; 36:14–20.

44. Hernegger GS, Moore HG, Guille JG. Attenuated familial adenomatous polyposis: an evolving and poorly understood entity. Dis Colon Rectum 2002; 45:127–134; discussion 134–126.

45. Giardiello FM, Brensinger JD, Luce MC, et al. Phenotypic expression of disease in families that have mutations in the 5′ region of the adenomatous polyposis coli gene. An Int Med 1997; 126:514–519.

46. Gardner RJ, Kool D, Edkins E, et al. The clinical correlates of a 3′ truncating mutation (codons 1982–1983) in the adenomatous polyposis coli gene. Gastroenterology 1997; 113:326–331.

47. Brensinger JD, Laken SJ, Luce MC, et al. Variable phenotype of familial adenomatous polyposis in pedigrees with 3′ mutation in the APC gene (see comments) Gut 1998; 43:548–552.

48. Soravia C, Berk T, Madlensky L, et al. Genotype–phenotype correlations in attenuated adenomatous polyposis coli. Am J Hum Gen 1998; 62:1290–1301.

49. Rozen P, Samuel Z, Shomrat R, Legum C. Notable intra familial phenotypic variability in a kindred with familial adenomatous polyposis and APC mutation in exon 9. Gut 1999; 45:829–833.

50. O'Sullivan MJ, McCarthy TV, Doyle CT. Familial adenomatous polyposis from bedside to benchside. Am J Cli Pathol 1998; 109:521–526.

51. Olschwang S, Tiret A, Laurent-Puig P, Muleris M, Parc R, Thomas G. Restriction of ocular fundus lesions to a specific sub group of APC mutations in adenomatous polyposis coli patients. Cell 1993; 75:959–968.

52. Wallis YL, Macdonald F, Hultén M, et al. Genotype–phenotype correlation between position of constitutional APC gene mutation

and CHRPE expression in familial adenomatous polyposis. Human Genetics 1994; 94:543–548.

53. Saurin JC, Ligneau B, Ponchon T, Lepretre J, Chavaillon A, Napoleon B, Chayvaille JA. The influence of mutation site and age on the severity of duodenal polyposis in patients with familial adenomatous polyposis. Gastrointest Endosc 2002; 55 342–347.

54. Caspari R, Olschwang SWF, Mandl M, Boisson C, Boker T, Augustin A, Kadmon M, Moslein G, Thomas G, Propping P. Familial adenomatous polyposis desmoid tumors and lack of ophthalmic lesions (CHRPE) associated with APC mutations beyond codon. 1995; 1:444.

55. Betario L, Russo A, Sala P, et al. Genotype and phenotype factors as determinants of desmoid tumors in patients with familial adenomatous polyposis Int J Cancer 2001; 95:102–107.

56. Vasen HFA, vander Luijt RB, Slors JFM, et al. Molecular genetic tests as a guide to surgical management of familialadenomatouspolyposis. Lancet 1995; 348:433–435.

57. Wu JS, Paul P, McGannon EA, Church JMAPC. Genotype polyp number and surgical options in familial adenomatous polyposis. Ann Surgery 1998; 227:57–62.

58. Friedl W, Caspari R, Sengteller M, et al. Can APC mutation analysis contribute to the rapeutic decisions in familial adenomatous polyposis. Experience from 680 FAP families. Gut 2001; 48:515–521.

59. Jones S, Emmerson P, Maynard J, et al. Biallelic germ line mutations in MYH predispose to multiple colorectala denoma and somatic G:C to T:A mutations. Hum Molec Genet 2002; 11:2961–2967.

60. Sieber OM, Lipton L, Crabtree M, et al. Multiple colorectal adenomas classica denomatouspolyposis and germ-line mutations in MYH. N Engl J Med 2003; 348:791–799.

61. Venesio T, Molatore S, Cattaneo F, Arrigoni A, Risio M, Ranzani GN. High frequency of MYH gene mutations in a subset of patients with familial adenomatous polyposis. Gastroenterology 2004; 126:1681–1685.

62. Dunlop MG. Guidance on gastro intestinal surveillance for hereditary nonpolyposis colorectal cancer familial adenomatous polyposis juvenile polyposis and Peutz-Jeghers syndrome. Gut 2002; 51:v21-v27.

63. Heiskanen I, Luostarinen T, Jarvinen HJ. Impact of screening examinations on survival in familial adenomatous polyposis. Scand J Gastroenterol 2000; 35:1284–1287.

64. Bulow S, Bjork J, Christensen IJ, Fausa O, Jarvinen H, Moesgaard F, Vasen HF. Duodenal adenomatosis in familial adenomatous polyposis. Gut 2004; 53:381–386.

65. Spigelman AD. Screening modalities in familialadenomatouspolyposis and hereditary nonpolyposiscolorectal cancer. Gastrointestinal Endoscopy Clin North Am 1997; 7:81–6.

66. Alacorn FJ, Burke CA, Church JM, van Stolk RU. Familial adenomatous polyposis efficacy of endoscopic and surgical treatment for advanced duodenaladenomas. Dis Colon Rectum 1999; 42: 1533–1536.

67. Heiskanen I, Kellokumpu I, Jarvinen H. Management of duodenal adenomas in 98 patients with familial adenomatous polyposis Endoscopy 1999; 31:412–416.

68. Norton ID, Geller A, Petersen BT, Sorbi D, Gostout CJ. Endoscopic surveillance and ablative therapy for periam pullary adenomas. Am J Gastroenterol 2001; 96:101–106.

69. de Vostot N, Ederveen Cappel WH, Jarvinen HJ, et al. World wide survey among polyposis registries of surgical management of severe duodenal adeno matosisin familial adenomatous polyposis. Br J Surg 2003; 90:705–710.

70. Betario L, Russo A, Radice P, et al. Genotype and phenotype factors as determinants forrectal stump cancer in patients with familial adenomatous polyposis. Ann Surg 2000; 231:538–543.

71. Wu JS, McGannon EA, Church JM. Incidence of neoplastic polyps in theileal pouch of patients with familial adenomatous polyposis after restorative proctocolectomy. Dis Colon Rectum 41:552–556; discussion 1998; 556–557.

72. van Duijvendijk P, Vasen HFA, Betario L, et al. Cumulative risk of developing polypsormalignancy attheileal pouch-analana stomos is in patients with familialadenomatouspolyposis. J Gastrointest Surg 1999; 3:325–330.

73. Giardiello FM, Hamilton SR, Krush AJ, et al. Treatment of colonic and rectaladenomas with sulindac in familial adenomatous polyposis. N Engl J Med 1993; 328:1313–1316.

74. Steinbach G, Lynch PM, Phillips RK, et al. The effect of celecoxiba cyclooxygenase-2 inhibitor in familial adenomatous polyposis. N Engl J Med 2000; 342:1946–1952.

75. Giardiello FM, Yang VW, Hylind LM, et al. Primary chemo prevention of familialaenomatouspolyposis with sulindac N Engl J Med 2002; 346:1054–1059.

76. Cruz-Correa M, Hylind LM, Romans KE, Booker SV, Giardiello FM. Long-term treatment with ulindac in familialadenomatouspolyposis a prospective study. Gastroenterology 2002; 122: 641–645.

77. Utech M, Bruwer M, Buerger H, Tubergen D, Senninger N. (Rectal carcinoma in a patient with familial adenomatous polyposis coli after colectomy with ileo rectal anastomosis and consecutive chemo prevention with sulindac suppositories). Chirurg 2002; 73:855–858.

78. Jeghers H, McKusick VA, Katz KH. Generalized intestinal polyposis and melan in spots of the oral mucosa lips and digits asyndrome of diagnostic significance. N Engl J Med 1949; 241:993–1005.

79. McGarrity TJ, Kulin HE, Zaino RJ. Peutz-Jeghers Syndrome. Am J Gastroenterol 2000; 95:596–604.

80. Bartholomew LG, Dahlin DC, Waugh JM. Intestinal polyposis associated with muco cutaneous melanin pigmentation (Peutz-Jeghers syndrome). Review of the literature and repor to six cases with special reference to pathologic findings. Gastroenterology 1957; 32:434–451.

81. Foley TR, McGarrity TJ, Abt A, Peutz-Jeghers syndrome a 38 year follow up of the "Harrisburg Family." Gastroenterology1988; 95: 1535–1540.

82. Utsunomiya J, Gocho H, Miyanaga T, Hamaguchi E, Kashimure A. Peutz-Jeghers syndrome its natural course and management. Johns Hopkins Med J 1975; 136:71–82.

83. Boardman LA, Thibodeau SN, Schaid DJ, et al. Increased risk for cancer in patients with the Peutz-Jegherssyndrome. Ann Int Med 1998; 128:896–899.

84. Giardiello FM, Brensinger JD, TersmetteAC, Goodman SN, Petersen GM, Booker SV, Cruz-Correa M, Offerhaus JA. Veryhigh risk of cancer in familial Peutz-Jeghers syndrome Gastroenterology, 2000; 119:1447–1453.

85. Perzin KH, Bridge MF. Adenomatous carcinomatous changes in hamartomatous polyps of the small intestine (Peutz-Jeghers syndrome). Report of a case and review of the literature Cancer, 1982; 49:971–983.

86. Jenne DE, Reimann H, Nezu J, et al. Peutz-Jeghers syndrome is caused by mutations in an ovelserine threoninekinase. Nat Genet 1998; 18:38–43.

87. Hemminki A, Markie D, Tomlinson I, et al. Aserine threoninek in as egenedefective in Peutz-Jegherssyndrome. Nature 1998; 391: 184–187.

88. Boardman LA, Couch FJ, Burgart LJ, et al. Genetic heterogeneity in Peutz-Jeghers syndrome. Hum Mutat 2000; 16:23–30.

89. Wirtzfeld DA, Petrelli NJ, Rodriguez-Bigas MA. Hamartomatous polyposis molecular genetics neoplastic risk and surveillance recommendations. Ann Surg Oncol 2001; 8.

90. Amaro R, Diaz G, Schneider J, Hellinger MD, Stollman NH. Peutz-Jeghers syndrome managed with a complete intra operative endoscopy and extensive polypectomy. Gastro in test Endosc 2000; 52:552–554.

91. Rubio CA, Jaramillo E, Lindblom A, Fogt F. Classification of colorectalpolyps guidelines for the endoscopist. Endoscopy 2002; 34:226–236.

92. Woodford-Richens K, Bevan S, Churchman M, Analysis of genetic and phenotypicheterogeneity in juvenilepolyposis. Gut 2000; 46:656–660.

93. Giardiello FM, Offerhaus JG. Phenotype and can cerrisk of the various polyposis syndromes. Eur J Cancer 1995; 31a:1085–1087.

94. Jarvinen H, Franssila KO. Familial juvenilepolyposis coli increased risk of colorectal cancer Gut, 1984; 25:792–800.

95. Howe JR, Mitros FA, Summers RW. The risk of gastrointestinal carcinoma in familial juvenilepolyposis. Ann Surg Oncol 1998; 5:751–756.

96. Howe JR, Roth S, Ringold JC, et al. Mutations in the SMAD4/DPC4 gene in juvenile polyposis (see comments). Science 1998; 280:1086–1088.

97. Houlston R, Bevan S, Williams A, et al. Mutations in DPC4 (SMAD4) cause juvenilepolyposis syndrome but only account for aminority of cases. Hum Mol Genet 1998; 7:1907–1912.

98. Woodford-Richens KL, Rowan AJ, Poulsom R, et al. Comprehensive analysis of SMAD4 mutations and protein expression in juvenile-polyposis evidence for a distinct path way and polypmorphology in SMAD4 mutation carriers Am J Pathol 2001; 159:1293–1300.

99. Takagi Y, Kohmura H, Futamura M, et al. Somatic alterations of the DPC4 gene in human colorectal cancers in vivo (see comments). Gastroenterology 1996; 111:1369–1372.

100. Olschwang S, Serova-Sinilnikova OM, Lenoir GM, Thomas G. PTEN germ line mutations in juvenile polyposis. Nat Genet 1998; 18:12–13.

101. Zhou XP, Woodford-Richens K, Lehtonen R, et al. Germline-mutations in BMPR1A/ALK3 cause a subset of cases of juvenile polyposis syndrome and of Bannayan-Riley-Ruvalcaba syndromes. Am J Hum Genet 2001; 69:704–711.

102. Burt RW. Polyposis syndromes. Clin Perspec Gastroenterol 2002; Jan/Feb:51–59.

103. Liaw D, Marsh DJ, Li J, et al. Germline mutations of the PTEN genein Cowden disease an inherited breast and thyroid cancer syndrome. Nat Genet 1997; 16:64–67.

104. Zigman AF, Lavine JE, Jones MC, Boland CR, Carethers JM. Localization of the Bannayan-Riley-Ruvalcaba syndrome gene-tochromosome 10q 23 Gastroenterology 1997; 113:1433–1437.

105. Ward EM, Wolfsen HC. Review article: the non-inherited gastrointestinal polyposis syndromes. Aliment Pharmacol Ther 2002; 16:333–342.

106. Rashid A, Houlihan S, Booker S, Petersen GM, Giardiello FM, Hamilton SR. Phenotypic and molecular characteristics of hyperplastic polyposis Gastroenterology 2000; 119:323–332.

107. Sumner HW, Wasserman NF, McClain CJ. Gianthy per plastic polyposis of the colon Dig Dis Sci 1981; 26:85–89.

108. Warner A, Glick ME, Fogt F, Multiple large hyperplastic polyps of the colonco incident with a denocarcinoma Am J Gastroenterol 1994; 89:123–125.

109. Cronkhite LW, Canada WJ. Generalized gastro intestinal polyposis unusual syndrome of polyposis pigmentational opecia and ony-chontrophia. N Engl J Med 1955; 252:1011–1015.

110. Burke AP, Sobin LH. The pathology of the Cronkhite-Canada polyps A comparison to juvenile polyposis. Am J Surg Pathol 1989; 13:940–946.

111. Russell DM, Bhathal PS, St. John DJ. Complete remission in the Cronkhite-Canada syndrome. Gastroenterology 1983; 85:180–185.

112. Rappaport LB, Sperling HV, Stavrides A. colon cancer in the Cronkhite-Canada syndrome. J Clin Gastroenterol 1986; 8: 199–202.

113. Malhorta R, Sheffield A. Cronkhite-Canada syndrome associated with coloncarcinoma and adenomatous changes in C-Cpolyps. Am J Gastroenterol 1988; 83:772–776.

114. Ward E, Wolfsen HC, Ng CS. Medical management of the Cronkhite-Canada syndrome. South Med J 2002; 95:272–274.

115. Kelly JK, Gabos S. The pathogenesis of inflammatory polyps. Dis Colon Rectum 1987; 30:251–254.

116. Fisher RL, Barwick KW. Fili form polyposis an un usual complication of inflammatory bowel disease. J Clin Gastroenterol 1985; 7:451–458.

117. Taylor BA, Wolff BG. Colonic lipomas. Report of two cases and review of the literature. Dis Colon Rectum 1987; 30:888–893.

118. Swain VA, Young WF, Pringle EM. Hypertrophy of the appendicese piploicae and lipomatous polyposis of the colon. Gut 1969; 10:587–589.

119. Ramirez JM, Ortego J, Deus J, Bustamante E, Lozano R, Dominguez M. Lipomatous polyposis of the colon. Br J Surg 1993; 80:349–350.

120. Ranchord M, Lewin KJ, Dorfman RF. Lymphoid hyperplasia of the gastrointestinaltract. Am J Surg Pathol 1978; 2:383–400.

121. Levendoglu H, Rosen Y. Nodularly mphoid hyperplasia of the gutin HIV infection. Am J Gastroenterol 1992; 87:1200–1202.

122. Bastlein C, Burlefinger R, Hlozberg E, Voeth C, Garbrecht M, Ottenjann R. Common variable immuno deficiency syndrome and nodularly mphoid hyperplasia in the small intestine. Endoscopy 1988; 20:272–275.

123. Lynch HT, Swmyrk TC, Watson P, et al. Genetics natural history tumor spectrum and pathology of hereditary nonpolyposis colorectal cancer an updated review Gastroenterology 1993; 104:1535–1549.

124. PonzdeLeon M, Sassatelli R, Benatti P, Roncucci L. Identification of hereditary nonpolyposis colorectal cancer in the general population The 6 year experience of a population-based registry. Cancer 1993; 71:3493–3501.

125. Evans DG, Walsh S, Jeacock J, et al. Incidence of hereditary non-polyposis colorectal cancer in a population-based study of 1137 consecutive cases of colorectal cancer. Br J Surg 1997; 84:1281–1285.

126. Aaltonen LA, Salovaara R, Kristo P, et al. Incidence of hereditary nonpolyposis colorectal cancer and the feasibility of molecular screening for the disease (see comments). New Engl J Med, 1998; 338:1481–1487.

127. Ravnik-Glavac M, Potocnik U, Glavac D. Incidence of germline hMLH1 and hMSH2 mutations (HNPCCpatients) among newly diagnosed colorectal cancer sina Slovenian population. J Med Genetics 2000; 37:533–536.

128. Lynch HT, Smyrk T, Lynch JF. Overview of natural history pathology molecular genetics and management to HNPCC Lynch Syndrome. Int J Cancer 1996; 69:38–431.

129. Kinzler KW, Vogelstein B. Lessons from hereditary colorectal cancer. Cell 1996; 87:159–170.

130. Watanabe T, Muto T, Sawada T, Miyaki M. Flat adenoma as a precursor of colorectal carcinoma in hereditary non polyposis colorectal carcinoma. Cancer 1996; 77:627–634.

131. Rijcken FEM, Hollema H, Kleibeuker JH. Proximal adenomas in hereditary nonpolyposis colorectal cancer are proneto rapid malignant transformation. Gut 2002; 50:382–386.

132. Lindgren G, Liljegren A, Jaramillo E, Rubio C, Lindblom A. A denomap revalence and cancer risk in familial nonpolyposis colorectal cancer. Gut 2002; 50:228–234.

133. Vasen HF, Wijnen JT, Menko FH, et al. Cancer risk in families with hereditary nonpolyposis colorectal cancer diagnosed by mutation analysis (published erratum appears in Gastroenterology 1996 Nov 111(5)1402). Gastroenterology 1996; 110:1020–1027.

134. Dunlop MG, Farrington SM, Carothers AD, et al. Cancer risk associated with germline DNA mismatch repair gene mutations. Hum Mol Genet 1997; 6:105–110.

135. Aarnio M, Sankila R, Pukkala E, et al.. Cancer risk in mutation carriers of DNA mismatch repair genes. Int J Cancer 1999; 81:214–218.

136. Vasen HFA, Stormorken A, Menko FH, et al. MSH2 mutation carriers are at a higher risk of cancer than MLH1 mutation carriers a study of hereditary nonpolyposis colorectal cancer families. J Clin Oncol 2001; 19:4074–4080.

137. Jass JR, Smyrk TC, Stewart SM, Lane MR, Lanspa SJ, Lynch HT, Pathology of hereditary non-polyposis colorectal cancer. Anti-cancer Res 1994; 14:1631–1634.

138. Michael-Robinson JM, Biemere-Huttmann A, et al. Tumor in filtratingly mphocytes and apoptosis are independent features in colorectal cancer according to micro satellite instability status Gut 2001; 48:360–366.

139. Young J, Simms LA, Biden KG, et al. Features of colorectal cancers with high-level micro satellite in stability occurring in familial and sporadic settings parallel pathways of tumorigenesis. Am J Pathol 2001; 159:2107–2116.

140. Lynch HT, Smyrk T. Colorectal cancer survival advantage and hereditary nonpolyposis colorectal carcinoma. Gastroenterology 1996; 110:943–947.

141. Sankila R, Aaltonen LA, Järvinen HJ, Mecklin JP. Better survival rates in patients with MLH1-associated hereditary colorectal cancer (see comments). Gastroenterology 1996; 110:682–687.

142. Myrhøj T, Bisgaard ML, Bernstein I, Svendsen LB, Søndergaard JO, Bülow S. Hereditary non-polyposis colorectal cancer clinical features and survival. Results from the Danish HNPCC register. Scand J Gastroenterol 1997; 32:572–576.

143. Watson P, Lin KM, Rodriguez-Bigas MA, et al. Colorectal carcinoma survival among hereditary nonpolyposis colorectal carcinoma family members (see comments) Cancer 1998; 83:259–266.

144. Bertario L, Russo A, Sala P, et al. Survival of patients with hereditary colorectal cancer comparison of HNPCC and colorectal cancer in FAP patients with sporadic colorectal cancer. In J Cancer 1999; 80:183–187.

145. Watson P, Lynch HT. Extra colonic cancer in hereditary nonpolyposis colorectal cancer. Cancer 1993; 71:677–685.

146. Lynch HT, Smyrk T. Hereditary nonpolyposis colorectal cancer (Lynchsyndrome). An updated review. Cancer 1996; 78:1149–1167.

147. Park YJ, Shin KH, Park JG. Risk of gastric cancer in hereditary nonpolyposis colorectal cancer in Korea. Clin Cancer Res 2000; 6:2994–2998.

148. Kim JC, Kim HC, Roh SA, et al. hMLH1 and hMSH2 mutations in families with familial clustering of gastric cancer and hereditary nonpolyposis colorectal cancer. Cancer Detection Prevention. 2001; 25:503–510.

149. Suspiro A, Fidalgo P, Cravo M, Albuquerque C, Ramalho E, Leitão CN, CostaMira F. The Muir-Torre syndrome are variant of hereditary nonpolyposis colorectal cancer associated with hMSH2 mutation. Am J Gastroenterol, 1998; 93:1572–1574.

150. Kruse R, Rütten A, Lamberti C, et al. Muir-Torrepheno type has a frequency of DNA mismatch-repair-gene mutations similar to that in hereditary nonpolyposis colorectal cancer families defined by the Amsterdam criteria Am J Hu Gen, 1998; 63:63–70.

151. Vasen HF, Mecklin JP, Khan PM, Lynch HT. The International Collaborative Group on Hereditary Non-Polyposis Colorectal Cancer (ICG-HNPCC). Dis Colon Rectum 1991; 34:424–425.

152. Wijnen JT, Vasen HF, Khan PM, et al. Clinical findings with implications for genetic testing in families with clustering of colorectal cancer New Eng J Med, 1998; 339:511–518.

153. Syngal S, Fox EA, Li C, Dovidio M, Eng C, Kolodner RD, Garber JE. Interpretation of genetic test results for hereditary nonpolyposis colorectal cancer implications for clinical predisposition testing (see comments). JAMA 1999; 282:247–253.

154. Syngal S, Fox EA, Eng C, Kolodner RD, Garber JE. Sensitivity and specificity of clinical criteria for hereditary non-polyposis colorectal cancer associated mutations in MSH2 and MLH1. J Med Gen 37:641–645.

155. Terdiman JP, Gum JR, Jr, Conrad PG, et al. Efficient detection of hereditary nonpolyposis colorectal cancer gene carriers by screening for tumor micro satellite instability before germ line genetic testing Gastroenterology 2001; 120:21–30.

156. Vasen HF, Watson P, Mecklin JP, Lynch HT. New clinical criteria for hereditary nonpolyposis colorectal cancer (HNPCC Lynch-syndrome) proposed by the International Collaborative group on HNPCC. Gastroenterology 1999; 116:1453–1456.

157. Rodriguez-Bigas MA, Boland CR, et al. National Cancer Institute Workshop on Hereditary Nonpolyposis Colorectal Cancer Syndrome meeting highlights and Bethesda guide lines. J Natl Cancer Inst 1997; 89:1758–1762.

158. Umar A, Boland CR, Terdiman JP, et al. Revised Bethesda Guidelines for hereditary nonpolyposis colorectal cancer (Lynchsyndrome) and microsatellite instability J Natl Cancer Inst 2004; 96:261–268.

159. Cunningham JM, Kim CY, Christensen ER, et al. The frequency of hereditary defective mismatch repair in a prospective series of unselected colorectal carcinomas. Am J Hum Gen 2001; 69:780–790.

160. Leach FS, Nicolaides NC, Papadopoulos N, et al. Mutations of amut Shomolog in hereditary nonpolyposis colorectal cancer Cell, 1993; 75:1215–1225.

161. Papadopoulos N, Nicolaides NC, Wei YF, et al. Mutation of amut Lhomolog in hereditary coloncancer. Science 1994; 263: 1625–1629.

162. Bronner CE, Baker SM, Morrison PT, et al. Mutation in the DNA mismatch repair gene homologue hMLH1 is associated with hereditary non-polyposis colon cancer Nature 1994; 368:258–261.

163. Nicolaides NC, Papadopoulos N, Liu B, et al. Mutations of two PM Shomologues in hereditary nonpolyposis colon cancer Nature, 1994; 371:75–80.

164. Fishel R, Lescoe MK, Rao MR, Copeland NG, Jenkins NA, Garber J, Kane M, Kolodner R. The human mutator genehomolog MSH2 and its association with hereditary nonpolyposis colon cancer. Cell 1994; 77:167.

165. Miyaki M, Konishi M, Tanaka K, et al. Germline mutation of MSH6 as the cause of hereditary nonpolyposis colorectal cancer (letter). Nat Genet 1997; 17:271–272.

166. Peltomäki P, Vasen HF. Mutation spred is posing to hereditary non-polyposis colorectal cancer data base and result so facollaborative study The International Collaborative Group on Hereditary Nonpolyposis Colorectal Cancer. Gastroenterology 1997; 113: 1146–1158.

167. Kolodner RD, Tytell JD, Schmeits JL, et al. Germ-line msh6 mutations in colorectal cancer families. Cancer Res 1999; 59: 5068–5074.

168. Wu Y, Berends MJ, Mensink RG, et al. Association of hereditary nonpolyposis colorectal cancer-related tumors displaying low micro satellite in stability with MSH6 germ linemutations. Am J Hum Gen 1999; 65:1291–1298.

169. Wang Q, Lasset C, Desseigne F, et al. Prevalence of germline mutations of hMLH1 hMSH2 hPMS1 hPMS2 and hMSH6 genes in 75 French kind red swith nonpolyposis colorectal cancer. Human Genetics 1999; 105:79–85.

170. Plaschke J, Kruppa C, Tischler R, et al. Sequence analysis of the mismatch repair gene hMSH6 in the germline of patients with familial and sporadic colorectal cancer. In J Cancer 2000; 85: 606–613.

171. Huang J, Kuismanen SA, Liu T, et al. MSH6 and MSH3 are rarely involved in genetic predis position to nonpolypotic colon cancer. Cancer Res 2001; 61:1619–1623.

172. Wagner A, Hendriks Y, Meijers-Heijboer EJ, et al. Atypical HNPC Cowing to MSH6 germline mutations analysis of a large Dutch pedigree. J Med Genet 2001; 38:318–322.

173. Fishel R. The selection for mismatch repair defect sin hereditary nonpolypos is colorectal cancer syndrome (HNPCC) revising the mutator hypothesis. Cancer Res 2001; 61:7369–7374.

174. Heinen CD, Schmutte C, Fishel R. DNA repair tumorigenesis lessons from hereditary cancer syndromes. Cancer Biol Ther 2002; 1:477–485.

175. Parsons R, Li LGM, Longley MJ, et al. Hypermutability and mismatch repair deficiency in RER+ tumor cells. Cell 1993; 75: 1227–1236.

176. Peltomaki P, Lothe R A, Aaltonen LA, et al. Microsatellite instability is associated with tumors that characterize the hereditary non-polyposis colorectal carcinoma syndrome. Cancer Res 1993; 53: 5853–5855.

177. Aaltonen LA, Peltomaki P, Mecklin JP, et al. Replication errors in benign and malignant tumors from hereditary nonpolyposis colorectal cancer patients. Cancer Res 1994; 54:1645–1648.

178. Dietmaier W, Wallinger S, Bocker T, Kullmann F, Fishel R, Rüschoff J. Diagnostic microsatellite instability definition and correlation with mismatch repair protein expression. Cancer Res 1997; 57:4749–4756.

179. Boland CR, Thibodeau SN, Hamilton SR, et al. National Cancer Institute Workshop on Microsatellite Instability for cancer detection and familial predisposition: development of international criteria for the determination of microsatellite instability in colorectal cancer. Cancer Res 1998; 58:5248–5257.

180. Cawkwell L, Gray S, Murgatroyd H, et al. Choice of management strategy for colorectal cancer based on a diagnostic immunohistochemical test for defective mismatch repair (see comments). Gut 1999; 45:409–415.

181. Salahshor S, Koelble K, Rubio C, Lindblom A. Microsatellite instability and hMLH1 and hMSH2 expression analysis in familial and sporadic colorectal cancer. Lab Invest 2001; 81:535–541.

182. Wahlberg SS, Schmeits J, Thomas G, et al. Evaluation of microsatellite instability and immunohistochemistry for the prediction of germline MSH2 and MLH1 mutations in hereditary nonpolyposis colon cancer families. Cancer Res 2002; 62:3485–3492.

183. Christensen M, Katballe N, Wikman F, et al. Antibody-based screening for hereditary nonpolyposis colorectal carcinoma compared with microsatellite analysis and sequencing. Cancer 2002; 95:2422–2430.

184. Lin KM, Shashidharan M, Thorson AG, et al. Cumulative incidence of colorectal and extracolonic cancers in MLH1 and MSH2 mutation carriers of hereditary nonpolyposis colorectal cancer. J Gastrointest Surg 1988; 2:67–71.

185. Lin KM, Shashidharan M, Ternent CA, et al. Colorectal and extracolonic cancer variations in MLH1/MSH2 hereditary nonpolyposis colorectal cancer kindreds and the general population. Dis Colon Rectum 1988; 41:428–433.

186. Hendriks YM, Wagner A, Morreau H, et al. Cancer risk in hereditary nonpolyposis colorectal cancer due to MSH6 mutations: impact on counseling and surveillance. Gastroenterology 2004; 127:17–25.

187. Ramsey SD, Clarke L, Etzioni R, Higashi M, Berry K, Urban N. Cost-effectiveness of microsatellite instability screening as a method for detecting hereditary nonpolyposis colorectal cancer. Ann Intern Med, 2001; 135:577–588.

188. Burke W, Petersen G, Lynch P, et al. Recommendations for follow-up care of individuals with an inherited predisposition to cancer. I. Hereditary nonpolyposis colon cancer. Cancer Genetics Studies Consortium JAMA, 1997; 277:915–919.

189. de Vos tot Nederveen Cappel WH, Nagengast FM, Griffioen G, Menko F H, Taal BG, Kleibeuker JH, Vasen HF Surveillance for hereditary nonpolyposis colorectal cancer. A long-term study on 114 families. Dis Colon Rectum 2002; 45:1588–1594.

190. Winawer SJ, Fletcher RH, Miller L, et al. Colorectal cancer screening: clinical guidelines and rationale (published erratum appears in Gastroenterology 1997 Mar;112(3):1060). Gastroenterology 1997; 112:594–642.

191. Jarvinen H J, Aarnio M, Mustonen H, et al. Controlled 15-year trial on screening for colorectal cancer in families with hereditary nonpolyposis colorectal cancer. Gastroenterology 2000; 118:829–834.

192. Vasen HF, van Ballegooijen M, Buskens E, et al. A cost-effectiveness analysis of colorectal screening of hereditary nonpolyposis colorectal carcinoma gene carriers. Cancer 1998; 82:1632–1637.

193. Syngal S, Weeks JC, Schrag D, Garber J E, Kuntz KM. Benefits of colonoscopic surveillance and prophylactic colectomy in patients with hereditary nonpolyposis colorectal cancer mutations. Ann Intern Med 1998; 129:787–796.

194. Dove-Edwin I, Boks D, Goff S, et al. The outcome of endometrial carcinoma surveillance by ultrasound scan in women at risk for hereditary nonpolyposis colorectal carcinoma and familial colorectal carcinoma. Cancer 2002; 94:1708–1712.

195. Renkonen-Sinisalo L, Sipponen P, Aarnio M, et al. No support for endoscopic surveillance for gastric cancer in hereditary nonpolyposis colorectal cancer. Scan J Gastroenterol 2002; 37:574–577.

196. Church JM. Prophylactic colectomy in patients with hereditary nonpolyposis colorectal cancer. Ann Med, 1996; 28:479–482.

197. Rodríguez-Bigas MA, Vasen HF, Pekka-Mecklin J, Rectal cancer risk in hereditary nonpolyposis colorectal cancer after abdominal colectomy. International Collaborative Group on HNPCC. Ann Surg 1997; 225:202–207.

198. Lichtenstein P, Holm NV, Verkasalo PK, et al. Environmental and heritable factors in the causation of cancer—analyses of cohorts of twins from Sweden, Denmark, and Finland (see comments). N Engl J Med 2000; 343:78–85.

199. Winawer SJ, Zauber AG, Gerdes H, et al. Risk of colorectal cancer in the families of patients with adenomatous polyps. National Polyp Study Workgroup. N Engl J Med 1996; 334:82–87.

200. Fuchs CS, Giovannucci EL, Colditz GA, Hunter DJ, Speizer FE, Willett WC. A prospective study of family history and the risk of colorectal cancer. N Engl J Med 1994; 331:1669–1674.

201. Sandler RS. Epidemiology and risk factors for colorectal cancer. Gastroenterology. Clin North Am 1996; 25:717–735.

202. Laken SJ, Petersen GM, Gruber SB, et al. Familial colorectal cancer in Ashkenazim due to a hypermutable tract in APC. Nat Genet 1997; 17:79–83.

203. Woodage T, King SM, Wacholder S, et al. The APC I1307K allele and cancer risk in a community-based study of Ashkenazi Jews (see comments). Nat Genet 1998; 20:62–65.

204. Rex DK, Johnson DA, Lieberman DA, Burt RW, Sonnenberg A. Colorectal cancer prevention 2000: screening recommendations of the American College of Gastroenterology. American College of Gastroenterology. Am J Gastroenterol 2000; 95:868–877.

205. US Preventive Services Task Force. Screening for colorectal cancer: recommendation and rationale. Ann Intern Med 2002; 137: 129–131.

206. Petersen GM, Brensinger JD, Johnson KA, Giardiello FM. Genetic testing and counseling for hereditary forms of colorectal cancer. Cancer 1999; 86:2540–2550.

207. Eng C, Hampel H, de la Chapelle A. Genetic testing for cancer predisposition. Annu Rev Med 2001; 52:371–400.

208. Solomon CH, Burt RW. Current status of genetic testing for colorectal cancer susceptibility. Oncology 2002; 16:161–171.

209. Geller G, Botkin JR, Green MJ, Press N, Biesecker BB, Wilfond B, Grana G, Daly MB, Schneider K, Kahn MJ. Genetic testing for susceptibility to adult-onset cancer. The process and content of informed consent (see comments). JAMA 1997; 277:1467–1474.

210. Lerman C, Marshall J, Audrain J, Gomez-Caminero A. Genetic testing for colon cancer susceptibility: Anticipated reactions of patients and challenges to providers. Int J Cancer 1996; 69:58–61.

211. Statement of the American Society of Clinical Oncology: genetic testing for cancer susceptibility, Adopted on February 20, 1996. J Clin Oncol 14: 1730–1736; discussion 1737–1734, 1996.

212. Cromwell DM, Moore RD, Brensinger JD, Petersen GM, Bass EB, Giardiello FM Cost analysis of alternative approaches to colorectal screening in familial adenomatous polyposis. Gastroenterology 1998; 114:893–901.

213. ACMG/ASHG statement. Genetic testing for colon cancer: Joint statement of the American College of Medical Genetics and the American Society of Human Genetics. Genet Med 2000; 2: 362–366.

214. Giardiello FM, Brensinger JD, Petersen GM, Luce MC, Hylind LM, Bacon JA, Booker SV, Parker RD, Hamilton SR. The use and interpretation of commercial APC gene testing for familial adenomatous polyposis (see comments). N Engl J Med 1997; 336:823–827.

215. Giardiello FM. Genetic testing in hereditary colorectal cancer (clinical conference). JAMA 1997; 278:1278–1281.

216. Lamberti C, Kruse R, Ruelfs C, et al. Microsatellite instability—a useful diagnostic tool to select patients at high risk for hereditary non-polyposis colorectal cancer: a study in different groups of patients with colorectal cancer. Gut 1999; 44:839–843.

217. Steinbrecher KA, Mann EA, Giannella RA, Cohen MB. Increases in guanylin and uroguanylin in a mouse model of osmotic diarrhea are guanylate cyclase C-independent. Gastroenterology 2001; 121:1191–1202.

19 Endoscopic Colon Surveillance

Post-Polypectomy, Post-Colorectal Cancer Resection, and Inflammatory Bowel Disease

DOUGLAS B. NELSON, MD AND MANDEEP S. SAWHNEY, MD

CONTENTS

1. INTRODUCTION

Unlike screening, which is defined as the identification of unrecognized or asymptomatic disease in an average-risk population, endoscopic surveillance for colorectal cancer (CRC) is based on the premise that repeated evaluation of a high-risk population will identify patients either with cancer at an earlier, treatable stage, or those who are likely to develop cancer. The purpose of this chapter is to present the recommendations for endoscopic surveillance after colonoscopic polypectomy, CRC resection, and in the setting of inflammatory bowel disease, and to discuss the evidence on which these recommendations are based. Surveillance of these conditions in the setting of an inherited or familial CRC syndrome are not discussed here, but are reviewed in Chapter 18.

2. ENDOSCOPIC SURVEILLANCE AFTER COLONIC POLYPECTOMY

2.1. CURRENT GUIDELINES

2.1.1. American Society for Gastrointestinal Endoscopy (2000)

Surveillance should be tailored to number and type of polyps found. High-risk lesions (>1 cm, villous) should have more frequent surveillance than low-risk (small and tubular) lesions. Surveillance intervals should be individualized, but should be performed approximately every 3–6 yr. Patients with a large sessile polyp should undergo a repeat colonoscopy within 6 mo *(1)*.

2.1.2. American College of Gastroenterology (2003)

Patients at high risk for the development of metachronous adenomas (>2 adenomas, any adenoma <1 cm, villous histology/high-grade dysplasia [HGD], first-degree relative with CRC) should have repeat colonoscopy in 3 yr. Patients at low risk (1–2 tubular adenomas <1 cm, negative family history of CRC) should undergo repeat colonoscopy in 5 yr. After one negative surveillance colonoscopy, intervals should be increased to 5 yr. Large sessile adenomas should undergo repeat colonoscopy in 3–6 mo *(2)*.

2.1.3. US Multi-Society Task Force on Colorectal Cancer (2003)

Patients who have more than three advanced or multiple adenomas should have follow-up colonoscopy in 3 yr. Patients with one or two small (<1 cm) tubular adenomas should have follow-up colonoscopy in 5 yr *(3)*.

2.1.4. American Cancer Society (2003)

Patients with a single, small adenoma should have a repeat colonoscopy in 3–6 yr. Patients with large (>1 cm) adenoma, villous/HGD, or multiple adenomas should have repeat colonoscopy within 3 yr *(4)*.

Although long held to be true, there is now good evidence that endoscopic removal of colonic adenomas prevents the development of colon cancer and decreases mortality *(5–11)*. However, once an adenomatous polyp has been removed, 20–50% of these patients will develop a new (metachronous) adenoma *(2)*. There are a number of clinical issues: What is the optimal interval for subsequent surveillance of adenomas? Are all adenomas alike? We know from numerous colonoscopy screening studies that the prevalence of adenomas in average-risk, asymptomatic individuals over age 50 ranges from 30 to 40% *(12–18)*, yet the incidence of cancer is much lower;

clearly not all adenomas progress into cancer. Are there some clinical or histological features that can predict that patients are at higher risk of developing recurrent adenomas and/or cancer? These questions have led to the concept of the advanced adenoma (those adenomas >1 cm, or that contain villous features or HGD), toward which screening and surveillance strategies are now targeted.

A pair of studies from the Mayo Clinic retrospectively examined the subsequent risk of CRC in a cohort of patients after resection or fulguration of polyps from 1950 to 1969. Patients with polyps less than 1 cm had no increased incidence of cancer compared with the local population (19). However, the relative risk of colon cancer increased to 3.2 for those with polyps greater than 1 cm, and to 5.3 for those with more than one polyp (20). A long-term follow-up study by Atkin et al. of 1618 patients undergoing resection of rectosigmoid polyps reported no increase in the incidence of colon cancer for patients with a single polyp less than 1 cm. The relative risk of cancer increased to 3.6 if the adenoma contained a villous component or was larger than 1 cm, and increased to 6.6 for multiple adenomas. A study of 479 patients by the Polyp Prevention Study Group found that the presence of three or more adenomas, or the presence of villous histology increased the subsequent incidence of adenomas. However, there were no predictors of advanced adenomas (21). Results of the National Polyp Study have provided the best evidence to direct post-polypectomy surveillance intervals. The 1418 study patients were randomized to two surveillance arms after initial polypectomy, with one group receiving colonoscopy at 1 and 3 yr, and the second group undergoing colonoscopy at 3 yr. There was no difference between groups in the number of advanced adenomas found at 3 yr (approx 3%), demonstrating that a 3-yr surveillance interval was as effective as shorter intervals for the detection of clinically significant lesions. Furthermore, the study found that the risk of subsequent adenomas was increased for patients with more than three adenomas, polyps larger than 0.5 cm, or older than 60. The only factor predictive of subsequent advanced adenomas was the presence of more than three adenomas at baseline (22).

Recurring factors in the studies above associated with an increased risk of subsequent adenomas or cancer are polyp multiplicity, polyp size, and the presence of villous histology or HGD. Patients that have one or more of these risk factors are considered "high risk" for recurrence of adenomas, and should undergo surveillance colonoscopy at 3 yr. It has been suggested that patients lacking these risk factors could have surveillance colonoscopy deferred for at least 6 yr (23). Of interest, a computer model created with the National Polyp Study data suggests that the observed reduction in CRC incidence could largely be attributed to the initial effect of polypectomy. For the group as a whole, post-polypectomy surveillance colonoscopy begins to have a perceptible effect on cancer incidence only after 6 yr (24). This is consistent with earlier epidemiological studies suggesting that the protective effect of a single endoscopic screening procedure lasted 6–10 yr (8,11,25). Although there are no randomized, controlled trials comparing even longer surveillance intervals for low-risk

patients, current evidence suggests that 5–6 yr is a reasonable surveillance interval.

3. ENDOSCOPIC SURVEILLANCE FOR MALIGNANT POLYPS

3.1. CURRENT GUIDELINES

3.1.1. American Society for Gastrointestinal Endoscopy (2000)

The management of pedunculated malignant polyps should be individualized depending on the operative risk of the patient. The risk of lymphatic spread is less than the risk of colonic surgery for most patients if the polyp has been completely resected and meets favorable histological criteria (absence of high-grade carcinoma, vascular or lymphatic invasion, or involvement of the resection margin). Resection of the involved bowel is recommended when these criteria are not met, and may be justified in younger patients with good operative risk.

Patients with sessile malignant polyps should usually undergo surgical resection unless contraindicated by the condition of the patient (1).

3.1.2. American College of Gastroenterology (2000)

No further treatment is indicated provided the following criteria are met: complete resection, recovery, and adequate processing; favorable histological criteria (not poorly differentiated; absence of vascular or lymphatic involvement; and absence of margin involvement). For malignant sessile polyps, the area should be reexamined in about 3 mo to check for residual abnormal tissue. After a negative examination, the clinician can revert to standard surveillance (2).

3.1.3. National Comprehensive Cancer Network (2004)

For patients with pedunculated polyp with invasive cancer with unfavorable histological criteria (polypectomy margin <1 mm or not assessable, grades 3–4, or angiolymphatic invasion), colectomy is recommended.

For patients with sessile polyp with invasive cancer, colectomy is recommended (26).

Invasive carcinoma is found in approx 1–5% of all endoscopically resected neoplastic polyps; these are commonly referred to as "malignant polyps," and are something of an intermediate stage in the adenoma–carcinoma sequence (27–42). The most commonly encountered scenario is that after the removal of an often innocuous-appearing polyp, the endoscopist is notified by the pathologist that invasive cancer is present in the specimen. Thus, the first surveillance question is whether polypectomy alone is sufficient, or whether additional surgical resection is required.

The term "malignant polyp" indicates the presence of cancer invading the submucosa of the polyp, and must be distinguished from a polyp with HGD (previously called "carcinoma *in situ*" or "intramucosal carcinoma," terms that should be abandoned because they overstate the cancer risk). Regardless of how advanced these lesions may look, the abnormal cells have not penetrated the muscularis mucosae, and the absence of lymphatics above the level of the muscularis mucosae precludes the risk of lymphatic spread (43). When completely excised, these lesions should be treated like other advanced adenomas, and not as malignant polyps.

Before the advent of fiberoptic colonoscopy in 1969 (44), polyps beyond the reach of the rigid sigmoidoscope that were removed required surgical intervention for access. This could range from a colotomy followed by simple polypectomy (much like that performed during colonoscopy today), a wedge resection, or a formal segmental colectomy. If a colectomy was not performed, and the histology of the polyp revealed an invasive cancer in the polyp, surgeons were faced with the same dilemma facing endoscopists today: is local resection adequate therapy? Does the risk of death from residual disease or lymph node metastasis (which may not occur for several years) exceed the risk of immediate surgical mortality from colectomy (which may still not guarantee cure)? Several early surgical studies noted that in colectomy specimens with malignant polyps, the cancer was confined to the polyp itself and had not spread to regional lymph nodes. This led one center to adopt a policy of local excision for malignant polyps, with favorable results (45). In that study, 3 of the 91 patients with malignant polyps that were locally excised experienced a recurrence. Each of these cases also illustrates the range of possible outcomes when balancing the relative risks of locoregional recurrence and surgery. In the first patient, a local recurrence was diagnosed 5 yr later (raising the possibility that this was a metachronous lesion); the colectomy specimen revealed two involved lymph nodes. This patient was a long-term survivor (23 yr). In the second case, the patient developed multiple lung metastases 2 yr later without evidence of local recurrence, thus it is not clear that an immediate colectomy would have resulted in a different outcome. In the third case, a local recurrence was detected 2 yr later; unfortunately, the patient died postoperatively.

Since the advent of colonoscopic polypectomy, there have been 39 retrospective studies (although some are overlapping publications) that have evaluated the risk of locoregional recurrence from malignant polyps (30–42,46–72). These studies have been quite heterogeneous and are difficult to neatly group together. A major limitation of several of the studies is the inclusion of "focal carcinoma," "intramucosal carcinoma," or "carcinoma in situ," lesions that, as explained earlier, are not invasive cancers. Inclusion of these cases would tend to underestimate the risk of locoregional recurrence. Early studies often do not contain complete information regarding the specific endoscopic and histological criteria (mentioned later) that are now accepted as critical for the determination of metastatic potential. Selection bias might also play a role in those studies reporting results from both endoscopic polypectomy alone, and polypectomy followed by colectomy. As endoscopic polypectomy became more accepted as definitive therapy for selected polyps, it is likely that cases subsequently referred to surgery had subtle characteristics that might indicate a poor outcome. It could be argued that selection bias favors endoscopic polypectomy studies, and we would agree with this assessment. However, this reflects real world practice, in that endoscopic therapy is reserved for optimal cases that meet specified criteria, with the default being colonic resection if there is uncertainty. Although later studies that are restricted solely to endoscopic polypectomy are the most useful for the present discussion, some have

not had a sufficient follow-up period for residual disease or regional/distant metastases to become manifest. The assessment of recurrent disease is also complicated by the development of new, incident CRCs (metachronous) at a rate of approx 0.35% per year (73,74). In other words, after removal of a malignant polyp, is the subsequent detection of a cancer a metachronous lesion or a recurrence?

As alluded to previously, the cumulative experience with endoscopic resection of malignant polyps led to a gradual appreciation of various risk factors that were predictive of a favorable outcome. These generally accepted "favorable" criteria include (1) the endoscopic resection is macroscopically complete; (2) the specimen is submitted in toto, and is adequate for histological analysis; (3) the carcinoma is moderately or well-differentiated; (4) there is no lymphatic or vascular invasion; and (5) the resection margin is "free of carcinoma" (studies have variably defined this as a tumor-free margin ranging from 0 to 2 mm).

Despite these limitations, several reviews have attempted to summarize this body of literature. In the largest review to date, investigators from the Cleveland Clinic reviewed 20 studies comprising 858 malignant polyps, and reported an overall risk of locoregional recurrence after endoscopic resection of a malignant polyp meeting favorable histological criteria of 1% (68). Another review was able to further classify this risk based on polyp morphology and concluded that the risk of recurrence for a pedunculated polyp that met favorable histological criteria was 1%, whereas the risk for a malignant sessile polyp was 4.1% (75). Both of these studies used a similar methodology to arrive at these figures, simply by dividing the number of recurrences with favorable histological criteria by the sum of all the polyps in the series. However, because the denominator included polyps with unfavorable criteria (which should be excluded, just as recurrences with unfavorable criteria were excluded), this would tend to underestimate the risk of recurrence.

It is also of interest to note that, although infrequent, the majority of recurrences in these studies have been associated with malignant rectal polyps (63,69). Although perhaps of limited applicability, there has been debate in the surgical literature regarding the effectiveness of local excision for early rectal cancers. At least one surgical report describes these early cancers as "freely mobile lesions without fixation to the muscular wall," a description that could easily be applied to most malignant polyps (76). Several studies have suggested that the recurrence rate after local excision of early T1 lesions (with histological criteria similar to that used for malignant polyps) ranged from 18 to 24% (77–79). Although this has not been systematically studied regarding endoscopic resection of malignant rectal polyps, it could suggest these lesions may reflect the differential biological behavior of frank cancers in the rectum vs the colon (i.e., higher recurrence and lower cure rates) and might warrant a more aggressive (i.e., surgical) approach.

Although in the presence of favorable histological criteria the risk of locoregional recurrence is low (particularly for pedunculated lesions), it is not zero. Does this mean that endoscopic therapy is inadequate? To answer this question, we must consider the risk of the alternative: elective colectomy. Wilcox and Beck published an elegant decision analysis to answer this question. Their model used as a base case a 50-yr-old individual with a malignant polyp, an operative risk ranging from 0.2 to 2.0%, and a 4.5% rate of residual disease after polypectomy. Under these conditions, the authors concluded that life expectancy was always improved with a subsequent colectomy unless operative mortality exceeded 2% and age over 70 yr *(80)*. However, the results of a decision analysis are heavily dependent on the underlying assumptions, many of which are severely flawed. To predicate the base case on a 50-yr-old individual (the earliest age at which routine colorectal screening would normally be instituted) is not particularly generalizable. In the studies mentioned above, the mean age of patients with malignant polyps ranged from 61 to 69, with most studies clustering around 67 *(37–39,41,42,51,53–56,59–61,63–65,67–71)*. In these studies, operative mortality ranged as high as 8.2% *(41)*. Population-based estimates of operative mortality for colectomy range from 3.5 to 7.5% *(81–86)*, with rates of 1.3–3.3% for those less than age 65. Finally, the estimated rate of residual disease after endoscopic polypectomy of 4.5% does not take into consideration the well-established criteria discussed earlier, resulting in an overall risk of residual disease of 1% with favorable criteria (although arguably the estimated 4.5% recurrence rate might approximate that for malignant sessile polyps). It also assumes that cases with lymph node metastases, but not distant metastases (e.g., hepatic and pulmonary), will uniformly be cured by surgery, which is obviously an overoptimistic assumption.

In summary, the (delayed) risk of death from residual cancer or lymphatic metastasis must be weighed against the risk of immediate surgical mortality from colectomy (which also may not be curative). When favorable criteria are met, the risk of residual (local or regional lymphatic disease) is very low (1%, although likely higher for sessile lesions). The risk of death from surgery is dependent on age and comorbid conditions. On balance, the surgical risk of colectomy for pedunculated malignant polyps with favorable histology exceeds the low risk of residual disease after endoscopic polypectomy. Sessile malignant polyps appear to have a higher risk of residual disease, and surgery may provide a better chance of cure. If endoscopic polypectomy is the sole therapy for a sessile lesion, a repeat examination in 3 mo to evaluate for the presence of residual disease seems prudent. For most patients, however, surgical risk is likely to exceed the chance of residual cancer. The risks and benefits of surgery in addition to polypectomy should be addressed on an individual basis with each patient. The possibility that malignant polyps of the rectum may be potentially higher risk warrants further investigation.

Although there are no studies aimed specifically at follow-up intervals after the resection of a malignant polyp (whether treated by polypectomy alone, or followed by colonic resection), it seems reasonable that they should undergo periodic surveillance for metachronous disease similar to that recommended for other CRCs, which will be discussed in the next section.

4. ENDOSCOPIC SURVEILLANCE AFTER CRC RESECTION

4.1. CURRENT GUIDELINES

4.1.1. British Society of Gastroenterology and the Association of Coloproctology for Great Britain and Ireland (2002)

Colonoscopy 5 yr after surgery (in a "clean" colon), and every 5 yr thereafter until age 70 *(87)*.

4.1.2. European Society for Medical Oncology (2001)

Colonoscopy every 5 yr. Sigmoidoscopy (and endosonography, if available) every 6 mo for 2 yr for patients with distal sigmoid or rectal cancer *(88)*.

4.1.3. British Society for Gastroenterology (2002)

4.1.4. American Society for Gastrointestinal Endoscopy (2000)

After clearing colonoscopy (either pre-operatively or within 1 yr post-operatively), colonoscopy at 3–6 yr *(1)*.

4.1.5. US Multi-Society Task Force on Colorectal Cancer (2003)

After clearing colonoscopy (either pre-operatively or within 1 yr post-operatively), colonoscopy at 3 yr, then every 5 yr *(3)*.

4.1.6. American Society of Clinical Oncology (2000)

After clearing colonoscopy (either pre-operatively or within 1 yr postoperatively), colonoscopy every 3–5 yr. Periodic imaging of the rectum in rectal cancer patients that have not received pelvic radiation is recommend *(89,90)*.

4.1.7. American Society of Colon and Rectal Surgeons (2004)

After clearing colonoscopy or ACBE, colonoscopy every 3 yr. Periodic anastomotic evaluation is recommended after resection of rectal cancer *(91)*.

4.1.8. American Cancer Society (2003)

Colonoscopy at 1 yr, then 3 yr, then every 5 yr *(4)*.

4.1.9. National Comprehensive Cancer Network (2004)

Colonoscopy at 1 yr, repeat in 1 yr if abnormal or every 3 yr if negative *(26)*.

There are essentially three objectives for colon surveillance in patients after the resection of CRC. The first is to detect missed synchronous lesions (both cancers and advanced adenomas). To the extent that all the guidelines recommend a full colonoscopic examination either prior to the resection, or shortly thereafter, this objective is satisfied by all the guidelines. The second objective is to detect metachronous adenomas and cancers, which will occur in up to 50–75% and 10% of patients after resection of CRC, respectively *(92)*. Again, all of the guidelines recommend periodic surveillance that should be adequate for this purpose. The third objective of surveillance in these patients is to detect treatable recurrences. It is this final objective that results in the divergence of the guidelines regarding the need for a follow-up (not clearing) colonoscopy 1 yr after resection. Approximately 30–40% of patients who undergo potentially curative colonic resection will have recurrence of their cancer *(93)*. Several guidelines recommend a colonoscopic examination at 1 yr to detect recurrent disease. To justify this practice, the following questions need to be answered: How often does cancer recur intraluminally, i.e., detectable by colonoscopy? How often is this recurrence asymptomatic (i.e., not detected as a result of symptoms, or other surveillance modality such as fecal occult blood testing [FOBT] or carcinoembryonic antigen [CEA] levels that would result in a colonoscopy?) Once the recurrence is detected, is it amenable to curative resection? Most importantly, does this result in improved patient survival?

Unfortunately, there are no randomized controlled studies specifically evaluating colonoscopy surveillance intervals post-cancer resection. There have been six randomized controlled trials comparing intensive surveillance regimens with "conventional" or "minimal" follow-up, and because these studies have generally included frequent colonoscopy in the treatment arms, these results are worth reviewing. The study by Mäkelä et al. followed 106 patients undergoing resection of CRC with curative intent and randomized them to conventional or intensive follow-up groups. All patients received physical exams, complete blood count, FOBT, CEA, and chest radiographs (CXR) every 3 mo for the first 2 yr, and then every 6 mo for 3 yr (patients with rectosigmoid cancers also received rigid or flexible sigmoidoscopy at these visits). Patients in the conventional group had a barium enema at 3 mo and then yearly, whereas those in the intensive group received colonoscopy at the same intervals. The overall recurrence rate was 41%. There was no difference in 5-yr survival between groups. Of note, anastomotic recurrences occurred in only three patients (2.8%). In each case repeat resection was performed, although it is not clear that this led to any long-term survivors (94).

Ohlsson et al. randomized 107 patients undergoing potentially curative resection to no follow-up or "intense follow-up." Control patients were told to have their local health care provider perform FOBT every 3 mo for 2 yr, then yearly thereafter, as well as a recommendation to contact the surgery department with new symptoms. Those in the intensive group received a physical exam, laboratory testing, FOBT, CXR, and rigid proctosigmoidoscopy every 3 mo for 2 yr, then every 6 mo for 2 yr. Colonoscopy was performed at 3, 15, 30, and 60 mo. Overall tumor recurrence occurred in 35 patients (33%); there were no cases in which colonoscopy was the first modality to detect the recurrence. There was no significant difference in 5-yr survival between groups. Anastomotic recurrences were detected in four patients (3.7%). All four of these patients underwent repeat resection; cancer recurred locally in each (95).

In the largest study to date, Kjeldsen et al. randomized 597 patients to essentially no follow-up or frequent follow-up. Evaluations included a medical history, clinical examination, labs, digital rectal examination, FOBT, CXR, and colonoscopy. Patients in the former group had visits at years 5, 10, and 15, whereas those in the latter had them every 6 mo for the first 5 yr, then at years 10, 12.5, and 15. The recurrence rate (26%), and 5-yr survival rate did not differ between groups (96).

Shoemaker et al. randomized 395 patients to "standard" or "intensive" follow-up. All patients received a clinical examination, complete blood count, liver function tests, CEA, and FOBT every 3 mo for the first 2 yr, then every 6 mo. Patients in the intensive follow-up group also underwent annual CXR,

liver CT, and colonoscopy. The overall recurrence rate was 33%. There was no difference in 5-yr survival between groups. Colonoscopy detected eight recurrences (2%), of which only three were subsequently resected and alive at 5 yr. The intensive arm of the study required an additional 505 colonoscopies and 24 barium enemas to find the single recurrence in the trial without symptoms or other abnormal screening tests (97).

Pietra et al. randomized 207 to "conventional" or "intensive" follow-up groups. Those in the former group were evaluated every 6 mo for the first year, and yearly thereafter, whereas those in the latter group were seen every 3 mo for 2 yr, and yearly thereafter. The evaluations included clinical examination, CEA, and ultrasound. CXR and colonoscopy was performed yearly in both groups. There was a statistically significant improvement in 5-yr survival for those patients followed intensively (73.1 vs 58.3%). However, as there was no difference in the frequency of colonoscopy between groups, it cannot be attributed to endoscopic surveillance. Only two patients (1%) had anastomotic recurrences (98).

Secco et al. stratified 358 patients into either high- or low-recurrence risk groups. Each group was then subsequently randomized into a "risk-adapted" arm, or to minimal follow-up. High-risk patients in the risk-adapted arm received intensive follow-up (which decreased in frequency with time), consisting of frequent physician visits and CEA testing, abdominal and pelvic ultrasonography, CXR, and annual sigmoidoscopy for patients with rectal cancer. Low-risk patients in the risk-adapted arm underwent a similar protocol, although somewhat less frequently than the high-risk group. All patients in the minimal follow-up group (high- and low-risk) were told to contact the surgical team by telephone every 6 mo, with a clinical assessment by their primary care physician yearly (or when symptoms arose). Patients in each arm of the intensive follow-up groups had a statistically significant improvement in 5-yr survival compared with their counterpart arm (risk group) with minimal follow-up (99). It is important to note in this study that neither group (with the exception of rectal cancer patients) underwent scheduled colonoscopy unless indicated by symptoms and signs of recurrence. Again, this suggests that the improvement in mortality is not attributable to endoscopic surveillance (with the possible exception of rectal cancer).

Four meta-analyses have assessed the utility of intensive follow-up after a curative resection for CRC. The meta-analysis by Bruinvels et al. incorporated seven nonrandomized studies comprising 3283 patients, and found no significant improvement in 5-yr survival for patients undergoing intensive follow-up (usually incorporating frequent clinical, laboratory, radiological, and endoscopic surveillance). However, when only those studies incorporating a CEA assay were included, a survival benefit emerged (100). A meta-analysis by Rosen et al. subsequently evaluated 19 studies (again, largely comprised of nonrandomized studies) that included CEA monitoring and found a 16% improvement in 5-yr survival (101). Two subsequent meta-analyses restricted to the randomized controlled trials discussed previously both found a statistically significant improvement in 5-yr survival with intensive follow-up, ranging from 7 to 13%. Both studies largely attributed this survival benefit to CEA monitoring and hepatic imaging (102,103).

In summary, the main benefit of colonoscopic surveillance after curative resection for CRC is in the prevention and detection of metachronous lesions, rather than the detection of recurrences. In recognition of this evidence, the American Society of Colon and Rectal Surgeons no longer recommends a colonoscopy at 1 yr after resection (assuming that the colon was completely visualized either pre- or perioperatively) (91,104). The literature suggests that true anastomotic recurrences are very rare. Local recurrence typically represents extraluminal disease invading the lumen of the bowel, and often carries a poor prognosis. When cancer recurs after surgical resection for curative intent, there are virtually always other clinical or laboratory abnormalities that would predict this before colonoscopy. Although meta-analyses have suggested that intensive follow-up may result in a small prolongation in 5-yr survival, this has not been attributable to colonoscopy (and is likely a result of serial CEA testing and liver imaging). Together, these data do not support more intensive endoscopic surveillance than would otherwise be justified for detection of metachronous neoplasia.

4.2. RECTAL CANCER

There is a general consensus of opinion in the surgical literature that rectal cancer (defined as <12 cm from the anal verge) has a higher risk of recurrence, lower overall survival, and higher mortality after recurrence than comparably staged tumors of the colon (defined as >12 cm from the anal verge) (105,106). Because of the dismal prognosis after recurrence (5-yr mortality ranging as high as 96–98%) (107), and the fact that most recurrences appear within 2–3 yr, it is tempting to speculate that earlier diagnosis and treatment might lead to better outcomes. Guidelines from the European Society for Medical Oncology, the American Society of Clinical Oncology, and the American Society of Colon and Rectal Surgeons specifically recommend periodic surveillance of the anastomosis after resection of rectal carcinoma (88–90,108). However, there are few data that specifically address the utility of this surveillance. The studies discussed in the preceding section have tended to group both colon and rectal cancers together, and thus do not directly address this issue. A retrospective study by Secco et al. in contrast to their findings for CRC in general, failed to find improved survival with intensive surveillance after resection of rectal cancer (107).

Endoscopic ultrasound has emerged as a promising imaging modality for the early detection of local recurrence of rectal cancer. The advantage of endoscopic ultrasonography over conventional endoscopy is the ability to assess extraluminal disease. Although a number of studies have demonstrated that endoscopic ultrasound can detect early asymptomatic recurrences, allowing potentially curative surgery (109–114), one prospective study was unable to demonstrate an improvement in the rate of salvage surgery or survival (115). Prospective, randomized controlled trials specifically looking at surveillance modalities after rectal cancer resection are needed.

5. COLON CANCER SURVEILLANCE IN INFLAMMATORY BOWEL DISEASE

5.1. CURRENT GUIDELINES

5.1.1. British Society of Gastroenterology and the Association of Coloproctology for Great Britain and Ireland (2002)

- Regular surveillance should begin after 8–10 yr for pancolitis, and after 15–20 yr for left-sided disease.
- Screening intervals should decrease with increasing disease duration. For patients with pancolitis, colonoscopy should be conducted every 3 yr in the second decade of disease, every 2 yr in the third decade, and yearly by the fourth decade.
- Two to four random biopsy specimens should be taken every 10 cm, with additional samples of suspicious areas.
- Patients with primary sclerosing cholangitis (PSC) should undergo annual colonoscopy (116).

5.1.2. American Society for Gastrointestinal Endoscopy (2000)

- Individuals with long-standing ulcerative colitis (UC) or Crohn's colitis (pancolitis >8 yr or left-sided colitis >15 yr) should undergo surveillance with systematic biopsies every 1–3 yr.
- Adenomas located outside the segment of UC, or in the absence of dysplasia in the surrounding mucosa can be managed the same as adenomas found in patients without UC (1).

5.1.3. American Cancer Society (2003)

- For patients with UC or Crohn's disease (CD), colonoscopic surveillance with biopsies should begin 8 yr after the onset of pancolitis, or 12–15 yr after the onset of left-sided colitis (4).

5.1.4. US Multi-Society Task Force on Colorectal Cancer (2003)

- In patients with long-standing, extensive inflammatory bowel disease (UC and Crohn's colitis), surveillance colonoscopy with systematic biopsies should be considered. All patients should have surveillance colonoscopy beginning with 8–10 yr of disease. Biopsy specimens should be taken every 10 cm in all four quadrants.
- Patients with HGD or multifocal low-grade dysplasia (LGD) should be advised to undergo colectomy.
- Polyps can be removed by polypectomy with biopsy of adjacent flat mucosa to determine if dysplasia is present. A dysplasia-associated lesion or mass (DALM) is an indication for colectomy (3).

5.1.5. American College of Gastroenterology (2004)

- After 8–10 yr of colitis, annual, or biannual surveillance colonoscopy with multiple biopsies at regular intervals should be performed. The finding of HGD is an absolute indication, and LGD in flat mucosa a relative indication for colectomy.
- It is prudent to start colonoscopic surveillance as soon as co-existing diagnoses of UC and PSC are established.

• Colectomy is advisable for the finding of LGD in a mass lesion, or a stricture that is symptomatic/impassable during colonoscopy.

6. RISK OF CRC IN UC

There is general agreement that patients with long-standing UC are at increased risk for developing CRC, and develop cancer at an earlier age than the general population. Although there have been numerous studies examining this subject, the magnitude of this risk remains controversial. Some early studies reporting very high rates of cancer development were criticized because of highly selected patient populations with severe disease that were more likely to develop cancer, and also included patients referred specifically with the diagnosis of established cancer (117). Other studies with very low rates of cancer had substantial rates of colectomy, in effect censoring those patients that might be most likely to develop cancer (118–120). The best estimate is probably derived from a meta-analysis of 41 studies, which estimated a cumulative probability of developing cancer of 2% at 10 yr, 8% at 20 yr, and 18% at 30 yr (121).

Duration, extent of disease at diagnosis, and age at onset of disease are established risk factors for cancer (122). Development of cancer is unusual within the first decade of disease onset. After the first decade, cancer risk increases by 0.5 to 1% per year (123,124). Patients with pancolitis, defined as disease proximal to the hepatic flexure, are at the highest risk for cancer, whereas those with proctitis, defined as disease limited to the rectum, do not appear to be at any increased risk. Left-sided colitis appears to carry an intermediate risk, and is delayed approx 10 yr later than in patients with pancolitis (125). The standardized incidence ratio for risk of CRC is 1.7 (95% CI 0.8–3.2) for patients with proctitis, 2.8 (95% CI 1.6–4.4) for patients with disease extending to the hepatic flexure and 14.8 (95% CI 11.4–18.9) for patients with disease involving the entire colon (126). Younger age at onset of disease also increases the age-specific risk of cancer, independent of duration of disease (126). Other factors that have been associated with an increased risk of CRC include PSC (127–129), disease severity (130), a family history of sporadic colon cancer (131,132), and the presence of backwash ileitis (133). It is possible that these risk factors could be used to identify subgroups that might benefit from more intensive surveillance.

However, before discussing the specifics of endoscopic surveillance in long-standing UC, it is important to discuss the surgical alternative of prophylactic colectomy. Whereas there is indirect evidence suggesting a benefit of endoscopic surveillance for preventing CRC mortality (120,132), it is important to note that this has never been demonstrated with a randomized, controlled trial (and as has been discussed by numerous authors, for logistic and ethical reasons it is unlikely that one will ever be done). A decision analysis by Provenzale et al. found that prophylactic colectomy offered a greater improvement in survival than endoscopic surveillance (134). Proponents of colectomy justifiably point out that actual practices of surveillance colonoscopy vary widely in the community (135,136), which, along with patient compli-

ance, may have an impact on the efficacy of surveillance. Furthermore, variation in the diagnosis of dysplasia, the current basis of endoscopic surveillance, is substantial (even among experts) (137,138). Finally, endoscopic surveillance is imperfect; patients under endoscopic surveillance programs can develop CRC (139), which might otherwise have been prevented with a prophylactic colectomy. In fact, in studies with a relatively high rate of colectomy, mortality rates from CRC are similar to the general population (119,120). The surgery currently performed for UC, an ileal pouch with anal anastomosis, avoids the need for a permanent ostomy with good functional results (140). It is the authors' practice to discuss prophylactic colectomy as a reasonable alternative with patients before embarking on a program of endoscopic surveillance (although admittedly, few patients have chosen the surgical option). It is also important that patients understand the goal of endoscopic surveillance, and they should be willing to undergo colectomy should there be a positive finding, i.e., the risk and expense of surveillance is not warranted if it will not ultimately alter management.

6.1. COLONOSCOPIC SURVEILLANCE

Unlike most sporadic colorectal carcinomas, whose development involves sequential mutations of numerous genes involved with epithelial proliferation and differentiation and progresses slowly from adenomatous polyps to cancer over a period of years, the development of cancer in patients with UC is believed to arise more rapidly in a background of flat mucosal dysplasia (141). Thus dysplasia is the marker currently used during colonic surveillance to identify patients with an increased risk of either having or soon developing CRC. Dysplasia is defined as an unequivocal neoplastic alteration of the colonic epithelium that remains confined to the basement membrane of the gland within which it arose (142). Some confusion might arise because this also defines the histology of sporadic adenomatous polyps in noncolitic patients (which can also arise in UC patients, most of which have a far less ominous prognosis, and will be discussed in greater detail later).

All patients should undergo at least one colonoscopy after 8–10 yr of disease onset to accurately determine the extent of disease. It has been common practice, supported by most of the guidelines, to begin a surveillance program after 8–10 yr in patients with pancolitis, and after 12–15 yr for those with left-sided colitis. One organization has recommended that all patients should begin a surveillance program after 8–10 yr, regardless of the extent of disease. There is good evidence, however, to support a differential risk of CRC development based on the extent of disease (125,126,143,144). Furthermore, the cost-effectiveness of endoscopic surveillance in ulcerative pan-colitis drops precipitously as screening intervals decrease to the levels generally advocated in the guidelines (145). Although the overall cost-effectiveness may be similar to other accepted health practices, such as cervical cancer screening, it does not meet the generally accepted benchmark for a cost-effective practice (<$50,000/life/year saved). Thus, to recommend earlier surveillance of left-sided colitis does not appear to be justified.

There is more variability in recommendations for surveillance intervals. Because the risk of cancer increases with duration of disease, most experts suggest intervals of every 1 to 2 yr (with an implicit recommendation leaning toward annual surveillance in later stages of the disease). Another common strategy based on the progressive increase in cancer risk over time, formalized in the guidelines by Eaden and Mayberry (116), recommend progressively decreasing surveillance intervals with time (initially every 3 yr, dropping to biennial and finally annual surveillance with time).

6.2. SPECIFIC MANAGEMENT ISSUES: BIOPSY TECHNIQUE/RESULTS

Surveillance is best performed during disease remission to eliminate the difficulty of differentiating reactive inflammatory changes from dysplasia. Careful examination of the entire colonic mucosa should be performed. Random biopsies should be obtained in four quadrants at 10-cm intervals, as well as of suspicious areas (e.g., elevated lesions, irregular surfaces, strictures, and so on). It has been estimated that 33 biopsy specimens are needed to detect dysplasia (not cancer) with 90% confidence (146). Studies have reported that the majority of cancers associated with UC arise in the rectum and sigmoid colon. Based on this, it has been proposed that more frequent biopsies be taken from the recto-sigmoid (147).

According to a widely accepted classification, biopsy specimens are categorized as negative, indefinite, or positive for dysplasia (142). The negative category includes all inflammatory and regenerative lesions. The indefinite category is applied to epithelial changes that appear to exceed the limits of ordinary regeneration but are insufficient for an unequivocal diagnosis of dysplasia or are associated with other features that prevent such unequivocal diagnosis. The positive category is divided into two subcategories: HGD and LGD. LGD corresponds to histopathological findings that were previously classified as mild or moderate dysplasia. In general, it is desirable that the finding of dysplasia be confirmed by a second experienced pathologist.

This diagnosis of "indefinite for dysplasia" is usually made by pathologists when the concomitant presence of inflammation does not allow for a definitive alternative diagnosis. In such situations, the management of colitis should be optimized to reduce inflammation, and the patient should then undergo repeat colonoscopy with surveillance biopsies in 3–6 mo. In a study of 51 patients who were indefinite of dysplasia on initial colonoscopy, 9 (18%) were later found to have HGD, DALM, or cancer (137). Therefore, patients with this diagnosis warrant heightened surveillance.

There is uniform consensus amongst experts and the various guidelines that patients with HGD should undergo colectomy. These recommendations are based on the observation that a significant number of patients with HGD were in fact found to have unsuspected invasive cancer at colectomy, ranging from 42 to 67% (137,148).

The optimal management of LGD remains controversial, largely because of the debate regarding the predictive value of LGD for advanced pathology. In general there has been a shift towards recommending colectomy for patients diagnosed with LGD, even if found in a single biopsy specimen. Proponents of this position point to a meta-analysis published in 1994 by Bernstein et al. Ten studies comprising 1225 patients were selected for analysis. Of the 69 patients with LGD on initial colonoscopy, 29% progressed to HGD, DALM, or cancer. Of the seven cancers diagnosed in the group, two were Duke's stage B and two were Duke's stage C (data on other patients is not available). Of the 1225 patients, 210 (17%) developed LGD at some point during surveillance. Of these, 17 (8%) progressed to cancer (137). Another center reviewed their experience with 46 UC patients diagnosed with flat LGD. In all, 7 out of 46 patients (15%) developed colon cancer, of which 5 were stage II or higher. On an actuarial basis, the authors calculated the rate of neoplastic progression for LGD to be 53% at 5 yr (149). The high rate of progression over the short follow-up period of these studies have led many (including the authors) to conclude that LGD should be treated with the same degree of concern as HGD.

An alternative strategy is to follow patients with LGD with intensive colonoscopic surveillance every 6 mo, and recommend colectomy only if progression to HGD or cancer is detected. Two studies support this approach. The first followed 60 patients with chronic colitis and LGD for a mean of 10 yr (range 1–22 yr). Only 2 of 60 patients (3.3%) progressed to advanced neoplasia. Both of these patients developed DALMs with HGD, underwent colectomy, and were cancer-free at 2 and 4 yr, respectively (150). In the second study, Lim et al. were able to trace 126 of 128 patients (with intact colons) who had participated in an earlier colonoscopy surveillance study. They identified 29 patients with LGD, and 97 patients without dysplasia served as controls. Out of 29 patients with LGD, 3 (10%) and 4 of 97 (4%) controls had developed colon cancer or HGD. Kaplan–Meier analysis from 1991 to death or colectomy showed no statistically significant difference between the two groups (log rank test $p = 0.63$). However, this may simply be an underpowered study. Patients who are reluctant to undergo surgery should be made aware of their increased risk for carcinoma and undergo more intensive surveillance as outlined earlier.

6.3. MANAGEMENT OF POLYPS

In the setting of UC, dysplasia can be either characterized as flat (endoscopically invisible but detected in a mucosal biopsy specimen) or raised (endoscopically visible) in which case it is generally termed DALM (151). The term DALM was first used by Blackstone and colleagues in a paper published in 1981 (152). They reported 12 patients with chronic UC and one or more mass lesions in the colon. Multiple surface biopsies of the lesions showed dysplasia without evidence of cancer. At colectomy, 7 of 12 (58%) patients were found to have an invasive cancer. A number of subsequent publications have confirmed the high association of DALM with invasive cancer, again underscoring the fact that even though a large percentage of these mass lesions are already malignant, biopsy specimens obtained from the surface reveal only dysplasia (153,154). DALM is therefore considered a strong indication for colectomy.

Unfortunately, patients with UC are not protected from developing sporadic colorectal adenomas. The dilemma faced by endoscopists is not how to manage patients with DALM, but how to differentiate a DALM from a sporadic adenoma. Sporadic adenomas are by definition polypoid dysplastic lesions. They are common findings at colonoscopy in average-risk, non-UC individuals, with a prevalence estimate as high as 30–40% in patients over the age of 50 *(16)*. Although adenomatous polyps are potentially premalignant, it is widely accepted that they can be removed definitively by colonoscopy *(7)*. In contrast to DALM, surgery for sporadic adenoma is reserved for those rare situations in which a polyp cannot be resected endoscopically. Despite the difference in the approach, the two lesions can be indistinguishable pathologically and must therefore be differentiated largely on clinical grounds. Are there any criteria that can help the endoscopist discern when a protuberant mass belongs to the DALM category (a cause for alarm and a strong indication for colectomy) or when it should be considered "simply a run of the mill sporadic adenoma" (can be adequately treated with endoscopic polypectomy)? The literature addressing this important distinction is based on relatively small case series. The Lahey clinic reported on five patients with UC and pedunculated polyps. No associated flat dysplasia was noted in the remainder of the colon. All polyps were resected endoscopically and patients were cancer-free at a follow-up of 3–11 yr *(155)*. In another study of eight patients with adenomatous lesions, multiple biopsies were obtained from the adjacent mucosa. In three patients, dysplasia was present in the adjacent mucosa and all patients were eventually developed cancer. Five patients without adjacent dysplasia underwent polypectomy and were cancer free at a 2- to 13-yr follow-up *(148)*. Suzuki et al. from Japan divided 27 patients with dysplastic mass lesions in two groups based on the presence of adjacent flat dysplasia (DALM). Out of 16 patients, 9 pre-operatively classified as DALMs were found to have an invasive cancer; 2 of 11 patients originally classified as adenomas were later found to have DALM, highlighting the difficult of differentiating between these two lesions *(156)*. Using the same definition, Engelsgjerd et al. identified 24 patients with UC and adenomas within the diseased segment of the colon. All patients underwent colonoscopic polypectomy and at a mean follow-up of 3.5 yr no patient had progressed to cancer. The authors also reported on 10 patients with adenomas outside of the colitic segment of the colon. These patients were also treated with colonoscopic polypectomy and did not develop cancer *(157)*. Rubin et al. reported their data on 48 patients with 70 dysplastic polyps without associated flat dysplasia, all of whom underwent colonoscopic polypectomy. Patients with polypectomy specimens still positive for dysplasia underwent repeat surveillance colonoscopy every 2–6 mo until all dysplasia was eradicated. At an average follow-up of 4.1 yr, no cancer was found. An additional 10 patients with polyps outside the colitic segment were also successfully treated endoscopically *(158)*. Based on the above data it has been suggested that for pedunculated polyps within the area of chronic colitis, and for all polyps outside the area of colitis, a simple polypectomy with close

follow-up is adequate therapy *(159)*. Sessile polyps within the area of chronic colitis require a more cautious approach. For these lesions, it may be reasonable to perform a colonoscopic polypectomy and extensive biopsies of the adjacent mucosa. If biopsies from the surrounding mucosa show any degree of dysplasia, the lesion is likely to be a DALM and colectomy is recommended. If no dysplasia is found and the polyp has been completely resected, patients need not undergo a colectomy. It is, however, imperative that these patients be carefully followed with repeat surveillance colonoscopy.

6.4. SURVEILLANCE FOR PATIENTS WITH CD

There is growing evidence that the tumor biology of CRC associated with CD is similar to that of UC *(160,161)*. Further, large and small bowel cancers in patients with CD are associated with dysplasia in the adjacent mucosa, suggesting a similar dysplasia–carcinoma sequence *(162)*. Numerous studies have concluded that patients with CD are also at an increased risk for developing CRC *(163–167)*. The majority of cancers associated with CD have been reported in patients with endoscopically apparent colonic involvement; those with disease limited to the small bowel do not appear to be at an increased risk. As with UC, the duration and extent of colonic involvement affects cancer risk; patients with longstanding, extensive colitis are at highest risk *(165)*. Although most of the data on which guidelines for surveillance in inflammatory bowel disease are based derive from the UC literature, because the risk of CRC is similar, most guidelines suggest that surveillance recommendations apply equally to patients with extensive Crohn's colitis *(1,3,4,116)*. One center, reporting their experience with surveillance colonoscopy in 259 patients with extensive, long-standing Crohn's colitis, found that the yield for neoplasia was comparable to that found in UC *(168)*.

7. CONCLUSION

Recommendations from various professional organizations vary widely for recommended surveillance intervals after polypectomy, CRC resection, and in the setting of inflammatory bowel disease. The evidence best supports the following surveillance practices. For post-polypectomy surveillance, patients with more than three advanced or multiple adenomas should have follow-up colonoscopy in 3 yr, whereas those with two or fewer tubular adenomas should be followed up in 5 yr. After the resection of a malignant polyp, the risk of surgery must be weighed against the likelihood of residual disease. For malignant pedunculated polyps, unless the patient is a young, optimal surgical candidate, polypectomy is likely sufficient. For those with malignant sessile polyps, the decision for surgery should be individualized. After curative CRC resection (assuming that the entire colon has been visualized pre-or postoperatively to rule out synchronous disease), the patient should undergo surveillance for metachronous neoplasms at 3 yr, and every 5 yr thereafter (subject to the findings at colonoscopy that might mandate a shorter interval). Finally, in the setting of longstanding colitis from either UC or CD, colectomy should be discussed with patients as an alternative to surveillance. Surveillance should be initiated after eight years of pancolitis, or 15 yr of left-sided colitis, and should comprise four quadrant biopsies at 10-cm intervals. The finding of flat dysplasia, whether low- or high-grade, or a DALM, should prompt a recommendation for colectomy. Finally, polypectomy appears to be adequate for adenomatous polyps outside the area of colitis, or within the colitic segment if not associated with surrounding flat dysplasia, although close follow-up is recommended.

REFERENCES

1. Eisen G, Chutkan R, Goldstein JL, et al. ASGE Guidelines for colorectal cancer screening and surveillance. Gastrointest Endosc 2000; 51:777–782.
2. Bond JH. Polyp guideline: diagnosis, treatment, and surveillance for patients with colorectal polyps. Am J Gastroenterol 2000; 95:3053–3063.
3. Winawer S, Fletcher R, Rex D, et al. Colorectal cancer screening and surveillance: clinical guidelines and rationale-update based on new evidence. Gastroenterology 2003; 124:544–560.
4. Smith RA, Cokkinides V, Eyre HJ. American Cancer Society guidelines for the early detection of cancer, 2003. CA Cancer J Clin 2003; 53:27–43.
5. Gilbertsen VA, Nelms JM. The prevention of invasive cancer of the rectum. Cancer 1978; 41:1137–1139.
6. Murakami R, Tsukuma H, Kanamori S, et al. Natural history of colorectal polyps and the effect of polypectomy on occurrence of subsequent cancer. Int J Cancer 1990; 46:159–164.
7. Winawer SJ, Zauber AG, Ho MN, et al. Prevention of colorectal cancer by colonoscopic polypectomy. N Engl J Med 1993; 329:1977–1981.
8. Müller AD, Sonnenberg A. Prevention of colorectal cancer by flexible endoscopy and polypectomy. Ann Intern Med 1995; 123:904–910.
9. Inadomi JM, Sonnenberg A. The impact of colorectal cancer screening on life expectancy. Gastrointest Endosc 2000; 51:517–523.
10. Citarda F, Tomaselli G, Capocaccia R, Barcherini S, Crespi M, Group TIMS. Efficacy in standard clinical practice of colonoscopic polypectomy in reducing colorectal cancer incidence. Gut 2001; 48:812–815.
11. Brenner H, Arndt V, Stürmer T, Stegmaier C, Ziegler H, Dhom G. Long-lasting reduction of risk of colorectal cancer following screening endoscopy. Br J Cancer 2001; 85:972–978.
12. Lieberman DA, Smith FW. Screening for colon malignancy with colonoscopy. Am J Gastroenterol 1991; 86:946–951.
13. DiSario JA, Foutch PG, Mai HD, Pardy K, Manne RK. Prevalence and malignant potential of colorectal polyps in asymptomatic, average-risk men. Am J Gastroenterol 1991; 86:941–945.
14. Rex DK, Lehman GA, Ulbright TM, et al. Colonic neoplasia in asymptomatic persons with negative fecal occult blood tests: influence of age, gender, and family history. Am J Gastroenterol 1993; 88:825–831.
15. Rogge JD, Elmore MF, Mahoney SJ, et al. Low-cost, office-based, screening colonoscopy. Am J Gastroenterol 1994; 89:1775–1780.
16. Lieberman DA, Weiss DG, Bond JH, et al. Use of colonoscopy to screen asymptomatic adults for colorectal cancer. N Engl J Med 2000; 343:162–168.
17. Mehran A, Jaffe P, Efron J, Vernavay A, Liberman A. Screening colonoscopy in the asymptomatic 50- to 59-year-old population. Surg Endosc 2003; 17:1974–1977.
18. Betés M, Muñoz-Navas MA, Duque JM, et al. Use of colonoscopy as a primary screening test for colorectal cancer in average risk people. Am J Gastroenterol 2003; 98:2648–2654.
19. Spencer RJ, Melton LJ, Ready RL, Ilstrup DM. Treatment of small colorectal polyps: a population-based study of the risk of subsequent carcinoma. Mayo Clin Proc 1984; 59:305–310.
20. Lotfi AM, Spencer RJ, Ilstrup DM, Melton LJ. Colorectal polyps and the risk of subsequent carcinoma. Mayo Clin Proc 1986; 61:337–343.
21. Van Stolk RU, Beck GJ, Baron JA, Haile R, Summers R. Adenoma characteristics at first colonoscopy as predictors of adenoma recurrence and characteristics at follow-up. Gastroenterology 1998; 115:12–18.
22. Winawer SJ, Zauber AG, O'Brien MJ, et al. Randomized comparison of surveillance intervals after colonoscopic removal of newly diagnosed adenomatous polyps. N Engl J Med 1993; 328:901–906.
23. Zauber AG, Winawer SJ. Initial management and follow-up surveillance of patients with colorectal adenomas. Gastroenterol Clin North Am 1997; 26:85–101.
24. Zauber AG, Winawer SJ, Loeve F, Boer R, Habbema D. Effect of initial polypectomy versus surveillance polypectomy on colorectal cancer incidence reduction: micro-simulation modeling of National Polyp Study data. Gastroenterology 2000; 118:A187.
25. Selby JV, Friedman GD, Quesenberry CP, Weiss NS. A case–control study of screening sigmoidoscopy and mortality from colorectal cancer. N Engl J Med 1992; 326:653–657.
26. Engstrom PF, Benson III AB, Choti MA, et al. Colon Cancer: version 2.2004. Available at: http://www.nccn.org/professionals/physician_gls/PDF/colon.pdf. Accessed June 8, 2004.
27. Grinnell RS, Lane N. Benign and malignant adenomatous polyps and papillary adenomas of the colon and rectum. An analysis of 1,856 tumors in 1,335 patients. International Abstracts of Surgery 1958; 106:519–538.
28. Enterline HT, Evans GW, Mercado-Lugo R, Miller L, Fitts Jr WT. Malignant potential of adenomas of colon and rectum. JAMA 1962; 179:322–330.
29. Kurzon RM, Ortega R, Rywlin AM. The significance of papillary features in polyps of the large intestine. Am J Clin Pathol 1974; 62:447–454.
30. Wolff WI, Shinya H. Definitive treatment of "malignant" polyps of the colon. Ann Surg 1975; 182:516–525.
31. Nivatvongs S, Goldberg S. Management of patients who have polyps containing invasive carcinoma removed via colonoscope. Dis Colon Rectum 1978; 21:8–11.
32. Coutsoftides T, Sivak Jr. MV, Benjamin SP, Jagelman D. Colonoscopy and the management of polyps containing invasive carcinoma. Ann Surg 1978; 188:638–641.
33. Colacchio TA, Forde KA, Scantlebury VP. Endoscopic polypectomy: inadequate treatment for invasive colorectal carcinoma. Ann Surg 1981; 194:704–707.
34. Kodaira S, Ono S, Puri P, et al. Endoscopic polypectomy of the large bowel: management of cancer-bearing polyps. Int Surg 1981; 66:311–314.
35. Rossini FP, Ferrari A, Spandre M, Coverlizza S. Colonoscopic polypectomy in diagnosis and management of cancerous adenomas: an individual and multicentric experience. Endoscopy 1982; 14:124–127.
36. Bartnik W, Butruk E, Orlowska J. A conservative approach to adenomas containing invasive carcinoma removed colonoscopically. Dis Colon Rectum 1985; 28:673–675.
37. Cranley JP, Petras RE, Carey WD, Paradis K, Sivak Jr. MV. When is endoscopic polypectomy adequate therapy for colonic polyps containing invasive carcinoma? Gastroenterology 1986; 91:419–427.
38. Eckardt VF, Fuchs M, Kanzler G, Remmele W, Stienen U. Follow-up of patients with colonic polyps containing severe atypia and invasive carcinoma: compliance, recurrence, and survival. Cancer 1988; 61:2552–2557.
39. Rossini FP, Ferrari A, Coverlizza S, et al. Large bowel adenomas containing carcinoma—a diagnostic and therapeutic approach. Int J Colorect Dis 1988; 3:47–52.
40. Muto T, Sawada T, Sugihara K. Treatment of carcinoma in adenomas. World J Surg 1991; 15:35–40.
41. Chantereau MJ, Faivre J, Boutron MC, et al. Epidemiology, management, and prognosis of malignant large bowel polyps within a defined population. Gut 1992; 33:259–263.
42. Whitlow C, Gathright Jr. JB, Hebert SJ, et al. Long-term survival after treatment of malignant colonic polyps. Dis Colon Rectum 1997; 40.
43. Fenoglio C, Kaye GI, Lane N. Distribution of human colonic lymphatics in normal, hyperplastic, and adenomatous tissue. Gastroenterology 1973; 64:51–66.

44. Wolff WI, Shinya H. Polypectomy via the fiberoptic colonoscope. N Engl J Med 1973; 288:329–332.

45. Morson BC, Bussey HJR, Samoorian S. Policy of local excision for early cancer of the colorectum. Gut 1977; 18:1045–1050.

46. Cooper HS. Surgical pathology of endoscopically removed malignant polyps of the colon and rectum. Am J Surg Pathol 1983; 7:613–623.

47. Lipper S, Kahn LB, Ackerman LV. The significance of microscopic invasive cancer in endoscopically removed polyps of the large bowel: a clinicopathologic study of 51 cases. Cancer 1983; 52.

48. Christie JP. Malignant colon polyps—cure by colonoscopy or colectomy? Am J Gastroenterol 1984; 79:543–547.

49. Fried GM, Hreno A, Duguid WM, Hampson LG. Rational management of malignant colon polyps based on long-term follow-up. Surgery 1984; 96:815–821.

50. Langer JC, Cohen Z, Taylor BR, Stafford S, Jeejeebhoy KN, Cullen JB. Management of patients with polyps containing malignancy removed by colonoscopic polypectomy. Dis Colon Rectum 1984; 27:6–9.

51. Morson BC, Whiteway JE, Jones EA, Macrae FA, Williams CB. Histopathology and prognosis of malignant colorectal polyps treated by endoscopic polypectomy. Gut 1984; 25:437–444.

52. Haggitt RC, Glotzbach RE, Soffer EE, Wruble LD. Prognostic factors in colorectal carcinomas arising in adenomas: implications for lesions removed by endoscopic polypectomy. Gastroenterology 1985; 89:328–336.

53. Fucini C, Wolff BG, Spencer RJ. An appraisal of endoscopic removal of malignant colonic polyps. Mayo Clin Proc 1986; 61:123–126.

54. Conte CC, Welch JP, Tennant R, Forouhar F, Lundy J, Bloom GP. Management of endoscopically removed malignant colon polyps. J Surg Oncol 1987; 36:116–121.

55. Richards WO, Webb WA, Morris SJ, et al. Patient management after endoscopic removal of the cancerous colon adenoma. Ann Surg 1987; 205:665–670.

56. Speroni AH, Meiss RP, Calzona C, et al. Early colorectal cancer: followup after endoscopic polypectomy. Endoscopy 1988.

57. Christie JP. Polypectomy or colectomy? Management of 106 consecutively encountered colorectal polyps. Am Surg 1988; 54:93–99.

58. Muller S, Chesner IM, Egan MJ, et al. Significance of venous and lymphatic invasion in malignant polyps of the colon and rectum. Gut 1989; 30:1385–1391.

59. Sugihara K, Muto T, Morioka Y. Management of patients with invasive carcinoma removed by colonoscopic polypectomy. Dis Colon Rectum 1989; 32:829–834.

60. Russell JB, Chu DZJ, Russell P, Chan CH, Thompson C, Schafer RF. When is polypectomy sufficient treatment for colorectal cancer in a polyp. Am J Surg 1990; 160:665–668.

61. Geraghty JM, Williams CB, Talbot IC. Malignant colorectal polyps: venous invasion and successful treatment by endoscopic polypectomy. Gut 1991; 32:774–778.

62. Kyzer S, Bégin LR, Gordon PH, Mitmaker B. The care of patients with colorectal polyps that contain invasive adenocarcinoma: endoscopic polypectomy or colectomy? Cancer 1992; 70:2044–2050.

63. Pollard CW, Nivatvongs S, Rojanasakul A, Reiman HM, Dozois RR. The fate of patients following polypectomy alone for polyps containing invasive carcinoma. Dis Colon Rectum 1992; 35:933–937.

64. Cunningham KN, Mills LR, Schuman BM, Mwakyusa DH. Long-term prognosis of well-differentiated adenocarcinoma in endoscopically removed colorectal adenomas. Dig Dis Sci 1994; 39:2034–2037.

65. Moore JWE, Hoffman DC, Rowland R. Management of the malignant colorectal polyp: the importance of clinicopathological correlation. Aust N Z J Surg 1994; 64:242–246.

66. Cooper HS, Deppisch LM, Gourley WK, et al. Endoscopically removed malignant colorectal polyps: clinicopathologic correlations. Gastroenterology 1995; 108:1657–1665.

67. Hackelsberger A, Frühmorgen P, Weiler H, Heller T, Seeliger H, Junghanns K. Endoscopic polypectomy and management of colo-rectal adenomas with invasive carcinoma. Endoscopy 1995; 27:153–158.

68. Volk EE, Goldblum JR, Petras RE, Carey WD, Fazio VW. Management and outcome of patients with invasive carcinoma arising in colorectal polyps. Gastroenterology 1995; 109:1801–1807.

69. Kikuchi R, Takano M, Takagi K, Fujimoto N, Nozaki R, Fujiyoshi T, et al. Management of early invasive colorectal cancer: risk of recurrence and clinical guidelines. Dis Colon Rectum 1995; 38:1286–1295.

70. Netzer P, Binek J, Hammer B, Lange J, Schmassmann A. Significance of histologic criteria for the management of patients with malignant colorectal polyps and polypectomy. Scand J Gastroenterol 1997; 32:910–916.

71. Netzer P, Forster C, Biral R, et al. Risk factor assessment of endoscopically removed malignant colorectal polyps. Gut 1998; 43:669–674.

72. Doniec JM, Löhnert MS, Schniewind B, Bokelmann F, Kremer B, Grimm H. Endoscopic removal of large colorectal polyps: prevention of unnecessary surgery? Dis Colon Rectum 2003; 46: 340–348.

73. Cali RL, Pitsch RM, Thorson AG, et al. Cumulative incidence of metachronous colorectal cancer. Dis Colon Rectum 1993; 36: 388–393.

74. Green RJ, Metlay JP, Propert K, et al. Surveillance for second primary colorectal cancer after adjuvant chemotherapy: an analysis of intergroup 0089. Ann Intern Med 2002; 136:261–269.

75. Cranley JP. Proper management of the patient with a malignant colorectal polyp. Gastrointest Endosc Clin N Am 1993; 3:661–671.

76. Ramamoorthy SL, Fleshman JW. Surgical treatment of rectal cancer. Hematol Oncol Clin North Am 2002; 16:927–946.

77. Garcia-Aguilar J, Mellgren A, Sirivongs P, Buie D, Madoff RD, Rothenberger DA. Local excision of rectal cancer without adjuvant therapy: a word of caution. Ann Surg 2000; 3.

78. Lamont JP, McCarty TM, Digan RD, Jacobson R, Tulanon P, Lichliter WE. Should locally excised T1 rectal cancer receive adjuvant chemoradiation? Am J Surg 2000; 180:402–406.

79. Mellgren A, Sirivongs P, Rothenberger DA, Madoff RD, Garcia-Aguilar J. Is local excision adequate therapy for early rectal cancer? Dis Colon Rectum 2000; 43:1064–1074.

80. Wilcox GM, Beck JR. Early invasive cancer in adenomatous colonic polyps ("malignant polyps"): evaluation of the therapeutic options by decision analysis. Gastroenterology 1987; 92:1159–1168.

81. Khuri S, Daley J, Henderson W, et al. Relations of surgical volume to outcome in eight common operations: results from the VA National Surgical Quality Improvement Program. Ann Surg 1999; 230:414–432.

82. Longo WE, Virgo KS, Johnson FE, et al. Risk factors for morbidity and mortality after colectomy for colon cancer. Dis Colon Rectum 2000; 43:83–91.

83. Birkmeyer JD, Siewers AE, Finlayson EVA, et al. Hospital volume and surgical mortality in the United States. N Engl J Med 2002; 346:1128–1137.

84. Hannan EL, Radzyner M, Rubin D, Dougherty J, Brennan MF. The influence of hospital and surgeon volume on in-hospital mortality for colectomy, gastrectomy, and lung lobectomy in patients with cancer. Surgery 2002; 131:6–15.

85. Callahan MA, Christos PJ, Gold HT, Mushlin AI, Daly JM. Influence of surgical subspecialty training on in-hospital mortality for gastrectomy and colectomy patients. Ann Surg 2003; 238:629–639.

86. Tekkis PP, Poloniecki JD, Thompson MR, Stamatakis JD. Operative mortality in colorectal cancer: prospective national study. BMJ 2003; 327:1196–1201.

87. Scholefield JH, Steele RJ. Guidelines for follow-up after resection of colorectal cancer. Gut 2002; 51 (Suppl V):v3–v5.

88. ESMO minimum clinical recommendations for diagnosis, adjuvant treatment, and follow-up of colon cancer. Ann Oncol 2001; 12:1053, 1054.

89. Desch CE, Benson AB, Smith TJ, et al. Recommended colorectal cancer surveillance guidelines by the American Society of Clinical Oncology. J Clin Oncol 1999; 17:1312–1321.

90. Benson III AB, Desch CE, Flynn PJ, et al. 2000 update of American Society of Clinical Oncology colorectal cancer surveillance guidelines. J Clin Oncol 2000; 18:3586–3588.

91. Anthony T, Simmang C, Hyman N, et al. Practice parameters for the surveillance and follow-up of patients with colon and rectal cancer. Dis Colon Rectum 2004; 47:807–817.

92. Buie WD, Rothenberger DA. Surveillance after curative resection of colorectal cancer: individualizing follow-up. Gastrointest Endosc Clin N Am 1993; 3:691–713.

93. Berman JM, Cheung RJ, Weinberg DS. Surveillance after colorectal cancer resection. Lancet 2000; 355:395–399.

94. Mäkelä JT, Laitinen SO, Kairaluoma MI. Five-year follow-up after radical surgery for colorectal cancer: results of a prospective randomized trial. Arch Surg 1995; 130:1062–1067.

95. Ohlsson B, Breland U, Ekberg H, Graffner H, Tranberg K-G. Follow-up after curative surgery for colorectal carcinoma. Dis Colon Rectum 1995:619–626.

96. Kjeldsen B, Kronborg O, Fenger C, Jørgensen O. A prospective randomized study of follow-up after radical surgery for colorectal cancer. Br J Surg 1997; 84:666–669.

97. Shoemaker D, Black R, Giles L, Toouli J. Yearly colonoscopy, liver CT, and chest radiography do not influence 5-year survival of colorectal cancer patients. Gastroenterology 1998; 114:7–14.

98. Pietra N, Sarli L, Costi R, Ouchemi C, Grattarola M, Peracchia A. Role of follow-up in management of local recurrences of colorectal cancer: a prospective, randomized study. Dis Colon Rectum 1998; 41.

99. Secco GB, Fardelli R, Gianquinto D, et al. Efficacy and cost of risk-adapted follow-up in patients after colorectal cancer surgery: a prospective, randomized and controlled trial. Eur J Surg Oncol 2002; 28:418–23.

100. Bruinvels DJ, Stiggelbout AM, Kievit J, van Houwelingen HC, Habbema JDF, van de Velde CJH. Follow-up of patients with colorectal cancer: a meta-analysis. Ann Surg 1994; 219:174–182.

101. Rosen M, Chan L, Beart RW, Vukasin P, Anthone G. Follow-up of colorectal cancer: a meta-analysis. Dis Colon Rectum 1998; 41:1116–1126.

102. Renehan AG, Egger M, Saunders MP, O'Dwyer ST. Impact on survival of intensive follow-up after curative resection for colorectal cancer: systematic review and meta-analysis of randomised trials. BMJ 2002; 324:813–816.

103. Figueredo A, Rumble RB, Maroun J, et al. Follow-up of patients with curatively resected colorectal cancer: a practice guideline. BMC Cancer 2003; 3:26.

104. Simmang CL, Senatore P, Lowry A, et al. Practice parameters for detection of colorectal neoplasms. Dis Colon Rectum 1999; 42:1123–1129.

105. Sagar PM, Pemberton JH. Surgical management of locally recurrent rectal cancer. Br J Surg 1996; 83:293–304.

106. Nelson H, Petrelli N, Carlin A, et al. Guidelines 2000 for colon and rectal cancer surgery. J Natl Cancer Inst 2001; 93:583–596.

107. Secco GB, Fardelli R, Rovida S, et al. Is intensive follow-up really able to improve prognosis of patients with local recurrence after curative surgery for rectal cancer. Ann Surg Oncol 2000; 7:32–37.

108. Anthony T, Fleming JB, Bieligk SC, et al. Postoperative colorectal cancer surveillance. J Am Coll Surg 2000; 190:737–749.

109. Mascagni D, Corbellini PU, Di Matteo G. Endoluminal ultrasound for early detection of local recurrence of rectal cancer. Br J Surg 1989; 76:1176–1180.

110. Ramirez JM, McC.Mortensen NJ, Takeuchi N, Smilgin Humphries MM. Endoluminal ultrasonography in the follow-up of patients with rectal cancer. Br J Surg 1994; 81:692–694.

111. Novell F, Pascual S, Viella P, Trias M. Endorectal ultrasonography in the follow-up of rectal cancer: is it a better way of to detect early local recurrence? Int J Colorect Dis 1997; 12:78–81.

112. Rotondano G, Esposito P, Pellecchia L, Novi A, Romano G. Early detection of locally recurrent rectal cancer by endosonography. British Journal of Radiology 1997; 70:567–571.

113. Löhnert MSS, Doniec JM, Henne-Bruns D. Effectiveness of endoluminal sonography in the identification of occult local rectal cancer recurrences. Dis Colon Rectum 2000; 43:483–491.

114. Hünnerbein M, Totkas S, Moesta KT, Ulmer C, Handke T, Schlag PM. The role of transrectal ultrasound-guided biopsy in the postoperative follow-up of patients with rectal cancer. Surgery 2001; 129:164–169.

115. de Anda EH, Lee S-H, Finne CO, Rothenberger DA, Madoff RD, Garcia-Aguilar J. Endorectal ultrasound in the follow-up of rectal cancer patients treated by local excision or radical surgery. Dis Colon Rectum 2004; 47:818–824.

116. Eaden JA, Mayberry JF. Guidelines for screening and surveillance of asymptomatic colorectal cancer in patients with inflammatory bowel disease. Gut 2002; 51 (Suppl V):v10–v12.

117. Devroede G, Taylor WF, Sauer WG, Jackman RJ, Stickler GB. Cancer risk and life expectancy of children with ulcerative colitis. N Engl J Med 1971; 285:17–21.

118. Hendriksen C, S K, Binder V. Long-term prognosis in ulcerative colitis—based on results from a regional patient group from the county of Copenhagen. Gut 1985; 26:158–163.

119. Stonnington CM, Phillips SF, Zinsmeister AR, Melton III LJ. Prognosis of chronic ulcerative colitis in a community. Gut 1987; 28:1261–1266.

120. Langholz E, Munkholm P, Davidsen M, Binder V. Colorectal cancer risk and mortality in patients with ulcerative colitis. Gastroenterology 1992; 103:1444–1451.

121. Eaden JA, Abrams KR, Mayberry JF. The risk of colorectal cancer in ulcerative colitis: a meta-analysis. Gut 2001; 48:526–535.

122. Eaden J, Mayberry JF. Colorectal cancer complicating ulcerative colitis: a review. Am J Gastroenterol 2000; 95:2710–2719.

123. Sachar DB, Greenstein AJ. Cancer in ulcerative colitis: good news and bad news [editorial]. Ann Intern Med 1981; 95:642–644.

124. Ransohoff DF. Colon cancer in ulcerative colitis. Gastroenterology 1988; 94:1089–1091.

125. Greenstein AJ, Sachar DB, Smith H, et al. Cancer in universal and left-sided ulcerative colitis: factors determining risk. Gastroenterology 1979; 77:290–294.

126. Ekbom A, Helmick C, Zack M, Adami H-O. Ulcerative colitis and colorectal cancer: a population-based study. N Engl J Med 1990; 323:1228–1233.

127. D'Haens GR, Lashner BA, Hanauer SB. Pericholangitis and sclerosing cholangitis are risk factors for dysplasia and cancer in ulcerative colitis. Am J Gastroenterol 1993; 88:1174–1178.

128. Kornfeld D, Ekbom A, Ihre T. Is there an excess risk for colorectal cancer in patients with ulcerative colitis and concomitant primary sclerosing cholangitis? A population based study. Gut 1997; 41:522–525.

129. Pardi DS, Loftus Jr. EV, Kremers WK, Keach J, Lindor KD. Ursodeoxycholic acid as a chemopreventative agent in patients with ulcerative colitis and primary sclerosing cholangitis. Gastroenterology 2003; 124:889–893.

130. Rutter M, Saunders B, Wilkinson K, et al. Severity of inflammation is a risk factor for colorectal neoplasia in ulcerative colitis. Gastroenterology 2004; 126:451–459.

131. Askling J, Dickman PW, Karlén P, et al. Family history as a risk factor for colorectal cancer in inflammatory bowel disease. Gastroenterology 2001; 120:1356–1362.

132. Eaden J, Abrams K, Ekbom A, Jackson E, Mayberry J. Colorectal cancer prevention in ulcerative colitis: a case–control study. Aliment Pharmacol Ther 2000; 14:145–153.

133. Heuschen UA, Hinz U, Allemeyer EH, et al. Backwash ileitis is strongly associated with colorectal carcinoma in ulcerative colitis. Gastroenterology 2001; 120:841–847.

134. Provenzale D, Kowdley KV, Arora S, Wong JB. Prophylactic colectomy or surveillance for chronic ulcerative colitis? A decision analysis. Gastroenterology 1995; 109:1188–1196.

135. Bernstein CN, Weinstein WM, Levine DS, Shanahan F. Physician's perceptions of dysplasia and approaches to surveillance colonoscopy in ulcerative colitis. Am J Gastroenterol 1995; 90:2106–2114.

136. Eaden J, Ward BA, Mayberry JF. How gastroenterologists screen for colonic cancer in ulcerative colitis: an analysis of performance. Gastrointest Endosc 2000; 51:123–128.

137. Bernstein CN, Shanahan F, Wcinstein WM. Are we telling patients the truth about surveillance colonoscopy in ulcerative colitis? Lancet 1994; 343:71–74.

138. Eaden J, Abrams K, McKay H, Denley H, Mayberry J. Interobserver variation between general and specialist gastrointestinal pathologists when grading dysplasia in ulcerative colitis. J Pathol 2001; 194:152–157.

139. Ahnen DJ. Gastrointestinal malignancies in inflammatory bowel disease. In: Inflammatory Bowel Disease, 5 ed. Kirsner JB, ed. Philadelphia: WB Saunders; 2000:379–396.

140. Cima RR, Pemberton JH. Early surgical intervention in ulcerative colitis. Gut 2004; 53:306, 307.

141. Judge TA, Lewis JD, Lichtenstein GR. Colonic dysplasia and cancer in inflammatory bowel disease. Gastrointest Endosc Clin N Am 2002; 12:495–523.

142. Riddell RH, Goldman H, Ransohoff DF, et al. Dysplasia in inflammatory bowel disease: standardized classification with provisional clinical applications. Hum Pathol 1983; 14:931–968.

143. Gilat T, Fireman Z, Grossman A, et al. Colorectal cancer in patients with ulcerative colitis: a population study in central Israel. Gastroenterology 1988; 94:870–877.

144. Gyde SN, Prior P, Allan RN, et al. Colorectal cancer in ulcerative colitis: a cohort study of primary referrals from three centres. Gut 1988; 29:206–217.

145. Provenzale D, Onken J. Surveillance issues in inflammatory bowel disease: ulcerative colitis. J Clin Gastroenterol 2001; 32: 99–105.

146. Rubin C, Haggitt RC, Burmer GC, et al. DNA aneuploidy in colonic biopsies predicts future development of dysplasia in ulcerative colitis. Gastroenterology 1992; 103:1611–1620.

147. Choi PM. Predominance of rectosigmoid neoplasia in ulcerative colitis and its implication on cancer surveillance (letter). Gastroenterology 1993; 104:666,667.

148. Connell WR, Lennard-Jones JE, Williams CB, Talbot IC, Price AB, Wilkinson KH. Factors affecting the outcome of endoscopic surveillance for cancer in ulcerative colitis. Gastroenterology 1994; 107:934–944.

149. Ullman T, Croog V, Harpaz N, Sachar D, Itzkowitz S. Progression of flat low-grade dysplasia to advanced neoplasia in patients with ulcerative colitis. Gastroenterology 2003; 125:1311–1319.

150. Befrits R, Ljung T, Jarmarillo E, Rubio C. Low-grade dysplasia in extensive, long-standing inflammatory bowel disease. Dis Colon Rectum 2002; 45:615–620.

151. Odze RD. Adenomas and adenoma-like DALMs in chronic ulcerative colitis: a clinical, pathological, and molecular review. Am J Gastroenterol 1999; 94:1746–1750.

152. Blackstone MO, Riddell RH, Rogers BHG, Levin B. Dysplasia-associated lesion or mass (DALM) detected by colonoscopy in long-standing ulcerative colitis: an indication for colectomy. Gastroenterology 1981; 80:366–374.

153. Willenbucher R. Inflammatory Bowel Disease. Seminars in Gastrointestinal Disease 1996; 7:94–104.

154. Torres C, Antonioli D, Odze RD. Polypoid dysplasia and adenomas in inflammatory bowel disease: a clinical, pathologic, and follow-up study of 89 polyps from 59 patients. Am J Surg Pathol 1998; 22:275–284.

155. Nugent FW, Haggitt RC, Gilpin PA. Cancer surveillance in ulcerative colitis. Gastroenterology 1991; 100:1241–1248.

156. Suzuki K, Muto T, Shinozaki M, Yokoyama T, Matsuda K, Masaki T. Differential diagnosis of dysplasia-associated lesion or mass and coincidental adenoma in ulcerative colitis. Dis Colon Rectum 1998; 41:322–327.

157. Engelsgjerd M, Farraye FA, Odze RD. Polypectomy may be adequate treatment for adenoma-like dysplastic lesions in chronic ulcerative colitis. Gastroenterology 1999; 117:1288–1294.

158. Rubin PH, Friedman S, Harpaz N, Goldstein E, Weiser J, Schiller J, et al. Colonoscopic polypectomy in chronic colitis: conservative management after endoscopic resection of dysplastic polyps. Gastroenterology 1999; 117:1295–1300.

159. Bernstein CN. ALMs versus DALMs in ulcerative colitis: polypectomy or colectomy. Gastroenterology 1999; 117:1488–1491.

160. Hamilton SR. Colorectal carcinoma in patients with Crohn's disease. Gastroenterology 1985; 89:398–407.

161. Choi PM, Zelig MP. Similarity of colorectal cancer in Crohn's disease and ulcerative colitis: implications for carcinogenesis and prevention. Gut 1994; 35:950–954.

162. Petras RE, Mir-Madjlessi SH, Farmer RG. Crohn's disease and intestinal carcinoma: a report of 11 cases with emphasis on associated epithelial dysplasia. Gastroenterology 1987; 93:1307–1314.

163. Weedon DD, Shorter RG, Ilstrup DM, Huizenga KA, Taylor WF. Crohn's disease and cancer. N Engl J Med 1973; 289:1099–1103.

164. Greenstein AJ, Sachar DB, Smith H, Janowitz HD, Aufses Jr. AH. A comparison of cancer risk in Crohn's disease and ulcerative colitis. Cancer 1981; 48:2742–2745.

165. Ekbom A, Helmick C, Zack M, Adami H-O. Increased risk of large-bowel cancer in Crohn's disease with colonic involvement. Lancet 1990; 336:357–359.

166. Gillen CD, Walmsley RS, Prior P, Andrews HA, Allan RN. Ulcerative colitis and Crohn's disease: a comparison of the colorectal cancer risk in extensive colitis. Gut 1994; 35:1590–1592.

167. Bernstein CN, Blanchard JF, Kliewer E, Wajda A. Cancer risk in patients with inflammatory bowel disease. Cancer 2001; 91: 854–852.

168. Friedman S, Rubin PH, Bodian C, Goldstein E, Harpaz N, Present DH. Screening and surveillance colonoscopy in chronic Crohn's colitis. Gastroenterology 2001; 120:820–826.

20 Endoscopic Ultrasound for Staging Rectal and Anal Cancer

Deepak V. Gopal, MD, FRCP(C), FACP

Contents

1. BACKGROUND

Rectal endoscopic ultrasound (RUS) has proven very beneficial in the staging of malignant neoplasm in the anus and rectum *(1,2)*. Typically, imaging is performed using an adult standard radial ultrasound endoscope, commonly used in evaluation of the upper gastrointestinal tract *(3)*. Based on RUS, the normal rectal wall architecture consists of a mucosal layer (muscularis mucosa and lamina propria—also referred to as superficial and deep layers), submucosa, muscularis propria, and surrounding perirectal fat tissue without a serosa/adventiaa layer *(2)*. Carcinoma appears as a hypoechoic mass lesion with partial or total destruction of the normal wall layer. RUS has also been useful in examining for tumor invasion in the surrounding regional organs: which in males would include evaluating the bladder, seminal vesicles, prostate, and internal anal sphincters (IASs)/external anal sphincters (EASs); and in females would include evaluation of the bladder, uterus/vagina, and IASs/EASs *(1,2)*. Moreover, RUS is very helpful in evaluation of malignant lymphadenopathy. All of these features are useful in the pre-operative staging of rectal and anal carcinomas *(1,2)*.

2. INTRODUCTION

Colorectal cancer is the second leading cause of cancer deaths in North America and affects men and women in equal proportions *(4)*. It is estimated that more than 135,000 people are diagnosed with colorectal cancer annually in the United States alone and it occurs in approx 6% of the population during their lifetimes *(2,4)*. Within the large bowel, approx 69% of cancers are in the colon and 31% are in the rectum or at the

From: *Endoscopic Oncology: Gastrointestinal Endoscopy and Cancer Management.* Edited by: D. O. Faigel and M. L. Kochman © Humana Press, Totowa, NJ

recto-sigmoid junction *(4)*. The incidence or rectal cancer is 14.6 per 100,000 population and in comparison with colon cancer, rectal cancer is more common in men with a male-to-female ratio of 1.5–2:1. Although most cancers in the colon are referred directly to surgery, it is important to accurately stage rectal cancers in order to determine the appropriate management regimen, which may include pre-operative chemotherapy and radiation therapy *(1,2,4)*.

RUS is very helpful in tumor (T) staging and nodal (N) staging and has several advantages over computed tomography (CT) and magnetic resonance imaging (MRI) techniques *(1,2,5–7)*. The endoscopic ultrasound (EUS) probe, which is a 360° radial echoendoscope, can be placed close to the area of interest (the tumor) and thus the quality of imaging and resolution is significantly enhanced *(1–3,5)*. The EUS unit is portable, cost-effective, and can be completed in a short time span without sedation and a longer recovery time. It is accurate for tumor and regional nodal staging, is accepted by most patients, and is relatively easy to perform. The sensitivity of RUS for staging of tumors and lymph nodes is approx 85 and 77%, respectively *(2,4)*. The technique of fine-needle aspiration (FNA), can also be utilized, and may help to increase diagnostic accuracy. If available, RUS can be used during the initial endoscopy visit, which can allow for immediate incorporation of the clinical data into the treatment plan. CT scan or MRI of the abdomen and pelvis is more beneficial to determine metastatic disease *(1,2,5,8)*.

3. ANATOMY OF THE ANORECTUM

Before discussion of the role of EUS in staging tumors of the rectum and anal canal, a basic understanding of anorectal anatomy is essential (Fig. 1) *(1)*. The rectum begins at the dentate line, which demarcates the transition zone between the

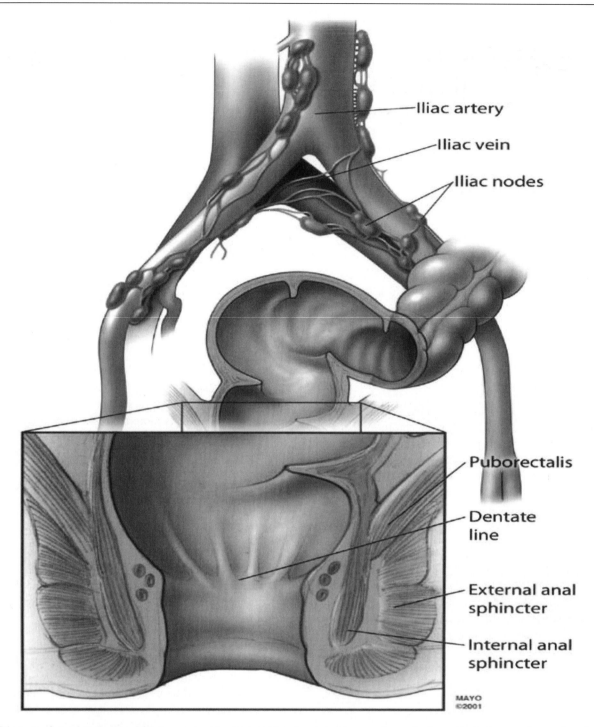

Fig. 1. Diagram of rectal anatomy, which is examined in most rectal endoscopic ultrasound examinations. Particular attention to the relationship between the iliac lymph nodes, rectum, and distal sigmoid colon should be noted. (Adapted from ref. 1.)

stratified squamous epithelium of the anal canal and the columnar mucosa of the rectum and colon, and extends to a distance of approx 15–20 cm from the anal verge (1,5,9). The venous drainage from the rectum is via the superior hemorrhoidal and inferior mesenteric veins to the portal vein or alternatively via the middle and inferior hemorrhoidal veins. In parallel with the vasculature, the lymphatic drainage follows a similar route and therefore knowledge of this anatomy is helpful in the staging of rectal cancer where inspection of the iliac vessels and their associated lymph nodes is necessary (1,5,9,10).

The anal canal is formed by two muscular cylinders: the IAS and the EAS (Fig. 2A). The IAS is formed by the downward continuation of the circular smooth muscle of the rectum and the EAS is formed by the downward extension of skeletal muscle of the puborectalis. The combined IAS/EAS sphincter complex is approx 4 cm in length and when examining them under EUS these sphincters appear as two discrete rings in pattern, where the IAS is hypoechoic and the EAS is hyperechoic, and a pattern of a "bulls-eye" target appears with EUS balloon in the center. The normal IAS is 2–3 mm in thickness and

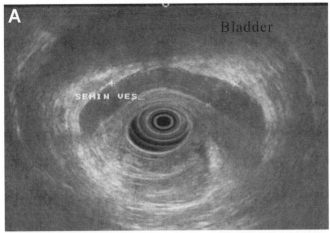

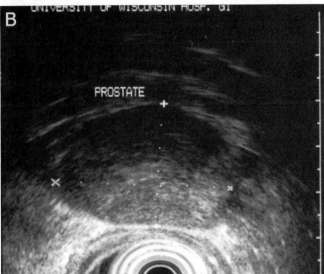

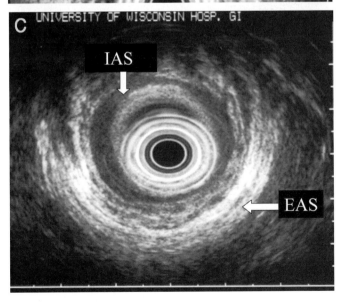

Fig. 2. (**A**) Normal rectal endoscope ultrasound (RUS) imaging of seminal vesicles and bladder in a male patient. (**B**) Normal RUS imaging of prostate. (**C**) Normal RUS imaging of IAS/EAS.

becomes thicker and more hyperechoic with age, reflecting collagen replacement. The EAS is 7–9 mm in thickness and tends to become thinner with increasing age *(1,5,9,10)*.

Because RUS has been useful in evaluating for cancer invasion into the surrounding regional organs, it is important, in males, to examine the bladder, seminal vesicles, prostate, and IAS and EAS (Fig. 2A–C); and in females, to examine the bladder, uterus, vagina, and IAS and EAS.

4. RUS EXAMINATION

Colonic preparation for anorectal endosonography is fairly straightforward and usually only requires laxative enemas similar to preparation for flexible sigmoidoscopy. Typically, no sedation is required, and most patients being referred for RUS for staging of anorectal cancers, already have had a complete colonoscopy, and biopsies of the primary tumor *(1,5,8)*.

Before the examination, informed consent must be obtained, and enough clinical detail should be available to predetermine if the case requires FNA. In the setting of anorectal cancer, most often a tissue diagnosis is easily obtained by forceps biopsies and in a few cases by partial endoscopic mucosal resection of the primary tumor. Only a few cases for staging of anorectal malignancy may require FNA (e.g., distal perirectal lymph node, cancer recurrence, or in cases where a tissue diagnosis has not been made and is deemed essential prior to proceeding with a treatment plan) *(1,2,8,11,12)*. If transrectal FNA is planned, one might consider using intravenous conscious sedation with monitoring (as FNA adds time to the procedure), a full colonic lavage, and postprocedure antibiotic therapy.

Before RUS, a flexible sigmoidoscopy examination should be routinely performed to assess the endoscopic location of the tumor, to assess the quality of the preparation to ensure that the recto-sigmoid lumen is free of stool to limit artifact and to improve accuracy of the procedure. Subsequently, the RUS is performed, most often at 7.5 and 12 MHz frequencies *(1–3,8)*. The EUS scopes can easily be inserted into the rectum, and advanced just slightly proximal to the recto-sigmoid junction to approx 30 cm above the anal verge. Usually it can be slightly difficult to advance to mid to proximal sigmoid colon owing to side-viewing optics. This distance is more than adequate to perform tumor staging, assess other organs in close proximity, and evaluate for regional lymphadenopathy. Rigid US probes can also be used, but they do not provide simultaneous endoscopic and ultrasound images and are only limited to the distal anorectum *(8)*. To examine the anal canal, the ultrasound balloon is minimally inflated and the EUS scope is then gripped with one hand up against the anus. This helps to stabilize the echoendoscope within the anal canal and reduce distortion of the anal canal to allow for more accurate imaging *(2,8,9)*.

5. RUS FOR RECTAL CANCER

5.1. RUS FOR T STAGING

The main criterion of tumor-node-metastasis (TNM) staging is the depth of cancer infiltration (Tables 1 and 2) *(13)*. Prior studies *(2,5,8,14)* have demonstrated an accuracy in T stage ranging from 73–94% with an overall accuracy of 83% *(1,2)*. T stage accuracy generally exceeds 90% for stages T1 (Fig. 3A,B), T3, and T4 (Table 3). T2 tumor stage has the lowest accuracy for RUS, approx 73%, owing to difficulty in detecting tumor invasion through the muscularis propria (Fig. 4A,B). Furthermore,

Table 1
TNM Staging for Rectal Cancer

T: Primary rectal tumor	Description
Tis (tumor *in situ*)	Tumor confined to mucosa layer
T1	Tumor invades through the lamina propria into the submucosa
T2	Tumor invades through the submucosa into the muscularis propria (MP layer intact)
T3	Tumor invades through the muscularis propria into the perirectal tissue
T4	Tumor invades adjacent Organs

N: Lymph nodes	
N0	No regional lymphadenopathy
N1	1–3 perirectal lymph nodes
N2	>3 perirectal lymph nodes
N3	Nodes along named vascular trunk
Nx	Regional lymph nodes cannot be assessed

M: Metastatic disease	
M0	No evidence of metastasis
M1	Metastasis present
Mx	Metastasis cannot be assessed

Adapted from ref. *13*.

Table 2
Staging System for Rectal Cancer

Stage	T (tumor)	N (nodal)	M (metastasis)	Duke's stage
I	T1	N0	M0	A
	T2	N0	M0	
II	T3	N0	M0	B
	T4	N0	M0	
III	Any T	N1	M0	C
		N2		
		N3		
IV	Any T	Any N	M1	–

Adapted from ref. *13*.

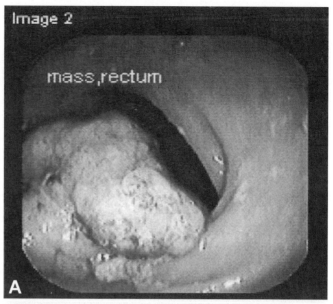

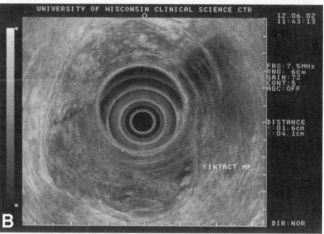

Fig. 3. **(A)** Endoscopic appearance of polypoid mass lesion. Biopsy demonstrates carcinoma arising from villous adenoma. **(B)** Rectal endoscopic ultrasound stages this tumor as a T1N0 cancer, with preservation of muscularis propria layer. Transanal excision was performed, and surgical stage c/w T1N0 rectal cancer.

depth of invasion beyond the fourth muscularis propria (MP) layer can be variable and one recent study has also suggested that determining the presence of advanced T3 disease (Fig. 5) from minimally invasive disease is important in prognosticating outcome *(14)*. Harewood et al. *(15)* used RUS to assess the depth of invasion beyond the MP layer and felt that this could predict tumor recurrence in patients with T3 rectal cancers. The authors evaluated patients with T3N × M0 rectal cancer, as determined by RUS, who underwent surgical resection without pre-operative chemoradiotherapy who were reviewed by two blinded endosonographers. The cancers, were subclassified by RUS as being minimally invasive (invasion ≤2 mm beyond MP) vs advanced T3 disease (invasion ≥2 mm beyond MP). In their study, of the 42 patients with T3 rectal cancer that underwent surgical resection without receiving neoadjuvant pre-operative chemoradiotherapy, 14 patients (33%) had minimally invasive T3 and 28 patients (67%) had advanced T3 rectal cancer based on the RUS criteria that were established. Cancer recurrence rates for minimally invasive vs advanced T3 rectal cancers were 14.3

vs 39.3%, respectively. Adjustment for nodal status and postoperative chemoradiation therapy using Cox proportional hazards model demonstrated advanced T3 disease to predict rectal cancer recurrence (Cox hazard ratio, 2.28 [95% confidence interval: 1.17–5.81]; $p = 0.01$). The authors concluded that not all T3 rectal cancers behave equally and that minimally invasive disease carries a more favorable prognosis. Therefore, it would be crucial to discriminate minimally invasive disease from advanced T3 cancer by pre-operative RUS and that this information would provide important prognostication and also enhance selection of patients to receive neoadjuvant, preoperative chemoradiation therapy *(15)*. The same is true for identifying, advanced T4 cancer (Fig. 6A,B), as these patients can be directed towards palliative therapies.

5.2. RUS FOR N STAGING

The overall accuracy of RUS for regional lymph node staging is less accurate than tumor staging, approximating a rate of 78%, with a range of 62–83% (Table 3) *(2,14)*. The accuracy is

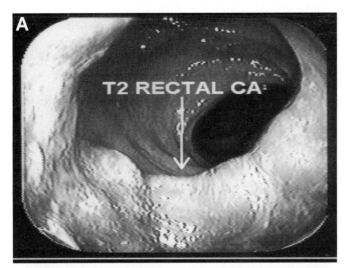

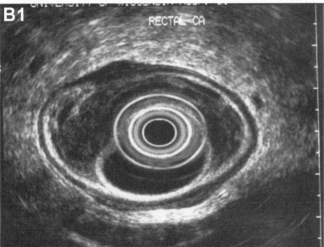

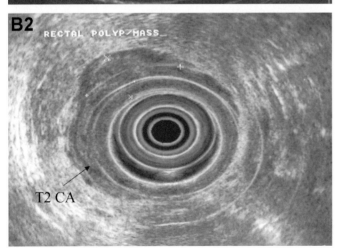

Fig. 4. (**A**) Endoscopic appearance, of rectal mass—biopsies confirms rectal adenocarcinoma. (**B**) Rectal endoscopic ultrasound (RUS) stages this tumor as T2N0. RUS imaging, at the pronimal margin of the rectal cancer, demonstrates initial appearance of tumor breaking through the submicosa into the muscularis propia layer (**B1**). Further imaging the maximum cross-sectional dimensions of the tumor clearly notes invasion into (→) but not through the muscularis propria (**B2**). This staging is confirmed after surgery.

Table 3
Staging Accuracy of Rectal Ultrasound Characterized by T and N-Stage

T stage	No. of patients	RUS stage accuracy (%)
T1	219	94
T2	214	73
T3	468	92
T4	56	94

N stage	No. of patients	RUS stage accuracy (%)
N0	503	79
N1	331	74

Adapted from ref. *14*.

less, as determining if lymph nodes inflammatory or malignant is based on pattern recognition *(2,14)*. Generally, lymph nodes that are hyperechoic, small, and have irregular margins tend to be benign, whereas lymph nodes that are round, hypoechoic, well demarcated, large (>1 cm), and adjacent to the leading edge of the tumor (Fig. 5C) are usually metastatic *(2,14)*.

The utilization of FNA technology using needle guidance with a curvilinear-array echoendoscope has perhaps also had an impact on increasing the accuracy of lymph node staging. In one study *(16)* reviewing 51 patients with rectal cancer who underwent RUS with FNA, 15 of 51 patients had FNA of perirectal lymph nodes and 45 of 51 patients underwent surgery. Surgery was considered the gold standard. Using RUS, the T stage was accurate in 36 of 45 (80%) patients with 9 patients being inaccurately staged, all being overstaged. FNA increased nodal staging with an overall accuracy of 87%. This facilitated neoadjuvant therapy in 22 of 51 patients. EUS with FNA of perirectal lymph nodes could be considered, if the lymph nodes are not adjacent to the tumor, and it has a higher accuracy compared with CT scan (which generally has an accuracy of 60–65%) *(2,16)*.

In another study by Parmar et al. *(11)*, the authors retrospectively reviewed 46 patients with rectal cancer. Of 46 patients, 12 had RUS with FNA with 8 of 12 (67%) undergoing lymph node sampling and 4 of 12 (33%) to evaluate areas suspicious for cancer recurrence. Of eight patients, five with positive malignant lymph nodes, four of these patients underwent preoperative chemo/external radiation therapy. Hence, RUS with FNA changed the management in about 75% of patients who were biopsied and FNA sampling was felt to increase staging accuracy and help select patients for primary surgical management vs preoperative chemo/radiotherapy.

Finally in subsequent recent study *(17)*, which was designed to determine the impact of EUS-FNA on the staging and management of rectal cancer and compare it to staging modalities such as CT, the findings demonstrated that RUS was a better staging modality than CT scan, especially for regional lymphadenopathy. Moreover, there was a trend with EUS-guided FNA demonstrating a more accurate nodal staging compared with routine RUS. Pre-operative staging with RUS changed the management of 38% of patients in this study, with EUS-guided FNA changing the management in 19% of patients who underwent lymph node sampling (especially of

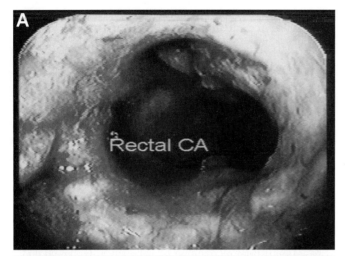

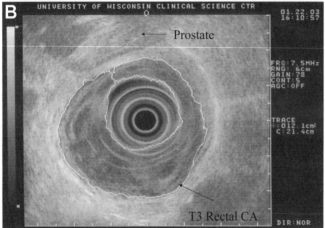

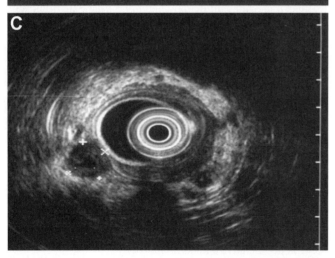

Fig. 5. (A) Endoscopic appearance of a friable, ulcerated rectal tumor with biopsy proven adenocarcinoma. (B) Rectal endoscope ultrasound appearance of this tumor suggests that this is a T3 Lesion. Note plane/interface between tumor and prostate. (C) There is regional malignant lymphadenopathy, making this tumor Nodal stage N1.

lymph nodes not directly juxtaposed against the tumor). However, EUS-guided FNA may not be routinely done for regional lymphadenopathy, because there is some controversy if this changes management, but some published data to suggests it increases diagnostic accuracy of nodal staging and that it may be considered (2,11,16,17).

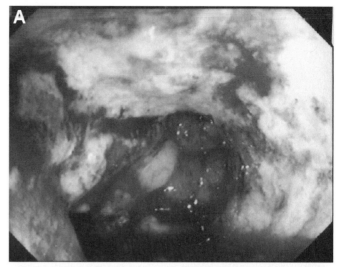

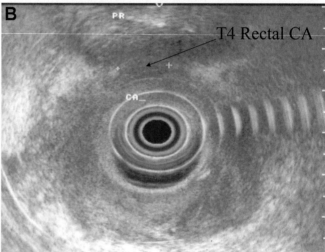

Fig. 6. (A) Endoscopic appearance, of large, circumferential, partially obstructing rectal cancer. (B) Corresponding rectal endoscopic ultrasound demonstrates that this tumor was invading the prostate gland anteriorly. This was confirmed on pelvic CT and is c/w T4 tumor stage.

5.3. RUS TO DIRECT THERAPY FOR RECTAL CANCER

RUS is useful in planning a treatment approach once rectal cancer has been staged. In an earlier study by Faigel and Lee (2), of 29 patients with rectal adenocarcinoma who were initially suggested to undergo low anterior resection or abdominoperineal resection (APR), 9 (31%) patients were able to undergo local excision once staged with EUS. This also impacted those patients who were originally to undergo neoadjuvant chemotherapy and radiation therapy. Of 29 patients, 6 initially planned to undergo chemo/radiotherapy, an additional 3 patients ($N = 9$ [31%]) underwent preoperative chemo/radiation after staging EUS. Similarly, Winde et al. (18) reviewed 50 patients with rectal adenocarcinoma, with EUS confirmed stage T1N0, who were randomized to operative treatment either with local surgical excision or low anterior resection. The 5-yr survival (96%) and local recurrence rate (4.2%) were equal in both surgical treatment arms. However, the number of hospital days was much less (5.7 vs 15.4 d, $p < 0.0001$) in the local excision group. Other factors that affected the local excision treatment arm were decreased

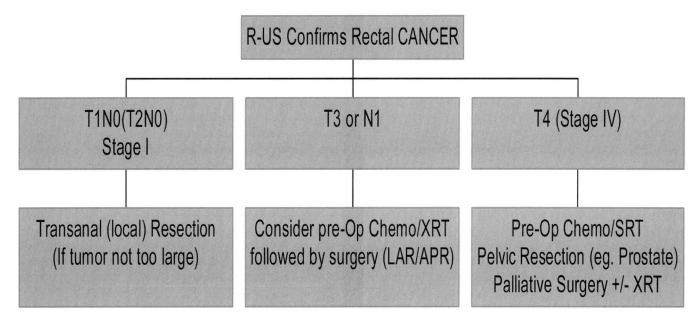

Fig. 7. Algorithm outlining treatment approaches for rectal adenocarcinoma based on staging via rectal endoscopic ultrasound. For T1 (and certain T2) rectal tumors without lymph nodes, local excision can be considered. For T3 or N1 rectal cancer, preoperative neoadjuvant chemo/radiation therapy can be considered before low anterior resection and abdomino perineal resection. (Adapted from ref. 2.)

blood loss, reduction in operation time, and reduced need for postsurgical narcotic analgesia *(2,18,19)*. Therefore, RUS may have a role in identifying patients for pre-operative neoadjuvant chemo/radiotherapy protocols and also modify the surgical approach in a subgroup of patients *(2,20)* (Fig. 7).

In a more recent study published by Harewood *(19)*, which discussed the clinical impact of EUS on rectal cancer, the aim was to assess the impact of EUS-FNA by comparing clinical outcomes of patients with rectal cancer before and after the introduction of RUS for staging at a single center institution. The outcomes of patients (*n* = 68) with *de-novo* nonmetastatic rectal adenocarcinoma evaluated in 1999 without EUS evaluation ("non-EUS" control group) were compared with patients (*n* = 73) staged and evaluated with RUS +/− FNA from 2000 to 2001 (the EUS group). Among the patients with advanced T or N stage, neoadjuvant therapy (chemo and/or radiotherapy), was administered to 45 patients in the RUS +/− FNA group (84.9%; pre-operative to 31 [58.5%] patients and postoperative to 14 [26.4%]) vs 37 patients in the "non-EUS" control group (78.7%; pre-operative to 7 [14.9%] and postoperative to 30 [63.8%]). Moreover, they demonstrated that staging of rectal cancer with RUS +/− FNA is associated with a reduction in tumor recurrence risk (Cox proportional hazard ratio: 0.72 [95% confidence interval: 0.52–0.97; *p* = 0.03]). This data also supports the fact that RUS staging of rectal adenocarcinoma appears to facilitate the appropriate utilization of pre-operative neoadjuvant therapy in those patients with advanced stage, and also offers a recurrence-free survival advantage *(19)*.

5.4. RUS FOR RESTAGING FOLLOWING NEOADJUVANT CHEMORADIATION THERAPY

Recent studies have demonstrated that EUS restaging of rectal cancer is inaccurate following neoadjuvant chemo/radiation therapy. In one study by Lin et al. *(21)*, 93 of 285 (34%) patients who had pre-operative staging with RUS were

examined over a decade. Of 93 patients, 56 (60%) underwent chemo/radiation therapy before restaging and 29 patients (31%) did not undergo pre-operative therapy. In their study population, in cases where restaging with EUS was performed, the overall RUS T stage accuracy was 42.9% in the chemo/ radiotherapy group vs 69% in the controls (*p* = 0.016). The overall RUS N status was 67.9% in the chemo/radiotherapy group vs 89% in the controls *(2,21)*.

In another study by Vanagunas et al. *(22)*, the authors also evaluated the accuracy of EUS for restaging rectal cancer following neoadjuvant chemo/radiotherapy by performing staging EUS before and after concurrent 5-fluorouracil and hyperfractionated radiotherapy in 82 patients with locally advanced rectal adenocarcinoma. These patients subsequently underwent surgical resection and final pathological staging. Postchemo/radiotherapy, there were 16 patients (20%) that had no residual disease at final staging (T0N0), but RUS predicted correctly the complete response in only 10 of 16 patients (63%). The overall accuracy of RUS postchemo/radiotherapy for pathological T stage was 48% (14% were understaged and 38% were overstaged) and for N status was 77%. The T stage was correctly staged before surgery in 23 of 56 responders (41%) and in 16 of 24 nonresponders (67%). These studies indicate that the RUS restaging accuracy is likely to be affected by local postradiation induced edema/fibrosis that distort ultrasound images and make it very difficult to accurately distinguish these changes from residual cancer *(2,22)*.

5.5. RUS FOR RECTAL ADENOCARCINOMA RECURRENCE

The current literature has suggested that the local recurrence of rectal adenocarcinoma may occur in 5–30% of all cases, after curative colorectal surgery *(4,16)*. It is essential to detect local recurrence, preferentially at a resectable stage, in order to have the opportunity for curative re-intervention, or to determine if the patient requires palliation for their symptoms owing to recurrence.

Conventional follow-up often fails to detect recurrence at an early stage as most local recurrences are extraluminal. They are usually picked up on another imaging such as CT scan or positron emission tomography scan that are being performed for evaluation of symptoms and follow-up. Lohnert et al. *(23)* performed a prospective study to assess the diagnostic potential of RUS to detect asymptomatic respectable local recurrence. Seven hundred and twenty-one RUS examinations were performed on 338 patients as a part of routine follow-up of rectal and left-sided colorectal cancer. Of 338 patients, 166 (34%) were found to have local recurrence diagnosed by RUS. In addition, EUS-guided FNA was useful in determining local cancer recurrence, in cases in which there were unclear perirectal structures that could not be verified by flexible endoscopy with biopsy. Other diagnostic modalities that could potentially detect local recurrence were surprisingly less satisfactory. Digital rectal examination (DRE) failed to detect local recurrence in 91 patients, flexible sigmoidoscopy failed to detect local recurrence in 80 patients, and tumor marker levels were normal in 25 patients. Both DRE and flexible sigmoidoscopy failed to detect local recurrence in 33 of 116 cases. Furthermore, in their study there were 25 EUS positive cases that underwent potential curative resection, where DRE, flexible endoscopy, and carcinoembryonic antigen levels were normal. Of 25 patients, 21 (84%) were free from disease and all 25 were alive at the conclusion of the study. The authors therefore concluded that postoperative RUS was able to identify local recurrence at an earlier and asymptomatic stage, could be verified by FNA techniques (if necessary), and its routine use may raise the ratio of curative retreatment by early detection of extramural local recurrence *(2,23)*.

In a recent surgical study by Hernandez de Anda et al. *(24)*, the role of a scheduled follow-up protocol using rectal ultrasonography for the diagnosis of local cancer recurrence after local excision and radical surgery was performed was evaluated. There was a selected group of 275 patients with invasive rectal adenocarcinoma followed prospectively by RUS after "curative-intent" local excision (*n* = 108) or radical surgery (*n* = 167). In order to evaluate the radical surgery group, these patient results were compared to a group of 176 colorectal cancer patients who had similar operations during the same period, but were not entered into a follow-up protocol. The exclusion criteria included: patients with invasive cancers removed by snare excision, male patients treated by APR, and patients treated by endocavitary radiation. The results of this study demonstrated, that of the patients in the local excision group, 32 of 108 patients (30%) developed local recurrence (26 patients [81%] were asymptomatic, and 10 patients [31%] were diagnosed only by RUS). However, in this subgroup, there was no difference in the rates of salvage surgery or survival between patients diagnosed of recurrence by RUS or other diagnostic methods. In the radical surgery subgroup, 12 of 167 patients (7%) developed local recurrence (5 [42%] were asymptomatic, and 4 patients (33%) were diagnosed only by RUS). In the follow-up subgroup, more patients with isolated local cancer recurrence (4/9; 44%) underwent salvage surgery compared with patients that did not have a follow-up protocol RUS examination (3/13; 23%). However this difference was not statistically significant. They concluded that follow-up RUS per protocol examination identified 33% of

asymptomatic local recurrences that were missed by DRE or flexible sigmoidoscopy. However, the authors noted that although this number maybe clinically significant, the impact of earlier diagnosis in patient survival can only be determined by larger, prospective, multicenter, randomized control trials *(2,24)*.

On the other hand, other reports argue that one significant disadvantage of RUS imaging postsurgery, is that it could be difficult to distinguish postsurgical changes and effects of chemotherapy and radiation, from small subtle recurrence. EUS images the anastomosis, which is characterized by diffuse thickening of the rectal wall. Postsurgery, the transmural inflammatory infiltration disappears gradually over time and the sonographic layer structure is subsequently reconstructed *(1,2,6)*. If recurrence is detected, it usually appears as a hypoechoic, heterogeneous lesion with transmural infiltration and loss of normal layer pattern. However, if radiation or chemotherapy was administered either as neoadjuvant or postoperative the index surgery, then diffuse thickening may still reflect benign post-therapy changes. In this setting FNA may be useful for diagnosis of recurrence but this needs to be further studied *(1,2,6,11)*.

5.6. US IN ANAL CANCER

The staging of anal cancer also uses the TNM staging classification (*see* Tables 4 and 5), but compared with rectal cancer, staging of anal cancer involves primarily the size of the tumor as opposed to the depth of infiltration (Fig. 8) *(13)*. Until recently, there has been little data in the current literature regarding the staging of anal carcinoma using rectal endosonography. Magedburg et al. *(25)*, published a retrospective study, in which 30 consecutive patients (9 males, 21 females) with anal carcinoma were examined using RUS and staging was based on an earlier TNM classification. RUS was performed either prior to the treatment commencing (*N* = 15 patients); after the initial treatment in order to plan further treatment sessions or during follow up examinations to assess for response to treatment (15 patients). The following T stages were diagnosed: T0 = 4 cancer lesions, T1 = 7 cancer lesions, T2 = 7 cancer lesions, T3 = 9 cancer lesions, and T4 = 3 cancer lesions. Of 30 patients, 7 (23%) suspected malignant lymphadenopathy was also detected by RUS. The authors found that RUS had a direct impact on the treatment selected which included: surgery alone (four patients: one T1, one T2, and two T3), radiation therapy alone (five patients: three with T2, two T3), combined chemo/radiation therapy (eight patients: three T2, three T3, two T4), interstitial booster radiotherapy (four patients: three T1, one T3) or no therapy at all (six patients: four T0, one T3, one T4). In only two cases was the cancer understaged. Therefore, this study suggested that in the setting of anal cancer, RUS has a strong advantage of precisely staging the tumor as it accurately assesses depth of tumor infiltration, size, spread to adjacent tissue and regional lymphadenopathy. RUS would also allow for follow-up examinations to determine treatment response, decrease the performance of extensive surgery, aid in directing further choice of therapy and perhaps improve quality control of various treatment modalities *(1,2,25)*.

5.7. EUS IN THE FOLLOW-UP OF ANAL CANCER

The treatment strategy of anal cancer was changed in the early to mid-1980s when several authors reported excellent

Table 4
TNM Staging for Anal Carcinoma

T: Primary anal cancer	Description
T1	Tumor <2 cm in greatest dimension
T2	Tumor 2–5 cm in dimension
T3	Tumor >5 cm in greatest dimension
T4	Tumor invades adjacent organs

N: Regional lymph nodes	
N0	No regional lymph nodes
N1	Perirectal lymph nodes with tumor
N2	Unilateral internal iliac and/or inguinal lymph nodes
N3	Perirectal and inguinal lymph nodes and/or bilateral internal iliac nodes
Nx	And/or bilateral inguinal lymph nodes Regional nodes cannot be assessed

M: Distant metastasis	
M0	No distant metastasis
M1	Distant metastasis present (includes periportal lymph nodes and/or lymph nodes above the diaphragm)
Mx	Metastasis cannot be assessed

Adapted from ref. *13*.

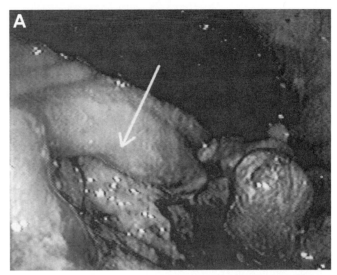
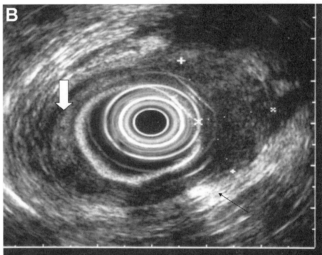
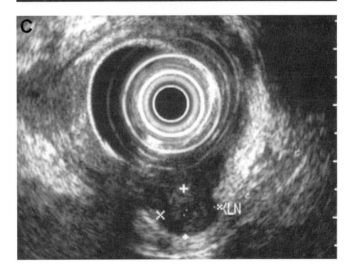

tumor control using radiation therapy as the basis of treatment. Until then, extensive surgery, using APR, which often resulted in impaired quality of life associated with rectal amputation, was considered the mainstay of therapy. Ultimately this change in treatment protocol has led to a shift towards a nonsurgical approach for anal cancer which presently includes chemotherapy combined with radiation therapy either preoperatively, or alone as the basis of treatment. This has led to overall 5-yr survival rates of approx 70–80% *(19,20,25)*.

RUS in the pretreatment staging of Anal cancer, has made a significant impact in directing therapy, but questions of its utility in the re-staging and follow up of anal carcinoma remain unanswered *(2,25)*. The treatment of anal cancer has a vigorous follow-up regimen and several experts in colorectal surgery and oncology have suggested the RUS is useful and a necessary part of a follow-up protocol. However, recently there have been some conflicting opinions to this theory. In a recently published Norwegian study by Lund et al. *(26)*, the authors retrospectively examined 82 patients with anal cancer that were treated over a 16-yr time period (1983–1999) with the main outcome measures being 5-yr survival, local recurrence rates, and how local anal cancer recurrence was detected. Their results in the follow-up of anal carcinoma, demonstrated overall 5-yr survival of 68%, with 14 of 82 patients (17%) developing local recurrence *(26)*. All of the local recurrences of anal carcinoma were first detected by DRE and visual flexible sigmoidoscopy examination despite approx 780 scheduled endoanal ultrasounds also being performed. Therefore the authors suggested, that with a careful clinical and physical examination, and flexible sigmoidoscopy, anal cancer recurrence can be detected and the addition of RUS adds to procedure costs and is unnecessary. However, long-term, multicenter prospective studies need to be performed

Fig. 8. **(A)** Endoscopic appearance of anal cancer, biopsies confirm squamous cell carcinoma. **(B,C)** Rectal endoscopic ultrasound confirms that this is T2N1 stage, with involvement of the internal anal sphinter (⇓), and disruption of the external anal sphinter anteriorly (→), and a single round, hypoechoic, malignant-appearing perirectal lymph node (anal cancer is seen to invoive the lymph node).

Table 5
Staging of Anal Cancer (From AJCC)

Stage	T (Tumor)	N (Nodal)	M (Metastasis)
I	T1	N0	M0
II	T2, T3	N0	M0
IIIA	T4	N0	M0
	T1,T2,T3	N1	M0
IIIB	T4	N1	M0
	Any T	N2, N3	M0
IV	Any T	Any N	M1

Adapted from ref. *13*.

to evaluate the role of follow-up RUS in the evaluation of anal cancer recurrence *(1,2,25,26)*.

6. CONCLUSION

In summary, RUS is easily performed and is an extremely useful modality for the evaluation and staging of anorectal malignancies. It can be done often without conscious sedation, and offers good staging accuracy of tumor because of its precise assessment of depth of infiltration of the cancer and helps to assess tumor extension and spread to adjacent organ tissue. It is also relatively helpful for nodal staging, and the technique of FNA, may be used in certain cases, to confirm malignant lymphadenopathy. This would help direct the therapeutic approach by facilitating the selection of stage-dependent treatment decisions including pre-operative chemo/radiation therapy. Furthermore, the role of RUS in staging rectal and anal carcinoma preoperatively may help to decrease extensive colorectal surgery thus improving the quality of life without sacrificing disease management and control.

The role of RUS in the restaging of anorectal malignancies after chemo/radiation therapy is less clear, as accuracy is markedly reduced owing to peritumor inflammatory and radiation changes. Similarly, routine RUS to evaluate recurrence of rectal and anal cancer, might not be as useful as once thought, again being affected by postoperative, radiation, and inflammatory changes. However, FNA may be helpful to assess disease recurrence if there is a well-defined mass, or recurrent lymphadenopathy *(27)*.

REFERENCES

1. Schwartz DA, Harewood GC, Wiersema MJ. EUS for rectal disease—review article. Gastrointest Endosc 2002; 56(1):100–109.
2. Gopal DV, Faigel DO. Rectal endoscopic ultrasound—a review of clinical applications. Practical Gastroenterol 2000; XXIV(12):24–34.
3. Bhutani M, Nadella P. Utility of an upper echoendoscope for endoscopic ultrasonography of malignant and benign conditions of the sigmoid/left colon and rectum. Am J Gastroenterol 2001; 96:3318–3322.
4. Baum AE. Overview of rectal cancer. The Resident Reporter 2001; 6(10):27–35.
5. Savides TJ, Hawes RH. Endoscopic ultrasound staging of rectal cancer. In Gastrointestinal Endosonography. Vandam & Sivak: WB Saunders; 1999:279–289.
6. Meyenberger C, Huch Boni RA, Bertschinger P, Zala GF, Klotz HP, Krestin GP. Endoscopic ultrasound and endorectal magnetic resonance imaging: a prospective, comparative study for preoperative staging and follow-up of rectal cancer. Endoscopy 1995; 27:469–479.
7. Waizer A, Powsner B, Russo I, et al. Prospective comparative study of magnetic resonance imaging versus transrectal ultrasound for preoperative staging and follow-up of rectal cancer. Preliminary report. Dis Colon Rectum 1990; 33:863–868.
8. Bhutani MS. Colorectal Endoscopic Ultrasonography. In: Gress FG and Bhattacharya I. Endoscopic Ultrasonography. Blackwell Science Inc. 2001: 126–135.
9. Rosch T, Classen M. Endosonography of the Colon and Rectum—Normal Anatomy using the Radial Scanning Echoendoscope. Gastrointestinal Endosonography. Vandam & Sivak. WB Saunders. 1999; (27):271–277.
10. Frudinger A, Bartrum CI, Halligan S, Kamm M. Examination techniques for endosonography of the anal canal. Abdominal Imaging 1998; 23:301–303.
11. Parmar KS, Fleming D, Waxman I. The Clinical impact of Endoscopic Ultrasound guided Fine Needle Aspiration in the Management of Colorectal Carcinoma. Gastrointest Endosc. 2000: Abstract#4572: AB 171.
12. Woodward T, Menke D. Diagnosis of recurrent rectal carcinoma by EUS-guided fine-needle aspiration. Gastrointest Endosc 2000; 51:223–225.
13. Colon and Rectum. American Joint Committee on Cancer. Manual for Staging of Cancer, 4th ed. Philadelphia: JB Lippincott; 1992:75–79.
14. Hawes RH. New Staging Techniques. Cancer (supplement) 1993; 71(12):4207–4213.
15. Harewood GC, Kumar KS, Clain JE, Levy MJ, Nelson H. Clinical implications of quantification of mesorectal tumor invasion by endoscopic ultrasound: All T3 rectal cancers are not equal. J Gastroenterol Hepatol. 2004; 19(7):750–755.
16. Park HH, Nguyen PT, Tran Q, Chang KJ. Endoscopic ultrasound—guided fine needle aspiration in the staging of rectal cancer. Gastrointest Endosc 2000: Abstract No. 4572:AB171.
17. Shami VM, Parmar KS, Waxman I. Clinical impact of endoscopic ultrasound and endoscopic ultrasound-guided fine-needle aspiration in the management of rectal carcinoma. Dis Colon Rectum 2004; 47(1):59–65.
18. Winde G, Nottberg H, Keller R, Schmid KW, Bunte H. Surgical cure for early rectal carcinomas (T1). Transanal endoscopic microsurgery vs anterior resection. Dis Colon Rectum 1996; 39(9): 969–976.
19. Harewood GC. Assessment of clinical impact of endoscopic ultrasound on rectal cancer. Am J Gastroenterol 2004; 99(4):623–627.
20. Swedish Rectal Cancer Trial. Improved survival with preoperative radiotherapy in resectable rectal cancer. N Engl J Med 1997; 336:980–987.
21. Lin DE, Vanagunas A, Stryker S. Endoscopic ultrasound restaging of rectal caner is inaccurate following neoadjuvant chemo-radiation therapy. Gastrointest Endosc 2000: Abstract No. 4574: AB172.
22. Vanagunas A, Lin DE, Stryker SJ. Accuracy of endoscopic ultrasound for restaging rectal cancer following neoadjuvant chemoradiation therapy. Am J Gastroenterol. 2004; 99(1):109–112.
23. Lohnert MS, Doniec JM, Henne-Bruns D. Effectiveness of endoluminal sonography in the identification of occult local rectal cancer recurrences. Dis Colon Rectum 2000; 43(4):483–491.
24. Hernandez de Anda E, Lee S-H, Finne CO, Rothenberger DA, Madoff RD, Garcia-Aguilar J. Endorectal Ultrasound in the Follow-up of Rectal Cancer Patients treated by local excision or radical surgery. Dis Colon Rectum 2004; 47:818–824.
25. Magdeburg B, Fried M, Meyenberger C. Endoscopic ultrasonography in the diagnosis, staging and follow-up of anal carcinomas. Endoscopy 1999; 31(5):359–364.
26. Lund JA, Sundstrom SH, Haaverstad R, Wibe A, Svinsaas M, Myrvold HE. Endoanal Ultrasound is of Little Value in follow-up of Anal Carcinomas. Dis Colon Rectum 2004; 47:839–842.
27. Hunerbein M, Totkas S, Moesta KT, Ulmer C, Handke T, Shlag PM. The role of transrectal ultrasound-guided biopsy in the postoperative follow-up of patients with rectal cancer. Surgery 2001; 129:164–169.

21 Endoscopic Therapy of Colorectal Carcinoma

VAMAN JAKRIBETTUU, MD AND YANG K. CHEN, MD

CONTENTS

BACKGROUND
INTRODUCTION
MANAGEMENT OF CRC
REFERENCES

1. BACKGROUND

Colon cancer is a common but often preventable disease. Although surgery is the mainstay of therapy, endoscopic therapy is helpful in managing selected cases of early colorectal cancer (CRC) and may offer palliation in advanced CRC. The role of endoscopic mucosal resection (EMR), snare polypectomy, colonic stenting, argon plasma coagulation (APC), and photodynamic therapy (PDT) in colon cancer is discussed.

2. INTRODUCTION

2.1. EPIDEMIOLOGY

CRC is a common but often preventable disease. It is the fourth most common cancer worldwide and the third leading cause of cancer in the United States (1). More than two-thirds of new cases occur in developed countries (2). The lowest incidence rates (less than 10/100,000 inhabitants) are found in Africa, South America, and Asia, except in Japan, in which there is a very high incidence in men. CRC is a lethal disease accounting for approx 10% of all deaths as a result of cancer in the United States, which is second only to lung cancer. The incidence of CRC is estimated at 130,000 new cases per year with more than 50,000 deaths directly attributable to CRC. The mortality from CRC in countries such as Japan has increased markedly in recent years owing to Westernization of dietary habits. It is believed that mortality from CRC will overtake gastric cancer in the near future in Japan. Registered annual incidence of CRC is often higher in the male population. In the United States and Canada, when the population group is determined, the incidence is usually higher in African Americans than in Caucasians. Recently, there has been a slight decline in the incidence of CRC but incidence rate for right-sided CRC in women has slightly increased (3) and it has remained markedly elevated among African Americans (4).

From: *Endoscopic Oncology: Gastrointestinal Endoscopy and Cancer Management.* Edited by: D. O. Faigel and M. L. Kochman © Humana Press, Totowa, NJ

2.2. PATHOGENESIS

The exact cause of CRC are not known (Table 1).

- Age is a major risk factor for the development of sporadic CRC and a majority of the disease occurs in people over 50 yr old.
- Family history is associated with increased risk of CRC. There are rare inherited syndromes such as familial adenomatous polyposis (FAP) or hereditary nonpolyposis colon cancer (HNPCC) that result in cancer at an unusually young age.

FAP is caused by mutation on *APC* gene on chromosome 5, which is inherited in an autosomal-dominant manner. The prevalence of this disease is 1 in 10,000 people accounting for less than 1% of CRC. More than 90% of patients with FAP develop CRC by age 40 if prophylactic colectomy is not performed.

HNPCC is an autosomal-dominant disease that is caused by abnormality in mismatch repair genes. These patients develop CRC at the mean age of 44 yr. They are also at an increased risk of developing other cancers of the gastrointestinal tract and genitourinary tract. The Amsterdam and Bethesda criteria may be used to suspect HNPCC with a high degree of probability. The Amsterdam criteria require at least three relatives with CRC (one of whom is a first-degree relative of the other two), the involvement of two generations, and one patient diagnosed with CRC under the age of 50 yr. Molecular diagnostics may confirm the suspicion of HNPCC.

Personal history of inflammatory bowel disease (IBD) also increases the risk of developing CRC. In patients with ulcerative colitis (UC) the risk begins to increase approx 7 yr after the onset and increases with the duration of the disease. The risk of developing CRC in patients with chronic UC may be as high as 35% at 30 yr. The risk of developing CRC in patients with chronic Crohn's disease is less than UC but still elevated when compared with the general population. Surveillence is discussed in Chapter 19.

239

Table 1
Risk Factors for CRC

Age > 40 yr
Low-fiber, high-fat "Westernized" diet
Personal history of CRC or colonic polyps
Family history of
 – Colon cancer
 – Familial adenomatous polyposis
 – Hereditary non-polyposis colon cancer
 – Other polyposis syndromes
Inflammatory bowel disease
 – Ulcerative colitis
 – Crohn's disease

CRC, colerectal cancer.

According to epidemiological data, CRC appears to be associated with diets rich in fat and calories and low in fiber. However, prospective studies of low-fat and high-fiber diets have failed to show any protective effect. Among the micronutrients, only calcium has been shown to have a modest effect in reducing colonic adenomas, a surrogate biomarker for CRC (5).

CRC is thought to follow the adenoma–carcinoma sequence in which polyps are premalignant lesions and a vital step in the carcinogenic progression that eventually leads to CRC. This is supported by the National Polyp Study, which showed that removal of colonic adenomas during colonoscopy prevented further development of CRC (6), discussed in detail in Chapter 17. Also, the prevalence curves for adenomas and carcinomas are similar to each other with adenoma curves shifted 5–10 yr earlier than carcinomas. Less frequently, the CRC may arise *de novo*.

2.3. SCREENING AND SURVEILLANCE FOR CRC

Screening for CRC is recommended starting at the age of 50 yr in average risk asymptomatic people (7) discussed in detail in Chapter 17.

Postpolypectomy surveillance is discussed in detail in Chapter 19.

2.4. PATHOLOGY

Carcinomas of the proximal colon tend to be bulky, often outgrowing their blood supply and undergoing necrosis. In the distal colon and rectum, the lesions are circumferential producing an annular constriction. Occasionally, in the setting of IBD tumors are flat with intramural spread. Carcinomas of the large bowel are usually adenocarcinomas, some with "Signet-ring" cells. Fifteen percent of the tumors are colloidal in which large lakes of mucin contain scattered collections of tumor cells and are more frequently seen in the setting of HNPCC, IBD, and in patients whose cancer occurs at an early age. Scirrhous carcinomas are uncommon and are characterized by sparse gland formation with marked desmoplasia.

The risk for high-grade dysplasia increases with the size of the polyp (6). The risk of dysplasia is 1% in small adenomas (<5 mm), 6% in medium-sized adenomas (5–10 mm), and 21% in large adenomas (>1 cm). Size also correlates positively with the degree of villous histology; tubular adenomas are usually smaller than villous adenomas. Villous adenomas are at a higher risk of dysplasia.

Certain endoscopic features of the polyp may suggest a superficial tumor without deep invasion of submucosa and therefore indicate endoscopic resectability. These include absence of ulceration, induration on instrumentation, or friability and the presence of the "lifting sign," i.e., the ability of the lesion to lift with submucosal injection. Saito et al. evaluated 257 patients with laterally spreading colorectal tumors of which 170 were removed by EMR (8). Ninety of these tumors were adenomas and 160 were adenocarcinomas (152 well differentiated, the rest poorly differentiated). The mean size of the lesion was 23.7 mm. Submucosal invasion was found to be extremely low in those lesions with even nodules without depression and uneven nodules without depression. Presence of depression in a polyp at colonoscopy indicated submucosal invasion and potential spread to lymph nodes (LNs) (8).

2.5. CLINICAL FEATURES

Adenocarcinomas of the colon and rectum grow slowly and are often present for years before becoming symptomatic. Right-sided colonic tumors may present with constitutional symptoms such as fatigue, shortness of breath, or angina secondary to microcytic hypochromic anemia. Obstruction from a right colonic tumor is rare unless it involves the ileocecal valve. Cancers of the left colon often cause obstructive symptoms owing to a smaller lumen, constrictive nature of the tumor and solid consistency of the stools. Rectal cancers may cause tenesmus and may locally invade the bladder, vaginal wall, or surrounding nerves, resulting in perineal or sacral pain.

Patients who are symptomatic at diagnosis have a 5-yr survival rate of 49 vs 71% for asymptomatic patients (9–11). Obstruction and perforation carry a poor prognosis, independent of stage (11). Tumors presenting with hemorrhage have been thought to have a better prognosis because of their tendency to be diagnosed earlier (11).

2.6. DIFFERENTIAL DIAGNOSIS

The differential diagnosis of CRC includes diseases that cause mass lesions, strictures, and rectal bleeding including benign tumors, diverticular disease, ischemic colitis, IBD, hemorrhoids, and infections such as amebiasis. These are differentiated by endoscopy and histology of the biopsied tissue.

3. MANAGEMENT OF CRC

3.1. STAGING

The best determinant of prognosis in CRC is the stage at diagnosis. The Duke's classification for staging of CRC is simple and widely used (Table 2).

3.1.1. Endoscopic Ultrasound

Endoscopic ultrasound (EUS) is a well-established imaging modality for staging CRC (12–15). Accurate staging of rectal cancer and assessment of extent of involvement is particularly useful for selecting patients for sphincter-preserving surgery and for neoadjuvant chemotherapy. Although EUS cannot be used to differentiate between a villous adenoma and a T1 carcinoma, it can detect infiltration of the muscularis propria by an adenoma containing a T2 carcinoma with a negative mucosal biopsy (16). EUS is also useful for excluding invasive carcinoma in large colorectal polyps when EMR is being considered (Fig. 1A,B). However, patients are sometimes referred for EUS staging after a partial or complete polypectomy or

Table 2
Duke's Classification of CRC and Prognosis

Stage	Extent of the tumor	5-yr survival (%)
A	Limited to the mucosa	100
B1	Extends into muscularis propria	85
B2	Extends through the serosa	75
C1	1–4 regional lymph nodes	65
C2	>4 regional lymph nodes	45
D	Distant metastasis	5

EMR because of incidental cancer identified in the histological specimen. Cautery-induced hypoechoic changes in the gut wall have been reported to mimic T2 and T3 lesions, thus posing a potential dilemma in the use of EUS for restaging a tumor after EMR *(17)*. One should be cognizant of this potential pitfall when interpreting the EUS findings in this setting. In a study by Cho et al. *(18)* the accuracy rate of EUS in the diagnosis of the depth of CRC in 164 patients was 83%. However, in a prospective study of 60 patients by Hizawa et al. the accuracy of invasion was 59% for pure cancers without adenomatous components. Of 40 lesions that appeared to be confined to the mucosa in this study, 8 (20%) CRC had invaded into the submucosa or beyond *(19)*. Using standard echoendoscopes, accurate staging of CRC with adenomatous component is possible, but caution must be taken in interpretation of *de novo* cancers without adenomatous components.

High-frequency ultrasound (HFUS) probes have been shown to be superior to conventional EUS in evaluating superficial lesions *(20,21)*. They accurately determine the level of submucosal invasion (sm1, sm2, or sm3) by a tumor if endoscopic therapy is considered. Saitoh et al. *(22)* evaluated 49 cases of flat and depressed tumors with a 20 MHz HFUS probe and the invasion depth was correctly diagnosed in 88% *(22)*. Depth of invasion was also accurately predicted in 13 patients with colonic lesions using 20 MHz probes by Waxman et al. *(23)*.

The procedure is usually performed with the patient in a left lateral decubitus position but repositioning may help to place the lesion of interest in the dependent portion of the rectum. Conscious sedation is not mandatory and antibiotics may be given when fine-needle aspiration cytology is planned. In order to achieve acoustic coupling and avoid overstaging, minimal balloon compression is encouraged. The radial echoendoscope is inserted to 30 cm and slowly withdrawn back to assess for iliac adenopathy. Several studies have suggested that EUS is superior to computed tomography and magnetic resonance imaging for T staging of the cancer *(24–26)*. HFUS is performed by introducing the probe through the operating channel of a colonoscope under continuous water irrigation or through water-filled balloon catheter. Examination is then conducted in a similar manner noting the invasion depth and ultrasound characteristics.

3.1.2. Magnifying Endoscopy, Chromoendoscopy, and Optical Biopsy

Chromoendoscopy is a technique in which a chromogen is used for augmenting the architectural changes in an abnormal lesion. The chromogen, such as indigo carmine, cresyl violet, acetic acid, and methylene blue, is sprayed on the mucosal sur-

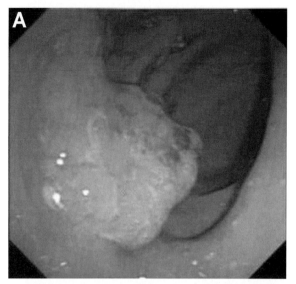

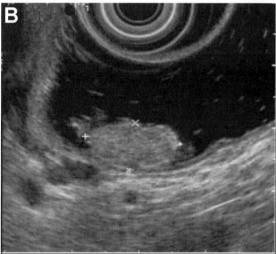

Fig. 1. **(A)** Endoscopic view of a polypoidal mass in a patient with rectal bleeding. **(B)** Endoscopic ultrasound view of the sessile polyp showing the lack of involvement of the deeper layers. Histology showed intramucosal cancer without involvement of muscularis mucosa.

face and precise morphological description of the lesion is obtained. In a study using this technique, 91% of deep submucosal invasion was identified correctly using characteristic colonoscopic findings of expansion surface, deep depression surface, irregular bottom of depression surface, and converging folds *(27)*.

Recently colonoscopes that have the ability to magnify images up to ×150 have become available. This is often combined with chromoendoscopy to highlight mucosal architecture and pit patterns. It has been able to reliably differentiate hyperplastic from adenomatous polyps and differentiate depressed-type cancers from other benign lesions *(28,29)*. However, one large study failed to predict invasion in neoplastic colonic lesions *(30)*. Techniques that utilize properties of light as it interacts with tissue such as light-induced fluorescence, optical coherence tomography, Raman spectroscopy, and light scattering are being investigated as tools for detecting dysplasia and cancer during endoscopy *(31)*.

3.2. TREATMENT
3.2.1. Surgical

Colon polyps with invasive carcinoma are traditionally treated with surgery if unfavorable criteria are present (Table 3) *(32–34)*. Endoscopic removal of a polyp with unfavorable characteristics is associated with 10–25% recurrence rate. Most surgeons include at least 2–5 cm resection margin. Despite potentially curative surgery and the use of modern adjuvant therapy, more than 40% of patients who present with stages II or III disease will have a disease recurrence following primary therapy *(35)*. The stage specific 5-yr survival rate of CRC is provided in the Table 2.

CRC detected at screening colonoscopy are at an earlier stage and potentially more amenable to endoscopic management *(36)*. When symptoms such as pain or obstruction occur at the time of presentation, the tumor is usually advanced.

3.2.2. Endoscopic
3.2.2.1. Endoscopic Mucosal Resection Techniques

EMR involves the lifting of a lesion from the deep muscle layer of the gut wall, either by injection and/or by suction of the lesion into a cap fitted to the tip of the endoscope, followed by snare removal of the lesion (Fig. 2). Complete removal of the lesion "*en bloc*" during a single therapeutic procedure is ideal because it allows for pathological examination with final staging and appropriate patient management. This is the advantage of EMR over other ablative techniques because EUS and HFUS cannot reliably distinguish between tumor infiltration and inflammation that might associated with a malignant lesion. Larger lesions of the colon, however, may require piecemeal resection. When feasible, a colonic lesion should be removed at one sitting, in order to minimize the risks and discomfort of multiple procedures and to avoid problems with scaring that follows partial removal of a lesion. If subsequent colonoscopy for piecemeal resection of residual polyp is planned, it should be repeated as soon as possible because fibrosis under any residual lesion becomes dense if the interval is longer than 2 wk *(37)*. This fibrosis may prevent elevation and separation of mucosa from the underlying layers during subsequent submucosal injection *(38)*.

Several EMR techniques have been described *(39–41)*:

1. Inject-and-cut technique.
2. Inject, lift, and cut technique.
3. EMR with ligation.
4. Cap-assisted EMR.

3.2.2.1.1. INJECT-AND-CUT TECHNIQUE

In the inject-and-cut technique, the lesion is lifted from the underlying muscularis propria by injecting a solution into the submucosal layer to produce a bleb beneath the lesion. The lesion is then captured and resected by using an electrosurgical snare (Fig. 3). The required volume of submucosal injection will vary according to the size of the lesion, provided the bleb is sufficient to ensure a good lift of the entire lesion so that it can be safely captured and resected.

One technical caveat is to perform the initial injection at the periphery and margins of the lesion farthest from the tip of the endoscope, followed by injection at the lateral margins

Table 3
Unfavorable Histological Criteria Requiring Surgery

Poorly differentiated histology
Lymphatic or venous invasion
Cancer at the resection or stalk margin
Invasion into the deep submucosa
Invasive carcinoma in a sessile polyp
Invasive carcinoma with incomplete polypectomy

and finally at the periphery of the lesion closest to the endoscope. This injection sequence minimizes the problem of obscuring the endoscopic view of the distal margins of the lesion yet to be injected. The submucosal bleb provides a pseudostalk for the snare and a protective cushion beneath the lesion, minimizing electrocautery injury to the deeper wall layers *(42)*. The colon should not be overinflated as this will thin the wall and increase the risk of perforation. The colonoscope should be rotated to keep the lesion at 6 o'clock position to facilitate endoscopic removal *(43)*. If the snare appears to entrap the muscularis propria, maneuvers such as pulling the snared tissue towards the lumen of the bowel to release the muscularis propria are performed. Carefully checking whether the snare wires are drawn back sufficiently and the snared lesion demonstrates good movement when the snare is gently moved back and forth help to ensure there is no entrapment of the muscle layer *(44)*. If piecemeal EMR is contemplated owing to a large size or difficult position of the lesion, some endoscopists recommend removal of the largest nodule of a sessile lesion first in order to diagnose pathological depth of invasion correctly *(8)*.

A variety of solutions are available for injection. Hypertonic saline-epinephrine is often used with the aim of decreasing the risk of bleeding *(45)*; other solutions have been utilized to obtain a more durable lift of the lesion *(46)*. Also, a variety of snares and currents (e.g., blended, ERBE) are preferred by different endoscopists. Barbed snares have been used to facilitate entrapment of the lesion by the electro-cautery snare *(47)*. Till date no human randomized trials have been conducted to compare the safety and effectiveness of different types of snares and injectants. Conio et al. *(42)* compared dissipation time of various submucosal fluids in porcine esophagus. The solutions compared were normal saline (NS), NS with epinephrine, 50% dextrose, 10% glycerine with 5% fructose in NS, and 1% rooster comb hyaluronic acid. The median time for dissipation was less than 3 min for NS and NS with epinephrine, 4–5 min for 50% dextrose and glycerine, and 22 min for hyaluronic acid. Tinting the fluid with a small amount of dye such as methylene blue or indigo carmine will allow better demarcation of the tumor boundaries especially in a flat lesion. Another way to delineate the lesion is to use cautery to mark the edges of the lesion *(38)*.

The advantage of the "inject and cut" technique is its simplicity and the fact that it does not require additional equipment. A disadvantage is that most solutions used to lift the lesion dissipate very rapidly thus making it difficult at times to safely capture the lesion with the snare. The early dissipation of the fluid and limited duration of mucosal "lift" can be prob-

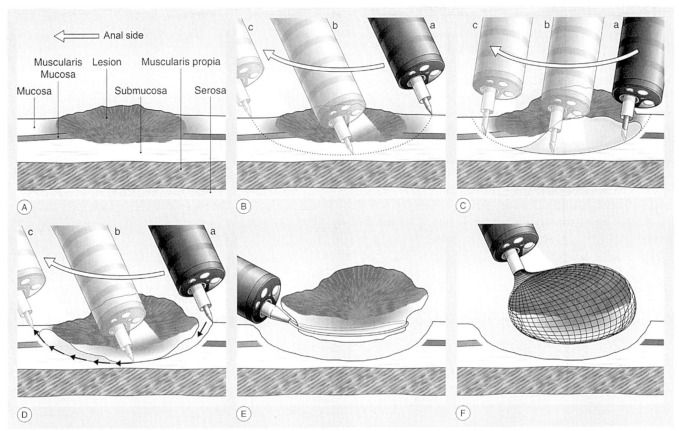

Fig. 2. *En-bloc* endoscopic mucosal resection. (**A**) Lesion involving the mucosal layer. (**B**) Marking of incision around lesion with needle knife from proximal (farther from the anus) to distal edge. (**C**) Submucosal injection of sodium hyaluronate below and around the lesion from proximal to distal edge. (**D**) Incision of marked area around lesion with needle knife from proximal to distal edge of the lesion. (**E**) Snare excision of entire lesion. (**F**) Retrieval of lesion with Roth net (Reprinted with permission from ref. *46a*.)

lematic during lengthy procedures such as EMR. Repeated injection is frequently needed during piecemeal resections to lift and separate the mucosa and prevent deep tissue injury.

3.2.2.1.2. INJECT, LIFT, AND CUT TECHNIQUE (STRIP BIOPSY)

In this technique the submucosal injection is performed in the standard manner, as already described. A snare and grasping forceps are passed through the operating channels of a dual-channel colonoscope. First the grasping forceps is captured by the open snare and the snare is closed over the forceps. Working as a unit the forceps is used to grasp the lesion, the snare is opened, and the lesion is pulled through the open snare. The snare is then closed over the lesion and resection of the lesion is performed *(48–50)* (Fig. 4). This technique is more cumbersome than the "inject and cut" technique, and requires a dual-channel colonoscope and two assistants to perform EMR.

3.2.2.1.3. EMR WITH LIGATION

In this technique, the lesion is removed with or without previous submucosal injection *(51–53)*. An endoscopic rubber band variceal ligation device is loaded over the tip of the endoscope. The lesion is ligated and snare polypectomy is then performed. The standard polypectomy snare is positioned immediately above or below the rubber band *(53)*. (Fig. 5A–C)

An advantage of this technique is that only conventional devices and instruments are required. Disadvantages include suboptimal visualization of the margins of the lesion when the variceal ligation device is loaded, and the need to reintubate after rubber band ligation. The band ligation devices are manufactured to fit the end of a gastroscope, which are generally of a smaller diameter than the colonoscope. This could lead to problems loading the device on the end of a colonoscope and a gastroscope could be used instead. As there are no case reports to date on the use of this technique in the colon, the authors recommend limiting this approach to rectal lesions only.

3.2.2.1.4. CAP-ASSISTED EMR

In this technique a specially designed transparent plastic cap is utilized *(54,55)*. The plastic cap is fitted over the tip of the endoscope and various cap sizes are available. Submucosal injection of the lesion is performed in the standard manner. A crescent-shaped snare is prelooped into the groove of the rim of the specialized cap by gently suctioning normal mucosa into the cap and opening the snare to allow it to rest along the inside groove of the rim of the cap (SD-221L-25 or SD-7P-1, Olympus America, Inc.). After prelooping the snare, the suction is turned off to release the normal mucosa. The cap is used to suction the lesion whereas maintaining constant vacuum. Once the lesion is trapped completely inside the cap, the snare is closed over the lesion. After the snare tightly strangulates the lesion, the suction is turned off and the lesion with the snare around it is allowed to leave the cap. Resection of the lesion is then performed with application of current. Gentle suction of the specimen into the cap will allow safe and com-

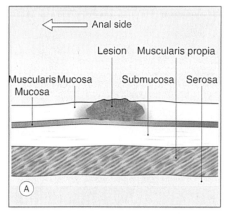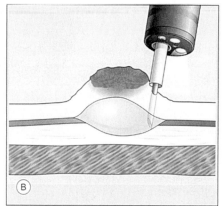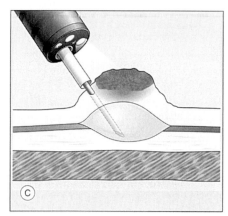
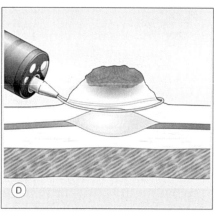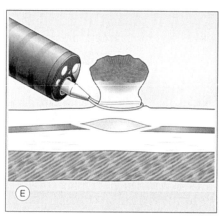

Fig. 3. Endoscopic mucosal resection inject-and-cut technique. (**A**) Lesion involving the mucosal layer. (**B**) Submucosal injection at proximal edge (farther from the anus) of the lesion. (**C**) Submucosal injection at the distal edge of the lesion. (**D**) Snaring of raised lesion. (**E**) Tightening of snare and excision of raised lesion. (Reprinted with permission from ref. *46a*.)

plete recovery of the specimen (Fig. 5). The resected specimen consists of the full thickness of the mucosal layer and upper one-third of the submucosal layer and may include surrounding normal mucosa.

For larger lesions greater than 3 cm some endoscopists have utilized a more viscous material, sodium hyaluronate, for submucosal injection. A small caliber tip transparent hood that accommodates a needle-knife or an insulated thermal knife with a ceramic cap is then used to cut around the lesion on its entire circumference. The final step is the complete removal of the lesion using a large snare *(56,57)*. Using a generous volume of fluid for submucosal injection and judicious use of suction with cap may help to reduce complications associated with this technique *(42)*.

This "suck and cut" method may have limitation in the removal of lesions located tangentially to an endoscope and for complete resection of large lesions. To overcome this limitation, Noda et al. *(58)* have described an EMR-C technique using partial transparent cap, grasping forceps, and electro-surgical current snare in the stomach and esophagus. Experience with this technique in colonic lesions is limited *(58)*.

3.2.2.2. EMR for CRC and Large Colorectal Adenomas

EMR can be a curative procedure for superficial CRC. Correct diagnosis of the depth of invasion and the absence of LN metastasis are crucial for achieving a cure with endoscopic therapy.

3.2.2.3. Preparation for Endoscopic Resection

Patients are prepped for colonoscopy using the standard bowel regimens. Some give antibiotics preoperatively for endocarditis prophylaxis when valvular heart disease is present or with prosthetic devices *(43)*.

3.2.2.3.1. PATIENT SELECTION

1. Well or moderately differentiated adenocarcinomas confined to the mucosa or superficial submucosa (sm1): Kudo classified tumor infiltration of the submucosa into sm1 (upper third), sm2 (middle third), and sm3 (lower third). The tumor category sm1 was further subdivided into sm1a, sm1b, and sm1c based on the horizontal extent of tumor invasion *(59)*. Any neoplasia that involves the middle third of the submucosa or the blood vessels needs additional surgery for LN dissection.
2. No evidence of metastasis: A superficially flat type tumor and laterally spreading variety of colonic neoplasia without depression are appropriate candidates for EMR *(8,60)*. These have a low incidence of LN metastasis. EUS maybe helpful in patient selection by delineating tumor invasion and LN involvement
3. Sessile polyps greater than 15 mm—several investigators have used EMR technique for sessile polyps greater than 15 mm *(38,47,61,62)*. Some endoscopists are of the opinion that EMR should be reserved for sessile polyps larger than 30 mm because simple piecemeal polypectomy can usually remove polyps 2–3 cm in size without complica-

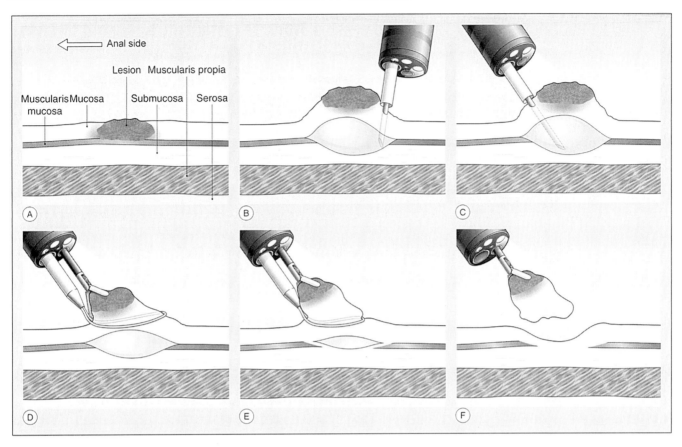

Fig. 4. Endoscopic mucosal resection inject, lift, and cut technique. **(A)** Lesion involving the mucosal layer. **(B)** Submucosal injection at proximal edge (farther from the anus) of lesion with double-channel endoscope. **(C)** Submucosal injection at distal edge of lesion. **(D)** Grasping forceps pulling lesion into open snare. **(E)** Tightening of snare and excision of lesion. **(F)** Mucosal defect created after removal of lesion. (Reprinted with permission from ref. *46a*.)

tions or residual tissue *(38)*. Similarly pedunculated lesions can be dealt with adequately by simple polypectomy techniques rather than EMR.

3.2.2.3.2. EXCLUSIONS
1. Poorly differentiated histology
2. Lymphatic or venous invasion
3. Cancer at the resection margin
4. Invasive carcinomas with incomplete polypectomy are indications for additional surgery
5. Absence of lift of the lesion with submucosal injection

Kato et al. *(63)* reviewed 94 cases of superficial CRC s that underwent EMR and classified the "lift" into four categories. These were lesions that "completely lifted and soft," "completely lifted and hard," "incompletely lifted," and "not lifted." All 44 tumors that were 'completely lifted and soft' were confined to the mucosa or sm1. Thirty two of the 37 tumors that were 'completely lifted and hard' were limited to the mucosa and sm1a/b. Five were of the of the sm1c or sm2 variety. Nine of the 15 'incompletely lifted' and all 8 of the 'not lifted' lesions were sm1c or deeper.

There have been several case series of patients undergoing EMR for colorectal polyps. These are summarized in Table 4. The techniques employed were cap assisted EMR or "inject and cut." The lesions ranged from 5 mm to more than 10 cm. Most investigators attempted to remove the lesion en bloc. The

residual tissue rate ranged from 0 to 40%. The residual polyps were managed successfully by repeat EMR in many instances. Some endoscopists used APC to treat residual tissue *(62,68)*. Surgical resection was generally performed if residual polyp tissue was noted after three endoscopic procedures. Patients with malignant infiltration into the deeper layers, poor differentiation, or unclear margins were often referred to surgery unless co-morbidities precluded operation. The complication, recurrence, and residual rates were similar for malignant polyps and large benign polyps.

Kudo et al. *(69)* did not have recurrences at 3 mo in 674 cases of early CRC managed with EMR or surgery for submucosal invasion. Kanamori et al. *(38)* in 1996, Tada et al. *(65)* in 1996 and Ahmad et al. *(61)* reported no recurrences in patients who underwent successful EMR of colonic polyps several of which were malignant. Ahmad et al. *(61)* reported a series of 101 patients who underwent EMR of the GI tract of whom 41 had colorectal neoplasms *(61)*. Nine lesions were in the cecum, 11 in the ascending colon, three in transverse colon, six in sigmoid colon and 12 in the rectum. The EMR technique utilized was "inject and cut" or "cap assisted EMR." Of these seven were adenocarcinomas, three were adenomas with high-grade dysplasia and the rest adenoma or uncertain pathology. Complete resection by EMR was achieved in 40 patients. One rectal cancer could not be resected completely and was sent to

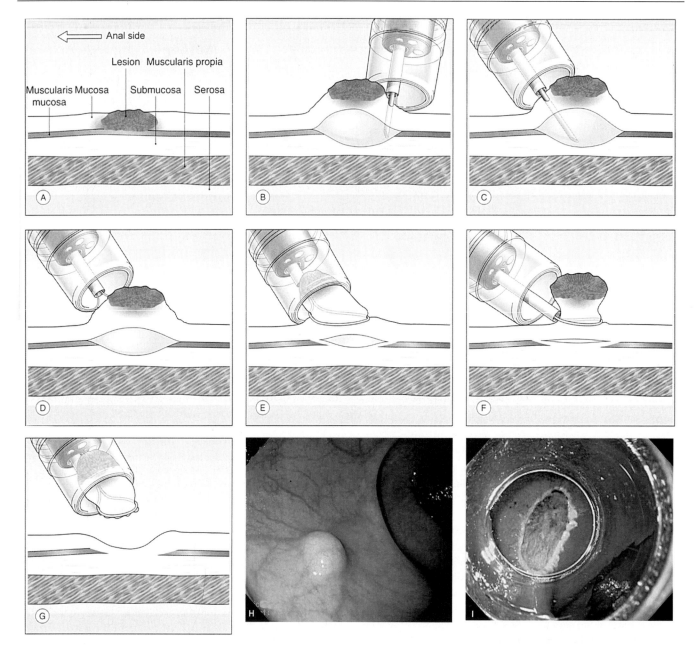

Fig. 5. (**A**) Endoscopic mucosal resection (EMR): cap-assisted EMR. Lesion involving the mucosal layer. (**B**) Submucosal injection at proximal edge (farther from the anus) of lesion. (**C**) Submucosal injection at distal edge of lesion. (**D**) Preloaded snare in groove of EMR cup. (**E**) Suction of lesion into EMR cup and capture of pseudostalk by snare. (**F**) Release of suction with continuous tight grasp of lesion by snare. (**G**) Suction of lesion into EMR cup for retrieval after snare excision. (Reproduced with permission from ref. *46a.*) (**H**) Endoscopic view of a subepithelial lesion in the colon. (**I**) Endoscopic view after cap assisted EMR showing exposed submucosa and muscularis propria. Note the bluish discoloration of the colon from methylene blue stain. Histopathologic examination revealed a carcinoid tumor. (Color versions of H and I appear in the color insert following p. 84.)

surgery. Conio et al. *(62)* performed EMR in 139 large sessile polyps, of which 58 were malignant or had high-grade dysplasia including 17 invasive cancers. All patients with invasive cancer were considered for surgery. The remaining polyps were considered to have been successfully removed by EMR. The average follow up was 12.3 mo but no follow up was available in 31 patients. Nine of 41 noninvasive malignant polyps recurred during follow up. Tanaka et al. *(47)* in 2001 reported using a barbed snare for EMR with good success *(47)*. The cap assisted EMR and inject and cut technique were utilized in the various studies and case series *(38,47,61,62,64–67)*.

3.2.2.4. Complications of EMR

Complications of EMR include adverse events secondary to sedation, as well as procedure-related complications which are specific but not exclusive to EMR.

3.2.2.4.1. BLEEDING

Bleeding is the most common complication of EMR. Extensive data are not available on the precise rate of post-polypectomy hemorrhage after EMR. Accurate prediction of delayed bleeding remains difficult. The reported incidence of bleeding after EMR has ranged between 1 and 15% *(61 62,64)*. The discrepancy may be owing to differences in definition of bleeding and to study methodology. Most institutions have reported the incidence of bleeding to be between 10 and 16%, although studies based on surveys have reported a much lower incidence. Most bleeding occurs during the procedure or within 24 h after EMR. There were a few instances of delayed bleeding occurring more than 24 h after an EMR (61,62). Among the patients who had early bleeding, 88% underwent endoscopic therapy and few required surgery or angiography (61,67). There was no extensive data on the location of the lesion in the colon and the risk for delayed post EMR bleeding. One randomized controlled study with 413 patients undergoing EMR had 3 out of 4 delayed post-EMR bleeds in the rectum (71). None of the bleeds, which occurred between 1 and 4 d post-EMR, were clinically significant and all were easily controlled by hemoclip application.

No maneuver has been shown to help prevent post-EMR bleeding, though blend current may be helpful (61). Fortunately bleeding during EMR usually stops spontaneously. Prophylactic application of hemoclips has not been found to be useful to reduce the rate of delayed post-EMR bleed, however the study excluded large polyps that were removed piecemeal (71). One group routinely bathed the base of post-EMR ulcer with thrombin solution (38). No randomized data is available to show benefits with this technique. If significant bleeding occurs, the standard methods of endoscopic hemostasis should be attempted. A few caveats are worth remembering when treating this complication endoscopically. Cautery should be applied cautiously keeping in mind that the site has already received a significant amount of energy. Vigorous delivery of additional coagulation current may result in a transmural burn or even a perforation. Injection of diluted epinephrine (1 in 10,000 or 1 in 20,000) can also be utilized to control the bleeding, either as the only measure or to prepare the bleeding site for another maneuver such as cauterization or placement of mucosal hemoclips (61,71). One potential advantage of the latter is that hemoclips do not cause additional colonic wall thermal injury to the EMR site. Detachable snares have also been used to control post-EMR bleeding (61). Hemoclip application was the preferred methodology in many case series.

Endoscopy is generally adequate to manage post-EMR bleeding. In the reported case series, patients were rarely sent to surgery or angiography for control of post-EMR bleeds.

3.2.2.4.2. PERFORATION

Perforation typically occurs when a portion of the muscularis propria is inadvertently resected in the specimen. Transmural burns secondary to aggressive cautery may also result in delayed perforation. The rate of EMR-induced perforation is highest for gastric lesions at 2.5–5%, compared with the colon at less than 1% (47,62). Reported rates of perforation are higher when performing EMR with an insulation-tipped knife (5.6%) compared with the endoscopic aspiration technique (0.8%) (30).

Some caveats may help to reduce the risk of perforation.

1. Avoid performing EMR in patients who have had prior attempts at endoscopic resection. This is because scarring

secondary to prior cauterization may prevent proper lifting of the lesion from the underlying muscularis propria during submucosal injection.
2. Proper technique and an adequate volume of submucosal injection are important to provide a margin of safety.
3. Avoid resnaring resected tissue.
4. Abort the procedure if patient experiences pain on closure of the snare as this may be an indication of full thickness capture by the snare.
5. If the snare appears to entrap the muscularis propria, maneuvers such as pulling the snared tissue towards the lumen of the bowel may help release the muscularis propria, whereas gently opening the snare.

Check if the snared lesion showing good movement when the snare is moved back and forth.

The earlier the diagnosis is established (within the first 6 h) the better the prognosis. The standard of care for management of a recognized perforation continues to be surgical. However if the perforation is small and the patient is asymptomatic, hemoclips may be utilized to close the defect but this should be performed early on (47,66,72). Patients should be placed nothing by mouth status and treated with broad spectrum antibiotics. The majority of perforations were sent to surgery in the early case series (64). In later case series, perforations were often managed conservatively and with hemoclip application (47,66).

3.2.2.4.3. TRANSMURAL BURN SYNDROME

Transmural burn syndrome occurs when thermal injury to the muscularis propria and serosa is produced by excessive electro coagulation during polypectomy or EMR. Transmural burn syndrome has been reported in 0.5–1% of colonic polypectomies but the exact incidence in EMR is still unknown.

Patients often present with symptoms and laboratory abnormalities that are indistinguishable from a perforation. Therefore it is extremely important to exclude a perforation immediately before resorting to conservative management. Once a perforation has been excluded patients should be placed on broad-spectrum antibiotics, intravenous hydration, and bowel rest. Serial abdominal X-rays should be ordered to monitor for the possibility of a late perforation. Most patients respond very well to conservative management (73).

3.2.2.4.4. LUMINAL STENOSIS

Luminal stenosis has been described as a delayed complication in patients who have had EMR mainly of an esophageal lesion (74). This complication tends to occur after extensive resection when the mucosa of more than three-fourths of the luminal circumference has been excised. This has not been described in colonic EMR.

3.2.2.5. Surveillance After an EMR

Most endoscopists repeated a colonoscopy at 3–6 mo for evaluation of polypectomy site after an EMR dependent on final histology (38,47,62,67). In the absence of a recurrence, the subsequent colonoscopies were planned at 12 mo after the EMR and every year from then on (47,62,66). We recommend that surveillance be individualized. If the polyp was partly removed, repeat the EMR as soon as possible for the goal of completing resection before dense fibrosis from scarring occurs. If there was a piecemeal resection of the colonic lesion,

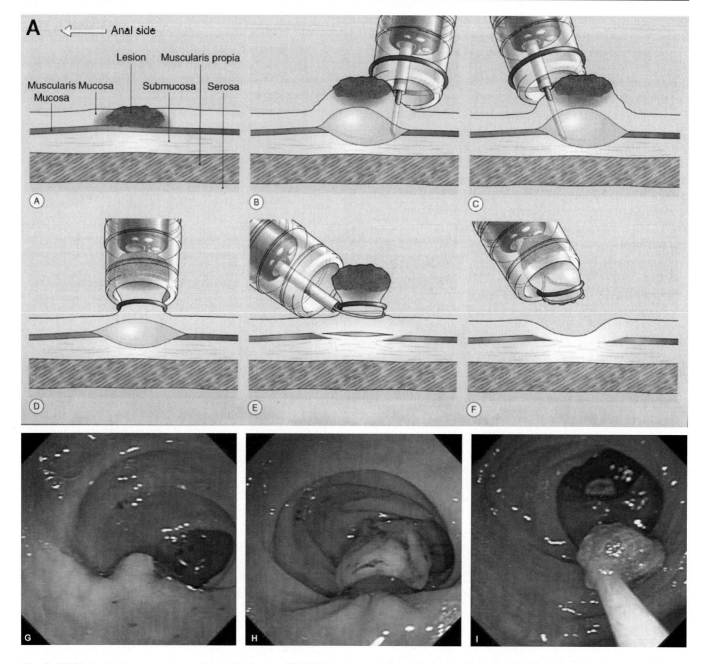

Fig. 6. (**A**) Endoscopic mucosal resection with ligation (EMRL). Lesion involving the mucosal layer. (**B**) Submucosal injection at proximal edge (farther from the anus) of lesion. (**C**) Submucosal injection at distal edge of lesion. (**D**) Suction of lesion into hood and ligation with rubber band. (**E**) Snaring and excision of lesion below the rubber band. (**F**) Mucosal defect created after removal of lesion. (Reprinted with permission from ref. *46a*.) (**G**) Sessile polyp in the colon raised by a submucosal injection containing methelene blue dye. (**H**) Band placed at the base of sessile polyp before EMR. (**I**) Resected sessile polyp being retrieved with a Roth net; polypectomy site in the background.

repeat colonoscopy in 3 mo to evaluate for residual polyp tissue.

3.2.2.6. Routine Snare Cautery Polypectomy

Snare cautery polypectomy without submucosal injection is routinely used for resection of pedunculated and small sessile colonic lesions. If the lesion cannot be removed *en bloc* owing to size (>20 mm) or difficult location, piecemeal resection is advocated. All procedures are performed on an outpatient basis, with colonic preparation as described under EMR section. Well-differentiated malignant polyps without invasion of

submucosa, lymphatics, or vasculature can be removed in the same fashion as benign polyps. The risk of nodal metastasis has been estimated by Waye to be 0.3% in pedunculated malignant polyps and 1.5% in sessile malignant polyps, which compares well with elective surgical resection *(75)*.

Technique: in order to remove a large pedunculated polyp, 1–3 cc of 1:10,000 concentration epinephrine may be injected at the base of the stalk to reduce the risk of postpolypectomy bleeding *(76)*. Then using a snare, complete entrapment of the stalk just underneath the polyp head is attempted. If unsuc-

Table 4
Selected Studies of Endoscopic Mucosal Resection of Colorectal Neoplasms

Author	No. of patients	No. of polyps	Polyp size mm (range)	Malignant lesions (%)	EMR initial success (%)	Complications	Follow up months	Recurrence of malignancy
Yokota (64)	282	337	5–21	46 (14)	283 (84)	3	NA	NA
Kanamori (38)	32	33	40 (35–80)	22 (66)	33 (100)	3	12	0
Tada (65)	25	NA	9.1 (5–45)	4	25 (100)	0	10.5 ± 4.2	0
Yoshikane (66)	23	NA	10–50	2	22 (96)	2		NA
Ishi (67)	56	56	20–50	38 (68)	49 (88)	4	34 (12–84)	NA
Tanaka (47)	NA	81	31–34 ± 20	7 (9)	81 (100)	14	61 ± 20	2
Ahmad (61)	41	41	5–70	7 (17)	40 (98)	6	14	0
Conio (62)	136	139	20-30 (15–100)	58 (42): 17 invasive, 41 non-invasive	122 (88)	20	12.3	9 of 41 noninvasive lesions

NA, data not available; EMR, endoscopic mucosal resection; f/u, follow up.

cessful, the polyp is trimmed in a piecemeal fashion until the snare can capture the entire polyp and its stalk. Sessile polyps can similarly be removed by capturing the entire lesion with the snare and shaving it off using snare cautery. If too big to be removed *en bloc*, piecemeal resection is performed. The colonoscope must be kept as straight as possible to preserve maneuverability of the endoscope. Reducing the sigmoid loop by "accordioning" the colon over the colonoscope with withdrawal motions and rotations often helps. Overdistention of the colon should be avoided and the endoscope rotated so that the polyp is viewed at the 6 o'clock position. Just as in EMR this technique is not suitable for polyps that are ulcerated or indurated or that cannot be satisfactorily visualized. Care should be taken not to capture normal mucosa that is proximal or distal to the polyp. Pulling the snared polyp to the center of the colonic lumen often helps release the trapped normal mucosa and avoids inadvertent deep tissue injury.

Using this technique, removal of colonic polyps up to 15 mm is technically feasible. Several endoscopists have described using this technique to remove polyps 30 mm or larger including malignant lesions. The rates of co-existing malignancy in these polyps were from 12 to 51% (76). Christie et al. (77) were able to successfully treat 58% of 80 polyps, size 2–6 cm, by snare cautery polypectomy . Nivatvongs et al. (78) were able to treat 28 patients with large sessile polyps successfully with snare cautery polypectomy. In this study five out of eight patients with malignancy who underwent surgical resection after polypectomy had no residual malignancy. Binmoeller et al. removed 176 polyps larger than 30 mm in 170 patients (76) of which 12% had co-existing malignancy. Bleeding complicated the procedure in 24% of the polypectomies of large polyps. Eight patients who had unfavorable criteria on histology underwent surgery after polypectomy. Only 19 patients with benign lesions had recurrences at follow-up. Only one of the seven patients with favorable malignant lesions had recurrence of malignancy and underwent surgery. Walsh et al. performed 132 polypectomies in 108 patients with a 30-mm mean polyp size; 23% had carcinoma *in situ* or carcinoma. Complications occurred in 3% with bleeding in 2% and the remainder being microperforations. More than one-fourth of the patients in this study had recur-

rence of adenomas that underwent subsequent endoscopic resection successfully. Endoscopic management was successful in 88% of the patients. Tung et al. (79) reported 338 colorectal lesions in 232 patients, 19 of which were malignant (79). All were treated endoscopically without recurrence. APC has been used in conjunction with simple snare polypectomy for complete removal and to reduce recurrence (68,80) in polyps larger than 20 mm. APC of the polypectomy base was found to be safe and useful when there is visible evidence of residual polyp.

An aggressive regimen of surveillance colonoscopy is warranted in these patients to detect and manage local recurrences and to remove subsequent adenomas. These may be done every 1–3 mo until all of the residual neoplasm is removed, then the surveillance interval may be increased to every year or more. The recurrence rate and the need for subsequent colonoscopy are greater for sessile polyps than pedunculated polyps (76). Most recurrences are detected within 9–12 mo (68).

3.2.2.6.1. COMPLICATIONS OF SNARE CAUTERY POLYPECTOMY

The complications are similar to the EMR and include bleeding, perforation, and transmural burn syndrome. Frank perforation occurs in 0.3–0.5 % and bleeding in 1–2% (81–83). The rate of complications from snare cautery polypectomy of large polyps (≥2 cm) are higher than the rate for removal of small polyps (43,76). These complications are managed in a similar manner as described under the EMR section. The post-polypectomy bleeding is usually controlled endoscopically.

3.2.2.7. Colonic Stenting

Self-expanding metal stents (SEMS) has been used in patients with advanced esophageal cancer, gastric cancer, and CRC (84–88). These patients are generally not candidates for surgery or alternative forms of therapy. In CRC, stenting has been used for palliation of a malignant obstruction and as a bridge to surgery. Pre-operative colonic decompression using SEMS has been shown in a number of studies to facilitate conversion of a conventional two-stage CRC resection surgery into a one-stage procedure in patients with colonic obstruction resulting from cancer (84).

3.2.2.7.1. TECHNIQUE OF COLONIC STENTING

Placement of SEMS requires access beyond the level of obstruction. Stent placement is achieved either through the endoscope (TTS) or by advancing a stent delivery system over a stiff guidewire with a floppy tip using fluoroscopic guidance. It is helpful to define the anatomy prior to the stent placement with a cautious barium enema or contrast computed tomography scan. The colon can be prepared in the absence of complete obstruction with enemas for distal lesions or with cautious oral preparation in partial obstruction. Prophylactic antibiotics are recommended if there is complete obstruction and/or marked colonic dilation because of the risks of microperforation and bacteremia from air insufflation. Commercially available colonic stents are all uncoated (Table 5), but coated esophageal stents have also been used in the distal colon and rectum for tumor ingrowth or for treatment of fistulas (88). The delivery system for most colonic stents is too large for introduction through the operating channel of an endoscope. Thus non-TTS stents are usually reserved for distal colonic/rectal lesions owing to the technical difficulty of advancing the stent delivery system into the proximal colon using only a guidewire and fluoroscopic guidance. The majority of CRCs are within the reach of a flexible sigmoidoscope or gastroscope; lesions proximal to the descending colon will require a longer SEMS delivery system small enough for deployment through the working channel of a colonoscope. Currently, the enteric Wallstent (Boston Scientific, Natick, MA) with a 10-Fr, 255-cm delivery system is the only FDA-approved SEMS that can be used for this purpose (Fig. 7A–C).

Typically the malignant stricture is traversed by the delivery system followed by stent deployment with fluoroscopic guidance. If the stricture cannot be traversed as in the case of high-grade or complete obstruction, a flexible guidewire (preferably with a hydrophilic tip) can be passed at least 20 cm beyond the stricture using gentle probing. The length of stent selected should account for stent foreshortening phenomenon upon deployment, and should be long enough to completely bridge the stricture leaving approximately 1–2 cm of stent at either end. Dilatation of the stricture before stent deployment may be performed but carries with it a slightly higher risk of perforation and stent migration. The distal end of the SEMS should be located at least 2 cm above the upper end of the anal canal. Dilation postdeployment should be reserved for stents that do not fully expand to at least two-thirds of the nominal stent diameter after 24 to 72 h. After the stent placement, generally a low-residue diet and laxatives are recommended.

3.2.2.7.2. Outcomes of Colonic Stenting

There are no prospective randomized trials comparing surgery vs pre-operative stenting for colonic decompression. Retrospective studies, and prospective cohort studies generally show that stenting effectively achieves colonic decompression, allowing for a one-stage operation, less total hospital days and number of days in the intensive care unit, and fewer surgical procedures. In a comprehensive review of publications reporting the outcomes of colonic stenting, endoscopic treatment was technically successful as a bridge to surgery in 85% of 223 patients, with one-stage operation possible in 95% (92). Similarly, there are no prospective randomized studies of surgery versus stenting for palliation of malignant obstruction. Several studies have shown that stenting is an effective pallia-

tion for up to 1 yr, with avoidance of surgery. In a comprehensive review of publications on colonic stenting for palliation, colostomy was avoided in 90% of 336 patients (92). Repici et al. (88) were able to successfully place covered colonic stents in 15 out of 16 people presenting with rectosigmoid obstruction with resolution of obstruction during the period of follow-up period of 21 wk (88). One patient had a perforation during stent placement that required surgery and two others had stent migration. Spinelli et al. placed metal stents for palliation of rectal cancer in 36 of 37 patients with no immediate complications and 3 events of late stent migration (89). Long-term luminal patency was maintained in 28 patients (78%). Meisner et al. placed 104 colonic stents in 96 patients with colonic obstruction for palliative treatment or postponement of emergent surgery. Clinical success was achieved in 82%. Of 38 patients presenting with acute obstruction, 29 were adequately decompressed and there were 3 perforations (90).

3.2.2.7.3. Complications of Colonic Stenting

1. Perforation: this is anywhere between 5 and 30% and more if balloon dilatation is performed and more likely in the distal colon (91). Urgent surgical management is warranted specially if the colon is not prepped.
2. Stent migration: migration of metal stents can occur in up to 25%. This is more so if the stricture has been dilated or small caliber stents are used. With esophageal and biliary stenting tissue hyperplasia occurs as a result of pressure necrosis by the stent against the wall and this helps to anchor the stent in place. With colonic stenting, the large diameter of the colonic lumen decreases this tissue reaction and thus stent migration may be more likely to occur. This complication is usually addressed by placement of a second stent of larger caliber if possible. Sometimes the new stent can be used to bridge the migrated stent and the stricture.
3. Bleeding may be caused by the jagged edges of the stent and also by friability of tumor tissue. Local endoscopic therapy such as epinephrine injection may be attempted for profuse bleeding and if unsuccessful angiographic embolization may be an option.
4. Stent occlusion: to avoid fecal impaction within the stent, stools should ideally be maintained at a soft consistency with a low-residue diet and laxatives. Other causes of obstruction such as tumor overgrowth and ingrowth require reintervention with a new stent placement or tumor debulking with thermal techniques.
5. Tenesmus, rectal pain and fecal incontinence may occur as a result of stent migration or malposition too low in the rectum.

3.2.2.8. Laser Ablation

Lasers (Light Amplification by Stimulated Emission of Radiation) are devices that produce a light energy that is focused into a unidirectional, single wavelength beam. The most common medical uses of lasers derive from the conversion of light to heat energy. The laser light beam can be used to cut, coagulate, or vaporize tissue depending on the wavelength of light, power density used to excite the lasing medium, and absorption and scattering. Neodymium/Yttrium-Aluminum-Garnet (Nd:YAG), CO_2, Nd:Holmium, and the

Table 5
Commercially Available Colonic Stents in the United States

Type	Delivery system (F)	Metal, design	Deployed shaft (mm)	Deployed length (cm)
Memoderm	14.5	Nitinol Wire mesh	30	6, 8, 10
Colonic Z-stent	31	Stainless steel Open wire spring	25	4, 6, 8, 10, 12
Enteral wallstent	10	Stainless steel Wire mesh	20–22	6, 9
Colonic ultraflex	21	Nitinol Wire mesh	25	5.7, 8.7, 11.7

argon ion laser are the most frequently used lasers in biomedical applications.

When performing laser therapy safety eyewear is used to avoid ocular damage to the patient and personnel. Adequate local exhaust ventilation and use of respiratory filter masks have been recommended to avoid respiratory exposure to aerosolized infectious pathogens resulting from vaporization of tissue (93). Endoscopic therapy using the neodymium-yttrium-aluminum-garnet (Nd:YAG) laser has been used to recanalize the rectum as palliative therapy in patients with obstructing rectal cancers who are poor surgical risks or who have advanced stages of malignant disease. Palliation generally has been satisfactory. Because of its limited portability, high cost, availability of less costly alternatives and the need for specific training, laser therapy is not widely used today for endoscopic treatment of colonic neoplasms.

3.2.2.8.1. ND:YAG LASER

Laser energy can be delivered through flexible optic fibers at wavelengths of 1320 and 1064 nm. Because the emission is invisible, a helium–neon aiming beam is used in conjunction with Nd:YAG to visualize the focal target area (94,95). To obtain photoablation an optical fiber is passed through the operating channel of the endoscope and the transmitted laser beam can be delivered in a contact or non-contact fashion. Tangential therapy is not possible with this technique so the location of some lesions may be more difficult to target (96).

3.2.2.8.2. LASER THERAPY AND CRC

Liozou et al. (97) treated 49 patients who had unresectable rectosigmoid carcinoma with endoscopic Nd:YAG laser treatment for palliation of symptoms and tumor eradication. In seven patients with tumors less than 3 cm in diameter, symptomatic improvement was achieved in all (mean follow-up 16 mo) and complete tumor eradication in three. In the remaining 42 patients with larger tumors (34 greater than two-thirds circumferential, mean length 5.5 cm), symptomatic improvement was achieved with repeated treatments (average 3.4) in 31 (74%) over a mean follow-up of 19 wk. Bowel perforation occurred in two patients (5%) but there was no treatment-related mortality. Brunetaud et al. (98) treated 272 patients for palliation of symptoms from rectosigmoid cancer. The immediate success rate and complication rate were 85 and 2%, respectively. Patients with an advanced cancer remained functionally improved during a 10.1 mo average period after initial improvement. Daneke et al. (99) subjected 37 patients to endo-scopic laser therapy sessions. In 84% of patients, patency was maintained during a median follow-up of 31.5 wk (range, 1–123). Morbidity and mortality were 2.5% (3/123) and 5% (1/37), respectively. Mandava et al. (100) retrospectively reviewed 27 patients with colorectal carcinoma treated with endoscopic Nd:YAG laser with palliative intent. The mean number of Nd:YAG laser treatments was three, with a range from one to nine. Of 27 patients, 4 (15%) developed complications. The success rate in terms of the relief of symptoms was 23 of 27 patients. Tan et al. (101) reported the results of treating 26 cases of inoperable CRC with Nd:YAG laser. Initial therapy improved quality of life in 92% of patients. Sixteen patients received follow-up maintenance therapy, with laser treatments performed over a mean interval of 7.3 (1–20) wk. Three patients (12%) suffered complications, with two deaths (8%). To summarize, laser therapy is reasonably effective in palliation of CRC but is tedious and associated with significant complications.

3.2.2.8.3. COMPLICATIONS OF LASER THERAPY

Bleeding is one of the most common complications of Nd:YAG laser therapy. A major bleeding rate of 12.5% after laser treatment has been reported (102). Perforations may occur in 1 to 9%, with a procedure-related mortality of up to 1%. Stricture formation as a late complication of laser therapy (Nd:YAG and PDT) has been observed in 5–13%.

3.2.2.9. Photodynamic Therapy

PDT delivers energy via flexible optic fibers. The laser light activates a photosensitizing agent, releasing toxic singlet oxygen, and causing tissue necrosis. The photosensitizer selectively accumulates in the target tissue, usually in a preferential manner. The only commercially available photosensitizer in the United States is porfimer sodium (Photofrin) (103). Other photosensitizes include 5-aminolevulinic acid (5-ALA), zinc II phthalocyanine, aluminum sulfonated phthalocyanine, benzoporphyrin, meta-tetrahydroxyphenylchlorin (mTHPC), N-aspartyl chlorine e6 (NPe6), and motexafin lutetium.

Among these different photosensitizers mTHPC, porfimer sodium, and ALA have been used extensively in gastroenterology. mTHPC is a potent, highly selective drug that has been used in the treatment of neoplasms, whereas ALA, which induces very superficial necrosis, has been used to treat Barrett's esophagus (104,105).

Porfimer sodium is administered at a recommended dose of 2 mg/kg intravenously, and activated 48 h later by a tunable dye laser at 630 nm (103). ALA is a heme pathway precursor

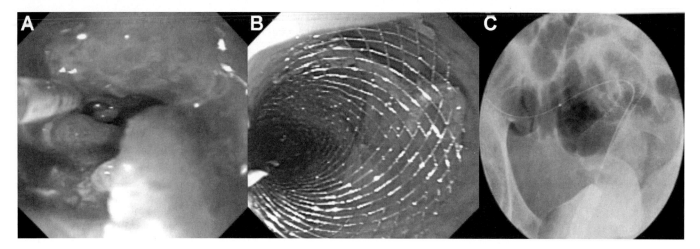

Fig. 7. (A) Endoscopic view of an obstructing colon cancer and use of a biliary catheter and guidewire to traverse the stricture. (B) Endoscopic view of self-expandable metal stent (Wallstent) placement. (C) Fluoroscopic view of Wallstent placement over a guidewire.

that can be given orally or intravenously. ALA is then converted to the endogenous photosensitized protoporphyrin IX that can be activated by red or green light.

PDT remains experimental and has been used to treat a small number of patients who are poor surgical risks with some success. Milkvy et al. *(106)* used PDT to treat large polyps (four duodenal and two colorectal) unsuitable for surgery in six patients with FAP. Patients were sensitized with ALA orally or intravenous porfimer sodium at 2 mg/kg. Laser treatment was performed 6 h after ALA or 48 h using a gold vapor laser. Necrosis was only superficial (up to 1.8 mm) using ALA but much deeper using porfimer sodium. The one malignant polyp (8-mm diameter in the colon) showed a complete response using porfimer. All healed safely with no complications. porfimer appeared to be efficacious, but caused cutaneous photosensitivity lasting up to 3 mo. ALA cleared within 2 d, but its use is limited by the superficial effect. Barr used PDT to treat 10 patients with CRC and achieved long-term remission in 2 patients with small tumors. One patient with a bulky CRC bled after therapy *(107)*. Kashatan et al. *(108)* conducted a pilot study using PDT in six patients with advanced, recurrent rectal cancer. Five patients had both clinical and radiological response to therapy. One patient developed a significant sunburn after discharge. There was no major toxicity of bleeding or sepsis. Loh et al. *(109)* treated eight patients with nine colosigmoid villous adenomas measuring 1–5 cm in length with PDT. Seven adenomas were eradicated. No local complications were seen. Substantial necrosis was produced in the other two adenomas, but they were not completely destroyed. One patient had photosensitivity but otherwise there were no complications. Photosensitization lasting up to 3 mo, and severe sunburn, have been reported in 5–7% of patients after PDT therapy *(104,110)*.

3.2.2.10. Argon Plasma Coagulation
APC is a simple, safe and versatile technique to deliver a high frequency current via ionized argon gas for coagulating tissue. In the early 1990s an APC delivery catheter that could be inserted through a flexible endoscope was invented by Farin and Grund *(111)*. The ionized argon gas (plasma) that flows

from the catheter tip provides a noncontact medium to deliver monopolar current to the mucosal surface. It can deliver a tangential current to uniformly coagulate a target lesion *(112)*. Initially introduced as a haemostatic device, the technology subsequently was utilized for ablation of Barrett's esophagus *(113,114)* and superficial neoplastic lesions and for debulking tumors.

The depth of injury correlates with the power setting, duration of burn and total energy delivery *(112)*. At lower power settings (45 watts) the depth of injury is limited due to tissue desiccation with consequent electric arcing to surrounding non-desiccated tissue. The depth of injury with APC is believed to be less than other modalities of coagulation.

The standard equipment consists of a high frequency generator and an automatically regulated argon source. The APC current and argon gas are delivered via a flexible probe introduced through the operating channel of the endoscope. Straight fire and side fire probes are available. The recommended settings for ablation of colonic lesions using the APC 300/ICC 200 electrosurgical system (ERBE USA Incorporated Surgical Systems, Marietta, GA) are, mode: auto coag; coagulation type: forced, and argon plasma flow rate: 1.0–2.0 L/min.

Power settings:

1. 45 watts for "touch up" coagulation of residual polyp tissue after piecemeal resection of large sessile colonic polyps.
2. 75–90 watts for tumor debulking

The VIO300D-APC2, a new second generation APC system recently released by the same manufacturer, achieves similar results at power settings at approximately half of the APC 300 unit.

3.2.2.10.1. APC IN CRC
APC has been used for endoscopic obliteration of superficial tumors and tumor debulking. It has been used in the fulguration of residual adenomas in patients with FAP and residual colonic polyp tissue after piecemeal polypectomy (Fig. 8A–C) *(68,80,115)*. In patients with apparent complete endoscopic snare resection of large sessile adenomas, post-polypectomy

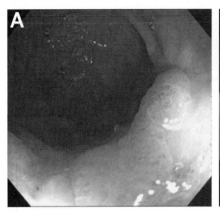 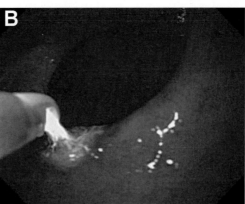 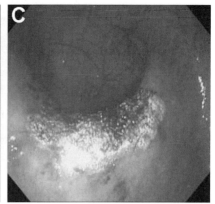

Fig. 8. (**A**) Endoscopic view of a sessile colonic polyp. (**B**) Argon plasma coagulation therapy of the polyp. (**C**) Post-treatment view of the sessile polyp.

applications of APC reduced adenomatous recurrence *(115)*. In the same study, 7 of 13 patients (9 with high-grade dysplasia) with incomplete snare polypectomy treated with APC, there was no recurrence at 3 mo follow-up colonoscopy. Four of the six patients with residual polyp tissue at 3 mo in this group had resolution with further applications of APC *(115)*. In another study, APC therapy in 77 patients with colorectal adenomas (7 malignant) had long-term resolution in 69 patients. Diagnosis of CRC was delayed owing to unsuccessful endoscopic therapy in two of these seven patients with malignancy *(68)*.

Owing to recurrences that are sometimes seen in patients undergoing APC ablation of large sessile tumors and lack of long-term controlled data, careful patient selection, and stringent endoscopic follow-up are necessary *(68,115)*.

3.2.2.10.2. COMPLICATIONS OF APC

Complications rates with APC are low compared with other methods of coagulation such as such as Nd:YAG laser, heat probe, and monopolar electrosurgery current. The morbidity is low and minor consisting of gas bloating and transient abdominal or anal pain in 10% of cases.

3.2.2.10.2.1. PERFORATION

This is the most severe complication but fortunately rare. The frequency was 0.27% in a study with 1062 patients *(116)*. It has been described with coagulation of right colon angiodysplasia and coagulation of adenomas in the rectal stump of a patient with FAP *(117)*. Using an animal model Norton et al. *(112)* showed that circular muscle damage was common during APC of the right colon. As total energy delivered tripled from 45 to 135 J, the circular muscle injury rose from 0 to 90%. The incidence of deep injury to the colon wall can be reduced by reducing the duration of application (short bursts or sweeping motion), lower power (45 watts instead of 60/75 watts) and using submucosal saline injection before APC application *(118)*.

3.2.2.10.2.2. MISCELLANEOUS

Rectovaginal fistula *(119)*, chronic rectal ulceration *(120)*, bowel explosion with certain bowel preparations *(121,122)*, and rectal stricture *(120)* have been described in patients undergoing APC application of radiation proctitis. Rigorous preparation of the colon using polyethylene glycol or phosphosoda and avoidance of colon preparation using only ene-

mas or fermentable agents before APC application will minimize bowel explosions.

REFERENCES

1. Jemal A, Tiwari RC, Murray T, et al. Cancer statistics, 2004. CA Cancer J Clin 2004; 54(1):8–29.
2. Parkin DM, Pisani P, Ferlay J. Estimates of the worldwide incidence of eighteen major cancers in 1985. Int J Cancer 1993; 54:594–606.
3. Weir HK, Thun MJ, Hankey BF, et al. Annual report to the nation on the status of cancer, 1975–2000, featuring the uses of surveillance data for cancer prevention and control. J Natl Cancer Inst 2003; 95:1276–1299.
4. Chow WH, Devesa SS, Blot WJ. Colon cancer incidence: recent trends in the United States. Cancer Causes Control 1991;2:419–425.
5. Bonithon-Kopp C, Kronborg O, Giacosa A, Rath U, Faivre J. Calcium and fibre supplementation in prevention of colorectal adenoma recurrence: a randomised intervention trial. European Cancer Prevention Organisation Study Group. Lancet 2000; 356: 1300–1306.
6. Winawer, SJ, Zauber, AG, O'Brien, MJ, et al. Randomized comparison of surveillance intervals after colonoscopic removal of newly diagnosed adenomatous polyps. The National Polyp Study Work Group. N Engl J Med 1993; 328:901.
7. Winawer SJ, Fletcher R, Rex D, et al. Colorectal cancer screening and surveillance: Clinical guidelines and rationale. Update based on new evidence. Gastroenterology 2003; 124:544.
8. Saito Y, Fujii T, Kondo H, Yokota T, Kozu T, Saito D. Endoscopic treatment for laterally spreading tumors in the colon. Endoscopy 2001; 33 (8):682–686.
9. Beahrs OH, Sanfelippo PM. Factors in prognosis of colon and rectal cancer. Cancer 1971; 28:213–218.
10. Copeland EM, Miller LD, Jones RS. Prognostic factors in carcinoma of the colon and rectum. Am J Surg 1968; 116:875–881.
11. Wolmark N, Wieand HS, Rockette HE, Fisher B. The prognostic significance of tumor location and bowel obstruction in Dukes B and C colorectal cancer. Findings from the NSABP clinical trials. Ann Surg 1983; 198:743–752.
12. Tio TL, Weijers O, Hulsman F, et al. Endosonography of colorectal diseases. Endoscopy 1992; 24:309–314.
13. Hizawa K, Suekane H, Aoyagi K, Matsumoto T, Nakamura S, Fujishima M. Use of endosonographic evaluation of colorectal tumor depth in determining the appropriateness of endoscopic mucosal resection. Am J Gastroenterol 1996; 91:768–71.
14. Ashihara T, Cho E, Hirano S, Yasuda K, Nakajima M. An ultrasonic probe in the diagnosis of colorectal lesions. Endoscopy 1992; 24:A657,A658.
15. Harada N, Hamada S, Kudo H, et al. Preoperative evaluation of submucosal invasive colorectal cancer using a 15-MHz ultrasound miniprobe. Endoscopy 2001; 33:237–240.

16. Boyce GA, Sivak MJ, Lavery IC, et al. Endoscopic ultrasound in the preoperative staging of rectal carcinoma. Gastrointest Endosc 1991; 38:468–477.

17. Chen YK, Powis ME. Pitfalls of endoscopic ultrasound staging after application of cautery. J Clin Gastroenterol 2004; 38: 1–5.

18. Cho E, Nakajima M, Yasuda K, Ashihara T, Kawai K. Endoscopic ultrasonography in the diagnosis of colorectal cancer invasion. Gastrointest Endosc 1993; 39:521–527.

19. Hizawa K, Suekane H, Aoyagi K, Matsumoto T, Nakamura S, Fujishima M. Use of endosonographic evaluation of colorectal tumor depth in determining the appropriateness of endoscopic mucosal resection. Am J Gastroenterol 1996; 91:768–771.

20. Yoshida M, Tsukamoto Y, Niwa Y, et al. Endoscopic assessment of invasion of colorectal tumors with a new high-frequency ultrasound probe. Gastrointest Endosc 1995; 41:587–592.

21. Hasegawa N, Niwa Y, Arisawa T, Hase S, Goto H, Hayakawa T. Preoperative staging of superficial esophageal carcinoma: comparison of an ultrasound probe and standard endoscopic Ultrasonography. Gastrointest Endosc 1996; 44:388–393.

22. Saitoh Y, Obara T, Einami K, et al. Efficacy of high frequency ultrasound probes for the preoperative staging of invasion depth in flat and depressed colorectal tumors. Gastrointest Endosc 1996; 44:34–39.

23. Waxman I, Saitoh Y. Clinical outcome of endoscopic mucosal resection for superficial GI lesions and the role of high frequency US probe sonography in an American population. Gastrointest Endosc 2000; 52:322–327.

24. Hildebrandt, U, Klein, T, Feifel, G, et al. Endosonography of pararectal lymph nodes. In vitro and in vivo evaluation. Dis Colon Rectum 1990; 33:863.

25. Thaler, W, Watzka, S, Martin, F, et al. Preoperative staging of rectal cancer by endoluminal ultrasound vs. magnetic resonance imaging. Preliminary results of a prospective, comparative study. Dis Colon Rectum 1994; 37:1189.

26. Rifkin, MD, Ehrlich, SM, Marks, G. Staging of rectal carcinoma: Prospective comparison of endorectal US and CT. Radiology 1989; 170:319.

27. Saitoh Y, Obara T, Watari J, et al. Invasion depth diagnosis of depressed type early colorectal cancers by combined use of videoendoscopy and chromoendoscopy. Gastrointest Endosc 1998; 48:362–370.

28. Kudo S, Tamure S. Nakajima T. Hirota S. Asano M. Ito O. Kusaka H. Depressed type of colorectal cancer. Endoscopy 1995; 27:54–57.

29. Hurlstone, DP, Brown, S, Cross, SS. The role of flat and depressed colorectal lesions in colorectal carcinogenesis: new insights from clinicopathological findings in high-magnification chromoscopic colonoscopy. Histopathology 2003; 43:413–426.

30. Hurlstone, DP, Cross, SS, Adam, I, et al. Efficacy of high magnification chromoscopic colonoscopy for the diagnosis of neoplasia in flat and depressed lesions of the colorectum: a prospective analysis. Gut 2004; 53:284–290.

31. Wagnieres GA, Star WH, Wilson BC. In vivo fluorescence spectroscopy and imaging for oncological applications: Invited Review. Photochem Photobiol 1998; 68:603–632.

32. Conte, CC, Welch, JP, Tennant, R, et al. Management of endoscopically removed malignant colon polyps. J Surg Oncol 1987; 36: 116–121.

33. Haggitt, RC, Glotzbach, RE, Soffer, EE, et al. Prognostic factors in colorectal carcinomas arising in adenomas: Implications for lesions removed by endoscopic polypectomy. Gastroenterology 1985; 89:328–336.

34. Wilcox, GM, Anderson, PB, Colacchio, TA. Early invasive carcinoma in colonic polyps: A review of the literature with emphasis on the assessment of the risk of metastasis. Cancer 1986; 57:160–171.

35. Desch, CE, Benson, AB III, Smith, TJ, et al. Recommended colorectal cancer surveillance guidelines by the American Society of Clinical Oncology. J Clin Oncol 1999; 17:1312.

36. Mandel JS, Bond JH, Church TR, et al. Reducing mortality from colorectal cancer by screening for fecal occult blood. Minnesota colon cancer control study. N Eng J Med 1993; 328:1365–1371.

37. Karita M, Tada M, Okita K. The successive strip biopsy partial resection technique for large early gastric and colon cancers. Gastrointest Endosc 1992; 38:174–178.

38. Kanamori T. Itoh M, Yokoyama Y, Tsuchida K. Injection incision assisted snare resection of large sessile colorectal polyps. Gastrointest Endosc 1996; 43:189–195.

39. Rembacken BJ, Gotoda T, Fujii T, Axon AT. Endoscopic mucosal resection. Endoscopy 2001; 33:709–718.

40. Inoue H, Tani M, Nagai K, et al. Treatment of esophageal and gastric tumors. Endoscopy 1999; 31:47–55.

41. Shim CS. Endoscopic mucosal resection. J Korean Med Sci 1996; 11:457–466.

42. Conio M, Rajan E, Sorbi D, et al. Comparative performance in the porcine esophagus of different solutions used for submucosal injection. Gastrointest Endosc 2002; 56:513–516.

43. Walsh RM, Ackroyd FW, Shellito PC. Endoscopic resection of large sessile colorectal polyps. Gastrointest Endosc 1992; 38:303–309.

44. Yoshikane H, Hidano H, Sakakibara A, Mori S, Takahashi Y, Niwa Y, Goto H. Endoscopic resection of laterally spreading tumours of the large intestine using a distal attachment. Endoscopy 1999; 31:426–430.

45. Hirao M, Masuda K, Asanuma T, et al. Endoscopic resection of early gastric cancer and other tumors with local injection of hypertonic saline–epinephrine. Gastrointest Endosc 1988; 34:264–269.

46. Yamamoto H, Yube T, Isoda N, et al. A novel method of endoscopic mucosal resection using sodium hyaluronate. Gastrointest Endosc 1999; 50:251–256.

46a. Antillon M, Cnen YK. Endoscopia therapy for gastic neoprisms. In: Ginsberg GG, Kochman ML, Norton I, Gostout CJ, eds. Clinical Gastrointestinal Endoscopy. Philadelphia: Elsevier; 2005:505–528.

47. Tanaka S, Haruma K, Oka S, et al. Clinicopathologic features and endoscopic treatment of superficially spreading colorectal neoplasms larger than 20 mm. Gastrointest Endosc 2001; 54:62–66.

48. Karita M, Tada M, Okita K, Kodama T. Endoscopic therapy for early colon cancer: the strip biopsy resection technique. Gastrointest Endosc 1991; 37:128–132.

49. Tada M, Murakami A, Karita M, Yanai H, Okita K. Endoscopic resection of early gastric cancer. Endoscopy 1993; 25:445–450.

50. Takekoshi T, Baba Y, Ota H, et al. Endoscopic resection of early gastric carcinoma: results of a retrospective analysis of 308 cases. Endoscopy 1994; 26:352–358.

51. Suzuki Y, Hiraishi H, Kanke K, et al. Treatment of gastric tumors by endoscopic mucosal resection with a ligating device. Gastrointest Endosc 1999; 49:192–199.

52. Suzuki H. Endoscopic mucosal resection using ligating device for early gastric cancer. Gastrointest Endosc Clin N Am 2001; 11: 511–518.

53. Ell C, May A, Gossner L, Pech O, et al. Endoscopic mucosal resection of early cancer and high-grade dysplasia in Barrett's esophagus. Gastroenterology 2000; 118:670–677.

54. Inoue H, Takeshita K, Hori H, Muraoka Y, Yoneshima H, Endo M. Endoscopic mucosal resection with a cap-fitted panendoscope for esophagus, stomach, and colon mucosal lesions. Gastrointest Endosc 1993; 39:58–62.

55. Tada M, Inoue H, Yabata E, Okabe S, Endo M. Feasibility of the transparent cap-fitted colonoscope for screening and mucosal resection. Dis Colon Rectum 1997; 40:618–621.

56. Yamamoto H, Kawata H, Sunada K, et al. Successful en-bloc resection of large superficial tumors in the stomach and colon using sodium hyaluronate and small-caliber-tip transparent hood. Endoscopy 2003; 35:690–694.

57. Ono H, Kondo H, Gotoda T, et al. Endoscopic mucosal resection for treatment of early gastric cancer. Gut 2001; 48:225–229.

58. Noda M, Kobayashi N, Kanemasa H, Endoscopic mucosal resection using a partial transparent hood for lesions located tangentially to the endoscope. Gastrointest Endosc 2000; 51:338–343.
59. Kudo S. Endoscopic mucosal resection of flat and depressed types of early colorectal cancer. Endoscopy 1993; 25:455–461.
60. Expert approaches to Endoscopic Mucosal resection. Clin P Gastro 2000; 178–185.
61. Ahmad NA, Kochman ML, Long WB, Furth EE, Ginsberg GG. Efficacy, safety and clinical outcomes of endoscopic mucosal resection: a study of 101 cases. Gastrointest Endosc 2002; 55:390–396.
62. Conio M, Repici A, Demarquay JF, Blanchi S, Dumas R, Filiberti R. EMR of large sessile colorectal polyps. Gastrointest Endosc 2004; 60:234–241.
63. Kato H, Haga S, Endo S, et al. Lifting of lesions during endoscopic mucosal resection of early colorectal cancer: Implications for the assessment of resectability. Endoscopy 2001; 33:568–573.
64. Yokota T, Sugihara K, Yoshida S. Endoscopic mucosal resection for colorectal neoplastic lesions. Dis Colon Rectum 1994; 37:1108–1111.
65. Tada M, Inoue H, Yabata E, Okabe S, Endo M. Colonic mucosal resection using a transparent cap-fitted endoscope. Gastrointest Endosc 1996; 44:63–65.
66. Yoshikane H, Hidano H, Sakakibara A, et al. Endoscopic resection of laterally spreading tumors of the large intestine using a distal attachment. Endoscopy 1999; 31:426–430.
67. Iishi H, Tatsuta M, Iseki K,et al. Endoscopic piecemeal resection with submucosal saline injection of large sessile colorectal polyps. Gastrointest Endosc 2000; 51:697–700.
68. Regula J, Wronska E, Polkowski M, et al. Argon plasma coagulation after piecemeal polypectomy of sessile colorectal adenomas: long term follow-up study. Endoscopy. 2003; 35:212–218.
69. Kudo S. Endoscopic mucosal resection of flat and depressed types of early colorectal cancer. Endoscopy 1993; 25:455–461.
70. Shioji K, Suzuki Y, Kobayashi M, et al. Prophylactic clip application does not decrease delayed bleeding after colonoscopic polypectomy. Gastrointest Endosc 2003; 57:691–694.
71. Okano A, Hajiro K, Takakuwa H, Nishio A, Matsushita M. Predictors of bleeding after endoscopic mucosal resection of gastric tumors. Gastrointest Endosc 2003; 57:687–690.
72. Tsunada S, Ogata S, Ohyama T, et al. Endoscopic closure of perforations caused by EMR in the stomach by application of metallic clips. Gastrointest Endosc 2003; 57:948–951.
73. Waye JD. Management of complications of colonoscopic polypectomy. Gastroenterologist 1993; 1:158–164.
74. Katada C, Muto M, Manabe T, Boku N, Ohtsu A, Yoshida S. Esophageal stenosis after endoscopic mucosal resection of superficial esophageal lesions. Gastrointest Endosc 2003; 57:165–169.
75. Waye JD. When is colonoscopic resection of an adenomatous polyp containing a "malignancy" sufficient? Am J Gastroenterol 1990; 85:1564–1566.
76. Binmoeller KF, Bobnacker S, Seifert H, Thonke F, Valdeyer H, Soehendra N. Endoscopic snare excision of giant colorectal polyps. Gastrointest Endosc 1996; 41:183–188.
77. Christie JP. Colonoscopic excision of large sessile polyps. Am J Gastroenterol 1977; 67:430–438.
78. Nivatvongs S, Snover DC, Fang DT. Piecemeal snare excision of large sessile colon and rectal polyps: is it adequate? Gastrointest Endosc 1984; 30:18–20.
79. Tung S, Wu C, Wu M, Su M. Endoscopic treatment of colorectal polyp and early cancer. Dig Dis Sci 2001; 46:1152–1156.
80. Zlatanic J, Waye JD, Kim PS, Baiocco PJ, Gleim GW. Large sessile colonic adenomas: use of argon plasma coagulator to supplement piecemeal snare polypectomy. Gastrointest Endosc 1999; 49:731–735.
81. Johnson SM. Colonoscopy and polypectomy. Am J Surg 1978; 136:313–316.
82. Webb WA, McDaniel L, Jones L. Experience with 1000 colonoscopic polypectomies. Ann Surg 1985; 5:626–632.
83. Nivatvongs S. Complications in colonoscopic polypectomy: lessons to learn form an experience with 1576 polyps. Am Surg 1988; 54:62–63.
84. Baron TH, Dean PA, Yates MR, Canon C, Koehler RE. Expandable metal stents for the treatment of colonic obstruction: techniques and outcomes. Gastrointest Endosc 1998; 47:277–86.
85. Tominaga K, Yoshida M, Maetani I, Sakai Y. Expandable metal stent placement in the treatment of a malignant anastomotic stricture of the transverse colon. Gastrointest Endosc 2001; 53:524–527.
86. Liberman H, Adams DR, Blatchford GJ, Ternent CA, Christensen MA, Thorson AG. Clinical use of self-expanding metallic stent in the management of colorectal cancer. Am J Surg 2000; 180:407–412.
87. Adler DG, Baron TH. Endoscopic palliation of malignant dysphagia. Mayo Clin Proc. 2001; 76: 731–738.
88. Repici A, Reggio D, De Angelis C, Barletti C, Marchesa P, Musso A, Carucci P, Debernardi W, Falco M, Rizzetto M, Saracco G. Covered metal stents for management of inoperable malignant colorectal strictures. Gastrointest Endosc 2000; 52: 735–740.
89. Spinelli P, Mancini A. Use of self-expanding metal stents for palliation of rectosigmoid cancer. Gastrointest Endosc 2001; 53:203–206.
90. Meisner S, Hensler M, Knop FK, West F, Wille-Jorgensen P. Self-expanding metal stents for colonic obstruction: experiences from 104 procedures in a single center. Dis Colon Rectum 2004; 47:444–450.
91. Mauro MA, Koehler RE, Baron TH. Advances in gastrointestinal intervention: the treatment of gastroduodenal and colorectal obstructions with metallic stents. Radiology 2000; 215:659
92. Khot UP. Lang AW. Murali K. Parker MC. Systematic review of the efficacy and safety of colorectal stents. Br J Surg 2002. 89:1096–1102.
93. Sliney DH. Laser safety. Lasers Surg Med 1995; 16:215–225.
94. Polanyi TG. Physics of surgery with lasers. Clin Chest Med 1985; 6:179–202.
95. Polanyi TG. Laser physics. Otolaryngol Clin North Am 1983; 16:753–774.
96. Hiki Y, Shimao J, Yamao Y, Kobayashi N, Kuranami M, Kikuchi S, et al. The concepts, procedures, and problems related in endoscopic laser therapy of early gastric cancer. A retrospective study on early gastric cancer. Surg Endosc 1989; 3:1–6.
97. Liozou LA, Grigg D, Boulos PB, et al. Endoscopic Nd:YAG laser treatment of rectosigmoid cancer. Gut 1990; 31:812–816.
98. Brunetaud JM, Maunoury V, Cochelard D. Lasers in rectosigmoid tumors. Semin Surg Oncol 1995; 11:319–327.
99. Daneker GWJ, Carlson GW, Hohn DC, et al. Endoscopic laser recanalization is effective for prevention and treatment of obstruction in sigmoid and rectal cancer. Arch Surg 1991; 126:1348–1352.
100. Mandava N, Petrelli N, Herrera L, et al. Laser palliation for colorectal carcinoma. Am J Surg 1991; 162:212–214.
101. Tan CC, Iftikhar SY, Allan A, et al. Local effects of colorectal cancer are well palliated by endoscopic laser therapy. Eur J Surg Oncol 1995; 21:648–652.
102. Mathus-Vliegen EM, Tytgat GN. Analysis of failures and complications of neodymium: YAG laser photocoagulation in gastrointestinal tract tumors. A retrospective survey of 18 years' experience. Endoscopy 1990; 22:17–23.
103. Patrice T, Foultier MT, Yactayo S, et al. Endoscopic photodynamic therapy with hematoporphyrin derivative for primary treatment of gastrointestinal neoplasms in inoperable patients. Dig Dis Sci 1990; 35:545–552.
104. Overholt BF, Panjehpour M, Halberg DL. Photodynamic therapy for Barrett's esophagus with dysplasia and/or early stage carcinoma: long-term results. Gastrointest Endosc 2003; 58:183–188.
105. Ell C, Gossner L, May A, Schneider HT, Hahn EG, Stolte M, et al. Photodynamic ablation of early cancers of the stomach by means

of mTHPC and laser irradiation: preliminary clinical experience. Gut 1998; 43:345–349.

106. Mikvy P, Messmann H, Debinski H, Regula J, Conio M, MacRobert A, Spigelman A, Phillips R, Bown SG. Photodynamic therapy for polyps in familial adenomatous polyposis — a pilot study. Eur J Cancer. 1995; 31:1160–1165.

107. Barr H. Krasner N. Boulos PB. Chatlani P. Bown SG. Photodynamic therapy for colorectal cancer: a quantitative pilot study. Br J Surg 1990; 77:93–96.

108. Kashtan H, Papa MZ, Wilson BC, Deutch AA, Stern HS. Use of photodynamic therapy in the palliation of massive advanced rectal cancer. Dis Colon Rectum 1991; 34:600–605.

109. Loh CS, Bliss P, Bown SG, Krasner N. Photodynamic therapy for villous adenomas of the colon and rectum. Endoscopy 1994; 26:243–246.

110. McCaughan JS, Jr., Ellison EC, Guy JT, Hicks WJ, Jones JJ, Laufman LR, et al. Photodynamic therapy for esophageal malignancy: a prospective twelve-year study. Ann Thorac Surg 1996; 62:1005–1009.

111. Canard JM, Vedrenne B. Clinical application of argon plasma coagulation in gastrointestinal endoscopy: has the time come to replace the laser? Endoscopy 2001; 33:353–357.

112. Norton ID, Wang L, Levine SA, Burgart LJ, Hofmeister EK, Yacavone RF, Gostout CJ, Petersen BT. In vivo characterization of colonic thermal injury caused by argon plasma coagulation. Gastrointest Endosc 2002; 55:631–636.

113. Van Laethem JL, Cremer M, Peny MO, Delhaye M, Deverie J. Eradication of Barrett's mucosa with argon plasma coagulation and acid suppression: immediate and midterm results. Gut 1998; 43:741–51.

114. Grade AJ, Shah IA, Medlin SM, Ramirez FC. The efficacy and safety of argon plasma coagulation therapy in Barrett's esophagus. Gastrointest Endosc 1999; 50:18–22.

115. Brooker JC, Saunders BP, Shah SG, Thapar CJ, Suzuki N, Williams CB. Treatment with argon plasma coagulation reduces recurrence after piecemeal resection of large sessile colonic polyps: a randomized trial and recommendations. Gastrointest Endosc 2002; 55:371–375.

116. Grund KE, Zindel C, Farin G. Argon plasma coagulation (APC) in flexible endoscopy. Experience with 2193 applications in 1062 patients (abstract). Gastroenterology 1998; 114:A603.

117. Prost B, Poncet G. Unusual complications of argon plasma coagulation. Gastrointest Endosc 2004; 59:929–932.

118. Norton ID, Wang LN, Levine SA, Bugart LJ, Hofmeister EK, Rumala et al. Efficacy of submucosal saline injection for the reduction of iatrogenic thermal injury. Gastrointest Endosc 2002; 56:95–99.

119. Silva RA, Correia AJ, Dias LM, Lomba Viana H, Lomba Viana R. Argon plasma coagulation therapy for hemorrhagic radiation proctosigmoiditis. Gastrointest Endosc 1999; 50:221–224.

120. Taieb S, Rolachon A, Cenni JC, Nancey S, Bonvoisin S, Descos L et al. Effective use of argon plasma coagulation in the treatment of severe radiation proctitis. Dis Colon Rectum 2001; 44:1766–1771.

121. Soussan EB, Mathieu N, Roque I, Antoneitti M. Bowel explosion with colonic perforation during argon plasma coagulation for hemorrhagic radiation-induced proctitis. Gastrointest Endosc 2003; 57:412–413.

122. Zinsser E, Will U, Gottaschalk P, Bosseckert H. Bowel gas explosion during argon plasma coagulation (abstract). Endoscopy 1999; 3:S26.

22 Radiological Imaging of the Lower Gastrointestinal Tract

Stephen E. Rubesin, MD

Contents

1. INTRODUCTION

This chapter focuses on radiological imaging of colonic neoplasia. Examination of the colon is most often performed with barium radiography and computed tomography (CT). Ultrasonography, positron emission tomography, and magnetic resonance imaging (MRI) have minor roles in colon imaging.

2. PREPARATION OF THE COLON FOR IMAGING STUDIES

When the clinician requests a study focusing on the colon, the colon should be clean and without feces. A wide variety of preparations have been devised to remove feces from the colonic lumen (1–3). None of the preparations devised to cleanse colons has proved perfect. In general, each preparation has a low-residue diet lasting 1–3 d before the examination to eliminate indigestible elements of food from reaching the colon. Most preparations then use a poorly absorbed liquid as a "radiator flush" of the small bowel and colon. Some preparations add one or two colonic irritants to stimulate colonic contraction to cleanse residual fecal debris and fluid from the colon. At our hospital, the preparation that we have found to be effective includes the following:

1. Clear liquids only the day before the examination.
2. 10–16 oz. of Magnesium citrate at 5 PM the day before the examination.
3. At least four 8-oz. glasses of water the day before of the examination.
4. Four 5-mg bisacodyl tablets taken with 8 oz. of water the evening before the examination.

From: *Endoscopic Oncology: Gastrointestinal Endoscopy and Cancer Management.* Edited by: D. O. Faigel and M. L. Kochman © Humana Press, Totowa, NJ

5. Nothing by mouth after midnight until after the examination.
6. A bisacodyl suppository, the morning of the examination.
7. When appropriate, reduce or eliminate insulin the morning of the examination.
8. After the examination patients are encouraged to drink water and take laxatives if they have colonic hypomotility.

An alternative preparation is to take two bottles of Fleets phosphasoda instead of the magnesium citrate and to forego taking the bisacodyl tablets and suppository. We do not use large-volume (4 L) lavage agents (such as Golytely) to prepare colons, because they leave a large fluid residue that impairs barium coating and leaves large pools of fluid on the dependent surface in patients undergoing virtual colonoscopy. We do not use cleansing enemas because they are time consuming, may not clear the right colon, and often leave residual fluid in the colon.

One-day colonic preparations are usually successful in healthy mobile outpatients who do not complain of constipation. Colonic preparations are often unsatisfactory in patients who have colonic hypomotility, such patients with diabetes or hypothyroidism, patients taking opiates or drugs with anticholinergic side effects, and postoperative patients who have an adynamic ileus. Bedridden patients often benefit from a 2-d preparation. If a clinician suspects colonic hypomotility, a 2-d preparation may be of value. The clinician should consider giving a patient a preparation before any CT in which symptoms or clinical history suggests the possibility of colonic disease.

3. CONTRAINDICATIONS TO VARIOUS IMAGING STUDIES

3.1. BARIUM ENEMA

A barium enema is contraindicated in those patients with suspected colonic perforation. If an enema must be performed in a patient with suspected colonic perforation, an ionic water-soluble contrast agent should be used. Perforation of the colon or rectum is a rare but serious complication of barium enema, occurring in less than 1 in 10,000 examinations *(4)*. The rectum is the most common site of perforation. Rectal perforations are usually owing to insertion of the enema tip or use of a retention balloon. Other portions of the colon may perforate in the presence of severe inflammatory disease or microscopic perforation, such as ulcerative colitis or diverticulitis, respectively.

There is a risk of colonic perforation if a barium enema is performed within 7 d of an endoscopic study that could have possibly disrupted the muscularis mucosae, including polypectomy, hot biopsy, or biopsy with large forceps at rigid sigmoidoscopy *(5,6)*. A small forceps biopsy of polyps via a flexible endoscope is not a contraindication to barium enema.

Hypersensitivity reactions during barium enema are extremely rare, and usually are mild, such as urticaria *(7)*. Anaphylactic reactions have been reported during barium enema *(8)*, but most were probably related to the use of latex balloons on enema tips *(9,10)*. Therefore, patients with a history of reaction during a prior barium study should probably undergo some other type of examination.

The risk of developing bacterial endocarditis during barium enema is unknown. Bacteremia associated with native colonic flora may occur during barium enema as well as endoscopy. Although barium sulfate itself is inert, flavorings, stabilizing agents, and barium suspension agents may be organic products capable of supporting bacterial growth *(11)*. Therefore, prophylactic antibiotics may be of value in patients with known endocarditis or prosthetic heart valves.

3.2. COMPUTED TOMOGRAPHY

There is almost no contraindication to CT itself. CT may be performed in pregnant patients with indications including serious conditions, such as trauma. Water-soluble oral contrast agents should be used in patients with suspected perforation, unless there is a history of allergy to iodinated contrast. Water-soluble contrast agents are minimally absorbed by the gastrointestinal tract and will be absorbed if they enter the peritoneal cavity or retroperitoneum. Therefore, in patients with a history of severe reaction to intravenously administered iodinated contrast, barium should be given as an oral contrast agent.

Intravascular contrast agents are used during most CT examinations, but not for virtual colonoscopy. Most radiologists use nonionic contrast agents that have a lower risk of adverse reactions. Steroid premedication should be considered for patients who have had a prior reaction to intravenous contrast, including urticaria, bronchospasm, laryngeal edema, vagal reaction, or anaphylactic shock.

3.3. MAGNETIC RESONANCE IMAGING

Patients with pacemakers or implanted defibrillators should not undergo MRI imaging and should not enter the portion of radiology that houses MRI scanners. Pacemaker or other electromagnetic device function can be altered when exposed to the electromagnetic field. The referring physician should alert patients (radiology) with implants or foreign bodies having high iron content. These objects may torque and move in the

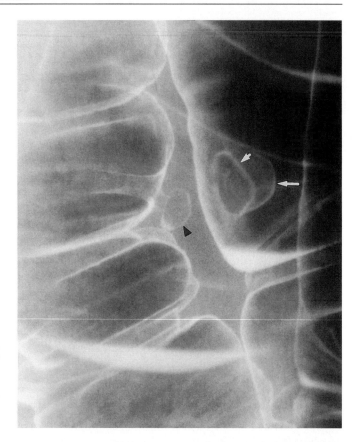

Fig. 1. Tubular adenoma of 0.8 cm in transverse colon. Coned-down image from a spot radiograph from a double-contrast barium enema shows a diverticulum in the ascending colon and a polyp in the adjacent proximal transverse colon. The diverticulum appears as a ring shadow (arrowhead) with a neck protruding outside of the expected luminal contour. The top of the polyp appears as a hemispheric barium-etched ring (long arrow). A barium-etched ring (short arrow) is present at the site where barium fills the space where the semipedunculated polyp is retracted against the adjacent colonic mucosa. This polyp has been described as resembling a hat (or Bowler hat). Colonoscopy 1 yr previous to this study was "normal."

magnetic field. Therefore, the MRI section should be consulted before examination in patients with cerebral aneurysm clips, neurostimulators, metallic heart values, intrauterine devices, various metallic orthopedic implants, and vena caval filters. Welders or other patients exposed to metal around the eyes should have radiography or orbital CT to exclude intraocular or extraocular metallic fragments before MRI.

Claustrophobia or inability to tolerate the supine position for a long time is a relative contraindication to MRI. Serious reactions to intravenously administered gadopentetate dimeglumine have about the same frequency as reactions to nonionic contrast agents used for CT.

4. RADIOGRAPHIC FINDINGS OF ADENOMAS

During a double-contrast barium enema, the radiologist instills barium and air via a rectal tube. The radiologist manipulates the barium pool to scrub feces and mucus off the mucosal surface and to coat the colonic wall with a thin layer of medium density barium *(12)*. Distension of the colon is achieved by

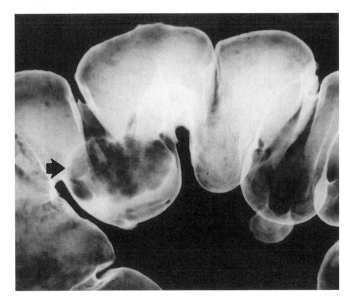

Fig. 2. Tubulovillous adenoma and sigmoid colon. Spot radiograph from double-contrast barium enema shows the fine lobulations in the surface of a 2.5-cm polyp (arrow) in the mid sigmoid colon. The fine lobulations mean that this polyp is somewhere in the spectrum from tubulovillous to villous adenoma with or without supervening adenocarcinoma. Overall, this polyp appears as a radiolucent filling defect in the barium pool.

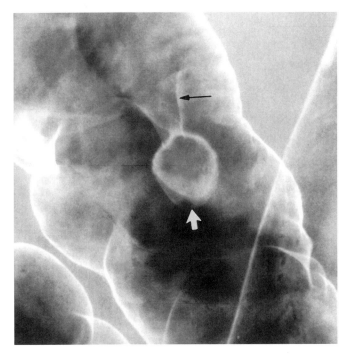

Fig. 3. Pedunculated tubular adenoma of 1.2 cm in sigmoid colon. Coned-down spot radiograph from double-contrast barium enema shows the head of the polyp as a barium-etched ring (white arrow) and the stalk of the polyp (black arrow) as a pair of converging lines.

insufflation of air or carbon dioxide. Intravenous glucagon is administered to make the examination more comfortable, achieving greater distensibility with less colonic spasm. The radiologist takes spot radiographs of each segment of the colon, turning the patient into the optimal position so the mucosal surface is coated,

the lumen is distended, and there is no overlap of colonic segments. The examination emphasizes fluoroscopically guided patient positioning and spot radiographs, not overhead radiographs performed by a technologist. The routine double-contrast barium enema takes about 10–20 min to perform and 5–10 min to interpret, dictate, and correct the report.

Radiographically, a polyp is a polyp is a polyp (Fig. 1). The radiologist assumes the worst-case scenario that a polyp is an adenomatous polyp until proven otherwise. Although hyperplastic polyps are usually small (0.5 cm), sessile rectal polyps, some hyperplastic polyps are larger, located anywhere in the colon and mimic pedunculated or sessile adenomas (13). Therefore, a radiologist cannot distinguish an adenomatous polyp from a hyperplastic polyp.

Size is by far and away the best radiological predictor of a polyp's malignant potential. One percent of tubular adenomas smaller than 1 cm are malignant, 10% of tubular adenomas 1–2 cm are malignant, and 35% of tubular adenomas larger than 2 cm are malignant (14). The surface of an adenomatous polyp may be smooth, finely lobulated, or reticular. When a polyp is viewed under a dissecting microscope, a pathologist can predict the amount of villous architecture by examining the number of surface lobulations. Tubular adenomas are either smooth or have 1–3 lobules and tubulovillous adenomas have 3–10 lobules (15). Villous adenomas have innumerable tiny lobules corresponding to the papillary fronds seen histologically. With proper technique, the radiologist can fill the interstices between tumor lobules with barium (Fig. 2) and to some degree predict an adenoma's histology based on its size and surface texture. If a polyp has more than several lobulations, the radiologist must suspect a tubulovillous adenoma or worse (see Fig. 2). As 9% of villous adenomas less than 1 cm and 10% of villous adenomas 1–2 cm harbor malignancy (14), the radiographic finding of a finely villous surface pattern implies that even a polyp smaller than 1 cm should be removed.

Macroscopically, a polyp may be sessile, pedunculated, or flat. The presence of a pedicle larger than 1 cm implies that a polyp will have a benign behavior (Fig. 3). Adenocarcinomas arising in pedunculated polyps are usually early cancers without deep invasion of the stalk (16). In one pathology study, no invasive cancers were found in polyps with a pedicle longer than 3 mm (17). The pedicle may be manifested as barium-etched lines or as a tubular or triangular radiolucency in the barium pool. Polyps that resemble "hats" (see Fig. 1) are usually pedunculated or semipedunculated polyps (18). If a sessile polyp larger than 1 cm has an irregular contour in profile, malignancy may be suspected (19), but this size adenoma has a 10% of malignancy anyway.

Some adenomas are relatively flat lesions that grow along the surface of the bowel forming a carpet of adenomatous tissue (20,21). Most carpet lesions are detected in the cecum, ascending colon, distal sigmoid colon (Fig. 4), and rectum (20). Most carpet lesions are usually tubulovillous or villous adenomas despite a large size. Some carpet lesions, however, will develop into adenocarcinoma (Fig. 5).

Flat, umbilicated adenomas are a different lesion. These are small tumors that have a small central depression within a flat

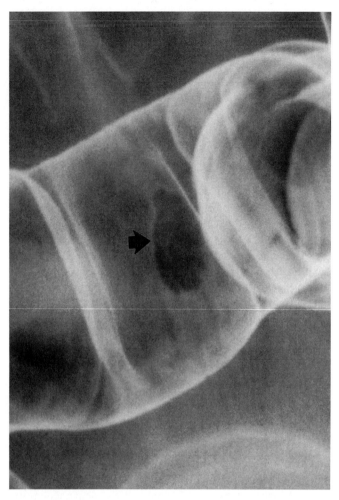

Fig. 4. Flat tubulovillous adenoma of the distal sigmoid colon. Spot radiograph from a double-contrast barium enema shows a 1.5-cm alteration (arrow) of the normally smooth mucosal surface. Barium fills the some of the interstices of the polyp.

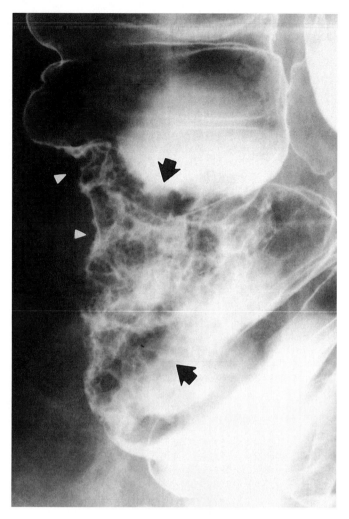

Fig. 5. Carpet lesion of the ascending colon. Spot radiograph from a double-contrast barium enema shows barium filling the interstices of a relatively flat lesion. The tumor lobules are sound or polygonal in shape. The tumor protrudes into the colon along the lateral wall (white arrows) at the site of adenocarcinoma arising in this tubulovillous adenoma.

or slightly raised lesion *(22,23)*. These are adenomas that so rapidly develop into adenocarcinoma that early reports termed these "*de-novo*" carcinomas. Fortunately, these tumors are uncommon in Western countries *(24)*. These small umbilicated lesions are probably the precursors of ulcerated, plaque-like colonic cancers, but this form of colonic cancer accounts for only about 5% of colonic adenocarcinomas *(25)*. At our hospital we have prospectively detected one 7-mm umbilicated cancer. Most of the umbilicated tumors we have detected are hyperplastic polyps (Fig. 6) *(26)*.

5. RADIOGRAPHIC AND CT FINDINGS OF COLONIC CARCINOMA

5.1. DISTRIBUTION

About 40–50% of colonic carcinomas are located in the right and transverse colon, out of reach of the flexible sigmoidoscope, in support of the proximal migration of colorectal neoplasia also noted at other centers. At our hospital, in a study of 152 patients with colon cancer, 27% of patients had cancers in the cecum and ascending colon and 17% had cancers in the

transverse colon. Only 51% of patients had cancers in the rectum or sigmoid colon.

5.2. MORPHOLOGY

The most common form of adenocarcinoma is the annular or semiannular lesion, accounting for about one-half of colon carcinomas *(25)*. Annular cancers are the end-stage of polypoid lesions that have spread circumferentially around the lumen of the bowel. This morphological type is usually found in the transverse, descending, and sigmoid colon. The annular narrowing is often asymmetric, thicker at the site of the original polypoid tumor *(27)*. The mucosal surface is nodular or ulcerated (Fig. 7). The margins of the tumor are sharp and shelf-like (Fig. 8). When an annular cancer is detected, there is a 98% chance of serosal invasion and a 50% chance of lymph node metastasis.

Polypoid tumors are the second most common morphologic type of colon cancer, accounting for 37% of carcinomas *(25)*. This is the most common morphological type of cancer in the cecum or rectum. By the time an adenomatous polyp becomes

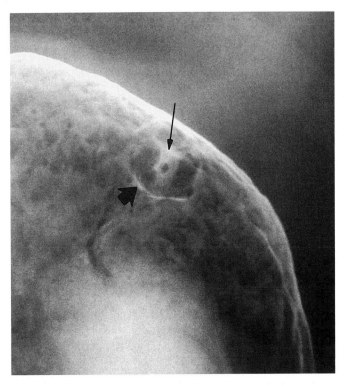

Fig. 6. Umbilicated polyp of the distal transverse colon. Spot radiograph from a double-contrast barium enema shows a relatively flat 1.3-cm polyp (arrow) with a central umbilication (arrow). This was a hyperplastic polyp.

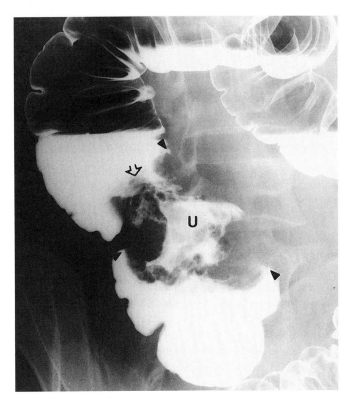

Fig. 7. Adenocarcinoma of proximal ascending colon. Spot radiograph from a double contrast barium enema shows a 6-cm annular lesion with abrupt, shelf-like margins (arrowheads), nodular mucosa (arrow), and a large barium-filled central ulcer (U).

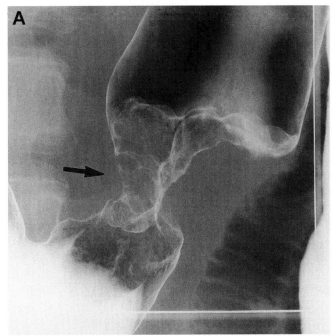

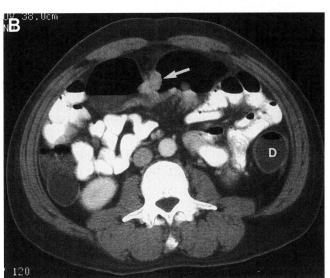

Fig. 8. Adenocarcinoma of the transverse colon arising in ulcerative colitis. (**A**) Spot radiograph from a double-contrast barium enema shows a 4-cm annular lesion (arrow). (**B**) Axial image from CT performed after the barium enema shows a mass (arrow) in the transverse colon. The colon is ahaustral. Fluid in the descending colon (D) is seen, an abnormal finding related to diarrhea associated with ulcerative colitis. This 54-yr-old man had greater than a 10-yr history of ulcerative colitis, but had been lost to follow-up for 4 yr and refused colonoscopy.

a cancer, the lesion is usually larger than 2 cm in size. Only 5% of polypoid cancers we detected were smaller than 2 cm (Fig. 9), the smallest about 1.5 cm. Polypoid morphology implies a better prognosis than an annular morphology. Only about 25% of patients with polypoid cancers have lymph node metastases (25).

About 5% of adenocarcinomas have a carpet-like morphology (see Fig. 5) and about 5% of cancers are plaque-like

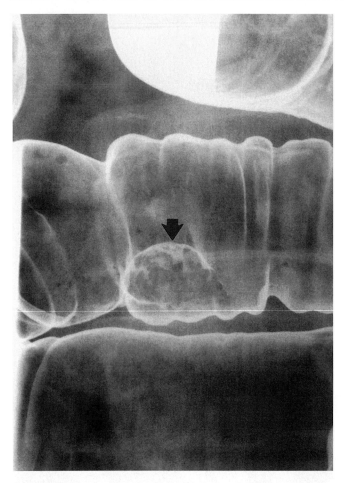

Fig. 9. Polypoid adenocarcinoma of 1.9 cm of transverse colon. Spot radiograph from a double-contrast barium enema shows a finely lobulated polypoid lesion (arrow).

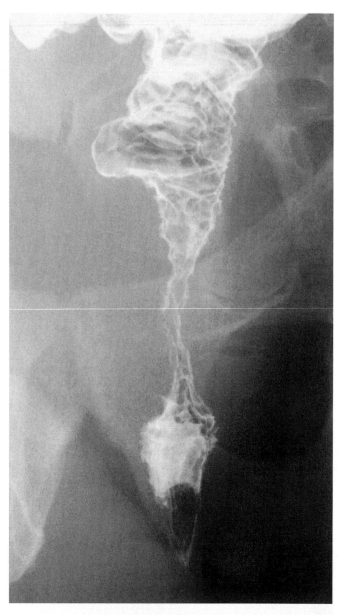

Fig. 10. Scirrhous adenocarcinoma of rectum. Spot radiograph from a double-contrast barium enema shows diffuse narrowing of the rectum. The mucosa is diffusely nodular.

tumors *(25)*. Small, flat adenocarcinomas average about 12 mm in Japanese series *(28)*, but are usually larger when detected in symptomatic patients. Rarely, colonic carcinomas have an infiltrative "linitis plastica"-type appearance (Fig. 10) *(29)*.

5.3. COMPUTED TOMOGRAPHY

Before virtual colonoscopy, about 70% of adenocarcinomas of the colon were retrospectively visible on CT studies in patients who were unprepped and in studies that were not tailored to detect adenocarcinomas. Most colon cancers are relatively large lesions (larger than 2 cm) and therefore are often detected by CT as a focal unilateral or circumferential thickening of the colonic wall (*see* Figs. 8A and 11).

5.4. THE VALUE AND PITFALLS OF BARIUM ENEMA, ENDOSCOPY, AND VIRTUAL COLONOSCOPY

A double-contrast barium enema is a powerful, safe tool for the detection of polyps larger than 1 cm, carcinomas, and other lesions of the colon. At our institution, in 1989, using a barium preparation much inferior to the one we use today, barium enema was equal to endoscopy in detection of colon cancer (93 vs 92%, respectively). This did not include cancers found in segments that the endoscopist did not reach.

The most common causes that polyps or cancers are missed at barium enema are perceptive errors (Fig. 12) and technically poor studies. The quality of the examination depends on the barium preparation (not all barium preparations are equal), the cleanliness of the colon, and the patient's rectal tone. Most missed colon cancers are seen in retrospect. Only 10% of "missed" colon cancers are not seen on good quality films *(30)*.

Barium enema has some advantages over endoscopy. Barium enema has a greater success rate in visualizing the whole colon. Colonoscopy is incomplete at our hospital in 9% of patients *(31)*. Neoplasms larger than 1 cm were detected on barium enema in 3% of patients who had incomplete colonoscopy at our institution *(31)*. Barium enema is about one-third to one-fourth as expensive as colonoscopy, has a much lower perforation rate (1 in 10,000 vs 1 in 1000), a much lower significant bleeding rate, and has no anesthesia risk *(32)*. It is superior to endoscopy in definitively demonstrating the

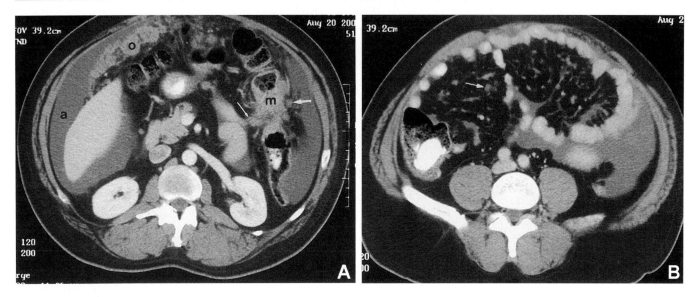

Fig. 11. Adenocarcinoma of splenic flexure with intraperitoneal metastases. **(A)** Axial image from CT scan performed for evaluation of an anterior abdominal wall hernia shows a circumferential soft tissue mass (m). Local invasion is manifested as stranding of the adjacent mesentery (thin arrow). Local lymphadenopathy is present (one node identified by thick arrow). Intraperitoneal metastasis is demonstrated as a "cake" of tumor in the greater omentum (o). Ascites (a) is present in the right perihepatic space and left paracolic gutter. **(B)** Axial image obtained inferior to A. shows diffuse ascites, most obvious in the left paracolic gutter. Nodules in the small bowel mesentery are owing to intraperitoneal metastasis to the small bowel mesentery (representative implant identified by arrow).

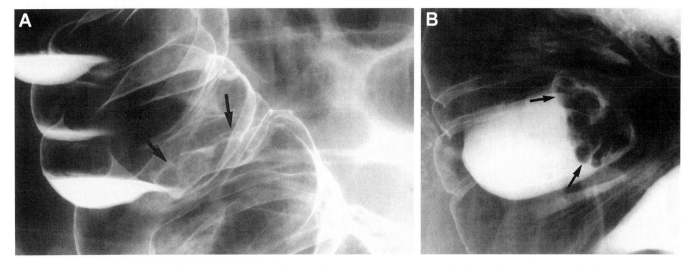

Fig. 12. Villous adenoma of ascending colon not perceived on double contrast barium enema. **(A)** Spot radiograph from a double-contrast barium enema shows a 3-cm lobulated lesion (arrows) etched in white by barium. **(B)** After 27 mo, a spot radiograph from a double-contrast barium enema shows minimal growth a coarsely lobulated mass on the medial wall of ascending colon.

location of the cancer and some complications, such as fistula formation (Fig. 13) or intraperitoneal metastasis (Fig. 14) that may alter the surgical approach. Barium enema is clearly inferior to endoscopy in the diagnosis of diminutive polyps less than 5 mm, because colons frequently have residual debris this size. Barium enema is slightly inferior to endoscopy in diagnosis of polyps 5–10 mm and approaches endoscopy in diagnosis of polyps larger than 1 cm. Barium enema may have difficulty distinguishing diverticulitis from an annular cancer in some patients (Fig. 15).

The major advantage of endoscopy is its ability to biopsy or remove lesions and to endoscopically mark lesions with a clip or tattoo for surveillance or later surgical removal. The small,

but finite risk of anesthesia is balanced by anesthesia's ability to ameliorate any discomfort felt during the examination. Endoscopy may miss flat lesions, small lesions (Fig. 16), lesions on the inner curve of a flexure and even annular lesions (Fig. 17). Endoscopy may not be able to examine the past a point of obstruction or herniation (Fig. 18).

Virtual colonoscopy has become a hot and controversial topic recently. Virtual colonoscopy has been used to examine colons proximal to obstructing lesions (33,34) or for screening for colonic carcinoma. Virtual colonoscopy has about one-fourth to one-tenth the spatial resolution of digitally performed barium enema, depending on the fluoroscopic magnification used. If a multidetector CT has a 1- to 1.25-mm resolution in

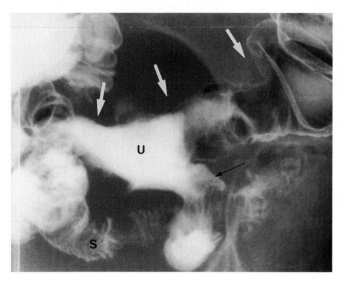

Fig. 13. Adenocarcinoma of sigmoid colon with invasion and fistula formation to adjacent pelvic ileum. Spot radiograph from a double-contrast barium enema shows a long (6 cm) annular lesion (arrows) of the sigmoid colon partly obscured by large barium filled ulceration (U). A fistula (arrow) has formed. Barium fills the adjacent small intestinal loop (S).

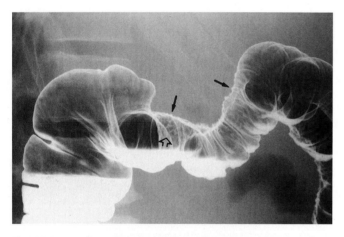

Fig. 14. Intraperitoneal metastasis to greater omentum and transverse colon by colonic carcinoma. Spot radiograph from a double contrast barium enema demonstrates a broad-based extrinsic mass involving the superior surface of the transverse colon at the site of attachment of the greater omentum. The contour is spiculated (arrows). En face, the mucosa has a polygonal appearance (open arrow) owing to tethering by tumor.

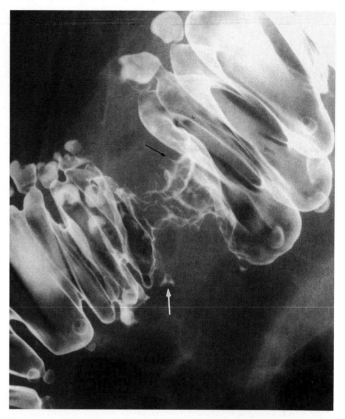

Fig. 15. Diverticulitis versus colon cancer. Spot radiograph of the distal descending colon shows a 3-cm annular lesion with shelf-like margins. It is difficult to determine whether the mucosal is nodular or thrown into folds by an adjacent inflammatory process. There are several deformed diverticula at the edge of the lesion (arrow on one deformed diverticulum). There is spiculation of the superior contour (arrow). The lesion in this 74-yr-old man with left lower quadrant pain was subsequently proven to be diverticulitis.

the z-axis, the result is a 2- to 2.5-mm line-pair resolution. In contrast, radiography has fluoroscopy has a resolution of 4–6 line-pairs per millimeter on a 1000 K fluoroscope at high magnification settings and a resolution of about 2 line-pairs per millimeter at middle magnification settings. Virtual colonoscopy cannot look at the mucosal surface en face by coating a lesion with barium. In a sense, virtual colonoscopy is a three-dimensional single-contrast barium enema. In a prospective, blinded study, experienced expert radiologists at the Mayo Clinic detected an average of 47% of polyps larger than 1 cm (35). There was such a wide variation in readers ability to detect polyps larger than 1 cm (32–73%) that it was recommend that

radiologists double read virtual colonoscopy (35). The best success rates for detection of polyps larger than 1 cm are about 90% under optimized conditions (36). Virtual colonoscopy may have trouble detecting carpet or plaque-like lesions (37). It is this radiologist's opinion that properly performed double-contrast barium enema is superior to virtual colonoscopy. It has better resolution, looks at the mucosal surface en face, the ability to optimally distend each segment of colon by turning the patient into various positions, and has the ability to move obscuring fecal debris in some patients.

No matter what the test used, a total examination of the colon should be performed, because flexible sigmoidoscopy will miss at least 40% of colonic carcinomas out of reach of the flexible sigmoidoscope. Furthermore, it may be advantageous to be screened by any modality, no matter what the examination. In the early 1990s, when we looked at our patients with colon cancer, almost all either had symptoms, bleeding, or signs of colon cancer (25). Only 5% of our patients with colon cancer had been detected by screening examination. This contrasts dramatically with the detection of colon cancer at our Veterans' Affairs hospital today, where many colon cancers are detected in patients who undergo screening for colonic carcinoma. In

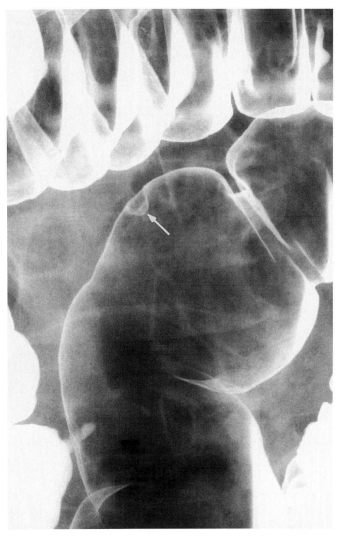

Fig. 16. Tubular adenoma of 6 mm missed at colonoscopy. A "bowler hat" (arrow) is seen in the distal sigmoid colon. One year previously, endoscopy was "normal." A subsequent polypectomy revealed a tubular adenoma.

summary, a strong case can be made to screen asymptomatic patients with double contrast barium enema as well as with colonoscopy *(38–40)*, as discussed in national consensus recommendations.

6. STAGING OF COLONIC CARCINOMA

Although this chapter is primarily about colonic imaging, a brief discussion of staging of colonic carcinoma will be presented here. For cancers of the rectum and anal region, pre-operative staging may help in selecting patients for pre-operative chemotherapy or radiation *(41,42)*. In cases where there is direct invasion of adjacent organs such as small intestine *(see* Fig. 13) or the urinary bladder, pre-operative staging may alert the surgeon to alter the surgical approach.

The radiologist evaluates the depth of invasion through the bowel wall, the presence of local or distant lymph node metastases and the presence of liver or other distant metastases *(42,43)*. CT, MRI, and endoscopic ultrasound are suboptimal at predicting the presence of serosal invasion, manifested as soft

tissue stranding in the pericolic fat *(see* Fig. 11) *(44–46)*. In fact, the gross morphology of the lesion itself is almost as good a predictor of serosal involvement, as is direct imaging by CT or MRI. When an annular lesion is detected, it is at such a late stage, that the chance of serosal invasion is 98% *(25)*. Polypoid tumors have a 50% chance of serosal invasion. CT and MRI are also mediocre at evaluating lymph node metastases, detecting about 60% of lymph node metastases *(41)*. CT misses metastases in lymph nodes that are not enlarged by CT criteria. Small groups of lymph nodes that are not enlarged by CT criteria but are clustered together adjacent to the tumor, however, are suspicious for metastases *(47)*. CT may also overcall metastases in lymph nodes that are enlarged by an inflammatory process *(48)*. The radiologist focuses on the site-specific lymphatic drainage areas for lymph node metastases: the periduodenal region and to the right of the superior mesenteric artery root for right-sided colon cancers; the region of the ligament of Treitz (left peri-aortic region near the superior mesenteric artery and inferior mesenteric artery origins) for left-sided colon cancers; the external iliac chains and left periaortic region for rectosigmoid cancer; and the external iliac chains and inguinal regions for distal rectal and anal cancer *(49)*.

Pre-operative detection of liver metastases may alter the surgical approach, because those patients with one to four liver metastases may benefit from resection of these lesions *(50)*. Both contrast enhanced CT and MRI are about 85% sensitive in detection of liver metastases *(41)*. The most sensitive test for detection of liver metastases is probably intraoperative ultrasound, with the transducer placed directly on the liver capsule. On CT, most hepatic metastases from colorectal carcinoma appear as mixed or low attenuation lesions (Fig. 19). Peripheral ring enhancement may be seen. Punctate calcification of mucinous metastases or treated metastases may be present. Positron emission tomography imaging may prove helpful in determining whether a lesion that is too small to biopsy is a metastasis (Fig. 20) *(51,52)*. CT and MRI are helpful, but not specific, in determining the possibility of a recurrence of rectal cancer (Fig. 21).

7. OTHER COLONIC TUMORS

7.1. LIPOMAS AND OTHER BENIGN LESIONS

Colonic lipomas are encapsulated masses of mature fat cells, predominately arising in the submucosa. Most lipomas (70%) are found in the cecum and ascending colon. Multiple lipomas are found in 25% of patients *(53)*. Radiographically, these tumors appear as smooth-surfaced pedunculated, semipedunculated, or sessile masses that change size and shape with compression and varying degrees of colonic distension *(54,55)* (Fig. 22). These tumors are not infrequently found incidentally at CT, appearing as smooth or lobulated masses of fat attenuation *(56)* (Fig. 23).

Arteriovenous malformations are flat vascular abnormalities that are not detectable by barium enema or CT. These lesions can only be demonstrated during colonoscopy or arteriography performed in patients who are acutely bleeding.

7.2. LYMPHOMA

Non-Hodgkin's lymphoma involves the colon in three ways: as a primary tumor, widely disseminated disease, or by direct

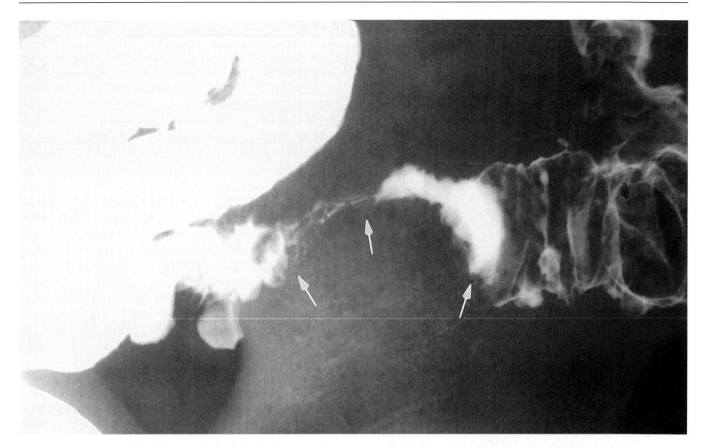

Fig. 17. Adenocarcinoma of the sigmoid colon missed at endoscopy. Spot radiograph of the mid sigmoid colon from a double contrast barium enema demonstrates a 4 cm annular lesion (arrows) with nodular mucosa. Sigmoidoscopy 5 mo previously was reportedly normal. The barium enema was performed for continuing heme-positive stool.

invasion from a contiguous nodal mass. Hodgkin's disease rarely involves the colon. Primary lymphomas usually involve the cecum, ascending colon, or rectum, whereas disseminated lymphoma may involve a long segment or the entire colon *(57)*. Primary colonic lymphomas are relatively unusual, often appearing as relatively long circumferential lesions with smooth-surfaced lobulated or effaced folds *(54,58)*. A lymphoma may also appear as a smooth-surfaced, slightly lobulated broad-based polypoid mass or as a cavitary lesion. Disseminated lymphoma may appear as isolated or multifocal submucosal-appearing mass lesions (Fig. 24) or as innumerable small submucosal nodules. In some patients, lymphomatous polyposis is a primary mantle cell lymphoma rather than disseminated disease.

7.3. METASTASES INVOLVING COLON

Tumors can secondarily involve the colon in a variety of ways: direct invasion by contiguous tumor (either primary or recurrence), spread via a mesentery, intraperitoneal metastases, or hematogenous metastasis *(59)*.

7.3.1. Direct Invasion

A wide variety of organs about the colon as it courses through the peritoneal space and retroperitoneum. Carcinomas of the gallbladder invade the superior border of the hepatic flexure. Carcinomas of the left kidney or recurrences of left kidney cancer invade the medial border of the splenic flexure. Cancers of the body and tail of the pancreas invade the mid

transverse colon and splenic flexure. Cancer of the prostate may directly invade the lower rectum via Denonvillier's fascia. More frequently, prostate cancer invades the seminal vesicles then the rectosigmoid junction *(60)*. Cancer of the cervix may directly invade the anterior wall of the rectosigmoid junction. On barium enema examination extrinsic mass effect (Fig. 25) cannot be distinguished from direct invasion if only a smooth-surfaced mass effect on the colonic wall is seen. However, spiculation of the colonic contour and tethering of mucosal folds *(61)* implies direct invasion of the colonic wall (Fig. 26).

7.3.2. Direct Invasion Via a Mesentery

Tumors from one organ can spread via a mesentery to the colon *(49)*. Cancers of the stomach can spread via the gastrocolic ligament to the midtransverse colon and splenic flexure. Cancer of the pancreas can spread via the transverse mesocolon to the transverse colon.

7.3.3. Intraperitoneal Metastasis

The peritoneal reflections direct flow of intraperitoneal fluid so that fluid pools within the ruffles of the right lower quadrant small bowel mesentery, in the sigmoid mesentery, in the pararectal fossae, and rectovesical space (male) or rectouterine space (female), along the right paracolic gutter, in Morison's pouch and in the right subdiaphragmatic space *(62)*. Thus, the most common sites of intraperitoneal implants are the pouch of Douglas/rectouterine space, the sigmoid colon, the medial

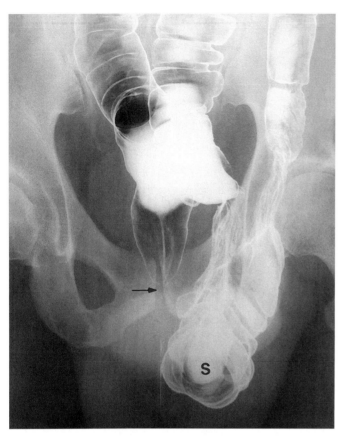

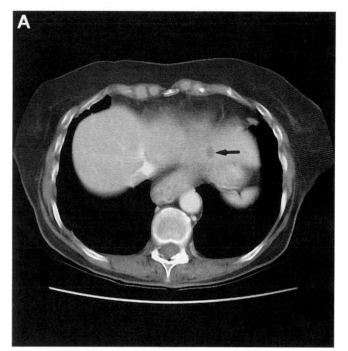

Fig. 18. Incomplete colonoscopy owing to inguinal hernia. This man had a progressive swelling of the scrotum during colonoscopy. Coned-down view from an overhead radiograph from a double contrast barium enema demonstrates the sigmoid colon (S) in a left inguinal hernia. The level of the anorectal junction and the symphysis pubis is identified (arrow).

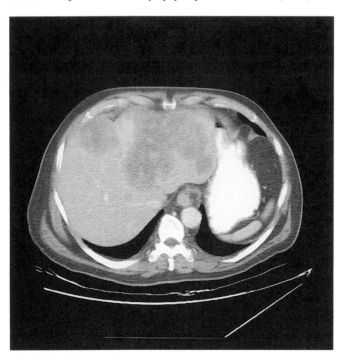

Fig. 19. Liver metastases demonstrated by CT. Axial image of liver shows many low and mixed attenuation mass in the left lobe of the liver, some less than 1 cm, another 4-cm lesion, and a conglomerate mass replacing much of the lateral left lobe. (Reproduced with permission from ref. *43*.)

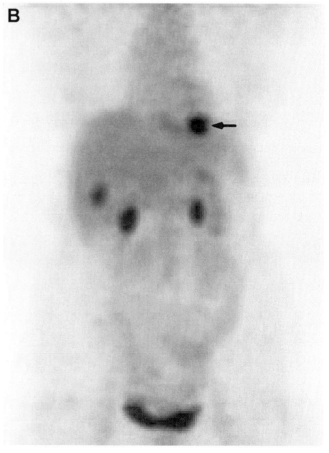

Fig. 20. Liver metastases confirmed by positron emission tomography imaging. **(A)** Axial computed tomography (CT) image through dome of liver shows a 9-mm low attenuation lesion in the lateral segment of the left lobe. A smaller, 7-mm nodule was seen in the liver tip. **(B)** Positron emission tomography image demonstrates uptake of 5-fluorodeoxyglucose in the lesion in the lateral segment of the liver lobe (arrow) and at the liver tip, corresponding to the tiny lesions detected at CT, findings highly suggestive that these lesions are metastases. The kidneys and urinary bladder are also demonstrated. (Reproduced with permission from ref. *43*.)

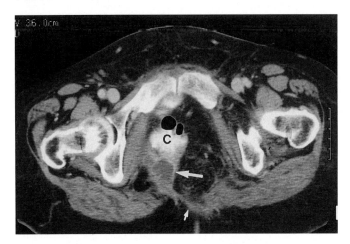

Fig. 21. CT demonstrating recurrent rectal cancer after abdomino-perineal resection. Axial image through pelvis shows 3 × 4 cm mass (large arrow) of mixed low and soft tissue attenuation posterior to a cecum (C) that has fallen into the empty pelvis. Stranding of subcoc-cygeal fat (small arrow) is owing to tumor infiltration. The right obtu-rator internus and cecum are invaded.

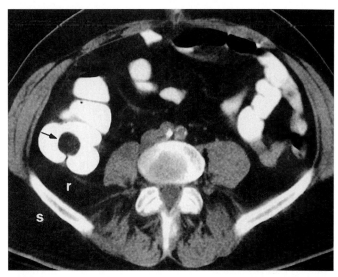

Fig. 23. Lipoma of the cecum on CT. Axial image through cecum demonstrates a 2-cm mass of fat attenuation in the contrast-filled cecum. Note that the attenuation of the mass is identical to retro-peritoneal (r) and subcutaneous (s) fat.

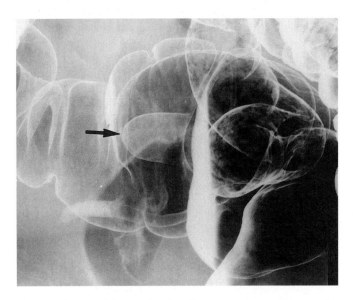

Fig. 22. Lipoma of ileocecal valve. Cone-down image from a right-sided down cross-table lateral decubitus view shows a smooth-surfaced polyp (arrow). The soft nature of the lesion is implied by the fact that it is elongated as it hangs inferiorly. The position of the patient is indicated by the air/barium levels.

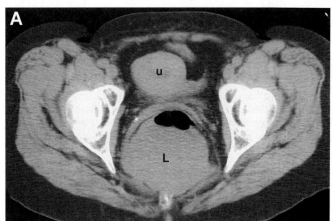

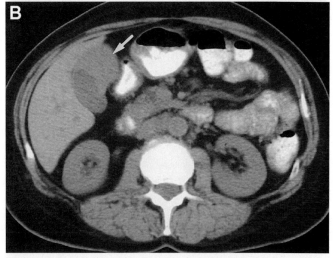

Fig. 24. Disseminated non-Hodgkin's lymphoma involving rectum and gallbladder. (A) Unenhanced axial image through the acetabulae shows a 5-cm soft tissue mass involving the posterior wall of the rec-tum. The uterus (u) is also identified. (B) Axial image through the tip of the right lobe of the liver shows a soft tissue mass (arrow) involv-ing the superior wall of the gallbladder.

border of the cecum/distal ileum, and the surface of the liver. Intraperitoneal metastases to the greater omentum and gastro-colic ligament result in secondary invasion of the transverse colon and greater curvature of the stomach (63,64). Tumors that abut the peritoneal space (ovary, colon, stomach, liver, and pancreas) are the most common tumors to seed the peritoneal space (65).

CT is the most sensitive radiological technique at determin-ing the presence of intraperitoneal metastasis. Ascites is present in 70% of cases. Soft tissue nodules involving the parietal peri-toneal surface, the surface of the liver, or abutting the colon or

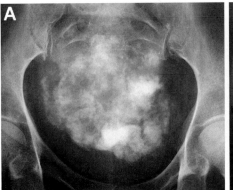
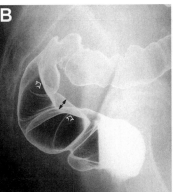
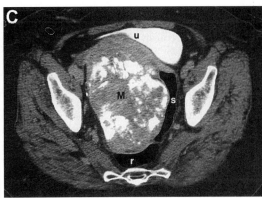

Fig. 25. Low-grade serous papillary adenocarcinoma of the ovary impressing the sigmoid colon. (A) Plain radiograph of the abdomen (a scout image) shows a densely calcified pelvic mass. The calcification is amorphous, not resembling the usual coarse, linear or "popcorn like" calcifications seen in uterine leiomyomas. (B) A cross-table lateral overhead view with the patient lying in the prone position demonstrates a smooth-surfaced extrinsic mass impression (arrows) at the rectosigmoid junction. Subtle signs of extrinsic mass effect are the double contour at the level of the arrows and increased density (double arrow) where the air-filled lumen has been compressed by extrinsic mass. The calcification seen on the plain radiograph is not as apparent as on the plain radiograph. (C) Axial computed tomography image through the pelvis shows a 15-cm calcified pelvic mass (M) compressing the rectum (r), sigmoid colon (s) and posterior wall of the urinary bladder (u).

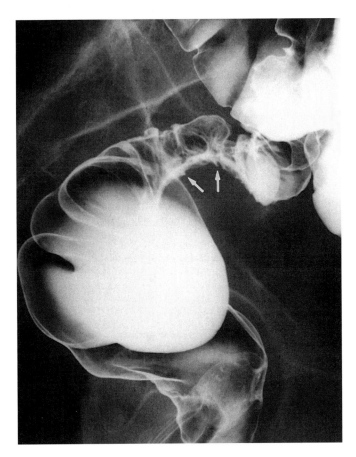

Fig. 26. Ovarian carcinoma invading the pouch of Douglas. Spot radiograph from a double contrast barium enema shows a 4 cm extrinsic mass impression on the anterior wall of the rectosigmoid junction. The contour is spiculated (arrows) due to invasion of the serosa.

small bowel may be detected (*see* Fig. 11) *(66)*. Direct involvement of bowel wall; however, is better demonstrated by barium studies of the stomach, small bowel, or colon. Radiographically, an extrinsic mass impression is present, associated with a spiculated contour and tethered mucosal folds (*see* Fig. 14).

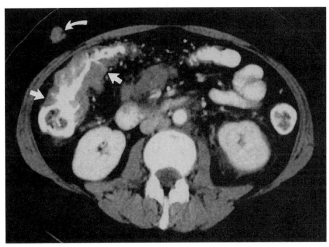

Fig. 27. Metastatic melanoma to hepatic flexure. Axial computed tomography image through level of mid kidneys shows circumferential marked focal thickening (arrows) of a long segment of the hepatic flexure. A subcutaneous metastasis is also identified (arrow).

7.3.4. Hematogenous Metastasis

The most common primary tumors that hematogenously metastasize to the colon are melanoma, breast cancer, and lung cancer. Unless extensive, these tumors rarely cause clinical symptoms. Radiographically, hematogenous metastases appear as submucosal nodules, eccentric strictures, or long circumferential narrowings, a linitis plastica appearance (Fig. 27).

REFERENCES

1. Fork ET, Ekberg O, Nilsson G, et al. Colon cleansing regimens. Gastrointest Radiol 1982; 7:383–389.
2. Gelfand DW, Chen YM, Ott DJ. Colonic cleansing for radiographic detection of neoplasia: efficacy of the magnesium citrate-castor oil-cleansing enema regimen. AJR 1988; 151:705–708.
3. Gelfand DW, Chen YM, Ott DJ. Preparing the colon for the barium enema examination. Radiology 1991; 178:609–613.
4. Williams SM, Harned RK. Recognition and prevention of barium enema complications. Curr Probl Diagn Radiol 1991; 20:123–151.

5. Maglinte DDT, Strong RC, Strate RW, et al. Barium enema after colorectal biopsies: experimental data. AJR 1982; 139.693–697.

6. Harned RK, Consigny PM, Cooper NB. Barium enema examination following biopsy of the rectum or colon. Radiology 1982; 145:11–16.

7. Janower ML. Hypersensitivity reactions after barium studies of the upper and lower gastrointestinal tract. Radiology 1986; 161:139–140.

8. Fezcko PJ, Simms SM, Bakirici N. Fatal hypersensitivity reaction during a barium enema. AJR 1989; 153:275–276.

9. Ownby DR, Tomlanovich M, Sammons N, et al. Anaphylaxis associated with latex allergy during barium enema examinations. AJR 1991; 156:903–908.

10. Gelfand DW. Barium enemas, latex balloons and anaphylactic reactions. AJR 1991; 156:1,2.

11. Skucas J. Contrast media. In: Gore RM, Levine MS, eds. Textbook of Gastrointestinal Radiology, 2nd ed. Philadelphia: WB Saunders; 2000:2–14.

12. Rubesin SE, Laufer I. Double contrast barium enema: technical aspects. In: Levine MS, Rubesin SE, Laufer I, eds. Double contrast gastrointestinal radiology, 3rd ed. Philadelphia: WB Saunders; 2000:331–356.

13. Levine MS, Barnes MJ, Bronner MP, et al. Atypical hyperplastic polyps on double-contrast barium enema. Radiology 1990; 175:691–694.

14. Muto T, Bussey HJR, Morson BC. The evolution of cancer of the colon and rectum. Cancer 1975; 36:2251–2270.

15. Thompson JJ, Enterline HT. The macroscopic appearance of colorectal polyps. Cancer 1981; 48:151–160.

16. Smith TR. Pedunculated malignant colonic polyps with superficial invasion of the stalk. Radiology 1975; 115:593–596.

17. Haggitt RC, Glotzbach RE, Soffer EE, Wruble WD. Prognostic factors in colorectal carcinomas arising in adenomas: implications for lesion removal by endoscopic polypectomy. Gastroenterology 1985; 89:328–336.

18. Youker JE, Welin S. Differentiation of the true polypoid lesions of the colon from extraneous material, a new roentgen sign. Radiology 1965; 84:610–615.

19. Ott DJ, Gelfand DW, Wu WC. Colonic polyp morphology on double contrast barium enema: its pathologic predictive value. AJR 1983; 141:965–970.

20. Rubesin SE, Sul SH, Laufer I, et al. Carpet lesions of the colon. Radiographics 1985; 5:537–552.

21. Iida M, Iwashita A, Yao T, et al. Villous tumor of the colon: correlation of histologic, macroscopic, and radiographic features. Radiology 1988; 167:673–677.

22. Matsumoto T, Iida M, Kohrogi N, et al. Minute nonpolypoid adenomas of the colon depicted with barium enema examination. Radiology 1993; 187:377–380.

23. Fujiya M, Maruyama M. Small depressed neoplasm of the large bowel: radiographic visualization and clinical significance. Abdom Imaging 1997; 22:325–331.

24. Bond JH. Small flat adenomas appear to have little clinical importance in Western countries. Gastrointest Endosc 1995; 42:184–186.

25. McCarthy PA, Rubesin SE, Levine MS, et al. Colon cancer: morphology detected by barium enema examination versus histopathologic stage. Radiology 1995; 197:683–687.

26. Cunnane ME, Rubesin SE, Furth EE, et al. Small flat umbilicated tumors of the colon: radiographic and pathologic findings. AJR 2000:175:747–749.

27. Rubesin SE, Stuzin N, Laufer I. Atlas of Colon Tumors. Seminars in Col & Rect Surg. 1993; 4:94–111.

28. Shimoda T, Ikegami M, Fujisaki J et al. Early colorectal carcinoma with special reference to its development de novo. Cancer 1989; 64:1138–1146.

29. Raskin MM, Viamonte M, Viamonte M Jr. Primary linitis plastica carcinoma of the colon. Radiology 1974; 113:17–22.

30. Kelvin FM, Gardiner R, Vas W, et al. Colorectal carcinoma missed on double contrast barium enema study: a problem in perception. AJR 1981; 137:307–313.

31. Chong A, Shah JN, Levine MS, et al. Diagnostic yield of barium enemas after incomplete colonoscopy. Radiology 2002; 223:620–624.

32. Habr-Gama A, Waye JD. Complications and hazards of gastrointestinal endoscopy. World J Surgery 1989, 13.193–201.

33. Fenlon HM, McAneny, Nunes DP, et al. Occlusive colon carcinoma: virtual colonoscopy in the preoperative evaluation of the proximal colon. Radiology 1999; 210:423–428.

34. Macari M, Berman P, Dicker M, et al. Usefulness of CT colonography in patients with incomplete colonoscopy. AJR 1999; 173:561–564.

35. Johnson CD, Harmsen LA, Wilson RL et al. Prospective blinded evaluation of computed tomographic colonography for screen detection of colorectal polyps. Gastroenterology 2003; 125:311–319.

36. Pineau BC, Paskett ED, Chen MA. Virtual colonoscopy using oral contrast compared with colonoscopy for the detection of patients with colorectal polyps. Gastroenterology 2003; 125:304–310.

37. Galdino GM, Yee J. Carpet lesion on CT colonography: a potential pitfall. AJR 2003; 180:1332–1334.

38. Eddy DM, Nugent FW, Eddy JF, et al. Screening for colorectal cancer in a high-risk population. Gastroenterology 1987; 92:682–692.

39. Glick S, Wagner JL, Johnson CD. Cost-effectiveness of double-contrast barium enema in screening for colorectal cancer. AJR 1998; 170:629–636.

40. Lieberman D. How to screen for colon cancer. Ann Rev Med 1998; 49:163–172.

41. Low RN, McCue, Barone R, et al. MR staging of primary colorectal carcinoma: comparison with surgical and histopathologic findings. Abdom Imaging 2003; 28:784–793.

42. Butch RJ, Stark DD, Wittenberg J, et al. Staging rectal cancer by MR and CT. AJR 1986; 146:1155–1160.

43. Dobos N, Rubesin SE. Radiologic imaging modalities in the diagnosis and management of colorectal cancer. Hem/Onc Clin NA 2002; 16:875–895.

44. Schnall MD, Furth EE, Rosato EF, et al. Rectal tumor stage: correlation of endorectal MR imaging and pathologic findings. Radiology 1994; 190:709–714.

45. Zagoria RJ, Schlarb CA, Ott DJ, et al. Assessment of rectal tumor infiltration utilizing endorectal MR imaging and comparison with endoscopic rectal sonography. J Surg Oncol 1997; 64:312–317.

46. Kim NK, Kim NJ, Yun SH, et al. Comparative study of transrectal ultrasonography, pelvic computerized tomography, and magnetic resonance imaging in preoperative staging of rectal cancer. Dis Colon Rectum 1999; 42:770–775.

47. Chintapalli KN, Esola CC, Chopra S, et al. Pericolic mesenteric lymph nodes: an aid in distinguishing diverticulitis from cancer of the colon. AJR 1997; 169:253–1255.

48. Farouk R, Nelson H, Radice E, et al. Accuracy of computed tomography in determining resectability for locally and advanced primary or recurrent colorectal cancers. AM J Surg 1998; 175:283–287.

49. Meyers MA. Dynamic radiology of the Abdomen: Normal and Pathologic Anatomy, 5th ed. New York: Springer, 2000.

50. Fong Y, Kemeny N, Paty P, et al. Treatment of colorectal cancer: hepatic metastases. Semin Surg Oncol 1996; 12:219–252.

51. Kim EE, Chung SK, Haynie TP, et al. Differentiation of residual recurrent tumors for post-treatment changes with F-18 FDG PET. Radiographics 1992; 12:269–279.

52. Tan TXL, Klein MY, Tabib VT, Turner C, Forde JM. Oncologic Applications of PET: An Updated Review. Applied Radiology 2000; 29:18–25.

53. Castro DB, Stearns MW. Lipomas of the gastrointestinal tract. Dis. Colon Rectum 1972; 15:441–444.

54. Rubesin SE, Furth EE. Other Tumors of the Colon. In Gore RM, Levine MS, eds. Textbook of Gastrointestinal Radiology, 2nd ed. Philadelphia: WB Saunders; 2001:1049–1074.

55. Hurwitz MH, Redleaf PD, Williams HJ, et al. Lipomas of the gastrointestinal tract. AJR 1967; 99:84–89.

56. Megibow AJ, Redmond PE, Bosniak MA, et al. Diagnosis of gastrointestinal lipomas by CT. AJR 1979; 133:743–745.

57. Williams SN, Berk RN, Harned RK. Radiologic features of multinodular lymphoma of the colon. AJR 1984; 143:87–91.

58. O'Connell DJ, Thompson AJ: Lymphoma of the colon. The spectrum of radiologic changes. Gastrointestinal Radiology 1978; 2:377–385.

59. Meyers MA, McSweeney J. Secondary neoplasms of the bowel. Radiology 1972; 105:1–11.

60. Becker JA. Prostatic carcinoma involving the rectum and sigmoid colon. AJR 1965; 94:421–428.

61. Rubesin SE, Levine MS, Bezzi M, et al. Rectal involvement by prostatic carcinoma: radiographic findings. AJR 1989; 152:53–57.

62. Meyers MA. Distribution of intra-abdominal malignant seeding: dependency on dynamics of flow of ascitic fluid. AJR 1973; 119:198–206.

63. Rubesin SE, Levine MS. Omental cakes: Colonic involvement by omental metastasis. Radiology 1985; 154:593–596.

64. Rubesin SE, Levine MS, Glick SN. Gastric involvement by omental cakes: Radiographic findings. Gastrointest Radiol 1986; 11:223–228.

65. Meyers MA. Intraperitoneal spread of malignancies and its effect on the bowel. Clin Radiol 1981; 32:129–146.

66. Pannu HK, Bristow RE, Montz FJ, Fishman EK. Multidetector CT of peritoneal carcinomatosis from ovarian cancer. RadioGaphics 2003; 23:687–701.

23 Current Status of Colorectal Cancer Therapy

*John Strother, md, Kevin G. Billingsley, md,
Arthur Y. Hung, md, and Charles D. Blanke, md*

Contents

1. INTRODUCTION

In 2004, the American Cancer Society estimated that approx 150,000 new cases of colorectal cancer would occur in the United States and that more than 57,000 Americans would die of the disease, making it the second most common cause of cancer-related death *(1)*. Despite improvements in screening techniques, 30–40% of patients with colorectal cancer present with locoregionally advanced or metastatic disease and are not candidates for potentially curative therapy. Overall, progress in the surgical and neoadjuvant/adjuvant management of locally confined colorectal cancer has been rapid and very encouraging over the past several years. In addition, median survival in advanced disease has improved almost fourfold, as several new and active salvage systemic agents have emerged and been rapidly integrated into first-line regimens.

2. SURGICAL PRINCIPLES

The ultimate goals of large-bowel cancer surgery include the excision of the tumor and adjacent colon or rectum, with resection of regional mesenteric lymph nodes, and, if necessary, *en bloc* resection of contiguously involved organs. New

From: *Endoscopic Oncology: Gastrointestinal Endoscopy and Cancer Management.* Edited by: D. O. Faigel and M. L. Kochman © Humana Press, Totowa, NJ

surgical developments have arisen from advances in technology and the procedures themselves, including the use of laparoscopy and minimally invasive techniques. Additional progress has come from developments in imaging technology, which provide surgeons with detailed staging and anatomic information.

2.1. EXTENT OF SURGERY FOR COLON TUMORS

Unlike esophageal or gastric cancer, colon cancer rarely spreads extensively within the gut wall. A series of meticulous clinicopathological studies demonstrated that colorectal tumors rarely spread more than a centimeter away from the margin of the primary lesion *(2,3)*. Achieving a 5-cm margin on either side of the lesion is thus adequate. Because lymphatics and regional lymph nodes are adjacent to the mesenteric vessels, it is necessary to perform a proximal ligation of the segmental blood supply to the colon to insure an adequate lymphadenectomy. In many cases proximal vascular ligation and lymphadenectomy devascularizes a larger area of colon and necessitates a more extensive bowel resection than would be required to obtain 5-cm margins on either side of the tumor.

Regional lymphadenectomy is performed for both therapeutic and staging purposes, because residual disease in regional nodes is a potential source of locoregional recurrence. Several studies show that obtaining between 12 and 14 mesenteric nodes is necessary to maximize the accuracy of lymph node staging

(4,5). To facilitate thorough lymphadenectomy, the mesenteric vasculature supplying the involved portion of the colon should be divided close to its origin at the superior mesenteric artery (for ascending and transverse colon lesions) or at its origin close to the inferior mesenteric artery (for descending colon lesions). Some have argued for division of the inferior mesenteric artery at its origin on the aorta for tumors of the descending colon or rectum *(6)*. Although this approach does afford a more complete lymphadenectomy, others have argued that patients with lymph node involvement at the level of the proximal inferior mesenteric artery rarely are cured regardless of the extent of lymphadenectomy *(7)*. The greatest benefit of high ligation is likely to be the mobility gained in the descending colon for tension-free bowel anastomosis in the pelvis.

2.2. LAPAROSCOPIC COLECTOMY

In recent years surgeons have gained increasing facility with complex laparoscopic procedures. The benefits of such a minimally invasive approach include a decrease in postoperative pain and a more rapid recovery. The first descriptions of laparoscopic colectomy emerged in the early 1990s *(8–10)*. The early results of laparoscopic colectomy for cancer were dominated by a number of concerning reports of recurrent disease in laparoscopic port sites *(11,12)*. As the procedure matured and both technique and instrumentation improved, port site recurrences have become increasingly rare.

The most significant question has been whether laparoscopic colectomy provides the same disease control as an open colectomy. The US Intergroup study of laparoscopic colectomy was recently reported *(13)*. This trial was a multicenter, prospective, randomized study of laparoscopic vs open colectomy for colon cancer. The study demonstrated that disease control provided by the two operative approaches was nearly identical. There was no evidence of excessive port site recurrences in the laparoscopic group. The other benefits of laparoscopic approach were modest, but measurable. The median hospitalization was reduced from 6 to 5 d with laparoscopy. The laparoscopic approach also decreased the postoperative use of narcotic pain relievers from a median of 4 d to a median of 3 d *(13)*. The data provided by this trial suggest that laparoscopic colectomy is an appropriate alternative for selected patients with colon cancer. However, there is clearly a learning curve to the procedure and significant surgical experience is necessary to obtain outcomes that approximate those reported in the intergroup trial. The issues of surgeon training and credentialing for laparoscopic colectomy for cancer remain unresolved.

2.3. SURGICAL APPROACHES FOR RECTAL CANCER

There are few areas in modern surgical oncology in which surgical experience and technique make as much of an impact on clinical outcome as they do in rectal cancer. The surgical approach to rectal tumors has evolved substantially in the past 20 yr. In the past, abdominoperineal resection, which involves the formation of a permanent end colostomy, was considered the "gold standard" for the treatment of the majority of patients with rectal cancer *(14)*. In the current era, a combination of technical developments as well as the selective utilization of neoadjuvant chemoradiotherapy has minimized the application of abdominoperineal resection and made sphincter-preserving surgery possible for most patients with rectal cancer *(15)*.

Recent years have shown that rectal cancer surgery requires experience and technical precision. A variety of studies demonstrate that increasing surgical volume is associated with decreased postoperative mortality and improved cancer survival *(16–19)*. Both short- and long-term outcomes, as well as sphincter preservation rates, are improved when patients receive care at an experienced rectal cancer center.

3. MANAGEMENT OF RECTAL CANCER BY LOCATION

Patients with tumors of the proximal and midrectum are generally treated with anterior or low anterior resection. This involves an abdominal approach with division of the sigmoid colon and resection of the sigmoid and proximal rectum. Rectal continuity is reestablished by forming an end-to-end stapled pelvic anastomosis with the use of an end-to-end stapler *(20)*. These staplers, which are introduced through the anus, allow surgeons to secure the anvil component of the devices in the proximal colon. The two pieces of colon are approximated and the surgeon deploys the staples. This technique allows precise approximation of the bowel even in the low pelvis, where visualization and access for a hand-sewn anastomosis would be difficult.

Tumors of the distal rectum require much more careful multidisciplinary decision making and sophisticated surgical techniques. The size and location of the tumor, as well as the potential involvement of adjacent organs are all critical elements that must be determined before making a judgment on the appropriate surgical approach. Computerized tomographic scans and endorectal ultrasound provide complementary, local staging information that assists with surgical decision making *(21,22)*.

The development of techniques of coloanal reconstruction *(23)* has enabled surgeons to offer a sphincter-preserving surgery to carefully selected patients with cancers of the low rectum. This procedure involves a complete dissection of the rectum down to the levator musculature using an abdominal approach. A transanal approach is then used perform a distal rectal mucosectomy. A hand-sewn anastomosis is then performed between colon and the anal mucosa at the dentate line. This approach is often coupled with neoadjuvant chemoradiotherapy to provide downstaging of the disease before operation *(24,25)*. In addition to coloanal anastomosis, it is also possible to perform stapled anastomoses in many patients with low tumors. One technical refinement that has been added to the procedure in recent years is the use of a colonic J-pouch to improve the reservoir function of the neorectum *(26)*.

In addition to technical precision, successful sphincter preservation in the patient with low rectal cancer requires meticulous patient selection *(27)*. The disease must be located in a position that allows the surgeon to obtain at least 1 cm of distal margin *(28,29)*. The tumor must not invade or overlie the sphincteric muscular complex *(15)*. In addition, the patient must have good sphincter function preoperatively. Abdominoperineal resection remains the appropriate procedure for patients with distal rectal cancer that do not meet these selection criteria *(30–33)*.

The functional outcomes from specialized centers with carefully selected patients indicate that most patients are pleased with their outcome and approx 70% describe their function as excellent or good (34). A small subset of these patients will have substantial difficulties with continence and bowel function, and some will eventually require conversion to colostomy.

4. LOCAL EXCISION

Patients with small tumors in the low rectum may also be treated with transanal excision. This approach avoids the morbidity and recovery associated with an abdominal incision, because the operation is performed entirely through the anus. Using an operating rectal speculum, the surgeon excises a full thickness portion of the rectal wall including the tumor. The rectal mucosa is then approximated using absorbable sutures. This method allows for complete resection of small tumors that are limited to the wall of the rectum and it provides an opportunity to accurately stage the depth of penetration through the wall. This technique, however, does not provide any information about the involvement of regional lymph nodes.

The transanal approach is appropriate for T1 tumors of the distal rectum in which the tumor does not involve more than one-third of the circumference of the rectum (35). The decision to perform a transanal resection vs a more traditional transabdominal resection with lymphadenectomy is often quite complex and it requires meticulous pathological assessment and locoregional staging, usually with endoscopic ultrasound. Controversy remains over the effectiveness of the transanal technique as a definitive surgical technique. Some large studies indicate very low local recurrence rates (36), although studies from other large institutions indicate that local recurrence rates can be as high as 26% for T2 tumors, even with adjuvant radiation therapy (37). In a series from the University of Minnesota the local recurrence rates without adjuvant radiation were 18 and 37% for T1 and T2 tumors, respectively (38). In all cases, preoperative local staging, particularly with endoscopic ultrasound, is essential for selecting the appropriate operative procedure. Unless patients have comorbid disease that prevents the utilization of a transabdominal resection, T3 tumors should not be treated with transanal excision. T2 tumors and possibly T1 patients with adverse prognostic features (lymphovascular invasion, poorly differentiated lesions) have significant likelihood of mesorectal lymph node involvement and should be considered for adjuvant therapy following transanal excision (39).

5. TOTAL MESORECTAL EXCISION

A series of detailed clinicopathological studies have shown that distal spread of rectal cancer within the bowel wall is generally quite limited, but tumor cells may spread laterally within the perirectal soft tissue. The presence of viable tumor cells at the radial resection margins is one of the most significant features associated with local cancer recurrence (3). There is, however, a fascial envelope that encloses all of the lymphatics of the mesorectum and this anatomic structure serves as a natural barrier to the spread of tumor if it is not violated in the course of surgical resection.

The understanding of the importance of preserving an intact mesorectal envelope has led to significant changes in the surgical approach to rectal cancer. Heald and others have developed and promoted the technique of total mesorectal excision (TME) (40,41). This approach involves a sharp dissection of the mesorectum under direct vision, which allows the surgeon to preserve the integrity of the mesorectum from the pelvic brim to the level of the levator ani. Blunt dissection in the posterior plane is assiduously avoided to prevent dissemination of tumor cells in the pelvis. Precise identification of the pelvic autonomic nerves (including the hypogastric plexus) and the sacral nerve roots in the pelvis is required and allows maintenance of erectile and ejaculatory function in male patients and vaginal lubrication in response to sexual stimulus in women (42).

A variety of large, prospective series demonstrate that total mesorectal excision may be performed with a very low rate of local disease recurrence, even in the absence of adjuvant radiation therapy (43). The Basingstoke Hospital series indicates local disease recurrence as low as 5% (44). Results from centers in North America are less clear, stemming from the fact that adjuvant radiation therapy has been the standard for T3 or node-positive tumors for well over 15 yr (45). However, studies from Memorial Sloan-Kettering Cancer Center and other tertiary care centers suggest that with meticulous technique, TME may be performed in selected patients without radiation therapy, with 5-yr local recurrence rate of 10% or less (46,47). A recent prospective, randomized trial from the Netherlands has attempted to clarify this issue (48).

The study involved the use of proctored surgery to insure technically sound TME for all study patients. A total of 1861 patients with non-fixed, potentially resectable rectal cancer underwent randomization to surgery alone vs a short course of neoadjuvant radiation followed by surgery. This study showed no difference in survival. The study did demonstrate, however, that with the addition of neoadjuvant radiation therapy to TME the local recurrence rate was reduced from 8.2 to 2.4%. In summary, although meticulous surgical technique may minimize local recurrence rates, in appropriately selected patients, the addition of adjuvant radiotherapy will also provide a substantial contribution to local disease control.

5.1. LAPAROSCOPIC RECTAL RESECTION

The laparoscopic approach to rectal resection is clearly feasible, but it has not undergone the scrutiny of a prospective, randomized clinical trial, as has occurred for colon cancer. Smaller institutional studies demonstrate that the procedure may be performed for carefully selected patients, with an acceptable local recurrence rate. The generalizability of these results to the widespread practice is uncertain. For the current time, open rectal resection for rectal cancer remains the standard of care.

6. CHEMOTHERAPY FOR COLORECTAL CANCER

Systemic therapy for colorectal cancer has dramatically changed over the last 10 yr. Many but not all agents are effective in both the adjuvant and metastatic settings.

6.1. FLUOROURACIL

Five-fluorouracil (5-FU) was first synthesized in 1957 (49). Its mechanism of action differs depending on the means of administration, and during the 40 yr in which it was the only available effective drug against colorectal malignancy, much effort was undertaken to identify and further develop the most efficacious route and schedules. With protracted intravenous infusion, 5-FU metabolites inhibit thymidylate synthase (TS), an enzyme required for DNA synthesis. However, when administered by bolus injection, inhibition of RNA synthesis predominantly contributes to its antitumor effect (50). A meta-analysis comparing intravenous 5-FU by continuous infusion or bolus injection found that toxicities were generally similar. However, the incidence of hand-foot syndrome was nearly doubled when 5-FU was administered by continuous infusion (34 vs 13%), whereas hematological toxicity (primarily neutropenia) occurred significantly more often in patients receiving bolus injections (31 vs 4%) (51).

Innumerable different doses and administration schedules of 5-FU have evolved. In Europe it is more common to administer 5-FU via continuous infusion over 24–48 h, but in the United States bolus injection five times daily or weekly has, until recently, been more popular. Bolus 5-FU is clearly more convenient and obviates the need for both a central venous catheter and an infusion pump and the associated risks, although peripherally inserted central venous catheters may be used in this situation. The meta-analysis discussed previously showed 5-FU administered by continuous infusion had a better toxicity profile and may also improve tumor response rate and survival time when compared with 5-FU bolus regimens.

Combining 5-FU with modulatory agents can also enhance efficacy. Leucovorin, the pharmacologically active form of folic acid (50), prolongs the TS-FdUMP interaction, leading to more effective inhibition of the enzyme (52). A meta-analysis of 18 trials comparing 5-FU to 5-FU/leucovorin in 2751 patients with advanced colorectal cancer and identified an increase in response rate (12 vs 23%, $p = 0.0001$) and a small but statistically significant survival benefit at 1 yr (43 vs 48%, $p = 0.003$) in favor of 5-FU/leucovorin (53). However, although improved by the use of leucovorin, median survival was only approx 11 mo in both treatment groups.

6.2. IRINOTECAN

Irinotecan, or CPT-11, is an antineoplastic agent derived from camptothecin. CPT-11 and its active metabolite, SN-38, inhibit topoisomerase I, leading to irreversible breaks in double-stranded DNA. Neutropenia and diarrhea are the dose-limiting toxicities of irinotecan, and late diarrhea can be life threatening if not treated promptly. A constellation of symptoms occurring within the first 24 h of administration (and resembling a cholinergic reaction) is common and includes abdominal cramps, diarrhea, diaphoresis, salivation, lacrimation, and bradycardia. Most or all symptoms respond to subcutaneous atropine (0.25–0.5 mg) (54,55). In addition, akathisia has also been reported when prochlorperazine is given as an antiemetic for irinotecan, preventing the administration of that agent within 24 h of irinotecan (56).

Initial studies in the United States focused on using single-agent irinotecan in patients with metastatic colorectal cancer refractory to 5-FU-based therapy; a response rate of 23% and median survival of 10.4 mo was reported in that setting

(56,57). Response rates of 19–32% in patients with previously untreated metastatic colorectal cancer were described in subsequent phase II studies (58,59). In 1998, two European randomized phase III studies definitively established the efficacy of single-agent irinotecan as second-line therapy in metastatic colorectal cancer. When compared with 5-FU/leucovorin or best supportive care, irinotecan improved median survival and 1-yr survival (60,61). Two landmark phase III studies published in 2000 also showed a benefit for irinotecan when used in the first-line setting for metastatic colorectal cancer. Irinotecan combined with bolus or infusional 5-FU improved response rate (39–49%) and median survival (14.4–17.6 mo) when compared directly with 5-FU/leucovorin (62,63). The US Food and Drug Administration (FDA) approved irinotecan with either bolus or infused 5-FU as the reference regimens for the indication of treatment for advanced colorectal cancer in the spring of 2000, although the IFL (or Saltz) regimen. CPT-11 with bolus 5-FU and leucovorin, was later nearly abandoned in the United States (see Section 7).

6.3. OXALIPLATIN

Oxaliplatin, a late-generation platinum, causes crosslinking adducts in DNA, blocking replication and transcription (64). In vitro, oxaliplatin potently inhibits colorectal tumor cell lines resistant to cisplatin and carboplatin (65) and it is the only platinum compound to show pre- or clinical activity in colorectal cancer. Unlike other platinum-based compounds, oxaliplatin does not cause nephrotoxicity; its toxicity profile includes neutropenia, nausea/vomiting, and a cumulative, usually reversible peripheral neuropathy (which can be dose-limiting). Patients may also develop a reversible, cold-induced acute pharyngolaryngeal neuropathy (66).

Three early phase II single-agent oxaliplatin studies in patients with metastatic colorectal cancer resistant to 5-FU identified a reproducible 10% response rate (67,68), and when oxaliplatin was used as a single agent in patients with previously untreated advanced colorectal cancer, response rates of 20–24% were reported (69,70) A substantial synergistic effect was seen when oxaliplatin was combined with 5-FU/leucovorin, and numerous phase II studies of oxaliplatin plus 5-FU/leucovorin in the second-line setting for metastatic colorectal cancer identified response rates of 20–46% (71–76). In 2000, de Gramont et al. randomized a total of 420 previously untreated patients to the combination of leucovorin (folinic acid), infusional 5-FU, and oxaliplatin (FOLFOX4) vs 5-FU and leucovorin alone. Patients treated on the oxaliplatin arm had a longer progression-free survival (9 vs 6.2 mo) and a better response rate (50.7 vs 22.3%). The observed improvement in overall survival (16.2 vs 14.7 mo); however, did not reach statistical significance in this study, which was powered to demonstrate a difference in time to progression. Patients treated with oxaliplatin had higher frequencies of grade 3/4 neutropenia and diarrhea and more neuropathy (77).

6.4. CAPECITABINE

Capecitabine is an oral prodrug that is absorbed intact through the intestinal wall and then converted to 5-FU in three sequential enzymatic reactions. The final enzyme is present in higher levels in tumors compared with normal tissues, providing a basis for enhanced selectivity *(78,79)*. Leucovorin is not used in combination with capecitabine because it mandates dose reduction of capecitabine without increasing efficacy *(80)*.

Two-phase III trials have compared capecitabine with 5-FU/leucovorin for the first-line treatment of patients with advanced colorectal cancer *(80,81)*. These trials were designed to demonstrate equivalency to 5-FU. On both studies, capecitabine was associated with a significantly higher response rate and a similar median time to progression and median survival. The incidence of grade 3/4 stomatitis and neutropenia was significantly less in the capecitabine groups, whereas hand-foot syndrome and (in one trial) hyperbilirubinemia were more common *(81)*.

Capecitabine has also been combined with both oxaliplatin and irinotecan. Phase II studies suggested response rates for capecitabine plus oxaliplatin (CapOx) and capecitabine plus irinotecan (CapIri) approach or exceed 50%. However, it is difficult to combine full-dose capecitabine with either drug without attenuating the dose of the fluoropyrimidine pro-drug. Phase III studies comparing capecitabine with oxaliplatin or irinotecan vs the same drugs with intravenous 5-FU as first-line treatment in advanced colorectal cancer have been started.

Capecitabine is currently approved in the United States for the first-line treatment of metastatic colorectal cancer in poor performance status patients or others who are not good candidates for combination therapy.

7. STANDARD FIRST-LINE THERAPY FOR METASTATIC DISEASE

Intergroup 9741 was a phase III trial that randomized 795 patients with untreated advanced colorectal cancer to oxaliplatin and irinotecan in combination (IROX), FOLFOX4, or bolus IFL (Table 1). The trial showed a statistically significant advantage for FOLFOX compared with bolus IFL, in terms of response rate (45 vs 31%), progression-free survival (8.7 vs 6.9 mo), and overall survival (19.5 vs 15 mo) *(82)*. However, the impact of the second-line therapies (more common after FOLFOX) and the infusional vs bolus 5-FU (the latter part of IFL while the former is used in FOLFOX) on overall survival must be considered *(83)*. Currently, FOLFOX represents the standard of care first-line option in the United States, whereas IFL is rarely used.

Tournigand et al. conducted an innovative randomized phase III trial of irinotecan plus infusional 5-FU/leucovorin (FOLFIRI) followed by FOLFOX at disease progression vs the reverse sequence. The most impressive result of this study was an overall survival exceeding 20 mo in both arms, which had not been previously reached in any randomized study of metastatic colorectal cancer therapy. Neither arm was superior, though toxicity profiles were different. In first-line therapy, grade 3/4 mucositis, nausea/vomiting, and grade 2 alopecia were more frequent with FOLFIRI, and grade 3/4 neutropenia and neurosensory toxicity were more frequent with FOLFOX. Interestingly, second-line response rate data was higher with FOLFOX (15%) than with FOLFIRI (4%) *(84)*. This trial suggests that the inferiority of IFL to FOLFOX in N9741 was not owing to the irinotecan, and that FOLFIRI represents a reasonable first-line choice for patients with metastatic disease.

Table 1
Systemic Therapy for Advanced Disease

Regimen	Response rate (%)	Median survival (mo)
Best supportive care *(144)*	Not applicable	6
5-FU/leucovorin	23	11
IFL *(62)*	39	14.8
IFL + bevacizumab *(95)*	45	20.3
FOLFIRI *(84)*	56	21.5
FOLFOX *(84)*	54	20.6

Finally, investigation of all three drugs in combination is underway. A phase II trial evaluated the triplet combination of irinotecan plus oxaliplatin plus continuous infusion 5-FU/leucovorin as first-line treatment in 31 patients with metastatic colorectal cancer. Overall response rate was 58% and the median time to progression was 13 mo. Predictable toxicities included grade 3/4 neutropenia in 45%, grade 3/4 diarrhea in 32%, and grade 3/4 neurotoxicity in 9% *(85)*. In order to assess whether triplet therapy will provide improved outcomes, phase III trials must be done to evaluate sequential doublet combinations against up-front triplet therapy.

7.1. CETUXIMAB

Cetuximab (C225; Erbitux) is a chimeric monoclonal antibody highly selective for the epidermal growth factor receptor (EGFR). EGF is important for colonic tumor cell proliferation, inhibition of apoptosis, angiogenesis, and metastasis, making EGFR a promising target in colon cancer *(86)*. Approximately 75% of colon cancers express EGFR. Preclinical models showed an additive effect of cetuximab to irinotecan even in irinotecan-resistant tumors.

Toxicities attributable to cetuximab include anaphylactoid reactions (1–2%) and an acne-like skin rash/folliculitis (approx 75%). Patients who develop the rash appear to survive longer than those who do not, and those with more intense rash survive the longest *(87–89)*. The rash may be a surrogate indicator of adequate receptor saturation by cetuximab. Future studies will take this possibility into consideration and target cetuximab doses to achieve a desired level of cutaneous toxicity to attempt to increase efficacy.

A phase II study that tested cetuximab in patients refractory to irinotecan demonstrated a response rate of 9%. Another, randomized, phase II trial in 329 patients failing irinotecan-containing therapy compared the combination of cetuximab and irinotecan to cetuximab alone and confirmed a significantly higher response rate (22.9 vs 10.8%) and longer progression-free survival (4.5 vs 1.5 mo) in favor of the combination, although overall survival was unchanged (8.6 vs 6.9 mo) *(90)*. Cetuximab has also been combined with FOLFOX in the first-line treatment of patients with metastatic disease, with a 70% response rate demonstrated in a phase II study *(91)*.

In 2004, cetuximab was approved by the FDA for treatment of metastatic, irinotecan-refractory colorectal cancer expressing EGFR in combination with irinotecan-based chemotherapy regimens. Although preclinical studies indicated that EGFR expression was necessary for cetuximab activity, this has not yet been demonstrated clinically, and some experts have questioned the need for EGFR expression.

7.2. BEVACIZUMAB

Bevacizumab is a recombinant humanized monoclonal antibody to vascular endothelial growth factor (VEGF). In addition to its direct antiangiogenic effects, bevacizumab may also improve the delivery of chemotherapy by altering tumor vasculature and decreasing the elevated interstitial pressure in tumors (92,93). In a phase II trial, 104 previously untreated patients with metastatic colorectal cancer were randomly assigned to 5-FU/leucovorin with or without bevacizumab (5 or 10 mg/kg every 2 wk). Response rates were higher with combined low-dose therapy (40 vs 17%) but not high-dose therapy, as was time to tumor progression (9 vs 5.2 mo) and median overall survival (21.5 vs 13.8 mo). Thrombosis was the most significant adverse event and was fatal in one person, and hypertension, proteinuria, and epistaxis were other side effects (94).

In a recent phase III trial, 813 patients with previously untreated advanced colorectal cancer were randomized to receive bolus IFL plus bevacizumab (5 mg/kg every 2 wk) or bolus IFL plus placebo. The addition of bevacizumab improved median overall survival (20.3 vs 15.6 mo), progression-free survival (10.6 vs 6.2 mo), and response rate (44.8 vs 34.8%) compared with bolus IFL alone. Grade 3 hypertension was more common during treatment with IFL plus bevacizumab than with IFL plus placebo (11 vs 2.3%) but was easily managed (95).

Based on the convincing proof of efficacy when added to IFL and bolus 5-FU/leucovorin as first-line treatment, bevacizumab was approved in 2004 for use in the first-line setting in combination with any intravenous 5-FU-based therapy. This surprisingly broad approval opened the door for a combination that has not yet been reported for first-line use: FOLFOX plus bevacizumab.

8. ADJUVANT THERAPY FOR LARGE-BOWEL CANCERS

Surgery remains the primary curative modality for treatment of colorectal cancers. However, many patients will relapse and die of recurrent colorectal cancer in spite of complete gross tumor removal. The risk of relapse following surgery correlates with stage of disease, and ranges from approx 20 to 30% for stage II disease (Tx, N0) to 50–80% for stage III disease (Tx, N+). For patients with rectal cancer, a recent meta-analysis demonstrated that local tumor recurrence was highly correlated with both the depth of tumor penetration and the number of regional lymph nodes involved by metastatic disease (96).

There is consensus that adjuvant therapy is indicated for most patients with stage III cancers of the colon or rectum and stage II cancers of the rectum. Opinion is divided whether patients with stage II colon cancer derive sufficient benefit to warrant adjuvant therapy on a routine basis, although a recent trial involving more than 3000 patients demonstrated a 3% absolute benefit in overall survival with chemotherapy compared with observation alone (97–99). The vast majority of tumor relapses occur in sites distant from the primary tumor following surgery for colon cancer. Therefore, the focus of adjuvant therapy for colon cancer is on systemic treatment aimed at eradicating micrometastatic disease.

In contrast, local tumor failure in the pelvis is a significant clinical problem for patients with rectal cancer treated with surgery alone, providing a rationale for regional adjuvant radiation therapy. Because distant metastasis is the principal mode of tumor relapse in patients with rectal cancer who receive aggressive local therapy, improved systemic therapy is also a key focus of rectal cancer adjuvant trials.

8.1. ADJUVANT CHEMOTHERAPY FOR COLON CANCER

Substantial advances have been made in the surgical adjuvant therapy of colon cancer in the past several years. Six months of 5-FU and leucovorin following resection of stage III colon cancer has become standard adjuvant therapy, credited with an approx 5–10% absolute improvement in 5-yr survival compared with surgery alone (100). For several years, levamisole, an antihelminthic whose beneficial effect is presumably immune-mediated, was standard treatment (with 5-FU) following resection of advanced colon cancer. A recent meta-analysis of 3302 patients with stages II and III colon cancer from seven randomized trials comparing 5-FU plus either leucovorin or levamisole to surgery alone demonstrated an improvement in 5-yr disease-free survival (67 vs 55%) and overall survival (71 vs 64%) with the use of adjuvant chemotherapy that was consistent across subsets of age, sex, location, T stage, nodal status, and grade (101). Adding levamisole was felt to increase toxicity over 5-FU/leucovorin alone without increasing efficacy, and its use has been abandoned (102).

Several newer agents have also been tested in adjuvant use, given their efficacy against metastatic disease. A randomized phase III trial comparing IFL to FL in resected stage III colon cancer showed IFL was associated with a greater degree of neutropenia, neutropenic fever, and death on treatment, with no associated clinical benefit. Whether an infusional 5-FU regimen combined with irinotecan would be of benefit is unknown (103).

More encouraging results were recently published from the MOSAIC trial, which evaluated oxaliplatin in combination with 5-FU and leucovorin (FOLFOX4) vs infusional 5-FU/leucovorin alone in stage II and III patients. This study demonstrated a significant improvement in 3-yr disease-free survival (78.2 vs 72.9%) for patients who received FOLFOX, although overall survival was not yet different between the two groups after just 3 yr of follow-up (87.7 vs 86.6%). Nevertheless, the FDA has not yet approved the use of oxaliplatin in the surgical adjuvant setting for patients with colon cancer.

Positive results for EGFR and VEGF inhibitors in metastatic disease provide a strong rationale for their study in the surgical adjuvant setting, but the failure of IFL despite its superiority in metastatic disease warns against off-label use now.

8.2. ADJUVANT IRRADIATION FOR COLON CANCER

Although postoperative chemotherapy is standard treatment for all stage III and selected phase II patients, the role of radiation therapy in any circumstance has been questioned. Local recurrences can, however, occur following resection of colon cancers. Retrospective assessment suggests T4 tumors and T3 N+ tumors are associated with local recurrence rates after surgery alone ranging from 31 to 53% (104). The addition of radiation reduces these rates to 7–30%, depending on the nodal status, with a possible 12% improvement in overall disease-free survival for T4 tumors. Confirmatory reports from the Mayo Clinic and the University of Florida have demonstrated local control rates of 90% with adjuvant radiation therapy following resection of locally advanced disease (105,106).

An Intergroup trial attempted to investigate whether the addition of radiation to an adjuvant chemotherapy regimen improved survival among patients at high risk of local-regional recurrence after complete resection of their colon cancer (107,108). Secondary objectives included evaluation of disease-free survival, patterns of recurrence, and toxicity. Local recurrence was not included as an end point. The chemotherapy consisted of weekly doses of fluorouracil 450 mg/m^2 iv with levamisole. For the patients who received radiation, the radiation was delivered to the pre-operative tumor volume, regional lymph nodes, and the adjacent para-aortic or pelvic lymph nodes to a total dose of 45 Gy, followed by a boost of 5.4 Gy if the small bowel could be safely excluded. The protocol closed early because of poor accrual with only 187 eligible patients, well short of the original goal of 700 patients.

With a median duration of follow-up of 6.6 yr, no differences were seen in survival, disease-free survival, and local control. Moreover, the study did demonstrate a significant increase in toxicity, specifically leukopenia, for patients treated with chemoradiation, most likely attributable to the para-aortic field. Although the study demonstrated similar outcomes between the two arms, the small number of patients makes it difficult to completely deny any benefit from the addition of radiation. Nevertheless, adjuvant radiation therapy following resection of colon cancer should be considered only in those patients in whom local recurrence is very likely.

8.3. ADJUVANT IRRADIATION FOR RECTAL CANCER

The role of radiation, in addition to surgery, has been fairly well established for distal large bowel cancers. The risk of local relapse after surgery alone ranges from 5 to 15% for stage I tumors and extends from 20 to 50% for stage III tumors (109–114). Radiation therapy is recognized as a nearly essential component of adjuvant therapy in all stages II and III tumors, as well as in stage I tumors when a major definitive resection of the bowel is not performed.

8.4. RADIATION TECHNIQUE

The primary goal of radiation is to lower the rates of locoregional recurrence. Lymphatic and venous drainage of rectal lesions depends on the level of the lesion. The upper rectum drains into the inferior mesenteric system via the superior hemorrhoidal vessels, and the middle and lower rectum can drain directly to the internal iliac and presacral nodes. Lesions that extend to the anal canal can spread to the inguinal nodes. With anterior extension of the tumor out of the rectum, the external iliac nodes become at risk. Review of treatment failure patterns indicates that the most common site for locoregional recurrences is in the presacral space, followed by the anastomotic site or perineum and the posterior aspect of anterior pelvic organs, including bladder or other genitourinary structures (110,115,116).

The radiation field depends on whether the patient is being treated pre- or postoperatively. The irradiated volume extends from the origin of the common iliac vessels to 3–5 cm distal of the tumor in a patient with an intact anal sphincter, or to the perineum after an abdominoperineal resection. Laterally, the radiation field encompasses the obturator and external iliac lymph nodes along the pelvic sidewall. If the tumor extends into the anal canal or lower third of the vagina, the field is widened to cover the inguinal lymph nodes. Posteriorly, the radiation field always encompasses at least the entire presacral space, if not the whole sacrum (in extensive tumors). Anteriorly, the radiation field may stretch to the pubic symphysis when external iliac lymph nodes are at risk. Otherwise, the majority of the bladder may be spared, and only the rectum is treated.

The tumor and lymph node beds are typically treated to 45–50 Gy in 5–6 wk at 1.8–2.0 Gy/d. At that point, the fields are reduced to treat only the tumor volume with a generous margin. An additional three to eight fractions are given to this "boost" field. Thus the total dose for treatments in the pre-operative setting is 50.4–54 Gy in 5.5–6 wk. In the postoperative setting, the doses range from 54 to 59.4 Gy in 6 to 6.5 wk.

The most common acute morbidity from irradiation is disturbed bowel movement function, for example, diarrhea and/or cramping. Local skin inflammation, cystitis, and myelosuppression can occur as well. Although some patients may require antidiarrheals and/or narcotics, interruptions of treatment are rare.

8.5. PRE- VS POSTOPERATIVE RADIATION THERAPY FOR RECTAL CANCER

The timing of radiation in relation to surgery has been extensively debated. The benefit from postoperative therapy has been demonstrated by the landmark trials of the Gastrointestinal Tumor Study Group (GITSG), National Surgical Adjuvant Breast and Bowel Project (NSABP), and North Central Cancer Treatment Group (NCCTG) (117–119). The principal argument for postoperative therapy is that the patient is accurately staged for the selection of adjuvant therapy. With pre-operative therapy, patients who are thought to be stage II or III but really have stage I disease are over-treated.

Pre-operative radiation has a compelling rationale for a number of clinical and biological reasons. For example, the tissues in the pelvis are better oxygenated before surgery. Tumor cells are significantly more sensitive to an equivalent dose of radiation in the presence of oxygen as opposed to hypoxic conditions (120). Pre-operative therapy may also "sterilize" tumor cells that during surgery could be inadvertently released into the regional tissues or bloodstream. Clinically, the volume of tissue that needs to be irradiated is smaller in the pre-operative setting. The tissue that is irradiated is resected, and thus the anastomosis remains naïve from the effects of radiation. The smaller treatment volume, lower radiation doses, and construction of the anastomosis with untreated bowel, leads to lower rates of acute and chronic toxicity with pre-operative therapy. Finally, pre-operative therapy can improve the resectability of tumors, allowing a sphincter-preserving procedure that would not have otherwise been possible. This response to preoperative therapy has been termed "downstaging" and allows sphincter preservation in almost 25% of patients who otherwise would have needed an abdominoperineal resection *(121–124)*.

Several European studies have used a pre-operative treatment regimen, whereas investigators in the United States have focused on postoperative radiation. The Swedish pre-operative regimen consists of 25 Gy over five fractions without chemotherapy, given 1 wk before surgery. This schedule obviously does not allow for tumor downstaging to occur, but it is the only radiation regimen that demonstrates an improvement in overall survival *(125,126)*. Because of the uniqueness of this schedule, it has been difficult to extrapolate the results to a more standard fractionation schedule that permits the addition of chemotherapy. Two trials attempted to answer the question of whether irradiation (with chemotherapy) was better in the pre- or postoperative setting were undertaken in the United States, including a study by the NSABP and an Intergroup collaborative effort by the RTOG and CALGB. Both trials had abysmal accrual and were closed early without meaningful results *(122)* (RTOG, unpublished).

The issue regarding timing may finally be resolved by the German collaborative study first reported in 2003 *(123)*. The protocol began accrual in 1994 and ultimately included 823 patients with ultrasound-determined UICC stage II or III disease. The patients were stratified by surgeon and randomized to combined modality therapy with radiation and 5-FU based chemotherapy either before or after a TME. At a median follow-up of 40 mo, the two arms were statistically equivalent for overall survival and disease-free survival. Local recurrences were seen half as often in the patients who were treated with the preoperative regimen (12 vs 6%, $p = 0.006$). Twenty percent of the patients who would have otherwise undergone an abdominoperineal resection were able to have a sphincter-preserving procedure.

Toxicity was a secondary endpoint of the German study. There was no evidence that the pre-operative therapy increased peri- or postoperative complications in terms of anastomotic leakage, postoperative bleeding, delayed wound healing, or the development of ileus or fistulas. As expected, the acute toxicities of combined modality therapy were significantly higher in the postoperative therapy arm. The chronic toxicities, usually related to anastomotic problems or changes in gastrointestinal function, were also significantly higher in the postoperative therapy arm, with World Health Organization grade 3 or 4 complications in 22.7 vs 9.6% of patients ($p = 0.04$). Overall, the benefits to pre-operative therapy thus included a 50% decrease in local failures, increased sphincter preservation, and significantly decreased morbidity.

9. ALTERNATIVES TO TRANSABDOMINAL RESECTION

In certain circumstances a patient may be able to undergo a more conservative procedure than a major operative procedure. For patients with small tumors, T1 or T2, the tumors may be resected with a transanal approach or treated with endocavitary radiation. The results of either treatment are comparable and with the addition of external adjuvant radiation to the pelvis in certain situations can result in local control rates of 80–95%. Two prospective, multi-institutional phase II trials have evaluated the results for local excision *(36,127)*. Both trials used adjuvant radiation for T2 tumors. The local control rates for T1 (surgery alone) and T2 tumors in a trial by the RTOG trial were similar, at 96 and 86%, respectively *(127)*. The CALGB reported on 110 patients with T1/ T2 tumors, with a failure-free survival rate of 78% at 6 yr.

As previously discussed, other investigators have reported results of local excision both with and without adjuvant irradiation, in general showing higher rates of failure than either prospective trial *(128,129)*. The differences in outcomes likely reflect the stringent work-up and enrollment criteria of the prospective trials, as both the RTOG and CALGB study required negative margins, with the RTOG additionally requiring that the margins be at least 4 mm, the histology be well or moderately differentiated, and that there be no evidence of lymphovascular invasion.

10. LOCALLY ADVANCED DISEASE/RECURRENT DISEASE

As with the primary presentation, surgery would ideally be the most important aspect of treatment for patients with locally advanced or recurrent rectal cancers. Although chemoradiation does induce a favorable tumor response with a complete pathological response seen in 20–30% of patients *(130–133)*, additional radiation doses do not result in sufficient long-term control without surgery. Because downstaging does occur with pre-operative therapy, the optimistic approach is to perform chemoradiation with the goal of rendering the disease resectable.

The outcomes for recurrent disease depend heavily on the original stage and what prior therapy was administered. For patients who were previously not irradiated, 5-yr survivals of 18–24% are achievable depending on the amount of residual disease after a salvage surgical operation *(134–136)*. With locally recurrent disease in patients who have already had radiation, additional doses of external beam radiation are limited by chronic toxicity. The potential benefit of intraoperative radiation and/or brachytherapy has been explored in this setting. With the former, the small bowel can be manually displaced, and the operative bed is exposed for treatment with electrons that have limited penetration. After intraoperative therapy for recurrent disease, single institution reviews report subsequent local failure rates of 11% *(134,135,137)*.

Brachytherapy involves placing radioactive sources directly over the pelvic wall or other area of concern, enabling treatment of the area without having as high amount of radiation doses to the surrounding bowel and tissues. Results from several institutions indicate that almost 30% of patients may be rendered disease-free with an aggressive approach combining surgery and brachytherapy *(138–140)*. The decision to undertake extensive therapy for recurrent disease needs to be carefully considered in a frank multidisciplinary discussion with the patient. Radical surgery with additional radiation is potentially debilitating and should be performed by centers with extensive experience.

11. COMBINED MODALITY ADJUVANT THERAPY OF RECTAL CANCER

Postoperative combined-modality therapy with chemotherapy and irradiation for patients with stages II or III rectal cancer has been recommended for decades, partly based on the results of randomized clinical trials performed by the GITSG, NSABP, and the NCCTG. The GITSG trial randomized 227 patients following surgical resection for rectal adenocarcinoma to one of four treatments: no adjuvant therapy, postoperative radiotherapy, postoperative chemotherapy (fluorouracil and semustine [methyl-CCNU]), or a combination of radiation therapy and chemotherapy. The recurrence rate was highest among the control patients (55%) and lowest among the patients receiving a combination of adjuvant radiation and chemotherapy (33%). Time to tumor recurrence was significantly prolonged by combined radiation and chemotherapy as compared with resection alone ($p < 0.009$), though overall survival did not differ significantly among the treatment groups *(117)*.

NSABP protocol R-01 randomized 555 postoperative patients to either no further treatment, postoperative chemotherapy with 5-FU, semustine, and vincristine (MOF), or postoperative radiation therapy alone. The chemotherapy group, when compared with the group treated by surgery alone, demonstrated an overall improvement in disease-free survival ($p = 0.006$) and in survival ($p = 0.05$). Postoperative radiation therapy reduced the incidence of locoregional recurrence, but it failed to affect overall disease-free survival and survival *(141)*. The NCCTG then randomized 204 patients following surgical resection of rectal adenocarcinoma to either postoperative radiation alone or to radiation plus fluorouracil, which was both preceded and followed by a cycle of systemic therapy with fluorouracil plus semustine. The combined therapy reduced local recurrence by 34% ($p = 0.0016$) and distant metastasis by 37% ($p = 0.011$). In addition, combined therapy reduced the rate of cancer-related death by 36% ($p = 0.0071$) and the overall death rate by 29% ($p = 0.025$) *(142)*.

NSABP protocol R-02 attempted to address whether the addition of radiotherapy to chemotherapy resulted in improved disease-free survival and overall survival. At total of 694 patients with stages II and III rectal adenocarcinoma were randomized to receive either postoperative adjuvant chemotherapy alone or chemotherapy with postoperative radiotherapy. Postoperative radiotherapy resulted in no beneficial effect on disease-free survival or overall survival, although it reduced the cumulative incidence of locoregional relapse from a relatively low 13% to an even lower 8% at 5-yr follow up *(118)*. Based on these results, it may be reasonable to treat patients felt to be at very low risk of locoregional relapse with chemotherapy alone.

Subsequent studies have established the superiority for infusional 5-FU over bolus, at least when administered during the irradiation *(143)*. Daily capecitabine has been combined with pre-operative irradiation, with preliminary results demonstrating it to be comparable with 5-FU. Randomized phase III trials are needed to confirm equivalency.

Planned cooperative group trials investigating adjuvant therapy for rectal cancer will focus on evaluating chemotherapeutics recently approved for use in metastatic large bowel malignancies. Specifically, an intergroup study coordinated by ECOG will examine whether the addition of either oxaliplatin or irinotecan to 5-FU/leucovorin (using FOLFOX or FOLFIRI) will decrease the rate of distant metastasis and improve long-term survival. Bevacizumab might also be combined with chemoradiotherapy in the pre-operative setting in an NSABP trial.

12. CONCLUSIONS

There have been recent and dramatic improvements in surgical and radiotherapeutic treatment of large-bowel malignancies. Similarly, the pace of drug development after many years of relative inactivity has been extraordinary. Median overall survivals reported in phase III trials of metastatic disease have almost quadrupled and are poised to break the 2-yr barrier. Hopefully, even small gains made in advanced disease will translate into large improvements in cure rates when similar regimens are combined with surgery and used in the adjuvant setting.

REFERENCES

1. Society AC. Estimated New Cancer Cases and Deaths by Sex for All Sites, US, 2004; Atlanta; 2004.
2. Williams NS, Dixon MF, Johnston D. Reappraisal of the 5 centimeter rule of distal excision for carcinoma of the rectum: a study of distal intramural spread and of patients' survival. Br J Surg 1983; 70(3):150–154.
3. Quirke P, Durdey P, Dixon MF, Williams NS. Local recurrence of rectal adenocarcinoma due to inadequate surgical resection. Histopathological study of lateral tumour spread and surgical excision. Lancet 1986; 2(8514):996–999.
4. Wong JH, Severino R, Honnebier MB, Tom P, Namiki TS. Number of nodes examined and staging accuracy in colorectal carcinoma. J Clin Oncol 1999; 17(9):2896–2900.
5. Tepper JE, O'Connell MJ, Niedzwiecki D, et al. Impact of number of nodes retrieved on outcome in patients with rectal cancer. J Clin Oncol 2001; 19(1):157–163.
6. Enker WE, Laffer UT, Block GE. Enhanced survival of patients with colon and rectal cancer is based upon wide anatomic resection. Ann Surg 1979; 190(3):350–360.
7. Grinnell RS. Results of Ligation of Inferior Mesenteric Artery at the Aorta in Resections of Carcinoma of the Descending and Sigmoid Colon and Rectum. Surg Gynecol Obstet 1965; 120:1031–1036.
8. Schlinkert RT. Laparoscopic-assisted right hemicolectomy. Dis Colon Rectum 1991; 34(11):1030,1031.
9. Wexner SD, Johansen OB. Laparoscopic bowel resection: advantages and limitations. Ann Med 1992; 24(2):105–110.
10. Milsom JW, Lavery IC, Church JM, Stolfi VM, Fazio VW. Use of laparoscopic techniques in colorectal surgery. Preliminary study. Dis Colon Rectum 1994; 37(3):215–218.
11. Wexner SD, Cohen SM. Port site metastases after laparoscopic colorectal surgery for cure of malignancy. Br J Surg 1995; 82(3):295–298.
12. Ramos JM, Gupta S, Anthone GJ, Ortega AE, Simons AJ, Beart RW, Jr. Laparoscopy and colon cancer. Is the port site at risk? A preliminary report. Arch Surg 1994; 129(9):897–899; discussion 900.
13. A comparison of laparoscopically assisted and open colectomy for colon cancer. N Engl J Med 2004; 350(20):2050–2059.
14. Miles W. A method of performing abdominoperineal resection for carcinoma of the rectum and of the terminal portion of the pelvic colon. Lancet 1908; 2:1812,1813.
15. Enker WE. New directions in rectal surgery: Conservative surgery for rectal cancer. Semin Surg Oncol 2000; 19(4):319–320.
16. Hodgson DC, Zhang W, Zaslavsky AM, Fuchs CS, Wright WE, Ayanian JZ. Relation of hospital volume to colostomy rates and survival for patients with rectal cancer. J Natl Cancer Inst 2003; 95(10):708–716.

17. Holm T, Johansson H, Cedermark B, Ekelund G, Rutqvist LE. Influence of hospital and surgeon related factors on outcome after treatment of rectal cancer with or without preoperative radiotherapy. Br J Surg 1997; 84(5):657–663.

18. Schrag D, Panageas KS, Riedel E, et al. Hospital and surgeon procedure volume as predictors of outcome following rectal cancer resection. Ann Surg 2002; 236(5):583–592.

19. Porter GA, Soskolne CL, Yakimets WW, Newman SC. Surgeon-related factors and outcome in rectal cancer. Ann Surg 1998; 227(2):157–167.

20. Beart RW, Jr., Kelly KA. Randomized prospective evaluation of the EEA stapler for colorectal anastomoses. Am J Surg 1981; 141(1):143–147.

21. Wiersema MJ, Harewood GC. Endoscopic ultrasound for rectal cancer. Gastroenterol Clin North Am 2002; 31(4):1093–1105.

22. Harewood GC, Wiersema MJ, Nelson H, et al. A prospective, blinded assessment of the impact of preoperative staging on the management of rectal cancer. Gastroenterology 2002; 123(1):24–32.

23. Parks AG, Percy JP. Resection and sutured colo-anal anastomosis for rectal carcinoma. Br J Surg 1982; 69(6):301–304.

24. Minsky BD, Cohen AM, Enker WE, Paty P. Sphincter preservation with preoperative radiation therapy and coloanal anastomosis. Int J Radiat Oncol Biol Phys 1995; 31(3):553–559.

25. Marks GJ, Marks JH, Mohiuddin M, Brady L. Radical Sphincter preservation surgery with coloanal anastomosis following high-dose external irradiation for the very low lying rectal cancer. Recent Results Cancer Res 1998; 146:161–174.

26. Hallbook O, Pahlman L, Krog M, Wexner SD, Sjodahl R. Randomized comparison of straight and colonic J pouch anastomosis after low anterior resection. Ann Surg 1996; 224(1):58–65.

27. Minsky BD. Multidisciplinary case teams: an approach to the future management of advanced colorectal cancer. Br J Cancer 1998; 77(Suppl 2):1–4.

28. Moore HG, Riedel E, Minsky BD, et al. Adequacy of 1-cm distal margin after restorative rectal cancer resection with sharp mesorectal excision and preoperative combined-modality therapy. Ann Surg Oncol 2003; 10(1):80–85.

29. Vernava AM, 3rd, Moran M, Rothenberger DA, Wong WD. A prospective evaluation of distal margins in carcinoma of the rectum. Surg Gynecol Obstet 1992; 175(4):333–336.

30. Guillem JG, Cohen AM. Current issues in colorectal cancer surgery. Semin Oncol 1999; 26(5):505–513.

31. Nissan A, Guillem JG, Paty PB, et al. Abdominoperineal resection for rectal cancer at a specialty center. Dis Colon Rectum 2001; 44(1):27–35; discussion 6.

32. Blumberg D, Paty PB, Picon AI, et al. Stage I rectal cancer: identification of high-risk patients. J Am Coll Surg 1998; 186(5):574–579; discussion 9–80.

33. Rothenberger DA, Wong WD. Abdominoperineal resection for adenocarcinoma of the low rectum. World J Surg 1992; 16(3):478–485.

34. Paty PB, Enker WE, Cohen AM, Minsky BD, Friedlander-Klar H. Long-term functional results of coloanal anastomosis for rectal cancer. Am J Surg 1994; 167(1):90–94; discussion 4,5.

35. Bleday R. Local excision of rectal cancer. World J Surg 1997; 21(7):706–714.

36. Steele GD, Jr., Herndon JE, Bleday R, et al. Sphincter-sparing treatment for distal rectal adenocarcinoma. Ann Surg Oncol 1999; 6(5):433–441.

37. Paty PB, Nash GM, Baron P, et al. Long-term results of local excision for rectal cancer. Ann Surg 2002; 236(4):522–529; discussion 9–30.

38. Garcia-Aguilar J, Mellgren A, Sirivongs P, Buie D, Madoff RD, Rothenberger DA. Local excision of rectal cancer without adjuvant therapy: a word of caution. Ann Surg 2000; 231(3):345–351.

39. Bleday R, Steele G, Jr. Current protocols and outcomes of local therapy for rectal cancer. Surg Oncol Clin N Am 2000; 9(4):751–758; discussion 9–61.

40. Heald RJ, Husband EM, Ryall RD. The mesorectum in rectal cancer surgery—the clue to pelvic recurrence? Br J Surg 1982; 69(10): 613–616.

41. Enker WE, Thaler HT, Cranor ML, Polyak T. Total mesorectal excision in the operative treatment of carcinoma of the rectum. J Am Coll Surg 1995; 181(4):335–346.

42. Enker WE. Potency, cure, and local control in the operative treatment of rectal cancer. Arch Surg 1992; 127(12).1396–1401, discussion 402.

43. MacFarlane JK, Ryall RD, Heald RJ. Mesorectal excision for rectal cancer. Lancet 1993; 341(8843):457–460.

44. Heald RJ, Moran BJ, Ryall RD, Sexton R, MacFarlane JK. Rectal cancer: the Basingstoke experience of total mesorectal excision, 1978–1997. Arch Surg 1998; 133(8):894–899.

45. NIH consensus conference. Adjuvant therapy for patients with colon and rectal cancer. JAMA 1990; 264(11):1444–1450.

46. Merchant NB, Guillem JG, Paty PB, et al. T3N0 rectal cancer: results following sharp mesorectal excision and no adjuvant therapy. J Gastrointest Surg 1999; 3(6):642–647.

47. Enker WE, Merchant N, Cohen AM, et al. Safety and efficacy of low anterior resection for rectal cancer: 681 consecutive cases from a specialty service. Ann Surg 1999; 230(4):544–552; discussion 52–54.

48. Kapiteijn E, Marijnen CA, Nagtegaal ID, et al. Preoperative radiotherapy combined with total mesorectal excision for resectable rectal cancer. N Engl J Med 2001; 345(9):638–646.

49. Heidelberger C, Chanakari NK, Danenberg PV. Fluorinated pyrimidines: A new class of tumor inhibitor compounds. Nature 1957; 179:663–666.

50. Sobrero A, Aschele C, Bertino J. Fluorouracil in colorectal cancer—a tale of two drugs: implications for biochemical modulation. J Clin Oncol 1997; 15:368–381.

51. Anonymous. Efficacy of intravenous continuous infusion of fluorouracil compared with bolus administration in advanced colorectal cancer. Meta-analysis Group in Cancer. J Clin Oncol 1998; 16(1):301–308.

52. Mini E, Trave F, Rustum YM, Bertino JR. Enhancement of the antitumor effects of 5-fluorouracil by folinic acid. Pharmacol Therapeut 1990; 47(1):1–19.

53. Piedbois P, Michiels S. Survival benefit of 5FU/LV over 5FU bolus in patients with advanced colorectal cancer: An updated meta-analysis based on 2751 patients. Am Soc Clin Oncol 2003; 22:294.

54. Saliba F, Hagipantelli R, Misset JL, et al. Pathophysiology and therapy of irinotecan-induced delayed-onset diarrhea in patients with advanced colorectal cancer: a prospective assessment. J Clin Oncol 1998; 16(8):2745–2751.

55. Gandia D, Abigerges D, Armand JP, et al. CPT-11-induced cholinergic effects in cancer patients. J Clin Oncol 1993; 11(1):196,197.

56. Rothenberg M, Eckardt J, Kuhn J, et al. Phase II trial of irinotecan in patients with progressive or rapidly recurrent colorectal cancer. J Clin Oncol 1996; 14(4):1128–1135.

57. Rothenberg ML, Kuhn JG, Burris HA, 3rd, et al. Phase I and pharmacokinetic trial of weekly CPT-11. J Clin Oncol 1993; 11(11): 2194–2204.

58. Conti JA, Kemeny NE, Saltz LB, et al. Irinotecan is an active agent in untreated patients with metastatic colorectal cancer. J Clin Oncol 1996; 14(3):709–715.

59. Rougier P, Bugat R, Douillard JY, et al. Phase II study of irinotecan in the treatment of advanced colorectal cancer in chemotherapy-naive patients and patients pretreated with fluorouracil-based chemotherapy. J Clin Oncol 1997; 15(1):251–260.

60. Rougier P, Van Cutsem E, Bajetta E, et al. Randomised trial of irinotecan versus fluorouracil by continuous infusion after fluorouracil failure in patients with metastatic colorectal cancer. (see comment) (erratum appears in Lancet 1998 Nov 14; 352(9140):1634). Lancet 1998; 352(9138):1407–1412.

61. Cunningham D, Pyrhonen S, James RD, et al. Randomised trial of irinotecan plus supportive care versus supportive care alone after fluorouracil failure for patients with metastatic colorectal cancer. (see comment). Lancet 1998; 352(9138):1413–1418.

62. Saltz LB, Cox JV, Blanke C, et al. Irinotecan plus fluorouracil and leucovorin for metastatic colorectal cancer. Irinotecan Study Group. (see comment). N Engl J Med 2000; 343(13):905–914.

63. Douillard JY, Cunningham D, Roth AD, et al. Irinotecan combined with fluorouracil compared with fluorouracil alone as first-line treatment for metastatic colorectal cancer: a multicentre randomised trial [erratum appears in Lancet 2000 Apr 15; 355(9212):1372]. Lancet 2000; 355(9209):1041–1047.

64. Woynarowski JM, Chapman WG, Napier C, Herzig MC, Juniewicz P. Sequence-and region-specificity of oxaliplatin adducts in naked and cellular DNA. Molecular Pharmacology 1998; 54(5):770–777.

65. Rixe O, Ortuzar W, Alvarez M, et al. Oxaliplatin, tetraplatin, cisplatin, and carboplatin: spectrum of activity in drug-resistant cell lines and in the cell lines of the National Cancer Institute's Anticancer Drug Screen panel. Biochemical Pharmacology 1996; 52(12):1855–1865.

66. Wilson RH, Lehky T, Thomas RR, Quinn MG, Floeter MK, Grem JL. Acute oxaliplatin-induced peripheral nerve hyperexcitability. J Clin Oncol 2002; 20(7):1767–1774.

67. Machover D, Diaz-Rubio E, de Gramont A, et al. Two consecutive phase II studies of oxaliplatin (L-OHP) for treatment of patients with advanced colorectal carcinoma who were resistant to previous treatment with fluoropyrimidines. Ann Oncol 1996; 7(1):95–98.

68. Levi F, Perpoint B, Garufi C, et al. Oxaliplatin activity against metastatic colorectal cancer. A phase II study of 5-day continuous venous infusion at circadian rhythm modulated rate. Eur J Cancer 1993; 29A(9):1280–1284.

69. Becouarn Y, Ychou M, Ducreux M, et al. Phase II trial of oxaliplatin as first-line chemotherapy in metastatic colorectal cancer patients. Digestive Group of French Federation of Cancer Centers. J Clin Oncol 1998; 16(8):2739–2744.

70. Diaz-Rubio E, Sastre J, Zaniboni A, et al. Oxaliplatin as single agent in previously untreated colorectal carcinoma patients: a phase II multicentric study. Ann of Oncology 1998; 9(1):105–108.

71. de Gramont A, Vignoud J, Tournigand C, et al. Oxaliplatin with high-dose leucovorin and 5-fluorouracil 48-hour continuous infusion in pretreated metastatic colorectal cancer. Eur J Cancer 1997; 33(2):214–219.

72. Andre T, Louvet C, Raymond E, Tournigand C, de Gramont A. Bimonthly high-dose leucovorin, 5-fluorouracil infusion and oxaliplatin (FOLFOX3) for metastatic colorectal cancer resistant to the same leucovorin and 5-fluorouracil regimen. Annals of Oncology 1998; 9(11):1251–1253.

73. deBraud F, Munzone E, Nole F, et al. Synergistic activity of oxaliplatin and 5-fluorouracil in patients with metastatic colorectal cancer with progressive disease while on or after 5-fluorouracil. Am J Clin Oncol 1998; 21(3):279–283.

74. Gerard B, Bleiberg H, Van Daele D, et al. Oxaliplatin combined to 5-fluorouracil and folinic acid: an effective therapy in patients with advanced colorectal cancer. Anti-Cancer Drugs 1998; 9(4):301–305.

75. Brienza S, Bensmaine MA, Soulie P, et al. Oxaliplatin added to 5-fluorouracil-based therapy (5-FU +/– FA) in the treatment of 5-FU-pretreated patients with advanced colorectal carcinoma (ACRC): results from the European compassionate-use program. Ann Oncol 1999; 10(11):1311–1316.

76. Andre T, Bensmaine MA, Louvet C, et al. Multicenter phase II study of bimonthly high-dose leucovorin, fluorouracil infusion, and oxaliplatin for metastatic colorectal cancer resistant to the same leucovorin and fluorouracil regimen. J Clin Oncol 1999; 17(11): 3560–3568.

77. de Gramont A, Figer A, Seymour M, et al. Leucovorin and fluorouracil with or without oxaliplatin as first-line treatment in advanced colorectal cancer. J Clin Oncol 2000; 18(16):2938–2547.

78. Miwa M, Ura M, Nishida M, et al. Design of a novel oral fluoropyrimidine carbamate, capecitabine, which generates 5-fluorouracil selectively in tumours by enzymes concentrated in human liver and cancer tissue. Eur J Cancer 1998; 34(8):1274–1281.

79. Schuller J, Cassidy J, Dumont E, et al. Preferential activation of capecitabine in tumor following oral administration to colorectal cancer patients. Cancer Chemother Pharmacol 2000; 45(4):291–297.

80. Van Cutsem E, Findlay M, Osterwalder B, et al. Capecitabine, an oral fluoropyrimidine carbamate with substantial activity in advanced colorectal cancer: results of a randomized phase II study. J Clin Oncol 2000; 18(6):1337–1345.

81. Hoff PM, Ansari R, Batist G, et al. Comparison of oral capecitabine versus intravenous fluorouracil plus leucovorin as first-line treatment in 605 patients with metastatic colorectal cancer: results of a randomized phase III study. J Clin Oncol 2001; 19(8):2282–2292.

82. Goldberg RM, Sargent DJ, Morton RF, et al. A randomized controlled trial of fluorouracil plus leucovorin, irinotecan, and oxaliplatin combinations in patients with previously untreated metastatic colorectal cancer. (see comment). J Clin Oncol 2004; 22(1):23–30.

83. Goldberg RM, Morton RF, Sargent DJ, et al. N9741: oxaliplatin (Oxal) or CPT-11 + 5-fluorouracil (5FU)/leucovorin (LV) or oxal + CPT-11 in advanced colorectal cancer (CRC). Updated efficacy and quality of life (QOL) data from an intergroup study. Am Soc Clin Oncol 2003; 252 (Abstract 1009).

84. Tournigand C, Andre T, Achille E, et al. FOLFIRI followed by FOLFOX6 or the reverse sequence in advanced colorectal cancer: a randomized GERCOR study. J Clin Oncol 2004; 22(2):229–237.

85. Souglakos J, Mavroudis D, Kakolyris S, et al. Triplet combination with irinotecan plus oxaliplatin plus continuous-infusion fluorouracil and leucovorin as first-line treatment in metastatic colorectal cancer: a multicenter phase II trial. J Clin Oncol 2002; 20(11):2651–2657.

86. Baselga J. The EGFR as a target for anticancer therapy—focus on cetuximab. Eur J Cancer 2001; 37(Suppl 4):S16–S22.

87. Saltz L, Kies M, Abbruzzese JL, Azarnia N, Needle M. The presence and intensity of the cetuximab-induced acne-like rash predicts increased survival in studies across multiple malignancies. Am Soc Clin Oncol 2003; p. 204 (abstr 817).

88. Gustafson NF, Saltz L, Cunningham D, Lenz H, Humphrey R, Adegbile IA. Safety profile of cetuximab in patients with metastatic colorectal cancer. In: ASCO Gastrointestinal Cancers Symposium; 2004; p. (abstr 237).

89. Saltz LB, Meropol NJ, Loehrer PJ, Sr., Needle MN, Kopit J, Mayer RJ. Phase II trial of cetuximab in patients with refractory colorectal cancer that expresses the epidermal growth factor receptor. [see comment]. J Clin Oncol 2004; 22(7):1201–1208.

90. Cunningham D, Humblet Y, Siena S, et al. Cetuximab Monotherapy and Cetuximab plus Irinotecan in Irinotecan-Refractory Metastatic Colorectal Cancer. N Engl J Med 2004; 351(4):337–345.

91. Tabernero JM, Van Cutsem E, Sastre J, et al. An international phase II study of cetuximab in combination with oxaliplatin/5-fluorouracil (5-FU)/folinic acid (FA) (FOLFOX-4) in the first-line treatment of patients with metastatic colorectal cancer (CRC) expressing Epidermal Growth Factor Receptor (EGFR). Preliminary results. Am Soc Clin Oncol 2004; p. (abstr. 3512).

92. Willett CG, Boucher Y, di Tomaso E, et al. Direct evidence that the VEGF-specific antibody bevacizumab has antivascular effects in human rectal cancer. [see comment][erratum appears in Nat Med 2004; 10(6):649]. Nature Medicine 2004; 10(2):145–147.

93. Jain RK. Normalizing tumor vasculature with anti-angiogenic therapy: a new paradigm for combination therapy. Nat Med 2001; 7(9):987–989.

94. Kabbinavar F, Hurwitz HI, Fehrenbacher L, et al. Phase II, randomized trial comparing bevacizumab plus fluorouracil (FU)/leucovorin (LV) with FU/LV alone in patients with metastatic colorectal cancer.[see comment]. J Clin Oncol 2003; 21(1):60–65.

95. Hurwitz H, Fehrenbacher L, Novotny W, et al. Bevacizumab plus irinotecan, fluorouracil, and leucovorin for metastatic colorectal cancer.[see comment]. N Engl J Med 2004; 350(23):2335–2342.

96. Gunderson LL, Sargent D, Tepper J, et al. Impact of TN stage and treatment on survival and relapse in adjuvant rectal cancer pooled analysis. Am Soc Clin Oncol; 2003; p. Abst 1008.

97. Mamounas E, Wieand S, Wolmark N, et al. Comparative efficacy of adjuvant chemotherapy in patients with Dukes' B versus Dukes' C colon cancer: results from four National Surgical Adjuvant Breast and Bowel Project adjuvant studies (C-01, C-02, C-03, and C-04)[see comment]. J Clin Oncol 1999; 17(5):1349–1355.

98. Buyse M, Piedbois P. Should Dukes' B patients receive adjuvant therapy? A statistical perspective. Seminars in Oncology 2001; 28(1 Suppl 1):20–24.

99. Gray RG, Barnwell J, Hills R, McConkey C, Williams N, Kerr D. QUASAR: A randomized study of adjuvant chemotherapy (CT) vs. observation including 3238 colorectal cancer patients. Am Soc Clin Oncol; 2004; p. Abst 3501.

100. Macdonald JS. Adjuvant therapy of colon cancer.[see comment]. Ca: a Cancer Journal for Clinicians 1999; 49(4):202–219.

101. Gill S, Loprinzi CL, Sargent DJ, et al. Pooled analysis of fluoro-uracil-based adjuvant therapy for stage II and III colon cancer: who benefits and by how much? [see comment]. J Clin Oncol 2004; 22(10):1797–1806.

102. Haller DG, Catalano PJ, Macdonald JS, Mayer RJ. Fluorouracil (FU), leucovorin (LV) and levamisole (LEV) adjuvant therapy for colon cancer: five-year final report of INT-0089 (Meeting abstract). Am Soc Clin Oncol; 1998; p. Abst 982.

103. Saltz LB, Niedzwiecki D, Hollis D, et al. Irinotecan plus fluoro-uracil/leucovorin (IFL) versus fluorouracil/leucovorin alone (FL) in stage III colon cancer (intergroup trial CALGB C89803). Am Soc Clin Oncol 2004; 2004. p. Abst 3500.

104. Willett CG, Fung CY, Kaufman DS, Efird J, Shellito PC. Postoperative radiation therapy for high-risk colon carcinoma. J Clin Oncol 1993; 11(6):1112–1117.

105. Schild SE, Gunderson LL, Haddock MG, Wong WW, Nelson H. The treatment of locally advanced colon cancer. Int J Radiat Oncol Biol Phys 1997; 37(1):51–58.

106. Amos EH, Mendenhall WM, McCarty PJ, et al. Postoperative radiotherapy for locally advanced colon cancer.[see comment]. Ann Surg Oncol 1996; 3(5):431–436.

107. Martenson JA, Shanahan TG, O'Connell MJ, et al. Phase I study of 5-fluorouracil administered by protracted venous infusion, leucov-orin, and pelvic radiation therapy. Cancer 1999; 86(4):710–714.

108. Martenson JA, Jr, Willett CG, Sargent DJ, et al. Phase III Study of adjuvant chemotherapy and radiation therapy compared with chemotherapy alone in the surgical adjuvant treatment of colon can-cer: results of intergroup protocol 0130. J Clin Oncol 2004; 22(16):3277–3283.

109. Rich T, Gunderson LL, Lew R, Galdibini JJ, Cohen AM, Donaldson G. Patterns of recurrence of rectal cancer after poten-tially curative surgery. Cancer 1983; 52(7):1317–1329.

110. Mendenhall WM, Million RR, Pfaff WW. Patterns of recurrence in adenocarcinoma of the rectum and rectosigmoid treated with sur-gery alone: implications in treatment planning with adjuvant radia-tion therapy. Int J Radiat Oncol Biol Phys 1983; 9(7):977–985.

111. Pilipshen SJ, Heilweil M, Quan SH, Sternberg SS, Enker WE. Patterns of pelvic recurrence following definitive resections of rec-tal cancer. Cancer 1984; 53(6):1354–1362.

112. Walz BJ, Green MR, Lindstrom ER, Butcher HR, Jr. Anatomical prognostic factors after abdominal perineal resection. Int J Radiat Oncol Biol Phys 1981; 7(4):477–484.

113. Randomized study on preoperative radiotherapy in rectal carci-noma. Stockholm Colorectal Cancer Study Group.[see comment]. Ann Surg Oncol 1996; 3(5):423–430.

114. Local recurrence rate in a randomised multicentre trial of preoperative radiotherapy compared with operation alone in resectable rectal carci-noma. Swedish Rectal Cancer Trial. Eur J Surg 1996; 162(5):397–402.

115. Gilbert SG. Symptomatic local tumor failure following abdomino-per-ineal resection. Int J Radiat Oncol Biol Phys 1978; 4(9,10): 801–807.

116. Gunderson LL, Sosin H. Areas of failure found at reoperation (sec-ond or symptomatic look) following "curative surgery" for adeno-carcinoma of the rectum. Clinicopathologic correlation and implications for adjuvant therapy. Cancer 1974; 34(4): 1278–1292.

117. Prolongation of the disease-free interval in surgically treated rectal carcinoma. Gastrointestinal Tumor Study Group. N Engl J Med 1985; 312(23):1465–1472.

118. Wolmark N, Wieand HS, Hyams DM, et al. Randomized trial of postoperative adjuvant chemotherapy with or without radiotherapy for carcinoma of the rectum: National Surgical Adjuvant Breast and Bowel Project Protocol R-02.[see comment]. J Nat Cancer Inst 2000; 92(5):388–396.

119. Krook JE, Moertel CG, Gunderson LL, et al. Effective surgical adjuvant therapy for high-risk rectal carcinoma. N Engl J Med 1991; 324(11):709–715.

120. Hall EJ. Radiobiology for the radiologist. 5th ed. Philadelphia: Lippincott Williams & Wilkins; 2000.

121. Janjan NA, Khoo VS, Abbruzzese J, et al. Tumor downstaging and sphincter preservation with preoperative chemoradiation in locally advanced rectal cancer: the M. D. Anderson Cancer Center experi-ence. Int J Radiat Oncol Biol Phys 1999; 44(5):1027–1038.

122. Hyams DM, Mamounas EP, Petrelli N, et al. A clinical trial to eval-uate the worth of preoperative multimodality therapy in patients with operable carcinoma of the rectum: a progress report of National Surgical Breast and Bowel Project Protocol R-03. Diseases of the Colon & Rectum 1997; 40(2):131–139.

123. Sauer R, Fietkau R, Wittekind C, et al. Adjuvant vs. neoadjuvant radiochemotherapy for locally advanced rectal cancer: the German trial CAO/ARO/AIO-94. Colorectal Disease 2003; 5(5):406–415.

124. Sauer R. Adjuvant versus neoadjuvant combined modality treat-ment for locally advanced rectal cancer: first results of the German rectal cancer study (CAO/ARO/AIO-94). Int J Radiat Oncol Biol Phys 2003; 57(2):S124–S125.

125. Frykholm GJ, Glimelius B, Pahlman L. Preoperative or postop-erative irradiation in adenocarcinoma of the rectum: final treat-ment results of a randomized trial and an evaluation of late secondary effects. Diseases of the Colon & Rectum 1993; 36(6): 564–572.

126. Anonymous. Improved survival with preoperative radiotherapy in resectable rectal cancer. Swedish Rectal Cancer Trial.[see com-ment][erratum appears in N Engl J Med 1997 May 22; 336(21): 1539]. N Engl J Med 1997; 336(14):980–987.

127. Russell AH, Harris J, Rosenberg PJ, et al. Anal sphincter conserva-tion for patients with adenocarcinoma of the distal rectum: long-term results of radiation therapy oncology group protocol 89-02.[see comment]. Int J Radiat Oncol Biol Phys 2000; 46(2): 313–322.

128. Garcia-Aguilar J, Mellgren A, Sirivongs P, Buie D, Madoff RD, Rothenberger DA. Local excision of rectal cancer without adjuvant therapy: a word of caution. Ann Surg 2000; 231(3):345–351.

129. Chakravarti A, Compton CC, Shellito PC, et al. Long-term follow-up of patients with rectal cancer managed by local excision with and without adjuvant irradiation.[see comment]. Ann Surg 1999; 230(1): 49–54.

130. Minsky BD, Coia L, Haller DG, et al. Radiation therapy for rec-tosigmoid and rectal cancer: results of the 1992–1994 Patterns of Care process survey. J Clin Oncol 1998; 16(7):2542–2547.

131. Videtic GM, Fisher BJ, Perera FE, et al. Preoperative radiation with concurrent 5-fluorouracil continuous infusion for locally advanced unresectable rectal cancer. Int J Radiat Oncol Biol Phys 1998; 42(2):319–324.

132. Minsky BD, Cohen AM, Kemeny N, et al. The efficacy of preoper-ative 5-fluorouracil, high-dose leucovorin, and sequential radiation therapy for unresectable rectal cancer. Cancer 1993; 71(11): 3486–3492.

133. Minsky BD, Cohen AM, Kemeny N, et al. Pre-operative combined 5-FU, low dose leucovorin, and sequential radiation therapy for unresectable rectal cancer. Int J Radiat Oncol Biol Phys 1993; 25(5):821–827.

134. Gunderson LL, Nelson H, Martenson JA, et al. Intraoperative elec-tron and external beam irradiation with or without 5-fluorouracil and maximum surgical resection for previously unirradiated, locally recurrent colorectal cancer. Diseases of the Colon & Rectum 1996; 39(12):1379–1395.

135. Gunderson LL, Nelson H, Martenson JA, et al. Locally advanced primary colorectal cancer: intraoperative electron and external beam irradiation +/- 5-FU. Int J Radiat Oncol Biol Phys 1997; 37(3): 601–614.

136. Gunderson LL, Haddock MG, Nelson H, et al. Locally recurrent col-orectal cancer: IOERT and EBRT +/-5-FU and maximal resection. Frontiers of Radiation Therapy & Oncology 1997; 31:224–228.

137. Sanfilippo NJ, Crane CH, Skibber J, et al. T4 rectal cancer treated with preoperative chemoradiation to the posterior pelvis followed by multivisceral resection: patterns of failure and limi-tations of treatment. Int J Radiat Oncol Biol Phys 2001; 51(1): 176–183.

138. Kuehne J, Kleisli T, Biernacki P, et al. Use of high-dose-rate brachytherapy in the management of locally recurrent rectal can-cer. Diseases of the Colon & Rectum 2003; 46(7):895–899.

139. Alektiar KM, Zelefsky MJ, Paty PB, et al. High-dose-rate intraoperative brachytherapy for recurrent colorectal cancer. Int J Radiat Oncol Biol Phys 2000; 48(1):219–226.

140. Temple WJ, Saettler EB. Locally recurrent rectal cancer: role of composite resection of extensive pelvic tumors with strategies for minimizing risk of recurrence. J Surg Oncol 2000; 73(1): 47–58.

141. Fisher B, Wolmark N, Rockette H, et al. Postoperative adjuvant chemotherapy or radiation therapy for rectal cancer: results from NSABP protocol R-01. J Nat Cancer Inst 1988; 80(1): 21–29.

142. Krook JE, Moertel CG, Gunderson LL, et al. Effective surgical adjuvant therapy for high-risk rectal carcinoma.[see comment]. N Engl J Med 1991; 324(11): 709–715.

143. O'Connell MJ, Martenson JA, Wieand HS, et al. Improving adjuvant therapy for rectal cancer by combining protracted-infusion fluorouracil with radiation therapy after curative surgery. N Engl J Med 1994; 331(8):502–507.

144. Scheithauer W, Rosen H, Kornek GV, Sebesta C, Depisch D. Randomised comparison of combination chemotherapy plus supportive care with supportive care alone in patients with metastatic colorectal cancer. BMJ 1993; 306(6880):752–755.

PANCREAS, BILE DUCTS, AND MEDIASTINUM

IV

24 Cystic Neoplasms of the Pancreas

William R. Brugge, MD

Contents

1. INTRODUCTION

Cystic neoplasms of the pancreas are an important entity for gastroenterologists and endoscopists because these lesions represent the best example of an early malignancy of the pancreas. In the past, cystic neoplasms of the pancreas were thought to be relatively rare, composing less than 10% of cancers of the pancreas. With the increasing use of cross-sectional imaging, an increasing number of these neoplasms are being seen. Cystic lesions of the pancreas are made up of a broad range of neoplastic cysts and inflammatory pseudocysts. The neoplastic cysts manifest a wide range of malignancy, from overtly malignant to premalignant lesions, and benign cystadenomas. Cystic neoplasms of the pancreas can be divided into two major categories, mucinous and nonmucinous lesions (Table 1) *(1)*. There are three types of mucinous lesions, benign mucinous cystadenomas, malignant mucinous cystic lesions, and intraductal papillary mucinous neoplasms (IPMNs). The nonmucinous lesions include microcystic serous cystadenomas and the cystic endocrine tumors.

2. EPIDEMIOLOGY

2.1. PREVALENCE

The prevalence of pancreatic cysts has been examined with autopsy studies performed in Japan. The prevalence of pancreatic cysts found at autopsies in Japan was about 73 of 300 autopsies (24.3%) cases *(2)*. The findings of cystic lesions at autopsy were related to the age of the subjects. The cysts were located throughout the pancreatic parenchyma and were not related to chronic pancreatitis. The epithelium of the cysts displayed a range of early malignancy, including atypical hyperplasia (16.4%) and carcinoma *in situ* (3.4%). The malignant epithelium was more commonly found in small cystic lesions,

rather than in larger lesions. In additional studies, a majority of the early malignancies of the pancreas arose from intraductal papillary mucinous tumors *(3,4)*.

The prevalence of pancreatic cysts in the United States has been estimated in patients undergoing magnetic resonance imaging (MRI) for a number of various medical problems *(5)*. This study revealed about 15–20% of 1444 patients had at least 1 pancreatic cyst. The type of cysts could not be determined in this study.

2.2. CLINICAL EPIDEMIOLOGY

Mucinous cystic neoplasms (MCNs) account for about 2–5% of all exocrine pancreatic tumors and are more common type of cystadenoma. Women are affected far more commonly than men (9:1 ratio), with a mean age at diagnosis in the fifth decade. IPMNs shares many of the features of MCNs. Their true incidence is uncertain, but estimates range from 1 to 8% of all pancreatic tumors. IPMNs affect men and women equally or men predominantly, depending on the reported series, and they tend to occur in an older age group than MCNs. Serous cystadenomas have been estimated to account for about 25% of all cystic neoplasms of the pancreas *(6)*. Serous cystadenomas were not established as an independent clinical or pathological cystadenoma until 1978 when the unique nonmucinous epithelial features that distinguish them from mucinous cystic tumors were accepted. Estimates of the incidence and prevalence vary. Using surgical pathology studies, it has been estimated that serous cystadenomas account for about 1 to 2% of all exocrine pancreatic neoplasms. Serous cystadenomas occur only in adults with a median age in the sixth or seventh decade. The vast majority of patients with serous cystadenomas are female *(7)*. Traditionally about half of the tumors are discovered as incidental findings during abdominal imaging or surgery or at autopsy.

2.3. RISK FACTORS FOR CYSTIC LESIONS

In the vast majority of patients with a cystic lesion, no risk factor is apparent. Von Hippel Lindau (VHL) syndrome is the

From: *Endoscopic Oncology: Gastrointestinal Endoscopy and Cancer Management*. Edited by: D. O. Faigel and M. L. Kochman © Humana Press, Totowa, NJ

Table 1
Key Characteristics of Common Pancreatic Cystic Lesions

Tumor type	Gender	Age	Location	Morphology	Type of epithelium
Mucinous cystadenoma	Female	Middle-aged	Tail	Unilocular	Mucinous
Mucinous cystic neoplasm	Female	Middle-aged	Tail	Associated mass	Malignant mucinous
Intraductal papillary mucinous tumor	Mixed	Elderly	Throughout	Unilocular, septated, associated dilated ducts	Papillary mucinous
Serous cystadenoma	Female	Middle-aged	Throughout	Microcystic	Serous (PAS positive for glycogen)
Cystic endocrine tumor	Mixed	Middle-aged	Throughout	Associated mass	Endocrine
Solid cystic pseudopapillary tumor	Female	Young	Throughout	Mixed solid and cystic	Endocrine-like

best-described inherited disorder associated with cystic lesions *(8)*. In the largest series to date, pancreatic involvement was observed in 122 of 158 patients (77.2%) and included true cysts (91.1%), serous cystadenomas (12.3%), neuroendocrine tumors (12.3%), or combined lesions (11.5%).

3. PATHOGENESIS

The pathogenesis of cystic neoplasms of the pancreas is poorly understood. Serous cystadenomas are strongly associated with mutations of the *VHL* gene, located on chromosome 3p25 *(9)*. The *VHL* gene is likely to play an important role in the pathogenesis of sporadic serous cystadenomas. In one study, 70% of the sporadic serous cystadenomas studied demonstrated loss of heterozygosity (LOH) at 3p25 with a *VHL* gene mutation in the remaining allele *(10)*. The mutations in the *VHL* gene probably affect most commonly the centro-acinar cell and result in hamartomatous proliferation of these small cuboidal cells. The expression of keratin in clear epithelial cells resembles that in ductal and/or centro-acinar cells and is most likely responsible for the fibro-collagenous stroma *(11)*.

The pathogenesis of MCNs and IPMNs is very different compared with serous cystadenomas. *K-ras* mutations are present only in MCNs but not in serous microcystic adenomas. In addition, LOH at 3p25, the chromosomal location of *VHL* gene, was present in 57% (8/14) of serous microcystic adenomas compared with 17% (2/12) of MCNs *(12)*. MCNs frequently contain mutations of the *K-ras* oncogene and *p53* tumor suppressor gene, and the frequency of these mutations increases with increasing degrees of dysplasia in the neoplasm. The frequency of *K-ras* mutation in MCNs is linearly related to the grades of atypia *(13)*. However, the degree of atypia in IPMT does not seem to correlate with the presence of *K-ras* mutations. LOH of the p16 gene was observed with increasing degrees of histological atypia in IPMN, whereas LOH of the *p53* gene was seen only in invasive carcinomas. The distribution of LOH in 9p21(p16) and 17p13(p53) of IPMT lesions is mostly clonal, without the

presence of the genetic alterations. The identical genetic statuses in the precursor lesions are consistent with the presence of clonal progression during the development of this tumor *(14)*.

4. PATHOLOGY

4.1. SEROUS CYSTADENOMAS

Serous cystadenomas (previously known as glycogen-rich cystadenomas) are benign, solitary, cystic tumors that arise from centro-acinar cells (Fig. 1). Although the majority of serous cystadenomas are microcystic, there are two other variants based on growth pattern: macrocystic and solid. Microcystic serous cystadenomas are made up of multiple small thin-walled cysts with a honeycomb-like appearance on cross-section. Microcystic serous cystadenomas may grow to a large diameter over the long-term and the large lesions often have a fibrotic or calcified central scar. Macrocystic serous cystadenomas are made up of far fewer cysts, and the diameter of each cyst varies from microcystic to large cavities *(15)*. The presence of discrete, large cystic cavities mimics the appearance of mucinous lesions. However, the cyst fluid from serous cystadenomas is nonviscous, clear, and contains no mucin.

The epithelial cells of all types of serous cystadenomas are similar. The cells are cuboidal and contain glycogen-rich, clear cytoplasm, and small centrally located nuclei *(16)*. Small surface microvilli are apparent on electron microscopy. The appearance of the surrounding stroma is variable and ranges from highly vascular to fibrotic MCNs (Fig. 2).

MCNs are made up of discrete individual locules that vary in diameter. MCNs are lined by mucin-producing cells in a columnar epithelium. The World Health Organization classification catalogues MCNs into three types, based on the degree of epithelial dysplasia: benign, borderline, and malignant. The degree of atypia of the tumor is classified according to the most advanced degree of dysplasia/carcinoma present.

MCNs of the pancreas often contain a unique, highly cellular (termed "ovarian") stroma. It occurs almost exclusively in female

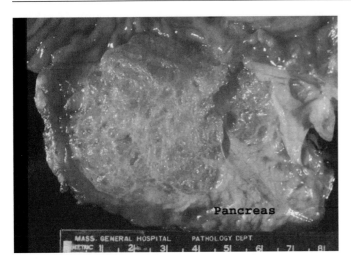

Fig. 1. Gross photograph of a serous cystadenoma.

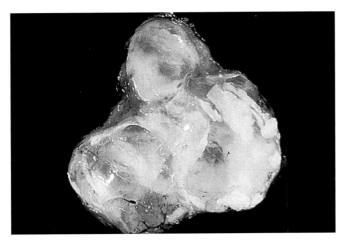

Fig. 2. Gross photograph of a MCN.

patients, although rare cases of MCNs with ovarian stroma in male patients have been encountered. Many authorities have restricted the very definition of MCNs to include only those cystic mucinous tumors that contain ovarian stroma. The cyst fluid from MCNs is often viscous and clear.

IPMNs are similar to MCNs in that they are cystic tumors that secrete mucin. However, IPMNs are characterized by a unique papillary epithelium and arise from ductal epithelium. The presence of a papillary neoplasm causes dilatation of the ducts as a result of tumor growth. The degree of ductal ectasia produced varies with degree of mucin production, but duct dilatation great enough to be seen on imaging studies or gross pathological examination is a *sine qua non* of the diagnosis. Mucin production may be so exuberant that extrusion from papilla of Vater is seen. The degree of dysplasia exhibited by the epithelium may range from mild to moderate to severe (carcinoma *in situ*), and the entire tumor is classified according to the greatest degree of dysplasia present.

4.2. CYSTIC ENDOCRINE NEOPLASMS

Cystic neoplasms that are made up of neuroendocrine elements are rare and comprise 0.5–4% of all primary pancreatic neoplasms. The classic neuroendocrine cystic tumor or islet cell tumor is a solitary lesion lined with small, granular cells that are stainable for immunoreactive hormones, chromogranin, and synaptophysin *(17)*. It is rare for the cystic endocrine tumors to produce sufficient hormones to be clinically active. Cystic endocrine tumors are seen in association with VHL syndrome *(18)*. A related cystic lesion, the solid pseudopapillary tumor is most commonly found in young woman *(19)*. The tumor often contains areas of hemorrhage and necrosis as well as cystic components. Myxoid stromal ball is the pathognomonic finding on cytology. Degenerative cystic changes are common, and the clinical presentation is often that of a cystic pancreatic tumor. Pathological features include solid, cellular, hypervascular regions without gland formation, and degenerative pseudopapillae. The cells contain eosinophilic granules rich in α-1-antitrypsin and the nuclei are typically grooved *(20)*. These neoplasms exhibit low-grade malignant behavior and have an excellent prognosis when resected.

4.3. CLINICAL PRESENTATION

Most patients with a pancreatic cystic lesion are symptom-free *(21)*. The cystic lesion is usually found with computed tomography (CT) or ultrasound imaging performed for the evaluation of another condition. When symptoms are present, the most common presentation is recurrent abdominal pain, nausea, and vomiting as result of mild pancreatitis. These symptoms often reflect the presence of a lesion causing ductal obstruction or a connection with the main ductal system. Chronic abdominal pain is a rare presentation of a benign cystic lesion and suggests a malignancy or a pseudocyst. Patients with a cystic malignancy will present with symptoms and signs similar to pancreatic cancer (i.e., pain, weight loss, and jaundice). Pseudocysts may arise after an episode of acute pancreatitis or insidiously in the setting of chronic pancreatitis and are associated with chronic abdominal pain. Large pseudocysts can compress the stomach, duodenum, or bile duct, causing early satiety, vomiting, or jaundice.

4.4. DIFFERENTIAL DIAGNOSIS

The finding of a cystic lesion of the pancreas by imaging exams presents the clinician with a wide range of possible diagnoses. The most important differentiation is between a cystic neoplasm and a pseudocyst. Although pancreatic pseudocysts usually arise in association with pancreatitis, the acute episode of pancreatitis may not have been clinically apparent or the patient may have mild chronic pancreatitis. Evidence of inflammatory changes or calcifications in the pancreas is suggestive of a pancreatic pseudocyst. However, in the acute setting of mild pancreatitis it may be difficult to differentiate between a cystic neoplasm that has caused pancreatitis and a small pseudocyst that has formed as a result of pancreatitis.

If a pancreatic pseudocyst can be excluded on the basis of a clinical history or imaging findings, attention should be focused on the differential between the types of cystic neoplasms. The principal differentiation is between mucinous and serous lesions because the fundamental difference in management is based on the neoplastic potential of mucinous lesions. Serous lesions are often diagnosed based on the characteristic microcystic morphology that is apparent on most imaging techniques. Once a serous lesion has been confidently diagnosed

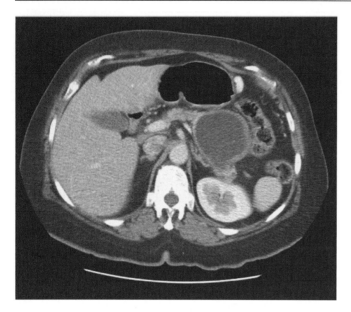

Fig. 3. Computed tomography scan of a mucinous cystic neoplasm.

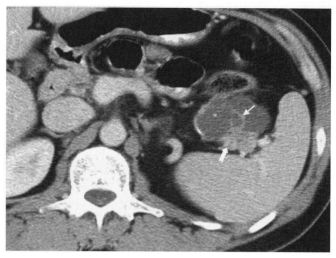

Fig. 4. Computed tomography scan of a mucinous cystadeno-carcinoma.

and if the patient has not suffered any complications of the serous cystadenoma, the lesion may not require resection. In contrast, mucinous cystic lesions are often resected because of the propensity toward growth and malignant degeneration. Under some clinical circumstances, such as in high-risk surgical patients, differentiation between benign and malignant mucinous lesions is important. Benign mucinous lesions in high-risk patients may in some circumstances be followed with serial imaging and not resected at diagnosis.

5. DIAGNOSTIC METHODS

CT is an excellent test for cystic lesions of the pancreas because of its widespread availability and ability to detect cysts *(22)* (Fig. 3). MRI is used increasingly because of the lack of radiation exposure and the ability to image the pancreatic duct with MR cholangiopancreatography *(23)*. Transabdominal ultrasonography may aid in differentiating between solid and cystic lesions, but complete evaluation of the pancreas is often difficult owing to overlying bowel gas.

Although seen in less than 20% of lesions, demonstration of a central scar by CT or MR is a highly diagnostic feature of a serous cystadenoma *(24)*. The honey-combed or microcystic appearance of the lesion is commonly used to provide a diagnosis. However, macrocystic serous cystadenomas are difficult to diagnose with cross-sectional imaging because of the morphological similarities with mucinous lesions *(15,25)*. Serous cystadenomas are often quite vascular and the finding of enhancement with intravenous contrast is used to differentiate between serous and mucinous cystic lesions. MCNs, in contrast, are commonly diagnosed with CT based on the unilocular or macrocystic characteristics *(26)*. Although not frequently seen, the finding of peripheral calcification by CT is specific for an MCN. The presence of a thickened wall, irregular septations, or an adjacent mass is suggestive of malignant degeneration.

IPMNs may involve the main pancreatic duct exclusively, a side-branch, or both. The finding of a dilated main pancreatic duct in conjunction with a cystic lesion is highly suggestive of IPMN by CT scanning. In addition, the finding of multiple cystic lesions is highly suggestive of an IPMN because serous cystadenomas and MCNs are usually solitary. Pancreatic calcifications are rarely seen in association with IPMN and the finding of parenchymal calcifications should suggest chronic pancreatitis. MR cholangiopancreatography can demonstrate the diagnostic findings of pancreatic duct dilation, mural nodules, and ductal connection better than endoscopic retrograde cholangiopancreatography *(27)*. Malignant degeneration of IPMN is difficult to detect, but the finding of a mural nodule is highly suggestive of a malignant IPMN.

Despite these imaging features, the ability to accurately diagnose a specific cystic lesion and to determine whether malignancy is present by CT and MR remains uncertain (Fig. 4). The diagnosis of a pancreatic pseudocyst is more dependent on the clinical history and the associated findings of chronic pancreatitis. Pancreatic pseudocysts appear as unilocular fluid-filled cavities associated with parenchymal changes such as calcifications and atrophy. The wall of a pancreatic pseudocyst is often thick and irregular, involving the serosa of the stomach, small bowel, or the colon. The fluid within a pancreatic pseudocyst may be heterogeneous, reflecting the presence of blood, inflammatory debris, or infection. High-grade infections of a pseudocyst may result in the presence of air in the cavity of a pseudocyst.

Recently endoscopy and endoscopic ultrasound (EUS) have been used to diagnose cystic lesions of the pancreas and guide fine-needle aspiration (FNA) *(28)*. Using the high-resolution imaging of EUS, the morphological features of various cystadenomas have recently been defined. However, the detailed imaging features of cystic neoplasms by EUS do not appear to be sufficiently accurate to differentiate between benign and malignant cystadenomas unless there is evidence of a solid mass or invasive tumor *(29)* (Fig. 5). EUS is also very sensitive for detecting IPMN lesions, but imaging alone may not be sufficient for differentiating between benign and malignant lesions *(30,31)*. Focal hypoechoic mass lesions in the pancreatic parenchyma are often seen in conjunction with IPMN and

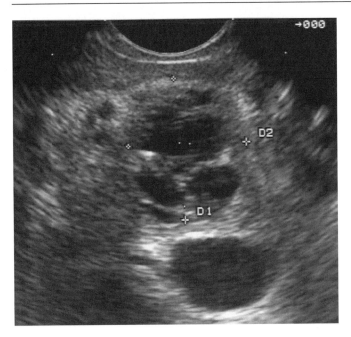

Fig. 5. Endoscopic ultrasound image of a mucinous cystadeno-carcinoma.

represent areas of focal, chronic pancreatitis. These lesions may be confused with malignant degeneration of IPMN.

The fluid contents of cystadenomas are often analyzed for cytology *(32)*. However, the low cellular content of cyst fluid has hampered the use of the cytological analysis of cyst fluid. Small, cuboidal cells in cytological specimens are diagnostic of serous cystadenomas. In contrast, mucinous cystadenoma may have large secretory epithelial cells with evidence of mucin secretion or atypia *(33)*. The finding of malignant cytology is highly diagnostic of a malignant mucinous cystic tumor but the sensitivity of cytology for the presence of malignancy is quite low, approx 30%. Similar cytological findings are seen in aspirants from IPMN lesions. Only inflammatory cells, such as macrophages, should be present in the fluid aspirated from pseudocysts.

A variety of cyst fluid tumor markers have been studied to help differentiate between the major types of cystic neoplasms. Several studies suggest that carcinoembryonic antigen (CEA) or CA 72-4 are useful for identifying mucinous lesions *(34)*. These carbohydrate antigens are secreted by the epithelium lining mucinous lesions and are present in high concentrations. Cyst fluid concentrations of CEA and CA 72-4 are very low in serous cystadenomas. Despite considerable overlap between mucinous and nonmucinous cysts, cyst fluid CEA remains the most accurate marker *(35)*.

IPMNs can be imaged with endoscopic retrograde cholangio-pancreatography or EUS *(36)*. The endoscopic appearance of mucin extrusion from a widely patent ampulla is diagnostic of an IPMN. Contrast retrograde pancreatography will demonstrate the characteristic findings of mucinous filling defects within the duct, diffuse ductal dilation, and cystic dilation of side branches. EUS may assist in the detection of malignancy arising from IPMNs by demonstrating wall invasion and guiding FNA. The demonstration of ductal communication with endoscopic retrograde cholangiopancreatography in serous and mucinous

cystadenomas is a rare finding. However, focal ductal invasion may be seen in malignant mucinous cystic lesions.

6. TREATMENT AND PREVENTION

6.1. CYSTIC NEOPLASMS

Surgical resection is the treatment of choice for premalignant cystic neoplasms. The decision to resect a lesion, however, is based on the presence or absence of symptoms, the risk of malignancy, and the surgical risk of the patient. High-risk patients with low-grade cystic neoplasms may be monitored with periodic CT/MRI scanning or EUS-FNA *(23)*.

The increasing safety of surgical resection has prompted the use of surgery for a wider range of lesions *(21)*. As most MCNs are located in the tail of the pancreas, a distal pancreatectomy is sufficient for these premalignant lesions. Although there are reports of enucleation of mucinous cystadenomas, the safety and the long-term outcome have not been well documented. Serous cystadenomas that require removal are resected with the involved portion of the pancreas: tail (tail resection), head (Whipple), or body (middle pancreatectomy). Unless invasive carcinoma is suspected or discovered at surgery, the spleen can often be preserved in tail resections. As the IPMNs invade the pancreas along ductal structures, it is important that frozen section histology be used during surgery to assure negative margins *(37,38)*. High-risk IPMNs involving the entire pancreas will require total pancreatectomy. These surgical approaches often require that the patients be managed in centers with considerable experience in cystic neoplasms of the pancreas.

6.2. PROGNOSIS

The prognosis for resected cystic neoplasms of the pancreas is excellent *(39)*. There are only rare reports of tumor recurrence if the lesion is completely resected and there is no evidence of malignant tissue in the resected specimen. Even for IPMNs containing carcinoma (which includes almost 60% of resected tumors) the 5-yr survival is more than 50% *(40)*. Similar survival rates are seen in patients with MCNs *(41)*. Side-branch lesions arising from IPMN have a better prognosis than main duct IPMN *(42)*. The worst prognosis is for advanced, transmural adenocarcinomas arising from mucinous lesions; the 5-yr survival is only 30% for resected lesions.

REFERENCES

1. Warshaw AL, Compton CC, Lewandrowski K, Cardenosa G, Mueller PR. Cystic tumors of the pancreas. New clinical, radiologic, and pathologic observations in 67 patients. Ann Surg 1990; 212: 432–443; discussion 444,445.
2. Kimura W, Nagai H, Kuroda A, Muto T, Esaki Y. Analysis of small cystic lesions of the pancreas. Int J Pancreatol 1995; 18:197–206.
3. Kimura W, Morikane K, Esaki Y, Chan WC, Pour PM. Histologic and biologic patterns of microscopic pancreatic ductal adenocarcinomas detected incidentally at autopsy. Cancer 1998; 82:1839–1849.
4. Kimura W. How many millimeters do atypical epithelia of the pancreas spread intraductally before beginning to infiltrate? Hepatogastroenterology 2003; 50:2218–2224.
5. Zhang XM, Mitchell DG, Dohke M, Holland GA, Parker L. Pancreatic cysts: depiction on single-shot fast spin-echo MR images. Radiology 2002; 223:547–553.
6. Compton CC. Serous cystic tumors of the pancreas. Semin Diagn Pathol 2000; 17:43–55.

7. Bassi C, Salvia R, Molinari E, Biasutti C, Falconi M, Pederzoli P. Management of 100 consecutive cases of pancreatic serous cystadenoma: wait for symptoms and see at imaging or vice versa? World J Surg 2003; 27:319–323.

8. Hammel PR, Vilgrain V, Terris B, et al. Pancreatic involvement in von Hippel-Lindau disease. The Groupe Francophone d'Etude de la Maladie de von Hippel-Lindau. Gastroenterology 2000; 119: 1087–1095.

9. Moore PS, Zamboni G, Brighenti A, et al. Molecular characterization of pancreatic serous microcystic adenomas: evidence for a tumor suppressor gene on chromosome 10q. Am J Pathol 2001; 158:317–21.

10. Vortmeyer AO, Lubensky IA, Fogt F, Linehan WM, Khettry U, Zhuang Z. Allelic deletion and mutation of the von Hippel-Lindau (VHL) tumor suppressor gene in pancreatic microcystic adenomas. Am J Pathol 1997; 151:951–956.

11. Yasuhara Y, Sakaida N, Uemura Y, Senzaki H, Shikata N, Tsubura A. Serous microcystic adenoma (glycogen-rich cystadenoma) of the pancreas: Study of 11 cases showing clinicopathological and immunohistochemical correlations. Pathol Int 2002; 52:307–312.

12. Kim SG, Wu TT, Lee JH, et al. Comparison of epigenetic and genetic alterations in mucinous cystic neoplasm and serous microcystic adenoma of pancreas. Mod Pathol 2003; 16:1086–1094.

13. Yoshizawa K, Nagai H, Sakurai S, et al. Clonality and K-ras mutation analyses of epithelia in intraductal papillary mucinous tumor and mucinous cystic tumor of the pancreas. Virchows Arch 2002; 441:437–443.

14. Wada K, Takada T, Yasuda H, et al. Does "clonal progression" relate to the development of intraductal papillary mucinous tumors of the pancreas? J Gastrointest Surg 2004; 8:289–296.

15. Khurana B, Mortele KJ, Glickman J, Silverman SG, Ros PR. Macrocystic serous adenoma of the pancreas: radiologic-pathologic correlation. AJR Am J Roentgenol 2003; 181:119–123.

16. Santos LD, Chow C, Henderson CJ, et al. Serous oligocystic adenoma of the pancreas: a clinicopathological and immunohistochemical study of three cases with ultrastructural findings. Pathology 2002; 34:148–156.

17. Kann P, Bittinger F, EngelbAch M, Bohner S, Weis A, Beyer J. Endosonography of insulin-secreting and clinically non-functioning neuroendocrine tumors of the pancreas: criteria for benignancy and malignancy. Eur J Med Res 2001; 6:385–390.

18. Marcos HB, Libutti SK, Alexander HR, et al. Neuroendocrine tumors of the pancreas in von Hippel-Lindau disease: spectrum of appearances at CT and MR imaging with histopathologic comparison. Radiology 2002; 225:751–758.

19. Ferlan-Marolt V, Pleskovic L, Pegan V. Solid papillary-cystic tumor of the pancreas. Hepatogastroenterology 1999; 46:2978–2982.

20. Klimstra DS, Wenig BM, Heffess CS. Solid-pseudopapillary tumor of the pancreas: a typically cystic carcinoma of low malignant potential. Semin Diagn Pathol 2000; 17:66–80.

21. Fernandez del Castillo CF, Targarona J, Thayer SP, Rattner DW, Brugge WR, Warshaw AL. Incidental pancreatic cysts: clinicopathologic characteristics and comparison with symptomatic patients. Arch Surg 2003; 138:427–434.

22. Curry CA, Eng J, Horton KM, et al. CT of primary cystic pancreatic neoplasms: can CT be used for patient triage and treatment? AJR Am J Roentgenol 2000; 175:99–103.

23. Irie H, Yoshimitsu K, Aibe H, et al. Natural history of pancreatic intraductal papillary mucinous tumor of branch duct type: follow-up study by magnetic resonance cholangiopancreatography. J Comput Assist Tomogr 2004; 28:117–122.

24. Torresan F, Casadei R, Solmi L, Marrano D, Gandolfi L. The role of ultrasound in the differential diagnosis of serous and mucinous cystic tumours of the pancreas. Eur J Gastroenterol Hepatol 1997; 9:169–172.

25. Chatelain D, Hammel P, O'Toole D, et al. Macrocystic form of serous pancreatic cystadenoma. Am J Gastroenterol 2002; 97:2566–2571.

26. Sahani D, Prasad S, Saini S, Mueller P. Cystic pancreatic neoplasms evaluation by CT and magnetic resonance cholangiopancreatography. Gastrointest Endosc Clin N Am 2002; 12:657–672.

27. Sugiyama M, Atomi Y, HAchiya J. Intraductal papillary tumors of the pancreas: evaluation with magnetic resonance cholangiopancreatography. Am J Gastroenterol 1998; 93:156–159.

28. Brugge WR. Evaluation of pancreatic cystic lesions with EUS. Gastrointest Endosc 2004; 59:698–707.

29. Ahmad NA, Kochman ML, Lewis JD, Ginsberg GG. Can EUS alone differentiate between malignant and benign cystic lesions of the pancreas? Am J Gastroenterol 2001; 96:3295–3300.

30. Brandwein SL, Farrell JJ, Centeno BA, Brugge WR. Detection and tumor staging of malignancy in cystic, intraductal, and solid tumors of the pancreas by EUS. Gastrointest Endosc 2001; 53:722–727.

31. Terris B, Ponsot P, Paye F, et al. Intraductal papillary mucinous tumors of the pancreas confined to Secondary ducts show less aggressive pathologic features as compared with those involving the main pancreatic duct. Am J Surg Pathol 2000; 24:1372–1377.

32. Centeno BA, Warshaw AL, Mayo-Smith W, Southern JF, Lewandrowski K. Cytologic diagnosis of pancreatic cystic lesions. A prospective study of 28 percutaneous aspirates. Acta Cytol 1997; 41:972–980.

33. Recine M, Kaw M, Evans DB, Krishnamurthy S. Fine-needle aspiration cytology of mucinous tumors of the pancreas. Cancer 2004; 102:92–99.

34. Frossard JL, Amouyal P, Amouyal G, et al. Performance of endosonography-guided fine needle aspiration and biopsy in the diagnosis of pancreatic cystic lesions. Am J Gastroenterol 2003; 98:1516–1524.

35. Brugge WR, Lewandrowski K, Lee-Lewandrowski E, et al. Diagnosis of pancreatic cystic neoplasms: a report of the cooperative pancreatic cyst study. Gastroenterology 2004; 126:1330–1336.

36. Telford JJ, Carr-Locke DL. The role of ERCP and pancreatoscopy in cystic and intraductal tumors. Gastrointest Endosc Clin N Am 2002; 12:747–757.

37. Gigot JF, Deprez P, Sempoux C, et al. Surgical management of intraductal papillary mucinous tumors of the pancreas: the role of routine frozen Section of the surgical margin, intraoperative endoscopic staged biopsies of the Wirsung duct, and pancreaticogastric anastomosis. Arch Surg 2001; 136:1256–1262.

38. Chari ST, Yadav D, Smyrk TC, et al. Study of recurrence after surgical resection of intraductal papillary mucinous neoplasm of the pancreas. Gastroenterology 2002; 123:1500–1507.

39. Harper AE, Eckhauser FE, Mulholland MW. Resectional therapy for cystic neoplasms of the pancreas. Am Surg 2002; 68:353–357; discussion 357,358.

40. Kanazumi N, Nakao A, Kaneko T, et al. Surgical treatment of intraductal papillary-mucinous tumors of the pancreas. Hepatogastroenterology 2001; 48:967–971.

41. Suzuki Y, Atomi Y, Sugiyama M, et al. Cystic neoplasm of the pancreas: a Japanese multiinstitutional study of intraductal papillary mucinous tumor and mucinous cystic tumor. Pancreas 2004; 28:241–246.

42. Kobari M, Egawa S, Shibuya K, et al. Intraductal papillary mucinous tumors of the pancreas comprise 2 clinical subtypes: differences in clinical characteristics and surgical management. Arch Surg 1999; 134:1131–1136.

25 Diagnosis and Evaluation of Pancreatic Ductal Adenocarcinoma

Kenneth H. Yu, MD and Nuzhat A. Ahmad, MD

Contents

1. INTRODUCTION

Pancreatic cancer is the fourth most common cause of cancer-related mortality in the United States *(1)*. The 5-yr survival rate is the lowest among all cancers, with estimates ranging from 0.4 to 4%. The only potentially curative treatment for pancreatic cancer is surgical resection. However, because the disease is generally advanced at presentation, only 10–20% of patients are eligible for attempted curative resection. In these patients who undergo pancreaticoduodenectomy, 5-yr survival is somewhat better, about 20% *(2)*. The epidemiology and clinical features of pancreatic cancer will be reviewed. A careful examination of current imaging technology in the staging, diagnosis, and evaluation of pancreatic adenocarcinoma will also be discussed.

2. EPIDEMIOLOGY

In 2003, an estimated 30,700 new cases of pancreatic cancer were diagnosed, and an estimated 30,000 patients died as a result of their disease *(3)*. Because of the aggressiveness of this cancer, the inability to diagnose it early, and the current lack of effective outcome altering therapies for advanced stage disease, mortality rates from pancreatic cancer are almost identical to incidence rates.

Age is clearly one risk factor for pancreatic cancer. Pancreatic cancer is rare before the age of 45 with the incidence rising sharply thereafter, and peaks with a 40-fold increased risk by the age of 80 *(4)*. Patients with chronic pancreatitis are at increased risk for developing pancreatic cancer.

From: *Endoscopic Oncology: Gastrointestinal Endoscopy and Cancer Management*. Edited by: D. O. Faigel and M. L. Kochman © Humana Press, Totowa, NJ

The most consistently attributable environmental risk factor for the development of pancreatic cancer is cigarette smoking. By one estimate, cigarette smoking is thought to account for 25–29% of pancreatic cancer cases. It has been theorized that the aromatic amines present in cigarettes are responsible for this increased risk. With much the same chemistry, occupational exposure to aromatic amines, for example, in chemists or petrochemical workers, may increase the risk of developing pancreatic cancer. Some plant components may inhibit the mutagenic effects of these amines, which could explain findings that diets high in fruits and vegetables may protect against development of pancreatic cancer *(5)*.

Genetic factors may also increase the risk of developing pancreatic cancer. Numerous genetic syndromes confer a higher relative risk of developing pancreatic cancer, including hereditary pancreatitis (cationic trypsinogen gene mutation), hereditary nonpolyposis colorectal cancer, ataxia-telangiectasia, Peutz-Jeghers syndrome, familial breast cancer, and familial atypical multiple mole melanoma (FAMMM) *(6)*.

3. PATHOLOGY

Ductal adenocarcinomas and its variants make up more than 90% of all malignant pancreatic exocrine tumors. The remaining 5–10% are mainly islet cell tumors. Other relatively uncommon tumors found in the pancreas include lymphoma, carcinoma metastatic from other organs, and cystic tumors. About 70% of ductal adenocarcinomas occur in the pancreatic head; the rest occur in the body or tail, or diffusely throughout the pancreas. Research into the molecular genetics of pancreatic cancer has resulted in a better understanding of how these tumors occur. Pancreatic adenocarcinoma is believed to be derived from pancreatic-ductular cells. One of the earliest genetic changes to occur is an activating mutation in the *K-ras* gene, found in virtually all pancreatic adenocarcinomas. Unfortunately, mutations in *K-ras* are not found exclusively in pancreatic cancers, having been discovered in the setting of benign pancreatic conditions and even in normal pancreas *(7)*. As lesions progress, other gene mutations commonly occur. One frequently altered gene is the tumor-suppressor *CDKN2A*. Inactivation of this gene is seen in 80–95% of pancreatic adenocarcinomas. Notably, some kindreds with FAMMM syndrome are associated with a germline mutation in *CDKN2A*, which confers a 13-fold increased risk of pancreatic cancer. Other important mutations commonly found in pancreatic cancers include inactivation of the *p53* tumor-suppressor gene and loss of the transcriptional regulator *SMAD4*. As our understanding of the molecular biology of pancreatic cancer improves, we may be able to develop better tumor markers and treatments.

4. CLINICAL PRESENTATION

Patients with pancreatic cancer commonly present with complaints of pain, weight loss, or jaundice. Symptoms at presentation can vary depending on the location and stage of the tumor. For tumors located in the head and body of the pancreas, symptoms are generally secondary to compression of surrounding structures; the bile duct, the pancreatic duct, duodenum, and/or celiac nerves. These symptoms usually bring the patient to medical attention. A small tumor in the head of the pancreas can produce symptoms of painless jaundice, resulting in an early diagnosis *(8)*. Tumors in the tail or body of the pancreas may cause pain and weight loss related to a large lesion with extension of the primary tumor. These tumors are usually more advanced at the time of diagnosis. Pain may be an indication of more advanced disease, and is seen in 80% of patients with locally unresectable disease, and in 85% of patients with advanced cancer *(9)*.

Other signs associated with pancreatic cancer include new-onset diabetes mellitus, malabsorption, pancreatitis, or migratory thrombophlebitis (Trousseau's syndrome). On physical exam, one might find an abdominal mass or ascites at presentation in a patient with pancreatic cancer. Other findings may include a palpable nontender gallbladder (Courvoisier's sign), often seen in patients with jaundice. In patients with widespread disease, left supraclavicular lymphadenopathy (Virchow's node) or a palpable rectal shelf metastasis may be demonstrated.

5. DIAGNOSIS AND STAGING

The two main issues in a patient with suspected pancreatic cancer are to establish the diagnosis and to determine whether the patient is a candidate for surgical resection. If the patient is deemed a surgical candidate, histological proof of malignancy is usually not required. However, in patients with unresectable disease (i.e., distant metastases or major vessel involvement on radiographic studies) or who are not operative candidates owing to comorbidities, a histological diagnosis is usually required before proceeding with any nonsurgical palliative therapy.

The tumor node metastasis (TNM) staging criteria for pancreatic cancer as defined by the American Joint Committee on Cancer (AJCC) was recently updated *(10)*. In 2002, the AJCC modified the tumor (T) staging system for pancreatic cancer to classify tumors invading the portal venous (superior mesenteric vein or portal vein) system as T3 (these were previously staged as T4) and tumors invading the celiac or superior mesenteric artery as T4. Based on pre-operative assessment, a resectable pancreatic cancer cannot involve the celiac axis or superior mesenteric artery. Involvement of the superior mesenteric vein or the portal venous confluence does not necessarily preclude resectability. Direct invasion of contiguous structures, such as bowel, spleen, kidney, or spine, and distant metastatic disease can preclude resectability.

A variety of studies are available for the diagnosis and staging of pancreatic cancer. High sensitivity and specificity are not the only important factors when assessing tools for preoperative staging. The ideal tools would be minimally invasive, safe, capable of obtaining tissue samples if needed, cost-effective, and widely available. Advances in technology have made available a wide range of imaging tools, such as helical computed tomography (hCT), magnetic resonance imaging (MRI), endoscopic ultrasound (EUS), endoscopic retrograde cholangiopancreatography (ERCP), and angiography. No consensus exists as to the best algorithm to use for staging and determining resectability. The strengths and weaknesses of these technique, and strategies for combining these techniques will be discussed.

5.1. TUMOR MARKERS

Several tumor markers for pancreatic cancer have been evaluated, but none has been shown to be particularly sensitive or specific in the diagnosis of pancreatic cancer. The most widely used tumor marker, cancer-associated antigen 19-9 (CA 19-9), has been found to have a sensitivity of 70–86% and a specificity of 87%, depending on the cutoff used *(11–13)*. CA 19-9 levels, however, may also be elevated in patients with biliary obstruction caused by lesions other than pancreatic cancer. One study demonstrated that serum concentrations above 37 U/mL had a sensitivity and specificity of 77 and 87%, respectively, for discriminating pancreatic cancer from benign pancreatic disease *(14)*. Although not useful as a diagnostic tool, serial CA 19-9 levels can be a useful way to monitor estimating response to therapy or disease progression.

Islet amyloid polypeptide (IAPP) is a candidate biomarker that has been shown to be elevated in the plasma of patients with pancreatic cancer, particularly those with concurrent diabetes *(15)*. IAPP appears to be secreted by pancreatic β-cells, and is associated with reduced insulin sensitivity. Recent studies, however, have shown IAPP to be an ineffective tumor marker. A recent study evaluated plasma IAPP levels in patients with pancreatic cancer compared with normal controls and patients with other pancreatic disease *(16)*. IAPP levels were elevated in pancreatic cancer patients, but overall IAPP was less sensitive than CA 19-9 (40 vs 75%) in diagnosing pancreatic cancer. In the patients enrolled in this study who had concurrent diabetes (46%), the sensitivity of IAPP was only 50%.

As previously discussed, activating *K-ras* mutations can be found in virtually all pancreatic cancers. Preliminary studies have demonstrated that *K-ras* mutations can be detected in plasma *(17)*, in pancreatic juice obtained by ERCP *(18)*, in duodenal juice obtained with secretin stimulation *(19)* and in stool *(20)*. Sensitivity is low with current techniques, and the implication of *K-ras* mutations in patients without overt pancreatic cancer is unknown.

5.2. HELICAL CT

CT of the abdomen should typically be the first diagnostic procedure performed when a pancreatic tumor is suspected. CT is useful in detecting pancreatic tumors, in assessing resectability and detecting distant metastases. Historically, sensitivity of conventional CT for detecting small pancreatic tumors (<3 cm) was as low as 53% *(21)*. With the advent of dual-phase hCT, this technique has proven to be far more accurate at identifying pancreatic masses and determining resectability.

In a prospective trial of 76 patients with suspected pancreatic cancer, in whom dual-phase hCT scan alone was used for evaluation and staging *(22)*, the positive predictive value of CT for resectability was determined to be 73.5%, and overall accuracy was determined to be 77%. Nine patients determined to be resectable by CT were found to actually be unresectable because of liver metastases, vascular encasement, or lymph node metastases. Liver metastases not seen by CT were found at time of surgery in 20.5% of the patients. CT accurately identified lymph node metastases in only 16.7% of patients.

In general, positive predictive values of hCT scan for surgical unresectability have been excellent, ranging from 89 to 95% *(23–26)*. Among patients with tumors judged potentially resectable on the basis of CT criteria, however, surgical results demonstrate that 60–91% of the tumors are resectable. The nonresectable patients had locally advanced tumors, lymph node metastases, or small peritoneal, omental, or hepatic metastases not identified by the pre-operative CT *(27–29)*. In particular, CT is not reliable in predicting nodal involvement in pancreatic cancer, and suspicious peripancreatic nodes on CT should not discourage resection *(30)*.

One of the most common causes of unresectability not detected by CT is vascular involvement by tumor. The sensitivities for vascular invasion are reported to be between 60 and 89% for hCT *(27,28)*. A relatively new CT technology (hCT or multi-detector CT [MDCT]) may improve detection of tumor infiltration of vascular structures. It will be interesting to see what impact multidetector CT has on improving resectability of pancreatic cancer.

5.3. ENDOSCOPIC ULTRASOUND

EUS is an imaging technique that combines endoscopy and ultrasonography. An ultrasound transducer is mounted on the tip of the endoscope, allowing accurate imaging of lesions located within and adjacent to the gastrointestinal wall. EUS is used routinely in the evaluation of numerous gastrointestinal disorders, including the diagnosis and staging of gastrointestinal tumors. During the last 10 yr, its applications have become more established, mainly because of improvements in the technology of endoscopes (e.g., video chip rather than fiberoptic) and ultrasound transducers. The applications of EUS have also expanded to include EUS-guided fine-needle aspiration (FNA) of lesions located within and outside the gastrointestinal wall.

The close proximity of the stomach and duodenum to the pancreas allows endosonography to provide high-resolution images of the pancreas and associated retroperitoneal vascular structures. The high resolution of EUS is particularly well suited to identify focal pancreatic neoplasms. A number of studies have evaluated the accuracy of EUS in the diagnosis and staging of pancreatic cancer. Direct comparison of these studies can be difficult because of differences in the inclusion criteria and the gold standard. EUS is very operator-dependent; the accuracy of EUS is clearly dependent on the experience of the operator. Accuracy is improved when endosonographers have performed at least 100 staging examinations *(31)*. Although the value of EUS in diagnosis of pancreatic cancer is recognized, significant controversy exists as to the exact role and timing of EUS in algorithms for staging pancreatic cancer. The role of EUS in the diagnosis and staging of pancreatic cancer will be reviewed in the following section.

5.3.1. Diagnosis of Pancreatic Cancer

There is ample evidence in the literature that EUS is the most sensitive method for detection of pancreatic tumors, with larger series demonstrating sensitivities in the range of 90% *(21,32–37)* (Fig. 1). When compared with CT scan, MRI, ERCP, and transabdominal ultrasound exam, EUS is more sensitive for detection of pancreatic carcinoma *(21,36)*. This superiority is particularly evident with respect to lesions smaller than 3 cm in diameter *(21,35,37–39)*. More recently, EUS has compared favorably with spiral CT for the detection of pancreatic tumors. Legmann and colleagues compared dual-phase spiral CT with endosonography in patients with suspected pancreatic tumors and found the two modalities equivalent in yield with a diagnostic sensitivity of 100% for EUS and 92% for spiral CT *(34)*.

5.3.2. Staging of Pancreatic Cancer

Staging of pancreatic cancer is considered one of the most difficult aspects of EUS. However, once a mass is identified in the pancreas, EUS, by virtue of its ability to determine local extension of the tumor and to predict vascular invasion and thereby potential resectability, provides useful staging information. In a recent review of EUS in pancreatic cancer *(40)*, an analysis of many of the largest series to date demonstrates a wide range in accuracy for TNM staging. Accuracy for T staging ranged from 78 to 94%, and nodal (N) staging ranged from 64 to 82%. However, more recent studies have described lower accuracy rates. In one series of 89 patients in whom EUS was compared with surgical and histopathological TNM staging using the 1997 TNM criteria, the overall accuracy of EUS for T and N staging was only 69 and 54%, respectively. Furthermore, only 46% of tumors that were believed to be resectable by EUS were actually found to be resectable during laparotomy. Similarly, in another recent retrospective study, sensitivity, specificity and accuracy of EUS for determining resectability of pancreatic cancer *(41)* were 66, 100, and 78%, respectively. The accuracy of vascular invasion and lymph node status were determined to be 85 and 71%, respectively. In 5 of the 10 false-negative cases, incorrectly determined by EUS to be resectable, the reason was understaged vascular invasion.

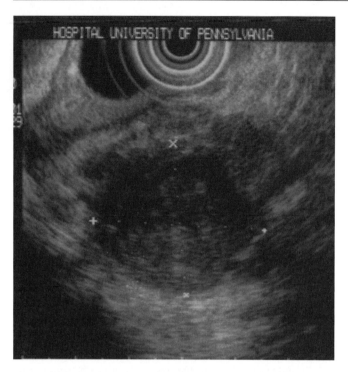

Fig. 1. Endosonographic image demonstrating a large hypoechoic mass in the head of the pancreas in a patient with obstructive jaundice.

These studies *(32,42,43)* suggest that EUS may be less accurate than previously thought at determining local stage and resectability. The changes in the new TNM staging system are expected to increase T staging accuracy. Several factors have been identified that could account for the decreased accuracy of EUS when compared to results from earlier studies *(41)*. Selection bias is one important factor. Most patients with pancreatic cancer are initially diagnosed by cross-sectional imaging. As these imaging techniques, particularly hCT, have become increasingly sensitive, patients with clearly resectable disease are often taken straight to surgery, and are not referred to EUS. Similarly, patients with obvious metastases or clearly unresectable disease often are not referred to EUS for further work-up. Thus, EUS is often used to image patients who have tumors that are difficult to stage accurately by any modality. Other possible factors include the small size of earlier studies, which included generally fewer than 40 patients, and the inconsistent use of surgical staging as a gold standard to judge the accuracy of EUS *(43,44)*. In addition, EUS can better detect vascular invasion in tumors that are smaller than 3 cm, which may be a factor in two studies that found EUS to be highly accurate in staging pancreatic cancer *(31,44)*; More than half of the patients had early T1 or T2 tumors. In contrast, two studies where tumors were predominantly T3 or T4 *(41,42)*, a more accurate reflection of clinical practice, EUS results were less impressive.

A recent study investigated the most effective way of combining imaging studies in the staging of pancreatic cancer *(45)*. A total of 62 patients with suspected pancreatic cancer were evaluated by EUS, CT, MRI, and angiography. All patients were taken to surgery. hCT was the most accurate modality when used by

itself for determining resectability (83%), as well as for determining surgical stage. An analysis was then performed to determine which combination of tests provided the greatest accuracy. The analysis determined that combining CT with EUS, in any sequence, resulted in the highest accuracy (87%) in predicting resectability. A selective strategy was also tested, where CT was performed in all patients, and in those patients who were deemed resectable, EUS was performed. Accuracy was preserved in this study. In a cost minimization analysis, this strategy also proved to be favorable, when the cost savings of avoiding unnecessary laparotomy were taken into account.

With the advances in cross-sectional imaging, the role of EUS can be more narrowly defined. EUS should be used in patients with suspected pancreatic cancer not well defined on dual-scan hCT. In patients with tumors felt to be resectable by CT, EUS can also be used to confirm this assessment and to search for distant lymph node metastases. In patients with unresectable tumors, EUS can be used for confirmation, and for tissue acquisition via FNA.

5.4. MAGNETIC RESONANCE IMAGING

MRI and magnetic resonance cholangiopancreatography (MRCP) are imaging technologies that can accurately assess pancreatic masses as well as both pancreatic and biliary ductal pathology. For routine staging, however, MRI has not been shown to be superior to dual-scan hCT. In a prospective trial of 62 patients who had CT and MRI performed to assess resectability of pancreatic cancer *(45)*, MRI was found to be inferior to CT regarding all parameters measured. The sensitivity, specificity, and accuracy of MRI were 57, 90, and 75%, respectively, as compared with 67, 97, and 83% for CT.

Studies have also compared MRI with EUS. In one study, 63 patients with pancreatic cancer who underwent both EUS and MRI were studied retrospectively *(46)*. Results were comparable. The sensitivity and positive predictive value of EUS for resectability were 61 and 69%, compared with 73 and 77% for MRI. Both imaging modalities predicted resectability in 18 patients, 16 (89%) of whom were found to be resectable on surgical exploration. Both imaging modalities predicted unresectability in 17 patients, of whom 4 (24%) were found to be resectable on surgical exploration. When both imaging modalities agreed on the likelihood of resectability or unresectability, the positive predictive value for resectability was 89%, and 76% for unresectability. The authors concluded that neither modality alone predicted resectability with great accuracy. The two studies could be used in combination, as tumors determined to be resectable by both modalities almost always were resectable on surgical exploration.

Another study compared the accuracy of EUS, MRI, and CT in 49 patients with lesions suspicious for pancreatic cancer *(21)*. MRI, compared with EUS, had a lower sensitivity (83 vs 94%), equivalent specificity (100% for both), and lower overall accuracy (84 vs 96%). As one would expect, EUS had a high sensitivity (93%) for detecting tumors less than 3 cm in size. MRI had a sensitivity of only 67% for detecting these lesions.

MRCP can be used to visualize biliary and pancreatic ducts, and may be useful in patients where ERCP is unsuccessful or nondiagnostic. MRCP was studied in 58 patients with failed or inadequate ERCP for the evaluation of suspected pancreatico-biliary disease *(47)*. MRCP was technically successful in 57 patients and resulted in a sensitivity, specificity, and diagnostic accuracy of 97, 100, and 98%, respectively. In a second study of 124 patients with suspected pancreatic cancer, MRCP had a sensitivity of 84% and a specificity of 97% with respect to diagnosing pancreatic cancer *(48)*. These values compared favorably to those of ERCP with a sensitivity and specificity of 70 and 94%, respectively. As MRI and MRCP technologies mature with the development of additional techniques, such as ultrarapid echoplanar imaging, these modalities may find a better-defined role in the evaluation of pancreatic cancers.

5.5. ENDOSCOPIC RETROGRADE CHOLANGIOPANCREATOGRAPHY

ERCP has no role in evaluating the resectability of pancreatic tumors. ERCP cannot evaluate vascular invasion, lymph node status, or metastatic disease. ERCP may be useful, however, in patients with suspected pancreatic cancer where cross-sectional imaging is unable to identify a mass. ERCP can more closely examine common bile and pancreatic ducts for evidence of malignant stricture or obstruction. Findings suggestive of a malignant tumor include the "double-duct sign" (Fig. 2), which signifies obstruction of the common bile and pancreatic ducts. Tissue for diagnosis can also be obtained by biopsy, sampling of pancreatic juice, or brushings. Palliation of pruritus and jaundice by placing an endoprosthetic in an obstructed duct may be performed. In patients where ERCP and stent placement are being considered, it has been suggested that cross-sectional imaging for staging be performed first. Inflammation caused by manipulation of the biliary tree or imaging artifacts induced by the presence of a stent could obscure visualization of small tumors and impede staging *(8)*. In addition, air artifact from a biliary stent can also alter accuracy of endosonographic staging of pancreatic cancer.

5.6. POSITRON EMISSION TOMOGRAPHY

18F fluorodeoxyglucose positron emission tomography (PET) works on the principle that malignant cells selectively take up and retain the positron emitting radiotracer 18F fluorodeoxyglucose, a glucose analog. Pancreatic adenocarcinomas, similar to other cancers, have increased glucose consumption when compared with normal pancreatic tissue. Several studies have found PET to be more accurate than other imaging modalities in the detection of pancreatic cancer. In small lesions, less than 2 cm in diameter, PET has been found to be more sensitive than CT *(49)*. In a range of studies, PET has a high level of accuracy in detecting pancreatic cancers, 85–91% *(50–54)*. Sensitivity (85–100%) and specificity (67–88%) are also relatively high and comparable to some competing technologies.

Despite excellent sensitivity for detecting pancreatic cancer, PET is unable to provide the accurate anatomical information needed to stage tumors. PET cannot accurately assess vascular invasion or invasion of adjacent visceral structures, and is therefore a poor tool for determining resectability. False-positive results can occur in the setting of active pancreatitis, autoimmune pancreatitis, or any other conditions that cause pancreatic inflammation *(49,55)*. False-positive results for

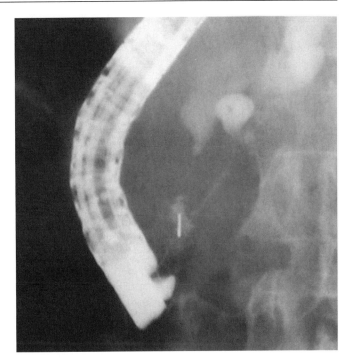

Fig. 2. ERCP image depicting stricture in the pancreatic and common bile duct, the so-called "double-duct sign," in a patient with a pancreatic head adenocarcinoma.

liver metastases have been reported in the setting of intrahepatic cholestasis *(56)*. False-negative results can occur in the setting of hyperglycemia. Of concern, some studies have also shown that false-negative results may occur in early-stage pancreatic cancers *(55,57)*.

One area where PET may be useful is in the detection of distant metastases not seen by CT. In one study, 17% of patients deemed resectable by CT and angiography were found to have distant metastases by PET *(58)*. The superiority of PET compared to CT and MRI in detecting distant metastases is confirmed in a recent study *(59)*. Given the current state of the technology, PET does not have a routine role in the staging of pancreatic cancer. With the development of new scanners, such as the hybrid PET–CT scanners, which combine the physiological information provided by PET and the morphological information provided by CT, a more useful role in the staging of pancreatic cancer might evolve.

6. TISSUE ACQUISITION

In patients with unresectable pancreatic cancer, it is necessary to have a histological diagnosis before a course of treatment can be initiated. Some surgeons and patients desire to have a pathological diagnosis, even if the tumor appears resectable. Historically, tissue from pancreatic lesions has been obtained percutaneously by CT-guided FNA, ultrasound-guided FNA, or laparoscopic-guided biopsy (Fig. 3). Evolution of techniques using EUS-FNA of targeted tissue provides several advantages over the older techniques. EUS-FNA can obtain tissue from lesions too small to be identified by CT or ultrasound. In addition, lesions encased by major vascular structures, which may not be amenable to a percutaneous

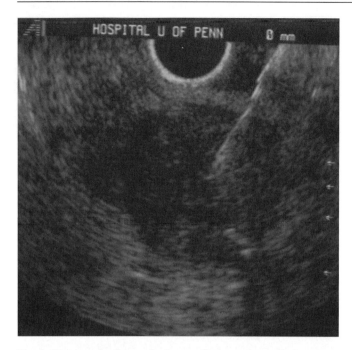

Fig. 3. Passage of a fine aspiration needle into a hypoechoic pancreatic mass under endosonographic guidance.

biopsy, can also be biopsied by EUS-FNA. The AJCC recommends EUS-FNA as the preferred modality for obtaining tissue from suspected pancreatic tumors.

Percutaneous biopsy techniques also introduce a real risk of tumor seeding along the needle track, a risk that is minimized with EUS-FNA. A recent retrospective study compared outcomes in 46 patients in whom a diagnosis of pancreatic cancer was made by EUS-FNA and 43 patients in whom the diagnosis was made by percutaneous FNA *(60)*. Tumor characteristics were similar between the two groups. In the EUS-FNA group, one patient developed peritoneal carcinomatosis compared with seven in the percutaneous FNA group (2.2 vs 16.3%). EUS-FNA is also less invasive and poses fewer risks than a laparoscopic biopsy. Though EUS-FNA introduces a small risk of bleeding, this risk is comparable to that of a diagnostic EUS.

A recent review found a wide range in the sensitivity of EUS-FNA for diagnosing pancreatic cancer as reported by many recent studies. Sensitivity ranged from 64 to 96% *(61)*. Specificity is generally very high (>85%), with the majority of studies reporting EUS-FNA to be nearly 100% specific.

In a review comparing nine studies with on-site pathologists to three studies without, there was a higher sensitivity in those studies with an on-site pathologist (85 vs 76%). In one retrospective study *(61)*, 80 patients with suspected pancreatic cancer had EUS-FNA performed. Of these, 34 patients subsequently underwent surgery or tissue biopsy. Overall, the study found EUS-FNA to have a sensitivity of 78% and a specificity of 100%. They further analyzed the 10 patients who had a negative EUS-FNA, but were found to have cancer. Half of these false-negative cases were felt to be the result of inadequate sampling. Having an on-site cytopathologist to ensure adequate sampling may have potentially eliminated these events.

EUS-FNA is a safe, minimally invasive technique for obtaining tissue for diagnosis in patients with suspected pancreatic cancer. The technique is both sensitive and specific, and results appear improved with utilization of an on-site cytopathologist.

7. RECOMMENDATIONS

Patients with pancreatic cancer usually present with jaundice, abdominal pain, weight loss, or an unexplained episode of pancreatitis. In all such patients, multidetector CT scan with both intravenus and oral contrast is the first diagnostic test of choice. Even in patients who present with painless jaundice, CT scan is recommended as the first diagnostic procedure rather than an ERCP. If a mass is not seen on CT scan and pancreatic pathology is still suspected, then EUS is indicated to assess for a small pancreatic mass. An ERCP may also be performed in patients with jaundice, if it is to assess for biliary strictures or choledocholithiasis, as well as to aid in the evaluation of selected ampullary lesions.

If a pancreatic mass is seen on CT scan, it is reasonable to conclude that a neoplasm is present. Tissue acquisition in such patients is not routinely helpful in a surgical candidate; if the clinical suspicion for a malignant process is high, management would still be surgical resection regardless of the biopsy result. Thus, at our institution, for resectable patients, surgery is routinely undertaken without prior tissue diagnosis.

The most important question for patients with a pancreatic mass is to determine resectability. Approaches to determining resectability vary across institutions and depend on availability of local expertise and the clinicians' comfort with one or the other radiological imaging modality. One approach is to perform a contrast-enhanced hCT scan. If the patient does not have distant metastases and no involvement or minimal involvement of the major vascular structures, then surgical resection is may be attempted, provided the patient is a candidate for surgery, usually accompanied by a preliminary laparoscopy in patients who do not require surgical bypass procedures. In patients with a mass in the body or tail of the pancreas, or in those who have partial involvement of major vessels, a staging laparoscopy is usually performed, which may occur as the prelude to a formal resection.

If the patient has equivocal findings on a quality hCT scan, then EUS with or without FNA should be the next logical step. Alternatively, an MRI may be obtained. The choice of these tests will depend on the available expertise. In cases where the patient has clearly unresectable disease on the initial CT scan, EUS-FNA may be performed before undertaking nonoperative therapy. The role of MRI in the staging work-up of pancreatic cancer is less clear. At our institution, we usually obtain an MRI, when the results of both CT and EUS are equivocal or when the results of these tests are conflicting.

8. CONCLUSION

Pancreatic adenocarcinoma remains a challenging problem into the 21st century. However, improvements in early detection and staging of patients will be expected to facilitate progress in the management of this disease, which relies heavily on surgical removal to effect a cure.

REFERENCES

1. Niederhuber JE, Brennan MF, Menck HR. The National Cancer Data Base report on pancreatic cancer. Cancer 1995; 76(9):1671–1677.

2. Ahrendt SA, Pitt HA. Surgical management of pancreatic cancer. Oncology (Huntington) 2002; 16(6):725–734.

3. Jemal A, Murray T, Samuels A, Ghafoor A, Ward E, Thun MJ. Cancer statistics, 2003. CA Cancer J Clin 2003; 53(1):5–26.

4. Bardeesy N, DePinho RA. Pancreatic cancer biology and genetics. Nat Rev Cancer 2002; 2(12):897–909.

5. DiMagno EP, Reber HA, Tempero MA. AGA technical review on the epidemiology, diagnosis, and treatment of pancreatic ductal adenocarcinoma. American Gastroenterological Association. Gastroenterology 1999; 117(6):1464–1484.

6. Hruban RH, Petersen GM, Ha PK, Kern SE. Genetics of pancreatic cancer. From genes to families. Surg Oncol Clin N Am 1998; 7(1):1–23.

7. Luttges J, Schlehe B, Menke MA, Vogel I, Henne-Bruns D, Kloppel G. The K-ras mutation pattern in pancreatic ductal adenocarcinoma usually is identical to that in associated normal, hyperplastic, and metaplastic ductal epithelium. Cancer 1999; 85(8):1703–1710.

8. Li D, Xie K, Wolff R, Abbruzzese JL. Pancreatic cancer. Lancet 2004; 363(9414):1049–1057.

9. Bakkevold KE, Arnesjo B, Kambestad B. Carcinoma of the pancreas and papilla of Vater: presenting symptoms, signs, and diagnosis related to stage and tumour site. A prospective multicentre trial in 472 patients. Norwegian Pancreatic Cancer Trial. Scand J Gastroenterol 1992; 27(4):317–325.

10. Exocrine pancreas. In: Greene FL, Page DL, Fleming DL, et al, eds. American Joint Committee on Cancer: AJCC Cancer Staging Manual. New York: Springer, 2002; 157–164.

11. Pleskow DK, Berger HJ, Gyves J, Allen E, McLean A, Podolsky DK. Evaluation of a serologic marker, CA19-9, in the diagnosis of pancreatic cancer. Ann Intern Med 1989; 110(9):704–709.

12. Posner MR, Mayer RJ. The use of serologic tumor markers in gastrointestinal malignancies. Hematol Oncol Clin North Am 1994; 8(3):533–553.

13. Safi F, Schlosser W, Falkenreck S, Beger HG. CA 19-9 serum course and prognosis of pancreatic cancer. Int J Pancreatol 1996; 20(3):155–161.

14. Kim HJ, Kim MH, Myung SJ, et al. A new strategy for the application of CA19-9 in the differentiation of pancreaticobiliary cancer: analysis using a receiver operating characteristic curve. Am J Gastroenterol 1999; 94(7):1941–1946.

15. Permert J, Larsson J, Westermark GT, et al. Islet amyloid polypeptide in patients with pancreatic cancer and diabetes. N Engl J Med 1994; 330(5):313–318.

16. Chari ST, Klee GG, Miller LJ, Raimondo M, DiMagno EP. Islet amyloid polypeptide is not a satisfactory marker for detecting pancreatic cancer. Gastroenterology 2001; 121(3):640–645.

17. Uemura T, Hibi K, Kaneko T, et al. Detection of K-ras mutations in the plasma DNA of pancreatic cancer patients. J Gastroenterol 2004; 39(1):56–60.

18. Watanabe H, Sawabu N, Ohta H, et al. Identification of K-ras oncogene mutations in the pure pancreatic juice of patients with ductal pancreatic cancers. Jpn J Cancer Res 1993; 84(9):961–965.

19. Iguchi H, Sugano K, Fukayama N, et al. Analysis of Ki-ras codon 12 mutations in the duodenal juice of patients with pancreatic cancer. Gastroenterology 1996; 110(1):221–226.

20. Caldas C, Hahn SA, Hruban RH, Redston MS, Yeo CJ, Kern SE. Detection of K-ras mutations in the stool of patients with pancreatic adenocarcinoma and pancreatic ductal hyperplasia. Cancer Res 1994; 54(13):3568–3573.

21. Muller MF, Meyenberger C, Bertschinger P, Schaer R, Marincek B. Pancreatic tumors: evaluation with endoscopic US, CT, and MR imaging. Radiology 1994; 190(3):745–751.

22. Valls C, Andia E, Sanchez A, et al. Dual-phase helical CT of pancreatic adenocarcinoma: assessment of resectability before surgery. AJR Am J Roentgenol 2002; 178(4):821–826.

23. Freeny PC, Marks WM, Ryan JA, Traverso LW. Pancreatic ductal adenocarcinoma: diagnosis and staging with dynamic CT. Radiology 1988; 166(1 Part 1):125–133.

24. Freeny PC, Traverso LW, Ryan JA. Diagnosis and staging of pancreatic adenocarcinoma with dynamic computed tomography. Am J Surg 1993; 165(5):600–606.

25. Megibow AJ, Zhou XH, Rotterdam H, et al. Pancreatic adenocarcinoma: CT versus MR imaging in the evaluation of resectability—report of the Radiology Diagnostic Oncology Group. Radiology 1995; 195(2):327–332.

26. Bluemke DA, Cameron JL, Hruban RH, et al. Potentially resectable pancreatic adenocarcinoma: spiral CT assessment with surgical and pathologic correlation. Radiology 1995; 197(2):381–385.

27. Zeman RK, Cooper C, Zeiberg AS, et al. TNM staging of pancreatic carcinoma using helical CT. AJR Am J Roentgenol 1997; 169(2):459–464.

28. Diehl SJ, Lehmann KJ, Sadick M, Lachmann R, Georgi M. Pancreatic cancer: value of dual-phase helical CT in assessing resectability. Radiology 1998; 206(2):373–378.

29. Lu DS, Reber HA, Krasny RM, Kadell BM, Sayre J. Local staging of pancreatic cancer: criteria for unresectability of major vessels as revealed by pancreatic-phase, thin-section helical CT. AJR Am J Roentgenol 1997; 168(6):1439–1443.

30. Roche CJ, Hughes ML, Garvey CJ, et al. CT and pathologic assessment of prospective nodal staging in patients with ductal adenocarcinoma of the head of the pancreas. AJR Am J Roentgenol 2003; 180(2):475–480.

31. Gress FG, Hawes RH, Savides TJ, et al. Role of EUS in the preoperative staging of pancreatic cancer: a large single-center experience. Gastrointest Endosc 1999; 50(6):786–791.

32. Akahoshi K, Chijiiwa Y, Nakano I, et al. Diagnosis and staging of pancreatic cancer by endoscopic ultrasound. Br J Radiol 1998; 71(845):492–496.

33. Baron PL, Aabakken LE, Cole DJ, et al. Differentiation of benign from malignant pancreatic masses by endoscopic ultrasound. Ann Surg Oncol 1997; 4(8):639–643.

34. Legmann P, Vignaux O, Dousset B, et al. Pancreatic tumors: comparison of dual-phase helical CT and endoscopic sonography. AJR Am J Roentgenol 1998; 170(5):1315–1322.

35. Rosch T, Lorenz R, Braig C, et al. Endoscopic ultrasound in pancreatic tumor diagnosis. Gastrointest Endosc 1991; 37(3):347–352.

36. Snady H, Cooperman A, Siegel J. Endoscopic ultrasonography compared with computed tomography with ERCP in patients with obstructive jaundice or small peri-pancreatic mass. Gastrointest Endosc 1992; 38(1):27–34.

37. Yasuda K, Mukai H, Fujimoto S, Nakajima M, Kawai K. The diagnosis of pancreatic cancer by endoscopic ultrasonography. Gastrointest Endosc 1988; 34(1):1–8.

38. Nakaizumi A, Uehara H, Iishi H, et al. Endoscopic ultrasonography in diagnosis and staging of pancreatic cancer. Dig Dis Sci 1995; 40(3):696–700.

39. Palazzo L, Roseau G, Gayet B, et al. Endoscopic ultrasonography in the diagnosis and staging of pancreatic adenocarcinoma. Results of a prospective study with comparison to ultrasonography and CT scan. Endoscopy 1993; 25(2):143–150.

40. Gress FG. The role of endoscopic ultrasound in the staging of pancreatic adenocarcinoma. In: Rose BD, editor. UpToDate. Wellesley, MA: 2004.

41. Yusoff IF, Mendelson RM, Edmunds SE, et al. Preoperative assessment of pancreatic malignancy using endoscopic ultrasound. Abdom Imaging 2003; 28(4):556–562.

42. Ahmad NA, Lewis JD, Ginsberg GG, Rosato EF, Morris JB, Kochman ML. EUS in preoperative staging of pancreatic cancer. Gastrointest Endosc 2000; 52(4):463–468.

43. Rosch T, Dittler HJ, Strobel K, R et al. Endoscopic ultrasound criteria for vascular invasion in the staging of cancer of the head of the pancreas: a blind reevaluation of videotapes. Gastrointest Endosc 2000; 52(4):469–477.

44. Rosch T, Braig C, Gain T, et al. Staging of pancreatic and ampullary carcinoma by endoscopic ultrasonography. Comparison with

conventional sonography, computed tomography, and angiography. Gastroenterology 1992; 102(1):188–199.

45. Soriano A, Castells A, Ayuso C, et al. Preoperative staging and tumor resectability assessment of pancreatic cancer: prospective study comparing endoscopic ultrasonography, helical computed tomography, magnetic resonance imaging, and angiography. Am J Gastroenterol 2004; 99(3):492–501.

46. Ahmad NA, Lewis JD, Siegelman ES, Rosato EF, Ginsberg GG, Kochman ML. Role of endoscopic ultrasound and magnetic resonance imaging in the preoperative staging of pancreatic adenocarcinoma. Am J Gastroenterol 2000; 95(8):1926–1931.

47. Varghese JC, Farrell MA, Courtney G, Osborne H, Murray FE, Lee MJ. Role of MR cholangiopancreatography in patients with failed or inadequate ERCP. AJR Am J Roentgenol 1999; 173(6):1527–1533.

48. Adamek HE, Albert J, Breer H, Weitz M, Schilling D, Riemann JF. Pancreatic cancer detection with magnetic resonance cholangiopancreatography and endoscopic retrograde cholangiopancreatography: a prospective controlled study. Lancet 2000; 356(9225): 190–193.

49. Friess H, Langhans J, Ebert M, et al. Diagnosis of pancreatic cancer by 2[18F]-fluoro-2-deoxy-D-glucose positron emission tomography. Gut 1995; 36(5):771–777.

50. Bares R, Klever P, Hauptmann S, et al. F-18 fluorodeoxyglucose PET in vivo evaluation of pancreatic glucose metabolism for detection of pancreatic cancer. Radiology 1994; 192(1):79–86.

51. Kato T, Fukatsu H, Ito K, et al. Fluorodeoxyglucose positron emission tomography in pancreatic cancer: an unsolved problem. Eur J Nucl Med 1995; 22(1):32–39.

52. Ho CL, Dehdashti F, Griffeth LK, Buse PE, Balfe DM, Siegel BA. FDG-PET evaluation of indeterminate pancreatic masses. J Comput Assist Tomogr 1996; 20(3):363–369.

53. Zimny M, Bares R, Fass J, et al. Fluorine-18 fluorodeoxyglucose positron emission tomography in the differential diagnosis of pancreatic carcinoma: a report of 106 cases. Eur J Nucl Med 1997; 24(6):678–682.

54. Delbeke D, Rose DM, Chapman WC, et al. Optimal interpretation of FDG PET in the diagnosis, staging and management of pancreatic carcinoma. J Nucl Med 1999; 40(11):1784–1791.

55. Kasperk RK, Riesener KP, Wilms K, Schumpelick V. Limited value of positron emission tomography in treatment of pancreatic cancer: surgeon's view. World J Surg 2001; 25(9):1134–1139.

56. Frohlich A, Diederichs CG, Staib L, Vogel J, Beger HG, Reske SN. Detection of liver metastases from pancreatic cancer using FDG PET. J Nucl Med 1999; 40(2):250–255.

57. Berberat P, Friess H, Kashiwagi M, Beger HG, Buchler MW. Diagnosis and staging of pancreatic cancer by positron emission tomography. World J Surg 1999; 23(9):882–887.

58. Bares R, Dohmen BM, Cremerius U, Fass J, Teusch M, Bull U. (Results of positron emission tomography with fluorine-18 labeled fluorodeoxyglucose in differential diagnosis and staging of pancreatic carcinoma). Radiologe 1996; 36(5):435–440.

59. Koyama K, Okamura T, Kawabe J, et al. Diagnostic usefulness of FDG PET for pancreatic mass lesions. Ann Nucl Med 2001; 15(3):217–224.

60. Micames C, Jowell PS, White R, et al. Lower frequency of peritoneal carcinomatosis in patients with pancreatic cancer diagnosed by EUS-guided FNA vs percutaneous FNA. Gastrointest Endosc 2003; 58(5):690–695.

61. Ylagan LR, Edmundowicz S, Kasal K, Walsh D, Lu DW. Endoscopic ultrasound guided fine-needle aspiration cytology of pancreatic carcinoma: a 3-year experience and review of the literature. Cancer 2002; 96(6):362–369.

26 Adenocarcinoma of the Pancreas
Endoscopic Palliation

GEORGIOS I. PAPACHRISTOU, MD, KEVIN MCGRATH, MD,
AND ADAM SLIVKA, MD, PhD

CONTENTS

BACKGROUND
INTRODUCTION
PALLIATION OF MALIGNANT BILIARY OBSTRUCTION
PALLIATION OF PAIN
PANCREATIC STENTING
ENDOSCOPIC ADJUVANT THERAPY
PALLIATION OF DUODENAL OBSTRUCTION
REFERENCES

1. BACKGROUND

Endoscopic approaches have revolutionized the palliation of advanced pancreatic cancer. The ideal management consists of a team approach involving surgeons, endoscopists, radiologists, and oncologists. Further technical improvements are needed to tackle the problem of stent occlusion. Concurrent advances in the fields of interventional radiology and laparoscopic surgical oncology need to be readdressed and directly compared with endoscopic approaches in novel randomized controlled trials.

2. INTRODUCTION

Approximately 32,000 new cases of pancreatic cancer were estimated to occur in the United States in 2004. Only a minority of these patients are eligible for curative resection at the time of diagnosis *(1)*. Those who undergo surgical resection have a long-term survival rate of approx 20% and a median survival of 13–20 mo. The main causes of unresectability include local or vascular invasion and metastatic disease. The 5-yr survival of pancreatic cancer is 4%, which is the lowest survival rate in comparison with all the other cancer sites *(2)*. Therefore, for the majority of pancreas cancer patients, palliative treatments constitute the cornerstone of care. Endoscopic therapy offers a non-invasive management option for the three major symptoms: obstructive jaundice resulting from neoplastic compression or invasion of the common bile duct (CBD), nausea, vomiting and inanition from gastric outlet obstruction (GOO), and pain resulting from neoplastic infiltration of adjacent nerve terminals, or from compression of the pancreatic duct (PD) with proximal PD

From: *Endoscopic Oncology: Gastrointestinal Endoscopy and Cancer Management.* Edited by: D. O. Faigel and M. L. Kochman © Humana Press, Totowa, NJ

dilation. Endoscopic biliary, enteral, and pancreatic stenting techniques, as well as endoscopic ultrasound (EUS)-guided celiac plexus neurolysis (CPN) have a remarkable efficacy with low morbidity and mortality. Endoscopic approaches are, therefore, considered first-line treatment for palliation in cases of inoperable or unresectable pancreatic tumors. Furthermore, endoscopic stenting can be used pre-operatively in patients with potentially resectable tumors and those who are candidates for neoadjuvant therapy with chemoradiation.

3. PALLIATION OF MALIGNANT BILIARY OBSTRUCTION

3.1. INDICATIONS

Before palliative biliary stent placement, it is important to confirm that the jaundice is resulting from biliary obstruction and not secondary to extensive intrahepatic metastatic disease. This can be assessed by several hepatic imaging studies, preferably by triphasic computed tomography (CT) or magnetic resonance imaging, which will also yield information regarding local unresectability and distant metastases *(3)*.

Quality-of-life improvement is the major goal of palliation. Therefore, it is important to assess if alleviating the jaundice is likely to provide true quality-of-life improvement to the patient. Prolonged biliary obstruction may result in pruritus, malabsorption, and consequent progressive malnutrition; recurrent attacks of cholangitis; and hepatic dysfunction. Moreover, relief of jaundice could provide a much-needed psychological boost to the patient and family members. However, up until recently, there were only scant objective data to support this concept. A recent study assessed prospectively the impact of endoscopic biliary decompression on the different physical, psychological, and social components of quality of life in patients with unresectable pancreatic cancer without liver

303

metastases *(4)*. In patients with baseline bilirubin under 14 mg/dL, biliary stenting resulted in improvement of the general and specific well being.

3.2. TECHNIQUE OF BILIARY STENTING

A complete cholangiogram to identify the location and extent of the stricture is the first step to effective biliary drainage. This information can be acquired before endoscopic retrograde cholangiopancreatography (ERCP) by magnetic resonance cholangiopancreatography (MRCP). This way, forceful contrast injection especially in strictures involving the main hepatic confluence or intrahepatic bile ducts during ERCP can be avoided, which decreases the risk of cholangitis.

ERCP is performed under moderate sedation. Deep selective cannulation of the CBD is achieved with a biliary catheter, a guidewire is manipulated across the stricture and advanced into the obstructed bile ducts to maintain access and facilitate exchange. Hydrophilic guidewires can expedite passage through tight and tortuous strictures when compared with Teflon-coated guidewires.

When indicated, tissue sampling (by endoscopic transpapillary wire-guided brush cytology, endoluminal forceps biopsy, or transductal fine-needle aspiration [FNA]) might be obtained from the stricture before stenting *(5,6)*. These techniques are usually performed under fluoroscopic guidance or occasionally under direct vision through per oral choledochoscopy *(7)*. The specificity and positive predictive value for these techniques approaches 100% *(8)*, indicating that a positive specimen is virtually diagnostic of malignancy. However, the sensitivity of tissue sampling is still relatively low, ranging from 15 to 70%; therefore, a negative result does not exclude malignancy. Combining a second or a third tissue sampling modality has shown to increase sensitivity *(9)*. For this reason, EUS with FNA, which has more than 80% sensitivity before ERCP is being routinely performed at many expert centers *(10)*, including our own. Catheter or balloon dilation of the stricture may be performed before stent placement, but is rarely needed *(11)*. Several techniques have been described for stent placement. The most widely used procedure involves advancing a stiff polyethylene inner catheter with radio-opaque markers (guide catheter) over the guidewire. The plastic biliary stent is then advanced over the complex guidewire/inner catheter using an outer pusher device as a three-layer system. The inner catheter and guidewire are then withdrawn leaving the stent in position. A single-assembly stent delivery system is available from several manufacturers. In a small, randomized trial, stent insertion appeared to be easier and faster with these systems compared with the standard three-layer system *(12)*. These procedures are performed under fluoroscopic guidance and a therapeutic duodenoscope that has an accessory channel of at least 3.8 mm is used. Biliary sphincterotomy is not generally required before stent insertion; however, it might be performed to facilitate future exchange or if placement of more than one stent is anticipated. Whether or not biliary sphincterotomy affects the risks of the procedure is controversial. A retrospective study suggested that the incidence of acute complications of biliary stent placement was higher in patients undergoing sphincterotomy and concluded that sphincterotomy

is not necessary *(13)*. In contrast, in a smaller case series, biliary sphincterotomy seemed to reduce the risk of post-ERCP pancreatitis in patients with malignant biliary obstruction requiring plastic stents 9 cm or longer *(14)*. Complex hilar strictures, involving the hepatic bifurcation, constitute a challenge for the endoscopist, but are rarely seen in pancreatic cancer. Ideally, stent placement should relieve both jaundice and cholestasis, which can be achieved by draining only one major segment *(15)*. In a retrospective study, patients with malignant hilar obstruction who had both the right and left systems opacified at ERCP but who then had only one system drained faired poorly compared with patients who had both lobes opacified and both lobes drained with bilateral stents and those had one lobe opacified and one lobe drained with a single stent *(16)*. However, in a randomized controlled trial of unilateral vs bilateral stenting for malignant biliary obstruction, De Palma and colleagues found less morbidity in patients randomized to unilateral drainage *(17)*. As a result of these findings, the authors have adopted the strategy of Hintze and colleagues in obtaining an MRCP before ERCP in all patients suspected of having biliary obstruction at the hilum *(18)*. This allows for pre-operative determination of the dominant obstructed segment, wire access to this segment avoiding contrast injection into other segments and targeted unilateral stent drainage.

The main causes of endoscopic failures include inaccessibility to the ampulla resulting from prior surgery or tumor infiltration of the duodenum, inability to cannulate the CBD, or to pass a guidewire through the stricture. In centers with adequate experience, endoscopic stent placement has a technical success of 90% or higher. Palliation of jaundice and pruritus should be expected in more than 80% of patients achieving a complete drainage of the bile ducts. Complications include acute pancreatitis, bleeding, cholangitis, and perforation. Acute cholangitis is seen with unsuccessful or incomplete drainage. When serum bilirubin remains persistently elevated, then the stent patency should be assessed by repeat ERCP.

3.3. TYPES OF BILIARY STENTS
3.3.1. Plastic Stents

In 1980, Soehendra and Reynders–Frederix described for the first time the endoscopic insertion of a 7-French (F) biliary stent to restore biliary flow in a distal CBD tumor *(19)*. For many years plastic stents had been the only available devices and today they still represent a valid therapeutic option (Fig. 1A). The most common configuration is a straight or curved stent with side flaps at each end to minimize the risk of proximal or distal migration, which may still occur up to 9% of patients *(13)* (Fig. 1B). The intent is to place the stent with the proximal flap located above the stricture and the distal flap just outside the papilla within the duodenal lumen.

The major problem encountered with the use of plastic stents is their tendency to occlude over time, leading to recurrent jaundice and cholangitis (Fig. 1C). Bile is ordinarily sterile. However, with the loss of the barrier function of the sphincter of Oddi, as occurs with stent placement, the biliary system is rapidly colonized with intestinal bacteria *(20)*. Clogging of plastic stents involves a complex mechanism starting with the formation of a biofilm on the inner surface of the stent. The

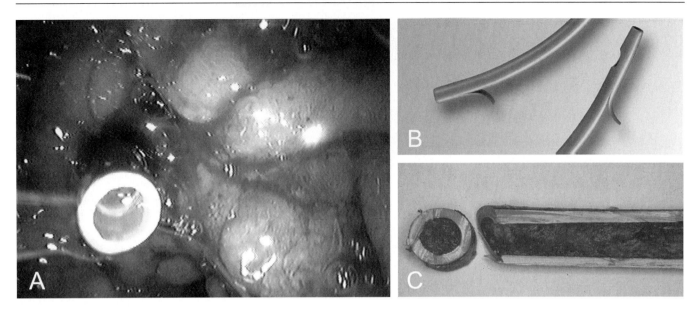

Fig. 1. **(A)** Endoscopy showing a plastic stent protruding from the ampulla which is infiltrated by pancreatic cancer. **(B)** The outer and inner tip of a plastic biliary stent with a single external and internal flap. **(C)** Longitudinal and transverse section of a plastic biliary stent occluded with sludge.

biofilm consists of cellular debris and microcolonies of bacteria in a matrix of extracellular anionic fibrillar material *(21)*. Once formed, it has been impossible to eliminate this biofilm from an indwelling stent. Stent function becomes impaired after weeks or months and results in the need to exchange stents in up to 30–60% of surviving patients *(22)*.

Many different approaches to prolong stent patency have been studied. Despite promising results in vitro, oral administration of mucolytic agents (i.e., aspirin), or choleretic agents (i.e., ursodeoxycholic acid) to alter the composition of bile combined with different antibiotics have not shown any consistent effects on preventing biliary stent occlusion in clinical practice *(23–25)*. Prevention of biofilm formation and adherence of bacteria was also tested by impregnating stents with bactericidal agents *(26)*, by designing stents that resist adherence and by making stents from ultrasmooth materials. It has been observed that larger amounts of sludge formation occurs around the stent side holes and flaps, most probably because of turbulent intraluminal bile flow *(27)*. Preliminary uncontrolled studies suggested a prolonged patency of Teflon stents without side holes compared with conventional plastic stents with side holes *(28)*. These results, however, were not confirmed by subsequent randomized trials *(29,30)*. In vitro studies using polyurethane covered with a hydrophilic polymer as stent material have shown an ultrasmooth surface with a very low friction coefficient that result in reduced bacterial adherence *(31)*. However, a significant longer patency of these polyurethane stents was not demonstrated in vivo when compared with standard plastic endoprostheses. This could be explained by the stent manipulation taking place during the endoscopic procedure that might damage the inner surface characteristics of the ultrasmooth material *(32,33)*.

The most direct approach to prolong patency is by increasing the diameter of the inserted plastic stent. In theory, a larger diameter stent provides greater flow through its lumen, leading to the notion that larger stents will decrease the rates of clogging (Poiseuille's law).

3.3.2. Poiseuille's Law

Laminar nonpulsatile flow $= \Delta P \times \pi \times r^4/8n \times L$

where r, radius of stent; L, length of stent; n, fluid viscosity.

There is clinical evidence that 10 French stents have significantly longer patency compared with 7- and 8-F stents *(34,35)*. However, 11.5-F stents have not shown prolonged patency compared with 10-F stents *(36)*. Therefore, 10-F stents are usually the preferred choice. The length of the stent is chosen according to the location of the stricture and may vary between 3 and 15 cm.

Stent occlusion may occur from days to several months after placement, with an average of 3–4 mo for 10-F stents. Removal and replacement of a clogged stent can be performed in an outpatient setting with repeat ERCP. Plastic stents can be extracted with a snare or basket through the endoscope channel whereas maintaining a cannulation position. Guidewire-assisted techniques allow the endoscopist to maintain access across the biliary stricture during stent removal *(37)*.

The optimal time interval for stent exchange is still debatable. Some experts practice regular elective stent exchange every 3 mo, whereas others proceed with stent exchange at the earliest clinical or laboratory signs of stent occlusion. The former practice carries the risk of performing more stent exchange procedures than necessary, whereas the latter option carries the risk of developing severe cholangitis secondary to stent occlusion. It is probably wise to "personalize" the endoscopic stent replacement strategy. Planned stent exchange is usually preferable in patients who are unable to maintain close follow-up, whereas compliant patients with easy access to the system may follow an "on demand" stent exchange strategy *(38)*.

Biliary stent migration can occur proximally or distally, at the time of insertion or at a later point of time. Factors that appear to be associated with stent migration include larger stent diameter,

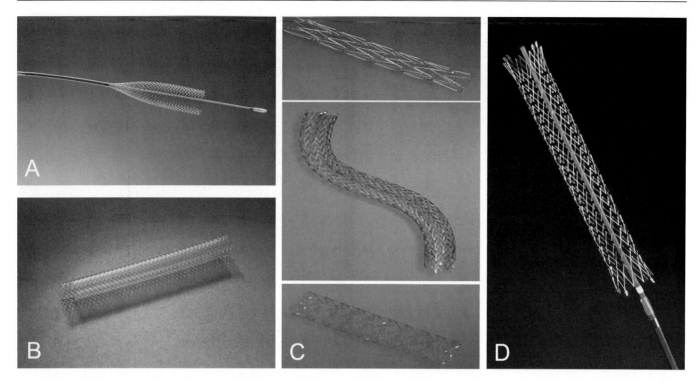

Fig. 2. Different types of metal stents. (**A**) Wallstent. (**B**) Covered Wallstent. (**C**) Z-stent, Zilver stent, and Za-stent. (**D**) Luminex.

proximal bile duct strictures and performance of sphincterotomy. The incidence of stent migration is 3–9% and most of the cases can be readily managed endoscopically *(13,39)*.

3.4. METAL STENTS

In search of a solution to the problem of plastic stent occlusion, self-expandable metal stents (SEMS) were introduced into clinical practice in early 1990s. Initially, they were deployed through the percutaneous transhepatic route, but have since been modified for endoscopic placement. Currently, several different types of metal biliary stents are available, varying in cell design and material. Examples include the Wallstent (Boston Scientific, Natick, MA), the Zilver Stent (Wilson-Cook Medical, Winston-Salem, NC) and the Luminex (Bard Inc., Billerica, MA) *(40)* (Fig. 2). All these types of stents are delivered in a collapsed configuration over a 7- or 8-F delivery catheter.

Most published experience has been gained with the Wallstent, which is a tubular mesh made from stainless steel alloy. The system is passed over a 0.035-in. guidewire and positioned across the malignant stricture under fluoroscopy with the aid of radiopaque markers on the delivery catheter. Controlled slow release of the Wallstent requires coordination between the endoscopist and assistant (Fig. 3). When fully expanded, the Wallstent can reach a diameter of 30 F. Because of its inherent expansible properties, it can shorten up to 30% to the designated length of 40, 60, or 80 mm. Once fully deployed, the Wallstent becomes embedded in the bile duct wall and the tissue beneath undergoes superficial necrosis. The inflammatory and fibrotic reaction progressively incorporates the stent, eliminating the possibility of its migration *(41)*.

Studies comparing the performance of different stents, which vary in material and cell design, have been performed. A retrospective comparison of Wallstent and Ultraflex Diamond (Boston

Scientific) stents (an open mesh metal stent popular in Europe), in patients with distal malignant biliary obstruction concluded that there were no differences in efficacy of biliary drainage nor in long-term stent patency *(42)*. However, a subsequent retrospective study showed higher patency rates for the Wallstent in comparison with the Diamond stent *(43)*. A recent randomized clinical trial compared the treatment with Wallstent vs spiral Z-stents for malignant biliary obstruction and found no differences in ease of placement, occlusion rates, and overall patency *(44)*.

The technical success of metal stent placement is very high and the early procedural morbidity is low. In addition, their ease of placement owing to a small and flexible delivery system and their increased luminal diameter makes SEMS a very appealing and safe alternative to the plastic stents. It is very important, however, to fully assess the resectability of the malignant stricture before their placement because metal stents cannot be removed once fully implanted. Therefore, if there is any doubt, a plastic stent is initially recommended with the possibility of metal stent placement, if indicated, at the time of first stent exchange.

Despite their larger diameter and the lower incidence of sludge and bacteria deposition, metal stent occlusion can still be seen in about 22–33% of patients *(45,46)*. It is a result of several factors, including tumor ingrowth through the interstices of the metal mesh, tumor overgrowth at either end of the stent, which was not previously encountered with the plastic stents, biliary epithelial hyperplasia, and sludge. Recanalization of occluded metal stents can be achieved endoscopically with the insertion of additional metal or plastic stents inside the clogged one *(47)*. Diathermic debulking of the obstructing tissue has been tested, but appears to carry a high risk of bleeding, ductal perforation, stent fragmentation and is only temporary, and therefore best avoided *(48,49)*. Covered metal stents have

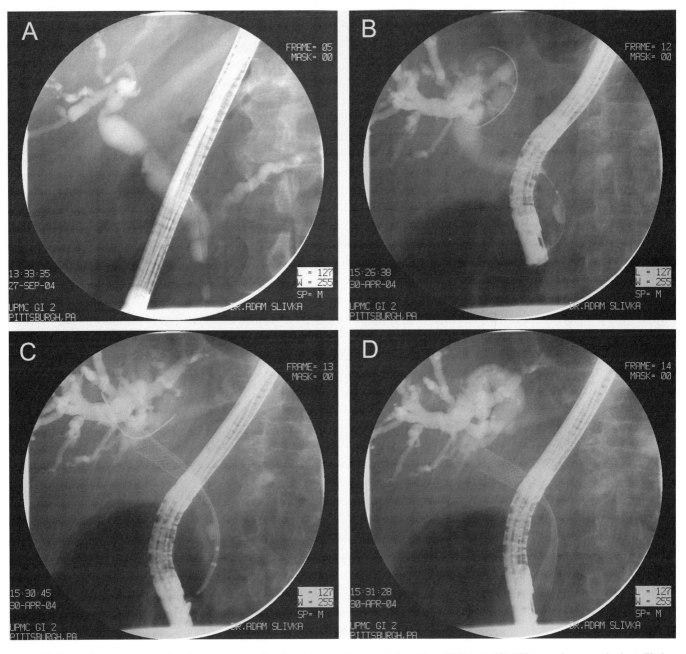

Fig. 3. Endoscopic retrograde cholangiopancreatography showing the placement of a biliary Wallstent. **(A)** Biliary and pancreatic duct dilation with distal stricture owing to pancreatic carcinoma (double duct sign). **(B)** Deep cannulation of the common bile duct and a guidewire advanced through the biliary stricture. **(C)** Controlled gradual release of the Wallstent. **(D)** The fully deployed stent.

been recently introduced aiming to protect against tumor ingrowth. In vitro studies have indicated that metal stents covered with a silicon membrane may be useful *(50)*. In a recent uncontrolled study, the polyurethane-covered Wallstent has shown a low occlusion rate of 14% *(51)*. Covered metal stents can also become occluded by bacterial adherence to the membrane coating. They may also be more prone to migrate. Long-term outcomes for covered metal stents have yet to be published.

3.5. OUTCOMES

3.5.1. Endoscopic vs Surgical vs Percutaneous Palliation for Malignant Biliary Obstruction

Complete surgical resection should always be considered in fit subjects with early pancreatic cancer because it is the only potential curative therapy. Patients with unresectable tumors or who are not candidates for a major surgery should be offered palliative decompression. Several randomized trials have compared surgical vs endoscopic palliation of malignant obstructive jaundice *(52–54)*. The procedure success rate and efficacy in relieving jaundice were comparable between both techniques at 90%. However, the procedure-related morbidity and mortality and the length of initial hospital stay were significantly lower in the endoscopic group. This initial benefit favoring endoscopy was balanced by the higher late complication rate mainly owing to stent dysfunction and subsequent need for frequent hospital visits. Although the 30-d mortality rate was lower for the endoscopic approach, there was no difference in terms of overall survival between the two groups.

A recent meta-analysis recommended the endoscopic approach for patients with a predicted survival of less than 6 mo, accounting for the vast majority of pancreas cancer patients, and palliative surgery in patients with longer life expectancy (55). These results should, however, be readdressed in light of recent stent advances. The current availability of SEMS favors the endoscopic approach owing to reduced stent occlusion rate in comparison to the plastic stents and the evolution of enteral stents to treat GOO nonoperatively. On the contrary, recent advances in laparoscopic biliary bypass with reduced immediate complication rate and lower length of initial hospitalization might favor the surgical approach.

Several studies have compared percutaneous transhepatic vs endoscopic stent placement in malignant biliary obstruction. The endoscopic route proved to be safer and more effective compared with the transhepatic technique when using plastic stents (56). There are no studies comparing endoscopic vs percutaneous metal stent placement. In most institutions that both techniques are available, an endoscopic approach is considered the preferred choice, with a percutaneous transhepatic route reserved for cases of endoscopic failure.

Overall, endoscopic placement of a biliary stent should be recommended in nonoperative subjects owing to large tumor burden or substantial comorbid illnesses. For those patients in the intermediate category in terms of tumor burden, general health status and expected survival, the decision is more complex. The patient and the physician should decide between a surgical approach, which is invasive, expensive, has a higher risk of immediate complications, but may be more effective on the long-term, vs an endoscopic approach which is quicker and safer method, but may need to be repeated in follow-up.

The use of biliary stents pre-operatively, in patients with resectable pancreatic cancer to reduce serum bilirubin levels and improve nutritional status is controversial. Multiple trials have reported inconsistent effects on operative morbidity and mortality (57–60). A recent meta-analysis of the available data concluded that there is no positive or negative effect of preoperative stent placement on the outcome of surgery in pancreatic cancer patients (61). However, in everyday practice, many patients continue to undergo preoperative biliary stenting (11). Our proposed algorithm for management of patients with suspected pancreatic cancer is summarized in Fig. 4.

3.5.2. Metal vs Plastic Stents

Plastic stents are inexpensive, effective, but have a limited patency with a mean occlusion interval of 3–4 mo. SEMS are more expensive, remain patent longer, but can also become clogged by tumor ingrowth and overgrowth. Moreover, metal stents are not removable. Four randomized controlled trials have been reported that directly compared SEMS to plastic stents (62–65). Overall, metal stents have shown significantly longer patency rates. Plastic stents are associated with a higher rate of cholangitis and occlusion and a more prolonged hospitalization in comparison with metal stents. Metal stents were found to be cost-effective in patients who survived beyond 3–4 mo because the overall number of ERCPs required for stent exchange was reduced by 28% (62). However, there was no significant difference in overall patient survival.

Keeping in mind the high cost of metal stents, it would be desirable to identify patients at risk for early metal stent occlusion. A recent study reported that the metal stent patency rate is not affected by tumor type, stricture morphology, length of the stent, age of patient, or initial bilirubin levels, whereas the ease of passage across the stricture of large-caliber devices before stent placement, and the adequate expansion of metal stents constitute predictors of longer patency (66). The patency rates between metal and plastic stents have been shown to run parallel during the first 3 mo (40). Thereafter, the curves diverge in favor of metal stents. Thus, insertion of a metal stent becomes cost-effective only in patients with a life expectancy that exceeds 3 mo. Another recent study demonstrated that the presence or absence of liver metastases can be used as an indicator of stent selection. Patients with liver metastases have a short life expectancy and should preferably receive plastic stents, whereas metal expandable stents would be more cost-effective in patients without tumor spread to the liver (67). In summary, advancement in techniques and technology of stent therapy to palliate malignant biliary obstruction have allowed for outpatient endoscopic management for the vast majority of patients with obstructive jaundice owing to pancreatic cancer.

4. PALLIATION OF PAIN

4.1. CELIAC PLEXUS NEUROLYSIS

The majority of pancreatic cancer patients have pain (68,69), therefore pain control and quality of life are of paramount importance in this unfortunate group of patients with limited life expectancy. Opioid administration is frequently necessary, however side effects such as constipation, nausea, vomiting, and drowsiness may limit dosing and effect. CPN, where the celiac plexus is ablated with a neurolytic agent, has additionally been offered to pancreatic cancer patients for pain control. Typically, alcohol or phenol have been injected into the celiac plexus in hopes of interrupting visceral afferent pain transmission. Traditionally, this has been performed via direct injection of the celiac plexus at the time of attempted resection, or percutaneously under fluoroscopic guidance by trained anesthesiologists using vertebral landmarks. Randomized studies have reported improved pain scores following CPN with both techniques, although opioid use is still generally necessary (70–72).

Given concern for neurological complications (paresis and paresthesia) with the fluoroscopically guided posterior approach, anterior approaches to CPN have been performed under ultrasound and CT guidance in the last decade with similar efficacy (73–77). Hollow-viscus and solid-organ puncture are concerns when the celiac plexus is accessed via the anterior percutaneous approach. Fortunately, major complications with both anterior and posterior percutaneous CPN are rare.

In 1995, EUS-guided CPN was first reported (78). Given the anatomic relation of the celiac plexus to the gastric lumen, this appears to be an ideal technique for improved localization of this targeted therapy. The celiac plexus is composed of an interconnecting network of ganglia and nerve fibers that surround the origin of the celiac trunk (79). Linear endosonographic imaging from the posterior lesser curve of the stomach allows easy identification of the celiac trunk as the first major branch from the

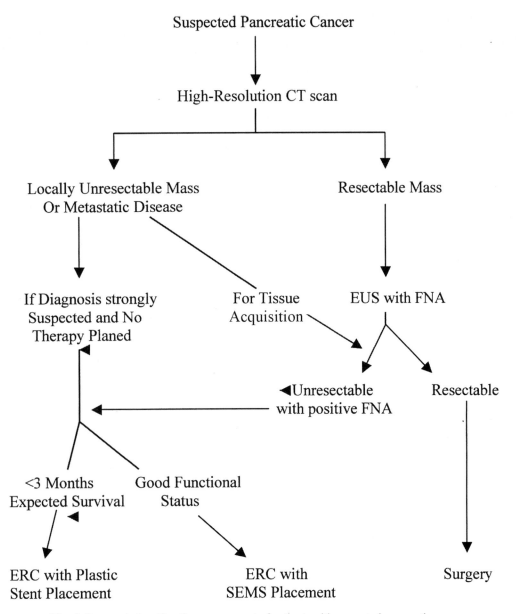

Fig. 4. Proposed algorithm for management of patients with suspected pancreatic cancer.

aorta (Fig. 5A). Under real-time EUS guidance, a saline-primed needle (22- or 19-gauge) can be advanced just anterior to the celiac trunk origin in the antecrural space (Fig. 5B,C). After an aspiration test to assure no blood return, varying amounts of 0.25% bupivicaine (6–20 mL) and 98% dehydrated alcohol (10–20 mL) are injected into the region of the celiac plexus (79–82). Alcohol injection results in an echogenic cloud that diffuses in the antecrural space surrounding the celiac plexus, providing neurolysis (Fig. 5D). Injection techniques vary as the total volume can be injected into a single site (anterior to the celiac origin) or bilaterally, with needle placement immediately lateral to the aorta at the level of the celiac trunk origin. To date, there have been no trials comparing the volume or technique of the neurolytic injection. Patients are monitored for 2 h before discharge, as complications of EUS-guided CPN are rare but include increased pain (9%), postural hypotension (20%), and diarrhea (17%), all of which are generally transient (81).

The largest experience with EUS-guided CPN reported significant improvement in pain scores following neurolysis. Of 58 patients, 45 (78%) experienced a decrease in pain score, with overall scores significantly lower 2 wk after CPN. Pain relief from concomitant adjuvant therapy increased over time, and opioid use was not altered. Multivariate analysis showed sustained pain relief for 24 wk independent of adjuvant therapy and opioid use (81). Although optimistic, this small-uncontrolled trial also reported that the benefit of CPN decreased at 8–12 wk in patients not receiving adjuvant therapy (79,81).

Larger randomized controlled trials evaluating the efficacy of EUS-guided CPN are warranted, as this technique must be subjected to the same rigorous evaluation as other CPN techniques. Extrapolation from the published literature shows that CPN improves pain relief in pancreatic cancer patients. Better localization of the neurolytic injection via EUS guidance may offer better efficacy, but this remains to be proven.

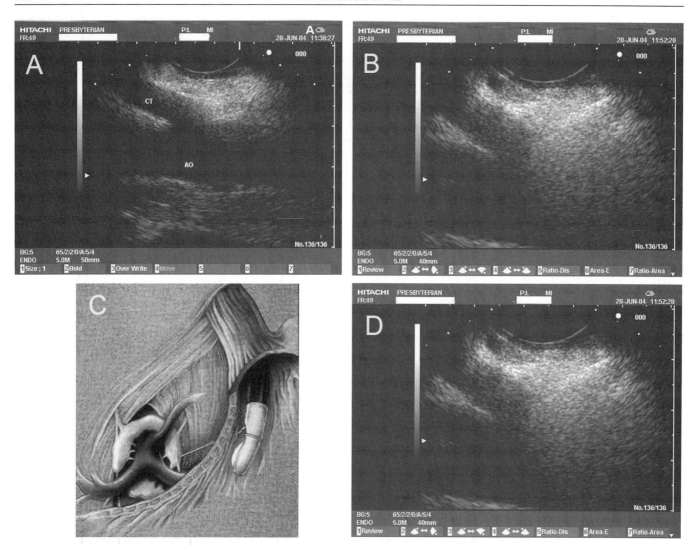

Fig. 5. (**A**) Linear EUS image of the celiac trunk origin from the aorta (CT, celiac trunk; AO, aorta). (**B**) A 22-gauge needle is guided immediately anterior to the celiac trunk origin. Small arrowhead marks the needle tip. (**C**) Illustration of EUS-guided CPN. Needle position is anterior and lateral to the celiac artery origin. (Courtesy of Jane Watson, CMI. Reprinted with permission from ref. *80.*) (**D**) An echogenic cloud from alcohol injection obscures the celiac trunk origin.

5. PANCREATIC STENTING

5.1. INDICATIONS

Pain related to PD obstruction occurs in about 15% of patients with advanced pancreatic cancer. This pain has an "obstructive" quality and is characterized by postprandial exacerbations and elevated pancreatic enzymes. At times it can be very severe and difficult to control with analgesic medications.

The principle of pancreatic stenting for palliation of pancreatic cancer pain is to relieve the neoplastic compression of the main PD and the upstream dilation. PD stents aim to traverse the ductal stricture, restore the impaired pancreaticoduodenal flow and subsequently reduce the ductal hypertension, which is considered a possible cause of pain in these patients. Before palliative pancreatic stent placement, it is important to confirm the PD obstruction with upstream dilation. This can be assessed similarly to the biliary obstruction by pancreatic protocol CT scan or MRCP.

5.2. TECHNIQUE OF PANCREATIC STENTING

The technique of pancreatic stenting is similar to that applied for biliary strictures. ERCP is performed under moderate sedation. A deep selective cannulation of the main PD is then attempted. A catheter is used and a hydrophilic guidewire is manipulated across the stricture and advanced to the tail of the pancreas to maintain access. At this point, the catheter is advanced over the guidewire and catheter dilation of the stricture is performed before the stent is placed. Five- to 7-F polyethylene stents are placed through the stricture. When obstructive jaundice co-exists, endoscopic insertion of biliary stents can be attempted during the same procedure either prior or after the pancreatic stent placement. Placement of a metal biliary stent may make pancreatic stent placement difficult.

5.3. OUTCOMES

Two recent studies have assessed the effect of pancreatic stenting in subjects with pancreatic cancer, "obstructive" pain, and dilation of the main PD beyond the ductal stricture and produced impressive results *(83,84)*. There were no procedure-related complications reported. About 50–60% of the subjects became symptom-free, and another 20–25% significantly reduced the amount of their analgesic consumption. Therefore, endoscopic pancreatic stenting should be considered an effective alternative for palliation of pancreatic cancer in selected patients with "obstructive" pain not responding to analgesics. The need for and timing of stent exchanges in this population are unknown and warrant further study.

6. ENDOSCOPIC ADJUVANT THERAPY

Biliary and pancreatic stents have also been used for administration of intraluminal brachy-radiotherapy (11). Preliminary results on intraluminal brachy-radiotherapy with 192 iridium in the biliary or PD are encouraging (85,86). It appears to be a safe method for delivery of high radiation doses to the tumor while sparing adjacent organs. However, larger experience is needed to assess the impact of intraluminal brachy-radiotherapy on survival and quality of life in patients with pancreatic cancer.

7. PALLIATION OF DUODENAL OBSTRUCTION

7.1. SELF-EXPANDABLE ENTERAL METAL STENTS

Pancreatic cancer is the most common malignancy causing GOO from direct duodenal invasion. Approximately 10–15% of subjects with pancreatic cancer develop GOO at some point before death. Before the development of enteral SEMS, surgical gastroenteric bypass (most commonly gastrojejunostomy) was the only way to restore luminal continuity from malignant obstruction in the duodenum. Surgical bypass is still considered the standard palliative approach and at present may be performed laparoscopically (87). In patients who are not considered candidates for palliative surgery, SEMS have provided an alternative option. SEMS primarily designed for palliation of gastrointestinal luminal obstruction are now available and can be deployed within the stomach, small bowel, and colon.

SEMS are placed by gastroenterologists under endoscopic and fluoroscopic guidance or by interventional radiologists under only fluoroscopic guidance. The advantages of endoscopic placement of SEMS include better accessibility to the duodenum and ability to pass the newer stents directly through the working channel of the endoscope. The principles of enteral stents are similar to those described for the biliary metal stents. They are composed by a variety of metal alloys and have several shapes and sizes depending on the individual manufacturer. Enteral stents with a covering membrane are being developed to prevent tumor ingrowth through the mesh wall (88).

In the United States, only the Enteral Wallstent (Boston Scientific) is approved as a palliative treatment of GOO. It is housed on a 10-F sheath, its diameter varies between 16 and 22 mm and comes in lengths of 6 and 9 cm. Commercially available esophageal stents and biliary stents have been used for GOO (88). The major advantage of the Enteral Wallstent is that can be advanced through the scope channel.

7.2. TECHNIQUE OF ENTERAL STENTING

An upper gastrointestinal contrast radiographic examination is the first step to assess the location and extent of the stricture. However, completing the examination might not be possible in the presence of complete obstruction. In general, a standard upper endoscope with a channel of 3.8 mm or larger is adequate. However, for lesions distal to the second portion of the duodenum, the use of a pediatric colonoscope may be required. Some endoscopists prefer enteral stent placement using a duodenoscope to allow wire and stent manipulation with the elevator. The procedure is usually performed under standard intravenous sedation. The patient is placed in the left lateral decubitus or prone position. The prone position results in a better view under fluoroscopy. A room equipped with fluoroscopy and the assistance of an experienced nurse is also required.

Initially, the endoscope is advanced to the site of obstruction. It is important to note that the procedure can be safely completed without passing the endoscope across the obstruction. Therefore, applying excessive force to the scope or aggressively dilating the stricture to facilitate its passage are unnecessary and increase the risk of perforation. At times, marking of the tumor margins with radiopaque contrast or markers can aid the fluoroscopic guidance.

If the endoscope passes through the obstruction, a stiff guidewire with a floppy tip is advanced through the scope channel beyond the point of obstruction. If the scope cannot pass across the stricture, a hydrophilic guidewire preloaded through a standard biliary catheter is used to traverse the stricture under endoscopic and fluoroscopic guidance. Once the guidewire has passed, the biliary catheter is advanced over the guidewire through the lesion. Water-soluble radiographic contrast can be injected to confirm both proper access and luminal patency. The hydrophilic guidewire is then exchanged for a stiff guidewire that provides stability during the stent placement.

The selected stent has to be at least 3–4 cm longer than the stricture to allow an adequate margin of stent on both sides of the obstructing tumor. The stent is passed over the guidewire, through the working channel, and is deployed from the distal end under direct endoscopic and fluoroscopic guidance, while maintaining its proximal position in the desired location. (Fig. 6). Once the stent is fully deployed, the ends of the stent should be inspected fluoroscopically. If either end is not fully expanded, then the stent's positioning has most likely not covered the entire length of the stricture. At this point, a second overlapping stent is required to adequately treat the stricture (88).

In patients with pancreatic cancer complicated by GOO, co-existent biliary obstruction can be present and usually occurs before the GOO. The bile duct may not be accessed endoscopically when a self-expandable metal duodenal stent has been placed across the papilla. Therefore, placement of a metal biliary stent should always be attempted in subjects with known or impending biliary obstruction before the duodenal stent placement (Fig. 7). When biliary obstruction develops after a duodenal stent placement across the papilla, percutaneous transhepatic is the usual approach for biliary decompression, although cases of ERCP through preplaced enteral stents have been reported.

The main causes of endoscopic failure of enteral stent placement include the inability to pass a guidewire across the stricture and inaccessibility of the obstruction owing to complicated postsurgical anatomy. At times, patients with widely spread pancreatic cancer and gastroduodenal obstruction may not improve after successful enteral stent placement because of other distal sites of malignant gastrointestinal obstruction,

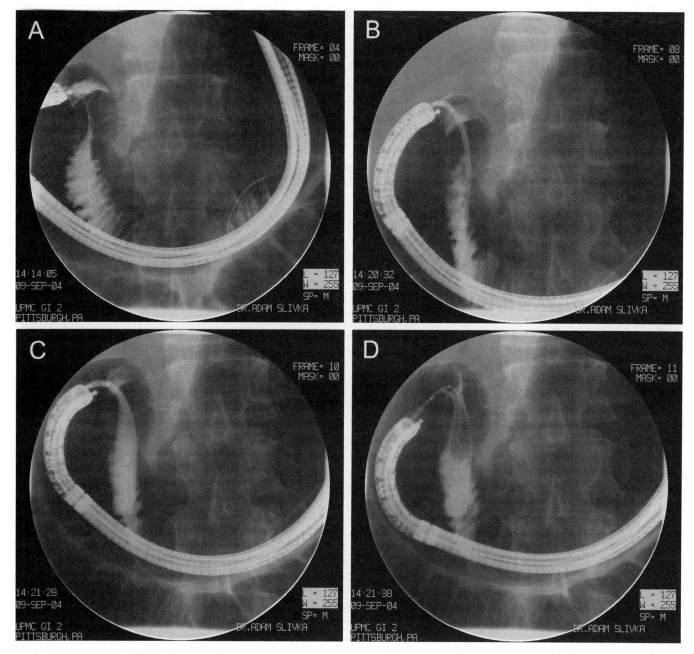

Fig. 6. Placement of a duodenal stent. (**A**) Guidewire advanced through the duodenal stricture. (**B**) Mechanical dilation of the stricture. (**C**) Controlled gradual release of the enteral Wallstent stent. (**D**) Full deployment of the stent.

diffuse peritoneal carcinomatosis with bowel encasement, or functional GOO from celiac neuronal infiltration by the tumor.

Intraprocedural complications include aspiration, stent malposition, perforation, and bleeding. Late complications include distal stent migration, bleeding, perforation, and fistula formation. Symptomatic stent occlusion from tumor ingrowth or overgrowth requires endoscopic intervention with placement of additional stents within the obstructed one.

7.3. OUTCOMES

Most of the published series of endoscopic SEMS placement as palliation for malignant GOO are retrospective with a variety of different stent types used (89–95).

Overall, the technical success rate was found between 90 and 100% with the clinical success rate, meaning subjects

being able to tolerate oral nutrition, to be approx 80–90%. The largest study involved 36 subjects and showed a significant improvement in dietary score following SEMS placement (93).

Two retrospective studies compared SEMS placement to surgical bypass. Duodenal stent placement appeared to result in lower costs and an earlier discharge from the hospital (91). Furthermore, more than half of the subjects in the gastrojejunostomy group developed delayed gastric emptying after surgery, whereas patients in the duodenal stent group were able to tolerate a soft diet the day after the procedure (95). The overall survival appeared to be similar in both groups (about 90 d). Thus, based on limited retrospective data, SEMS placement seems to provide shorter recovery time and be less expensive than palliative gastrojejunostomy and should probably considered the

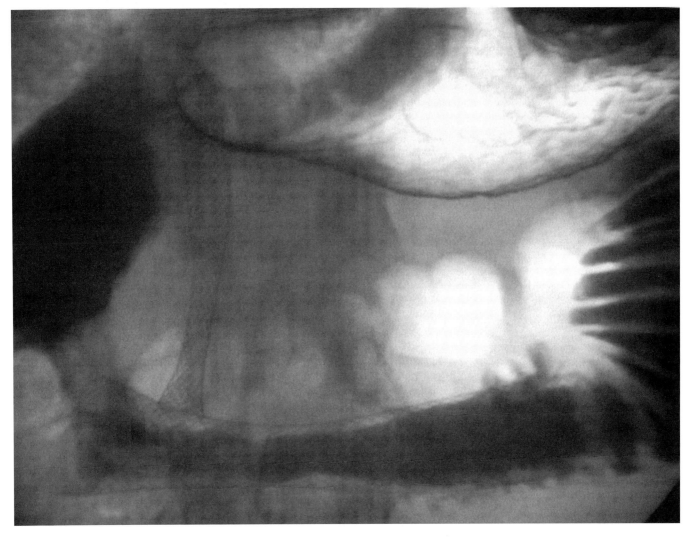

Fig. 7. Radiograph showing the presence of both biliary and duodenal metal stents.

procedure of choice in most patients with pancreatic cancer and malignant GOO.

Finally, in end-stage patients with GOO and very short-term survival who are not candidates for stent therapy, a venting gastrostomy tube placed endoscopically or percutaneously may provide welcome palliation from refractory vomiting.

REFERENCES

1. National Cancer Institute: Fact Book 2003, US Department of Health and Human Services.
2. SEER Cancer Statistics 1995-2000. National Cancer Institute. http://www.seer.cancer.gov.
3. Fuhrman GM, Charnsangavej C, Abbruzzese JL, et al. Thin-section contrast enhanced computed tomography accurately predicts resectability of malignant pancreatic neoplasms. Am J Surg 1994; 167:104.
4. Abraham NS, Barkun JS, Barkun AN. Palliation of malignant biliary obstruction: a prospective trial examining impact on quality of life. Gastrointest Endosc 2002; 56:835–84.
5. Kubota Y, Takaoka M, Tani K, et al. Endoscopic transpapillary biopsy for diagnosis of patients with pancreatobiliary ductal strictures. Am J Gastroenterol 1993; 88:1700–1704.
6. Howell DA, Parsons WG, Jones MA, Bosco JJ, Hanson BL. Complete tissue sampling of biliary strictures at ERCP using a new device. Gastrointest Endosc 1996; 43:498–502.
7. Neuhaus H. Cholangioscopy. Endoscopy 1992; 24:125–132.
8. Ferrari Jr AP, Lichtenstein DR, Slivka A, et al. Brush cytology during ERCP for the diagnosis of biliary and pancreatic malignancies. Gastrointest Endosc 1994; 140–45.
9. Jailwala J, Fogel EL, Sherman S, Gottlieb K, Flueckiger J, Bucksot LG, Lehman GA. Triple-tissue sampling at ERCP in malignant biliary obstruction. Gastrointest Endosc 2000; 51:383–390.
10. Eloubeidi MA, Chen VK, Eltoum IA, et al. Endoscopic ultrasound-guided fine needle aspiration biopsy of patients with suspected pancreatic cancer: diagnostic accuracy and acute and 30-day complications. Am J Gastroenterol 2003; 98:2663–2668.
11. Costamagna G, Pandolfi M. Endoscopic stenting for biliary and pancreatic malignancies. J Clin Gastroenterol 2004; 38:59–67.
12. Lawrie BW, Pugh S, Watura R. Bile duct stenting: a comparison of the One-Action Stent Introduction System with the conventional delivery system. Endoscopy 1996; 28:299–301.
13. Margulies C, Siqueira ES, Silverman WB, et al. The effect of endoscopic sphincterotomy on acute and chronic complications of biliary endoprostheses. Gastrointest Endosc 1999; 49:716–19.
14. Tarnasky PR, Cunningham JT, Hawes RH, et al. Transpapillary stenting of proximal biliary strictures: does biliary sphincterotomy reduce the risk of postprocedure pancreatitis? Gastrointest Endosc 1997; 45:46–51.
15. Polydorou AA, Cairns SR, Dowsett JF, et al. Palliation of proximal malignant biliary obstruction by endoscopic endoprosthesis insertion. Gut 1991; 32:685–689.

16. Chang WH, Kortan P, Haber GB. Outcome in patients with bifurcation tumors who undergo unilateral versus bilateral hepatic duct drainage. Gastrointest Endosc 1998; 47:354–362.

17. De Palma GD, Galloro G, Siciliano S, et al. Unilateral versus bilateral endoscopic hepatic duct drainage in patients with malignant hilar biliary obstruction: results of a prospective, randomised and controlled study. Gastrointest Endosc 2001; 53:547–553.

18. Hintze RE, Abou-Rebyeh H, Adler A, et al. Magnetic resonance cholangiopancreatography-guided unilateral endoscopic stent placement for Klatskin tumors. Gastrointest Endosc 2001; 53:40–46.

19. Soehendra N, Reynders-Frederix V. Palliative bile duct drainage: a new endoscopic method of introducing a transpapillary drain. Endoscopy 1980; 12:8–11.

20. Sung JY, Leung JW, Shaffer EA, et al. Ascending infection of the biliary tract after surgical sphincterotomy and biliary stenting. J Gastroenterol Hepatol 1992; 7:240–245.

21. Groen AK, Out T, Huibregtse K, et al. Characterization of the content of occluded biliary endoprostheses. Endoscopy 1987; 19:57–59.

22. Smith AC, Dowsett JF, Russell RC, et al. Randomized trial of endoscopic stenting versus surgical bypass in malignant low bile duct obstruction. Lancet 1994; 344:1655–1660.

23. Smit JM, Out MM, Groen AK, et al. A placebo-controlled study on the efficacy of aspirin and doxycycline in preventing clogging of biliary endoprostheses. Gastrointest Endosc 1989; 35:485–489.

24. Ghosh S, Palmer KR. Prevention of biliary stent occlusion using cyclical antibiotics and ursodeoxycholic acid. Gut 1994; 35:1757–1759.

25. Barrioz T, Ingrand P, Besson I, et al. Randomised trial of prevention of biliary stent occlusion by ursodeoxycholic acid plus norfloxacin. Lancet 1994; 344:581,582.

26. Leung JW, Liu Y, Desta TD, et al. In vitro evaluation of antibiotics prophylaxis in the prevention of biliary stent blockage. Gastrointest Endosc 2000; 51:296–303.

27. Coene PP, Groen AK, Cheng J, et al. Clogging of biliary endoprostheses: a new prospective. Gut 1990; 31:913–917.

28. Seitz U, Vadeyar H, Soehendra N. Prolonged patency with a new designed Teflon biliary prosthesis. Endoscopy 1994; 26:478–482.

29. Van Berkel AM, Boland C, Redekop WK, et al. A prospective randomised trial of Teflon versus polyethylene stents for distal malignant biliary obstruction. Endoscopy 1998; 30:681–686.

30. England RE, Martin DF, Sheridan MB, et al. A prospective randomised multicentre trial comparing 10 Fr Teflon Tannenbaum stents with 10 Fr polyethylene Cotton-Leung stents in patients with malignant common duct strictures. Gut 2000; 46:395–400.

31. Jansen B, Goodman LB, Rutien D. Bacterial adherence to hydrophilic polymer-coated polyurethane stents. Gastrointest Endosc 1993; 39:670–673.

32. Costamagna G, Mutignani M, Rotondano G, et al. Hydrophilic hydromer-coated polyurethane stents versus uncoated stents in malignant biliary obstruction: a randomized trial. Gastrointest Endosc 2000; 51:8–11.

33. Schilling D, Rink G, Arnold JC, et al. Prospective, randomised, single-center trial comparing 3 different 10F plastic stents in malignant mid and distal bile duct stricture. Gastrointest Endosc 2003; 58:54–58.

34. Speer AG, Cotton PB, MacRae KD. Endoscopic management of malignant biliary obstruction. Stents of 10 French gauge are preferable to stents of 8 French gauge. Gastrointest Endosc 1988; 34:412–417.

35. Pedersen FM. Endoscopic management of malignant biliary obstruction. Is stent size of 10 French gauge better than 7 French gauge? Scand J Gastroenterol 1993; 28:185–189.

36. Pereira-Lima J, Jakobs R, Maier M, et al. Endoscopic biliary stenting for the palliation of pancreatic cancer: results, survival predictive factors and comparison of 10 Fr with 11.5 Fr gauge stents. Am J Gastroenterol 1996; 91:2179–2184.

37. Tarnasky PR, Morris J, Hawes RH, Hoffman BJ, Cotton PB, Cunningham JT. Snare beside-a-wire biliary stent exchange: a method that maintains access across biliary strictures. Gastrointest Endosc 1996; 44(2):185–187.

38. Hawes RH. Diagnostic and therapeutic uses of ERCP in pancreatic and biliary tract malignancies. Gastrointest Endoscosc 2002; 56:S201–S205.

39. Johanson JF, Schmalz MJ, Geenen JE, et al. Incidence and risk factors for biliary and pancreatic stent migration. Gastrointest Endosc 1992; 38:341–346.

40. Das A, Sivak MV. Endoscopic palliation for inoperable Pancreatic cancer. Cancer Control 2000; 7:452–457.

41. Lichtenstein DR, Carr-Locke DL. Endoscopic palliation for unresectable pancreatic carcinoma. Surg Clin North Am 1995; 75:969–988.

42. Dumonceau JM, Cremer M, Auroux J, et al. A comparison of Ultraflex Diamond stents and Wallstents for palliation of distal malignant biliary strictures. Am J Gastroenterol 2000; 95:670–676.

43. Ahmad J, Siqueira E, Martin J, Slivka A. Effectiveness of the Ultraflex Diamond stent for the palliation of malignant biliary obstruction. Endoscopy 2002; 34:793–796.

44. Shah RJ, Howell DA, Desilets DJ, et al. Multicenter randomized trial of the spiral Z-stent compared with the Wallstent for malignant biliary obstruction. Gastrointest Endosc 2003; 57(7):830–836.

45. Davids PHP, Groen AK, Rauws EA, et al. Randomized trial of self-expanding metal stents versus polyethylene stents for distal malignant biliary obstruction. Lancet 1992; 340:1488–1492.

46. Knyrim K, Wagner HJ, Pausch J, et al. A prospective, randomised, controlled trial of metal stents for malignant obstruction of the common bile duct. Endoscopy 1993; 25:207–212.

47. Mixon T, Goldschmid S, Brady PG, et al. Endoscopic management of expandable metallic biliary stent occlusion. Gastrointest Endosc 1993; 39:82–84.

48. Cremer M, Deviere J, Sugai B, et al. Expandable biliary metal stents for malignancies: Endoscopic insertion and diathermic cleaning for tumor ingrowth. Gastrointest Endosc 1990; 36:451–457.

49. Ell C, Fleig WE, Hochberger J. Broken biliary metal stent after repeated electrocoagulation for tumor ingrowth. Gastroint Endosc 1992; 38:197–199.

50. Tsang TK, Pollack J, Chodash HB, et al. Silicone-covered metal stents: an in vitro evaluation of biofilm formation and patency. Dig Dis Sci 1999; 44:1780–1785.

51. Isayama H, Komatsu Y, Tsujino T, et al. Polyurethane-covered metal stent for management of distal malignant biliary obstruction. Gastrointest Endosc 2002; 55:366–370.

52. Shepherd HA, Royle G, Ross AP, et al. Endoscopic biliary endoprosthesis in the palliation of malignant obstruction of the distal common bile duct: a randomized trial. Br J Surg 1988; 75:1166–1168.

53. Andersen JR, Sorensen SM, Kruse A, et al. Randomised trial of endoscopic endoprosthesis versus operative bypass in malignant obstructive jaundice. Gut 1989; 30:1132–1135.

54. Smith AC, Dowsett JF, Russell RC, et al. Randomised trial of endoscopic stenting versus surgical bypass in malignant low bile duct obstruction. Lancet 1994; 344:1655–1660.

55. Taylor MC, McLeod RS, Langer B. Biliary stenting versus bypass surgery for the palliation of malignant distal bile duct obstruction, a meta-analysis. Liver Transpl 2000; 6:302–308.

56. Speer AG, Cotton PB, Russel RC, et al. Randomized trial of endoscopic versus percutaneous stent insertion in malignant obstructive jaundice. Lancet 1987; 2:57–62.

57. Lai ECS, Mok FPT, Fan ST, et al. Preoperative endoscopic drainage for malignant obstructive jaundice. Br J Surg 1994; 81:1195–1198.

58. Karsten TM, Allema JH, Reinders M, et al. Preoperative biliary drainage, colonisation of bile and postoperative complications in patients with tumors of the pancreatic head: a retrospective analysis of 241 consecutive patients. Eur J Surg 1996; 162:881–888.

59. Marcus SG, Dobryansky M, Shamamian P, et al. Endoscopic biliary drainage before pancreaticoduodenectomy for periampullary malignancies. J Clin Gastroenterol 1998; 26:125–129.

60. Heslin MJ, Brooks AD, Hochwald SN, et al. A preoperative biliary stent is associated with increased complications after pancreatoduodenectomy. Arch Surg 1998; 133:149–154.

61. Saleh MMA, Norregard P, Jorgensen HL, et al. Preoperative endoscopic stent placement before pancreaticoduodenectomy: a meta-analysis of the effect on morbidity and mortality. Gastrointest Endosc 2002; 56:529–534.

62. Davids PHP, Groen AK, Rauws EA, et al. Randomized trial of self-expanding metal stents versus polyethylene stents for distal malignant biliary obstruction. Lancet 1992; 340:1488–1492.

63. Knyrim K, Wagner HJ, Pausch J, et al. A prospective, randomised, controlled trial of metal stents for malignant obstruction of the common bile duct. Endoscopy 1993; 25:207–212.

64. Carr-Locke DL, Ball TJ, Connors PJ, et al. Multicenter randomized trial of Wallstent biliary endoprosthesis versus plastic stents. Gastrointest Endosc 1993; 39:310–316.

65. Prat F, Chapat O, Ducot B, et al. A randomized trial of endoscopic drainage methods for inoperable malignant strictures of the common bile duct. Gastrointest Endosc 1998; 47:1–7.

66. Kim HS, Lee DK, Kim HG, et al. Features of malignant biliary obstruction affecting the patency of metallic stents: a multicenter study. Gastrointest Endosc 2002; 55:359–365.

67. Kaassis M, Boyer J, Dumas R, et al. Plastic or metal stents for malignant stricture of the common bile duct? Results of a randomized prospective study. Gastrointest Endosc 2003; 57:178–182.

68. Kalser MH, Barkin J, MacIntyre JM. For the Gastrointestinal Tumor Study Group, Pancreatic Cancer: assessment of prognosis by clinical presentation. Cancer 1985; 56:397–402.

69. Grahm AL, Andren-Sandberg A. Prospective evaluation of pain in exocrine pancreatic cancer. Digestion 1997; 58:542–549.

70. Lillemoe KD, Cameron JL, Kaufman HS, et al. Chemical splanchicectomy in patients with unresectable pancreatic cancer: a prospective randomized trial. Ann Surg 1993; 217:447–457.

71. Polati E, Finco G, Gottin L, et al. Prospective randomized double-blind trial of neurolytic celiac plexus block in patients with pancreatic cancer. Br J Surg 1998; 85:199–201.

72. Wong GY, Schroeder DR, Carns PE, et al. Effect of neurolytic celiac plexus block on pain relief, quality of life, and survival in patients with unresectable pancreatic cancer: a randomized controlled trial. JAMA 2004; 291:1092–1099.

73. Das KM, Chapman AH. Sonographically guided celiac plexus block. Clin Radiol 1992; 45:401–403.

74. Gimenez A, Martinez-Noguera A, Donoso L, et al. Percutaneous neurolysis of the celiac plexus via the anterior approach with sonographic guidance. Am J Roentgenol 1993; 161:1061–1063.

75. Montero Matamala A, Vidal Lopez F, Inaraja Martinez L. The percutaneous anterior approach to the celiac plexus using CT guidance. Pain 1998; 34:285–288.

76. Lee MJ, Mueller PR, van Sonnenberg E, et al. CT-guided celiac ganglion block with alcohol. Am J Roentgenol 1993; 161:633–636.

77. Romanelli DF, Beckmann CF, Heiss FW. Celiac plexus block: efficacy and safety of the anterior approach. Am J Roentgenol 1993; 160:497–500.

78. Wiersema M, Sandusky D, Carr R, et al. Endosonography guided celiac plexus neurolysis (EUS CPN) in patients with pain due to intraabdominal (IA) malignancy. [Abstract] Gastrointest Endosc 1995; 4:15 (AB).

79. Levy MJ, Wiersema MJ. EUS-guided celiac plexus neurolysis and celiac plexus block. Gastrointest Endosc 2003; 57:923–930.

80. Wiersema MJ, Wiersema LM. Endosonography-guided celiac plexus neurolysis. Gastrointest Endosc 1996; 44:656–662.

81. Gunaratnam NT, Sarma AV, Norton ID, Wiersema MJ. A prospective study of EUS-guided celiac plexus neurolysis for pancreatic cancer pain. Gastrointest Endosc 2001; 54:316–324.

82. Hoffman BJ. EUS-guided celiac plexus block/neurolysis. Gastrointest Endosc 2002; 56(4 Suppl):S26–S28.

83. Costamagna G, Alevras P, Palladino F, et al. Endoscopic pancreatic stenting in pancreatic cancer. Can J Gastroenterol. 1999; 13:481–487.

84. Tham TC, Lichtenstein DR, Vandervoort J, et al. Pancreatic duct stents for "obstructive type" pain in pancreatic malignancy. Am J Gastroenterol. 2000; 95:956–960.

85. Montemaggi P, Morganti AG, Dobelbower Jr, RR et al. Role of intraluminal brachytherapy in extrahepatic bile duct and pancreatic cancers: is it just for palliation. Radiology 1996; 199:861–866.

86. Mutignani M, Shah SK, Morganti AG, et al. Treatment of unresectable pancreatic carcinoma by intraluminal brachytherapy in the duct of Wirsung Endoscopy 2002; 34:555–559.

87. Choi YB. Laparoscopic gastrojejunostomy for palliation of gastric outlet obstruction in unresectable gastric cancer. Surg Endosc 2002; 16:1620–1626.

88. Baron TH, Harewood GC. Enteral self-expandable stents. Gastrointest Endosc 2003; 58:421–433.

89. Feretis C, Benakis P, Dimopoulos C, Manouras A, Tsimbloulis B, Apostolidis N. Duodenal obstruction caused by pancreatic head carcinoma: palliation with self-expandable endoprostheses. Gastrointest Endosc 1997; 46:161–165.

90. Soetikno RM, Lichtenstein DR, Vandervoort J, Palliation of malignant gastric outlet obstruction using an endoscopically placed Wallstent. Gastrointest Endosc 1998; 47:267–270.

91. Yim HB, Jacobson BC, Saltzman JR, et al. Clinical outcome of the use of enteral stents for palliation of patients with malignant upper GI obstruction. Gastrointest Endosc 2001; 53:329–332.

92. Kim JH, Yoo BM, Lee KJ, et al. Self-expanding coil stent with a long delivery system for palliation of unresectable malignant gastric outlet obstruction: a prospective study. Endoscopy 2001; 33:838–842.

93. Adler DG, Baron TH. Endoscopic palliation of malignant gastric outlet obstruction using self-expanding metal stents: experience in 36 patients. Am J Gastroenterol 2002; 97:72–78.

94. Shand AG, Grieve DC, Brush J, Palmer KR, Penman ID. Expandable metallic stents for palliation of malignant pyloric and duodenal obstruction. Br J Surg 2002; 89:349–350.

95. Wong YT, Brams DM, Munson L, Sanders L, Heiss F, Chase M, et al. Gastric outlet obstruction secondary to pancreatic cancer: surgical vs endoscopic palliation. Surg Endosc 2002; 16:310–12.

27 Pancreatic Neuroendocrine Tumors

Erik-Jan Wamsteker, MD and James M. Scheiman, MD

Contents

1. BACKGROUND

Neuroendocrine tumors of the pancreas are uncommon neoplasms. They may occur as a sporadic lesion or as part of a genetic disease such as the multiple endocrine neoplasia type 1 (MEN-1) syndrome. Sporadic tumors usually arise as a single lesion, whereas those associated with familial disorders generally are multifocal. Tumors may be classified as functioning or nonfunctioning depending on whether or not there is excess hormone production correlated with a clinical syndrome. Clinical suspicion is based on development of the constellation of clinical symptoms characteristic of excess hormone production. In the case of a nonfunctioning tumor, its presence often becomes apparent because of symptoms from local tumor growth or metastatic disease. Once biochemical studies confirm the diagnosis and cross-sectional imaging exclude metastatic disease, endoscopic ultrasound (EUS) can localize the tumor and guide surgical management, providing potentially curative resection.

2. INTRODUCTION

Pancreatic neuroendocrine tumors (NETs) are uncommon neoplasms with a prevalence of less than 10 per million population *(1)*. They may occur as a sporadic tumor or as part of a genetic disease such as the MEN-1 or Von Hippel Lindau (VHL) syndrome. MEN-1 is a genetic disorder that leads to tumor development in the parathyroid, pancreatic islet cells, and pituitary gland *(2)*. VHL is a genetic disorder that predisposes patients to bilateral and multicentric retinal angiomas, hemangioblastomas in the central nervous system, renal cell carcinomas, pheochromo-

cytomas, islet cell tumors of the pancreas, endolymphatic sac tumors, and cysts of the kidney, pancreas, and epididymis *(3)*.

Sporadic NETs usually occur as a single lesion, whereas those associated with familial disorders generally are multifocal. They may be classified as functioning or nonfunctioning tumors depending on whether or not there is excess hormone production and an associated clinical syndrome. In general, the clinical suspicion of a NET is based on development of clinical symptoms characteristic of excess hormone production. In the case of a nonfunctioning tumor, its presence becomes apparent because of symptoms from local tumor growth or metastatic disease.

For patients with MEN-1, the lethality of the disease can be substantially attributed to disease burden from the pancreatic tumors. The cause of death in this patient population has been attributed directly to a complication of the neuroendocrine tumors in nearly 50% of patients, leading to an earlier age at death than those who did not die of MEN-1-related disease (47 vs 55 yr of age) *(4)*. Despite these grim statistics, the prognosis in patients with NETs is far better than in patients with pancreatic adenocarcinoma, and many patients can expect a cure with surgical resection *(5)*.

In the setting of a family history of MEN-1 or a personal history of VHL, screening programs may be employed, which may detect tumors prior to the onset of clinical symptoms *(6)*. This chapter will provide a general overview of NETs and concentrate on the role of endoscopy and EUS in the diagnosis, localization, and management of patients with these tumors.

3. CLINICAL PRESENTATION

Small tumors that present owing to symptoms of hormone excess might be diagnosed at an early and potentially surgically

From: *Endoscopic Oncology: Gastrointestinal Endoscopy and Cancer Management*. Edited by: D. O. Faigel and M. L. Kochman © Humana Press, Totowa, NJ

Table 1
Endocrine Tumor Syndromes

Tumor type	Clinical syndrome	Clinical	Diagnosis
Insulinoma	Insulinoma syndrome/ neuroglycopenic syndrome	Headaches, visual disturbances, irrational behavior, confusion, drowsiness	Glucose levels near or below 40 mg/dL, insulin levels > 6 micU/mL, elevated C-peptide levels
Gastrinoma	Zollinger-Ellison syndrome	Abdominal pain, peptic ulcer disease, diarrhea, reflux esophagitis	Elevated gastrin, positive secretin stimulation testing, gastric acid analysis
Glucagonoma	Glucagonoma syndrome	Necrolytic migratory erythema, diabetes, weight loss	Elevated glucagon
VIPoma	Verner-Morrison, pancreatic cholera	Secretory diarrhea >1 L/d, hypokalemia	Elevated VIP
Somatostatinoma	Somatostatinoma-inhibitory syndrome	Diabetes, steatorrhea, cholelithiasis	Elevated somatostatin

curable stage. If unrecognized early or as a consequence of aggressive tumor biology, patients may present later with symptoms resulting from metastatic disease. Depending on the dominant hormone (the hormone produced in excess), clinical presentations vary. The clinical syndromes that occur with functioning NETs are listed in Table 1.

The most common symptomatic NETs are insulinoma and gastrinoma (7). Insulinomas cause symptoms as a result of excess insulin production with resultant hypoglycemia. Prolonged fasting will precipitate central nervous system dysfunction leading to seizures, difficulty awakening, visual disturbance, confusion, lethargy, weakness, and transient motor deficits (8). The vast majority of insulinomas are sporadic tumors (90%), with approx 10% presenting as part of MEN-1. Sporadic insulinomas present most commonly as solitary tumors, whereas in the familial form, they might be multiple (9). Most insulinomas (85–90%) are benign. Of the insulinomas that are malignant, metastases will be present in 15–30% at the time of diagnosis (10).

Gastrinomas produce symptoms as a result of excess gastrin production. Hypersecretion of this hormone drives excess gastric acid production leading to peptic ulcer disease, abdominal pain, and diarrhea. Although the approach to hypergastrinemia cannot be exhaustively reviewed in this chapter, it is essential to establish the diagnosis of gastrinoma with appropriate biochemical testing prior to studies for tumor localization such as EUS.

Other hormone excess syndromes are summarized in Table 1. Nonfunctioning NETs do not produce a characteristic clinical syndrome although modest nonspecific elevation in gastrointestinal hormones may be seen in these patients (11).

In patients with a family history of MEN-1 or VHL, biochemical testing and screening with imaging studies may be performed on a routine basis. In carefully selected patients, intensive screening with EUS can detect pancreatic endocrine tumors (PETs) prior to clinical symptom production, which will be reviewed in detail later in this chapter.

4. DIAGNOSIS

4.1. SPORADIC PANCREATIC ENDOCRINE TUMORS

4.1.1. Insulinoma

Insulinomas are diagnosed by demonstrating elevation of plasma insulin and C-peptide levels in the setting of recurrent fasting hypoglycemia. The C-peptide assay is necessary to exclude factitious insulin administration (12). Provocation testing is sometimes necessary when insulinoma is suspected. Diagnostic testing can include an overnight fast as well as a 48–72 h supervised fast. Hypoglycemia needs to be present in order to interpret C-peptide and insulin levels and studies indicate that 100% of patients with insulinoma will be detected after a supervised 72-h fast (13). Biochemical testing to confirm the clinical diagnosis should precede any attempt to image the tumor with either cross-sectional imaging or EUS.

Once the diagnosis is confirmed, pre-operative localization is essential because it directs surgical management. Because these tumors are small, (90% are <2 cm, 40% are <1 cm), and the majority located in the head of the pancreas (which might be more difficult to palpate at the time of surgery), pre-operative localization is critically important (14).

4.1.2. Gastrinoma and the Zollinger-Ellison Syndrome (ZES)

Gastrinomas produce the ZES, named by the surgeons who described the clinical disorder resulting from excessive gastric acid production. The tumor should be suspected after recognition of the constellation of clinical symptoms that include "ulcer-like" abdominal pain (dyspepsia) with associated diarrhea. The endoscopic findings of peptic ulcer disease and concomitant esophagitis are a clue to the diagnosis. Profound acid hypersecretion leads to ulcerations throughout the upper gut, and the peptic ulcers may be in atypical locations such as the second, third, and fourth portions of the duodenum and jejunum (15).

Most gastrinomas present as solitary tumors (75%). Approximately 25% of patients with gastrinomas present as part of a familial syndrome, most commonly the MEN-1. This situation should be excluded by obtaining a serum calcium level reflecting the absence of associated parathyroid disease. The diagnosis of gastrinoma is based on an elevated serum gastrin level (generally levels >1000 pg/mL are felt diagnostic) with persistent peptic ulcer disease and a basal acid output (BAO) of greater than 15 mEq/h. When ZES is suspected, but the above criteria are not met, provocation testing with the secretin stimulation test is necessary to exclude other causes of hypergastrinemia. In normal individuals, secretin does not have a stimulatory effect on gastrin. In patients with ZES, secretin has a paradoxical effect resulting in a dramatic increase in gastrin level and acid secretion (16). In situations in which secretin is unavailable for clinical diagnostic testing, a calcium infusion study can be performed with an anticipated increase in gastrin of more than 400 pg/mL, however, this test lacks in both sensitivity and specificity compared with the secretin provocation test (17).

BAO more than 15 mEq/h is present in more than 90% of patients with ZES, but is also present in a small percentage of patients with common duodenal ulcer disease. The addition of a maximal acid output test, with the use of the secretegogue pentagastrin, would be expected not to result in a significant increase in gastric acid output in ZES because BAO is already felt to be near maximal in patients with ZES. Therefore, a BAO/MAO ratio of greater than 0.6 is highly suggestive of ZES. Although gastric acid analysis is not completely diagnostic, its importance is in allowing exclusion of patients that have elevated gastrin levels owing to hypo- or achlorhydria. This is a critical issue to differentiate given the frequent problem of hypergastrinemia in patients taking potent acid inhibitory medications, such as proton pump inhibitors (PPIs). Such patients, particularly those with concomitant atrophic gastritis, may have similar symptoms and marked hypergastrinemia. However, they have low acid output when formally tested and should not have the diagnostic changes in gastrin levels with secretin administration. Like insulinoma, it is essential to establish the diagnosis before imaging studies to localize tumor, for fear that a false-positive exam leading to inappropriate surgical exploration.

4.1.3. Glucagonoma

Glucagonomas are very rare tumors. They may present with weight loss, necrolytic migratory erythema (a painful, pruritic cutaneous eruption), cheilosis, diabetes mellitus, normochromic and normocytic anemia, venous thrombosis, and neuropsychiatric symptoms, as well as diarrhea. The most common presentation is diabetes, necrolytic migratory erythema, and imaging demonstrating an islet cell tumor. The diagnosis is most frequently made by obtaining a fasting glucagon level, which should be markedly elevated, followed by identification of a pancreatic islet cell tumor by imaging.

4.1.4. VIPoma

VIPomas are very rare tumors that are generally malignant and present with a large volume watery secretory diarrhea. Presenting symptoms may include hypokalemia and dehydration. The general approach to secretory diarrhea is documentation of persistence of diarrhea during fasting followed by stool characterization. If the stool quantity exceeds 1 L/d, this suggests that a VIPoma, rather than another neuroendocrine tumor, is most likely the source of the diarrhea (18). Direct measurement of a fasting VIP level confirms the diagnosis. VIPomas in children might occur in extrapancreatic locations, although generally primary VIPomas in adults are intrapancreatic (19).

4.1.5. Somatostatinomas

Somatostatinomas are the rarest of the neuroendocrine tumors, presenting with signs of inhibition of other endocrine hormone production. The syndrome consists of diabetes mellitus, gallbladder disease (cholelithiasis), weight loss, anemia, diarrhea, and steatorrhea, all felt to be owing to the inhibitory effects of somatostatin. The most common primary site is the pancreas followed closely by the duodenum. Somatostatinomas can occur in MEN-1 and in patients with neurofibromatosis (20). The diagnosis may be supported by the demonstration of an elevated fasting somatostatin level.

4.2. FAMILIAL FORMS OF PANCREATIC ENDOCRINE TUMORS

4.2.1. MEN-1

This syndrome is characterized by an autosomal-dominant inheritance pattern with variable penetrance. Before the genetic advances of the 1980s and 1990s, MEN-1 was diagnosed clinically in patients with polyglandular diseases, most commonly hyperparathyroidism with associated pancreatic islet cell tumors and less commonly anterior parathyroid tumors (two or more primary organ sites). Other diagnostic criteria include the presence of one or more primary organ site involvement plus a first-degree relative with MEN-1. The pancreatic tumors are often multifocal and may secrete several different hormones. With relatively recent genetic advances and the cloning of the gene for MEN-1 (menin) (21), genetic testing may allow for identification of those at risk for the disease.

4.2.2. Von Hippel Lindau

This syndrome is characterized by an autosomal-dominant pattern of inheritance with a high penetrance. There is no single pathognomonic finding. In patients with a family history of VHL, minimal clinical criteria include the presence of a single retinal or cerebral hemangioblastoma, renal cell carcinoma, or pheochromocytoma. In isolated cases, the diagnosis can be established in a person who has two or more retinal or central nervous system hemangioblastomas or a single hemangioblastomas and a characteristic visceral tumor. A high index of clinical suspicion with strong interdisciplinary collaboration among specialists is essential to make the diagnosis (22). As with MEN-1, the gene for VHL has been identified and may allow for early identification of disease carriers.

5. TUMOR LOCALIZATION

Imaging studies are important to establish the location of the primary tumor to guide surgical extirpation, and to evaluate for metastatic disease, which precludes surgery. Localization of NETs remains challenging. Multiple modalities including transcutaneous ultrasound, computed tomography (CT), magnetic resonance imaging (MRI), arteriography, intra-arterial stimulation with venous sampling, somatostatin receptor scintigraphy (SRS), EUS, and intra-operative ultrasound have been used for localization with variable success (23). Special attention will be given to EUS and SRS, relatively new approaches, which have had great impact in tumor localization strategies.

Transcutaneous ultrasound, CT, MRI, and diagnostic angiography fail to localize the primary tumor in 40–60% of cases, frequently missing lesions less than 2 cm in size (24). More invasive angiographic techniques, such intra-arterial calcium injection for stimulation of insulin release by the tumor at the time of angiography have been employed in some centers. Doppman and colleagues (25) reported a sensitivity of 88% for insulinoma localization using this technique, a result that surpassed ultrasound, CT, MRI, arteriography, and portal venous sampling with sensitivities of 9, 17, 43, 36, and 67%, respectively. However, in most centers these invasive techniques have been relegated to a supportive role given the accuracy of EUS for pre-operative localization.

5.1. SOMATOSTATIN RECEPTOR SCINTINGRAPHY

SRS is performed using a radiolabeled analog of the somatostatin analog octreotide, indium 111-penetreotide. Somatostatin receptor positive tumors might be localized following administration of the tracer. Images are captured with a γ-camera so that planar anterior and posterior images of the thorax, abdomen, and pelvis can be acquired at 4 and 24 h. SRS is of limited value for insulinoma, owing to a low rate of somatostatin receptor expression on the tumors. The test is of greatest value for the diagnosis of occult metastatic disease not seen on cross sectional imaging studies such as CT or MRI.

In a correlation study between EUS and SRS followed subsequently by surgery, sensitivity was calculated using pathology as the gold standard. Using EUS alone, the sensitivity for identification of insulinoma and gastrinoma, respectively, were 79 and 73%, respectively. Using SRS alone, the sensitivity for identification of insulinoma and gastrinoma were 60 and 75%, respectively. When the two modalities were combined, the sensitivity for detection of insulinoma and gastrinoma were 89 and 93%, respectively (26). EUS is limited to visualization of the pancreas and its immediate surroundings. SRS has excellent sensitivity but it is often not possible to differentiate uptake in pancreatic tissue vs an adjacent lymph node. It also may poorly localize a PET to a specific anatomical region of the pancreas (27). It therefore has been advocated that both techniques are useful for localization of these tumors and is often necessary (6).

5.2. ENDOSCOPIC ULTRASOUND

When EUS is performed, an echoendoscope is advanced to the descending duodenum beyond the major ampulla and slowly withdrawn from the duodenum to the stomach. Regional anatomy is verified by its relationship to the surrounding vessels and organs. The tumor's size, echotexture, location within the pancreas, involvement of the peripancreatic vessels, and the presence of regional lymph nodes are documented. Examinations may require approx 30–60 min, even in experienced hands. Generally, radial scanning instruments are most commonly used, by it is also possible to localize tumors with the linear array instruments used for fine-needle aspiration (FNA).

In experienced hands, EUS is ideal for localization of small tumors because of the ability to produce high-resolution images of the pancreas and surrounding structures. EUS correctly localizes NETs with a sensitivity as high as 93% (Table 2) (28). The "classical" EUS appearance of a NET is a hypoechoic to isoechoic homogeneous well-demarcated mass within the gland (Fig. 1). Cystic tumors uncommonly occur. The precise localization of the NET can be established by examining relationships with the large vessels and duct. At the University of Michigan, when insulinoma is biochemically confirmed, EUS may be the only localization technique used prior to taking a patient to the operating room based on its high sensitivity and positive predictive value of 28. FNA is generally not performed in the setting of a hormone excess syndrome, but can be used to confirm the diagnosis for nonfunctional sporadic tumors (Fig. 2).

Table 2
Localization of Pancreatic Neuroendocrine Tumors Using EUS: The University of Michigan Experience

	Gastrinoma N = 36	Insulinoma N = 36
Sensitivity	100%	88%
Specificity	94%	100%
PPV	95%	100%
NPV	100%	43%
Accuracy	97%	89%

PPV, positive predictive value; NPV, negative predictive value. Modified from ref. 28.

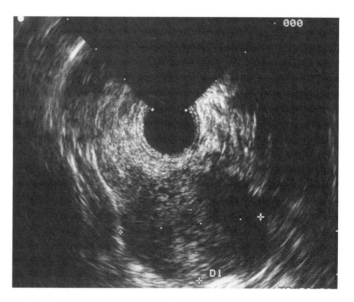

Fig. 1. Classical appearance of a pancreatic endocrine tumor imaged by the Pentax radial array echoendoscope.

It is important to consider the limitations of EUS given its pre-eminent role in tumor localization. First and foremost, it is operator-dependent, and experience likely is a key determinant to tumor localization. Pitfalls of the techniques may occur owing to differing echotextures of the tumor or the gland itself. Isoechoic tumors may be very difficult to visualize from surrounding pancreatic parenchyma and can be missed by an inexperienced operator (Table 3). The finding of a subtle hyperechoic rim surrounding the lesion may help to localize the tumor. In the setting of diffuse pancreatic parenchymal abnormalities seen with chronic pancreatitis, small tumors might be impossible to see.

When insulinoma is suspected, a "negative EUS" does not reliably exclude an intrapancreatic insulinoma, whereas when a gastrinoma is suspected, a "negative EUS" in experienced hands appears to reliably exclude an intrapancreatic gastrinoma. A detailed exam with a forward-viewing endoscope might also identify subepithelial duodenal tumors occasionally, and should be performed in all patients prior to EUS. We suspect that this might be owing to the very high percentage of hypoechoic gastrinomas as compared with insulinomas that may have a higher percentage of isoechoic lesions (Table 3).

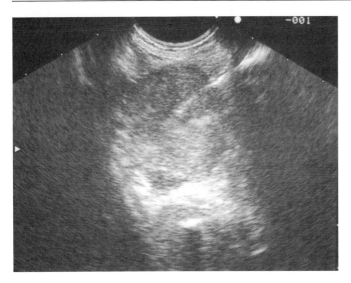

Fig. 2. Image of well-circumscribed pancreatic neuroendocrine tumor undergoing endosonographically guided fine-needle aspiration performed using a Pentax curved linear array echoendoscope.

Table 3
Ultrasonographic Features of the Pancreatic Endocrine Tumors Detected by Endoscopic Ultrasound

Feature	Number of tumors (%)
Insulinomas	25
Echogenic pattern	
Hypoechoic	17 (68)
Isoechoic	7 (28)
Hyperechoic	1 (4)
Ultrasonographic texture	
Homogenous	21 (84)
Inhomogeneous	4 (16)
Gastrinoma	47
Echogenic pattern	
Hypoechoic	45 (96)
Isoechoic	2 (4)
Hyperechoic	0
Ultrasonographic texture	
Homogenous	45 (96)
Inhomogeneous	2 (4)

Modified from ref. 28.

When EUS is negative, the intra-arterial calcium stimulation is the logical next step for insulinoma localization (25).

The use of EUS for diagnosis and localization of PETs is becoming routine. Compared with other highly accurate modalities, EUS is a low-risk procedure that is highly sensitive and accurate. In a case–control study, we demonstrated EUS to be highly cost-effective when used early in the pre-operative localization strategy, leading to reductions in pre-operative testing and intra-operative time (29).

5.3. SELECTIVE ANGIOGRAPHY WITH SECRETIN INFUSION

Another technique, selective angiography with secretin infusion (SASI), had also been used for tumor localization in patients

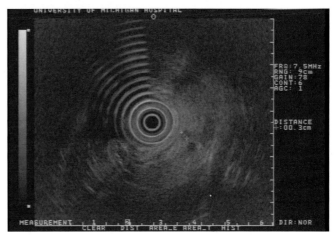

Fig. 3. Two small (3 mm) pancreatic endocrine tumors identified by screening in an asymptomatic patient with multiple endocrine neoplasia type-1 syndrome using the Olympus Radial Echoendoscope.

with suspected gastrinomas. This technique suffers from poor sensitivity (41%), however, higher specificity (98%) has been reported (30). Unfortunately another study examining the utility of SASI suggested a much lower specificity, of approx 12%, for this technique. In eight patients with suspected gastrinoma, SASI incorrectly suggested the presence of tumor in seven patients and was correctly negative in one patient (28). As a result of these conflicting studies, the role of SASI remains unclear.

5.4. TUMOR LOCALIZATION IN PATIENTS WITH MEN-1

There is no consensus on the approach to early diagnosis and management of NETs for patients with MEN-1. In MEN-1 kindreds, biochemical screening is often performed. Detection of tumors by biochemical screening and subsequent imaging may lead to diagnosis two decades before the disease becomes clinically overt. Recently, our group has pioneered the use of EUS (Fig. 3) to discover NETs in this population at an even earlier stage than imaging with cross-sectional imaging such as CT (31).

The timing of surgical treatment remains controversial for these patients. The lethality of MEN-1 is felt to be resulting from complications of excess hormone production and the metastatic potential for these tumors. Little controversy exists about surgical resection when patients present with a VIP or insulin secreting NET or when it is greater than 3 cm in size. The timing of surgery in MEN-1 patients with ZES remains controversial because of the use of PPIs, which can control nearly all the acid production and protect patients from the complications related to peptic ulcer disease (32).

At the University of Michigan, MEN-1 patients with pancreaticoduodenal disease are treated with aggressive surgical resection. This approach is based on the results of a series of 40 patients with MEN-1 and ZES where aggressive surgical resection was performed with only 1 patient developing a metachronous solitary liver metastasis with patients followed as long as 19 yr (33). Additionally, in a cohort (11 out of 48 patients) that was explored surgically, no correlation was found between tumor size and the presence of metastases (34). This finding suggests that tumor size alone cannot be used as a

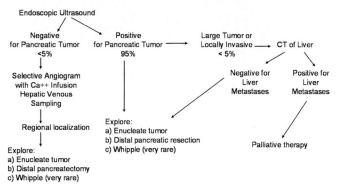

Fig. 4. Approach to patients with insulinoma.

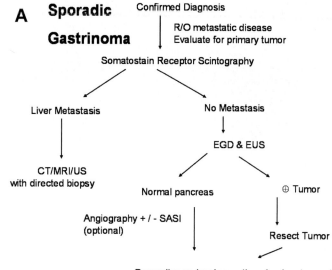

Fig. 5. (A) Algorithm for the approach to patients with biochemically confirmed gastrinoma/Zollinger-Ellison syndrome. (B) Algorithm for the approach to patients with multiple endocrine neoplasia type-1 and biochemically confirmed insulinoma.

pre-operative criterion for surgical exploration, and might support a more aggressive approach.

5.5. TUMOR LOCALIZATION IN VHL

Pancreatic lesions associated with VHL may be found in up to 75% of patients. Most pancreatic lesions are cysts and by nature are benign. At times, complete replacement of the pancreas with cystic change can lead to exocrine insufficiency. Solid lesions of the pancreas are less common and may be because of cystic neoplasms (serous cystadenomas) or neuroendocrine tumors. Because studies have demonstrated that neuroendocrine tumors in VHL can demonstrate malignant potential, it has been suggested that surveillance CT imaging be performed in patients with VHL (35). Because patients with VHL are at risk of multiple tumors, screening recommendations are provided by the National Institutes of Health. Ultrasound, CT, and MRI are currently used to screen for renal cell carcinoma as well as other abdominal organ complications of the disease. General recommendations are to screen starting at the age of 11 and repeat yearly or every other year (except CT, which screening starts at 20 yr and repeated yearly or every other year) (36). The role of EUS in VHL has not been defined. We speculate that the role of EUS might allow for the morphological differentiation of solid pancreatic masses. The differentiation of benign cystic neoplasms from neuroendocrine tumors could alter the surgical approach.

6. SURGICAL APPROACH TO SPORADIC NEUROENDOCRINE TUMORS

6.1. INSULINOMA

Surgical excision is the treatment of choice, and cure rates in the literature range from 77 to 100% (Fig. 4). The surgical procedure varies based on the anatomical position of the tumor as well as its size. The general approach is tumor enucleation whenever possible (37). Some surgeons employ intraoperative ultrasound if EUS or other imaging failed to identify the tumor location pre-operatively. When the tumor is located in the head, enucleation, or rarely a Whipple procedure, is performed (38). Blind distal pancreatectomy historically was performed when localization was not confirmed either pre- or intra-operatively. A review of 17 patients referred to the National Institutes of Health for failure to respond after blind distal pancreatec-

tomy, 5 patients had factitious hypoglycemia and the remaining 12 patients had the tumor eventually localized to the head, a finding that has resulted in this recommendation being reversed (39).

6.2. GASTRINOMA/ZES

Tumor excision is the goal for treatment. If pre-operative localization with EUS demonstrates that the pancreas appears normal, we assume there is a duodenal primary, and duodenotomy with transillumination with or without the use of intraoperative ultrasound is employed at the time surgical excision (Fig. 5). Duodenotomy added to surgical exploration for gastrinoma has been shown to improve outcomes both in the immediate postoperative cure rate as well as in the long-term cure rate (40). This is likely owing to the increased recognition of duodenal gastrinomas. The surgical approach to gastrinomas is directed with localization, and enucleation is favored over resection (41). If this is not possible, or multiple tumors are present in a particular location, then resection is performed

MEN-I Gastrinoma

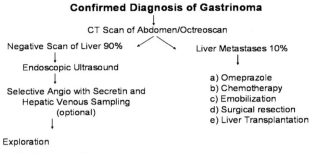

Fig. 6. Algorithm for the approach to patients with multiple endocrine neoplasia type-1 and biochemically confirmed gastrinoma/Zollinger-Ellison Syndrome.

either with a distal pancreatectomy for tumors in the body and tail or Whipple procedure for tumors in the head.

7. SURGICAL APPROACH TO FAMILIAL NEUROENDOCRINE TUMORS

7.1. MEN-1 INSULINOMA

Insulinomas in MEN-1 patients may be multicentric and therefore local tumor resection often is associated with disease recurrence (Fig. 6). Therefore, a different surgical approach in this patient population is advocated. The aim is distal subtotal pancreatectomy and enucleation of any tumor identified in the head of pancreas in patients with MEN-I and hyperinsulinemia (42).

7.2. MEN-1 GASTRINOMA/ZES

ZES in patients with MEN-1 will typically undergo a distal pancreatectomy to the level of the superior mesenteric vein, preserving the spleen when appropriate and feasible. Duodenotomy is only performed as part of this operation if MEN-1 ZES is suspected or in a patient with an elevated serum gastrin and a positive secretin test. Lymph node dissection is performed in the lymphatic distribution of a tumor that is located in the pancreas or small bowel because these are common locations of metastatic disease (43).

8. MEDICAL MANAGEMENT OF NETS

8.1. INSULINOMA

Chemotherapy is generally reserved for malignant islet cell tumors. Combination streptozocin with 5-fluorouracil or doxorubicin has response rates significantly better than with streptozocin alone (63 vs 36%) (44). The long-acting somatostatin analog octreotide might reduce hormone secretion as well as tumor proliferation in many patients (45). Specific medical treatments depend on the tumor type. Insulinomas may respond to the use of diazoxide, a drug that has been found to inhibit release of insulin and also has a peripheral hyperglycemic effect. In gastrinomas, medical therapeutics includes the use of intravenous H2 blockers and, more commonly, oral PPIs. Higher doses of PPIs may be required to completely

control excess acid production and prevent acid secretion induced side effects. Nearly 100% of patients can achieve complete control of acid production with this class of medications and in the few that cannot comply with medical management, or who have refractory disease, may undergo palliative total gastrectomy (46). Octreotide can also be used in patients who do not have a complete response to anti-secretory agents (47).

9. CONCLUSIONS

Endoscopic methods are primarily used in the pre-operative localization of NETs and have been shown to alter the surgical approach in patients with both sporadic and familial sources of NETs. The use of EUS is highly accurate and cost-effective. For patients with MEN-1 not only can EUS localize NETs in the head, which might alter the surgical approach, but EUS can identify PETs earlier than any other screening technique to date and can be used to monitor tumor size in surveillance programs (6).

The state of the art in the management of NETs is a multidisciplinary approach where EUS has an integral role, which, when used in combination with other limited localization techniques, facilitates the surgical management of patients with NETs.

REFERENCES

1. Jensen RT. Endocrine neoplasms of the pancreas. In: Yamada T, Alpers DH. Owyang, et al., eds. Textbook of Gastroenterology, 4th ed. Philadelphia: Lippincott Williams & Wilkins, 2003; 2108.
2. Glascock JM, Carty SE. Multiple endocrine neoplasia type 1: fresh perspective on clinical features and penetrance. Surgical Oncol 2002; 11:143–150.
3. Hes FJ, Feldberg MAM. Von Hippel-Lindau disease: strategies in early detection (renal-, adrenal-, pancreatic masses). Eur Radiol 1999; 9:598–610.
4. Doherty GM, Olson JA, Frisella MM, Lairmore TC, Wells SA, Nortton JA. Lethality of multiple endocrine neoplasia type 1. World J Surg 1998; 22:581–587.
5. Maton PN, Gradner JD, Jensen RT. Diagnosis and management of Zollinger-Ellison syndrome. Endocrinol Metab Clin North Am 1989; 18:519.
6. Wamsteker EJ. Gauger PG. Thompson NW. Scheiman JM. EUS detection of pancreatic endocrine tumors in asymptomatic patients with type 1 multiple endocrine neoplasia. Gastrointestinal Endosc 2003; 58:531–535.
7. Fraker DL, Jensen RT. Pancreatic endocrine tumors. In: DeVita VT, Hellman S, Rosenberg SA, eds. Cancer: Principles and practice of oncology. Philadelphia: Lippincott-Raven, 1997:1678–1704.
8. Norton JA. Pancreatic Islet Cell Tumors Excluding Gastrinomas. St Louis, Missouri: Mosby, 1998.
9. O' Riordain DS, O'Brien T, van Heerden JA, Service FJ, and Grant CS. Surgical management of insulinoma associated with multiple endocrine neoplasia type I. World J Surg 1994; 18:488–494.
10. Grant CS. Surgical management of malignant islet cell tumours. World J Surg 1993; 17:498–503.
11. Kent RB, Van Heerden JA, Weiland LH. Nonfunctioning islet cell tumors. Ann Surg 1981; 193:185.
12. Grumberger G, Weiner JL, Silvermar R, Taylor S and Gordon P. Factitious hypoglycemia due to surreptitious administration of insulin. Ann Int Med 1988; 108:252–257.
13. van Heerden JA. Insulinoma: diagnosis and management. Surgical Rounds 1980:40–51.
14. Bliss RD, Carter PB, Lennard TWJ. Insulinoma: a review of current management. Surgical Oncol 1997; 6:49–59.
15. Stage JG, Stadil F. The clinical diagnosis of the Zollinger Ellison syndrome. Scand J Gastroenterol 1979; 14(suppl 33):79.

16. Isenberg JI, Walsh JH, Passaro E Jr, Moore EW, Grossman MI. Unusual effect of secretin on serum gastrin, serum calcium and gastric acid secretion in a patient with suspected Zollinger Ellison syndrome. Gastroenterology 1972; 62:626.

17. Frucht H, Howard JM, Slaff JI, et al. Secretin and calcium provocative tests in the Zollinger-Ellison syndrome. Ann Intern Med 1989; 111:713.

18. Krejs GJ. VIPoma syndrome. Am J Med 1987; 82:37–48.

19. Verner JV, Morrison AB. Endocrine pancreatic islet disease with diarrhea. Arch Intern Med. 1974; 133:492–500.

20. Soga J, Yakuwa Y. Somatostatinoma/inhibitory syndrome: a statistical evaluation of 173 reported cases as compared to other pancreatic endocrinomas. J Exp Clin Cancer Res 1999; 18:13–22.

21. Chandrasekharappa SC, Guru SC, Manickamp P, et al. Positional cloning of the gene for multiple endocrine neoplasia-type 1. Science 1997; 276: 404–407.

22. Couch VMS, Lindor NM, Karnes PS, Michels VV. Von Hippel-Lindau Disease. 2000; 75: 265–272.

23. Chatziioannou A, Kehagias D, Mourikis D, Antoniou A, Limouris G, Kaponis A, Kavatzas N, Tseleni S, Vlachos L. Imaging and localization of pancreatic Insulinomas. J Clin Imag 2001; 25: 275–283.

24. Zimmer T, Ziegler K, Bader M, et al. Localisation of neuroendocrine tumours of the upper gastrointestinal tract. Gut 1994; 35:471–475.

25. Doppman JL, Chang R, Fraker, et al. Localization of Insulinomas to regions of the pancreas by intra-arterial stimulation with calcium. Ann Intern Med 1995; 123:269–73.

26. Proye C, Malvaux P, Pattou F, Filoche B, Godchaux JM, Maunorury V, Palazzo L, Huglo D, Lefebvre J, Paris JC. Noninvasive imaging of insulinomas and gastrinomas with endoscopic ultrasonography and somatostatin receptor scintigraphy. Surgery 1998; 124:1134–1144.

27. Nocaudie-Calzada M, Huglo D, Deveaux M, Carnaille B, Proye C, Marchandise X, Iodine-123-tyr-3-octreotide uptake in pancreatic endocrine tumors and in carcinoids in relation to hormonal inhibition by Octreotide. J Nucl Med 1994; 35:57–62.

28. Anderson MA, Carpenter S, Thompson NW, Nostrant TT, Elta GH, Scheiman JM. Endoscopic ultrasound is highly accurate and directs management in patients with neuroendocrine tumors of the pancreas. Am J Gastroenterol 2000; 95:2271–2277.

29. Bansal R. Tierney W. Carpenter S. Thompson N. Scheiman JM. Cost effectiveness of EUS for preoperative localization of pancreatic endocrine tumors. Gastrointest Endosc 1999; 49:19–25.

30. Gibril F, Doppman JL, Chang R, et al. Metastatic gastrinomas. Localization with selective arterial injection of secretin. Radiology 1996; 198:77–84.

31. Oberg K, Skogseid B. The ultimate biochemical diagnosis of endocrine pancreatic tumours in MEN-1. J Intern Med 1998; 243: 471–476.

32. Gauger PG, Thompson NW. Early surgical intervention and strategy in patients with multiple endocrine neoplasia type 1. Best Practice Res Clin Endocrinol Metabol 2001; 15(2):213–223.

33. Thompson NW. Current concepts in the surgical management of multiple endocrine neoplasia type 1 pancreatic-duodenal disease. Results in the treatment of 40 patients with Zollinger-Ellison syndrome, hypoglycemia or both. J Int Med 1998; 243:495–500.

34. Lowney JK, Frisella MM, Lairmore TC, Doherty GM. Pancreatic islet cell tumor metastasis in multiple endocrine neoplasia type 1: Correlation with primary tumor size. Surgery 1999, 125:1043–1049.

35. Lubutti SK, Choyke PL, Bartlett DL, Vargas H, McClellan W, Lubensky I, Glenn G, Linehan WM, Alexander HR. Pancreatic neuroendocrine tumors associated with von Hippel Lindau disease: Diagnostic and management recommendations. Surgery 1998; 124:1153–1150.

36. Choyke PL, Glenn GM, Walther MM, Patronas NJ, Linehan WM, Zbar B. von Hippel-Lindau disease: genetic, clinical and imaging features. Radiology 1995; 194:629–642.

37. Finlayson E, Clark OH. Surgical treatment of insulinomas. Surg Clin North Am 2004; 84:775–785.

38. Geoghegan JG, Jackson JE, Lewis MPN, Owen ERTC, Bloom SR, Lynn JA, Williamson RCN. Localization and surgical management or insulinoma. Br J Surg 1994; 81:1025–1028.

39. Hirshberg B, Libutti SK, Alexander HR, et al. Blind distal pancreatectomy for occult insulinoma, an inadvisable procedure. J Am Coll Surg 2002; 194:761–764.

40. Norton JA, Alexander HR, Fraker DL, Venzon DJ, Gibril F, Jensen RT. Does the use of routine duodenotomy affect rate of cure, development of liver metastases, or survival in patients with Zollinger-Ellison Syndrome? Ann Surg 2004; 239:617–623.

41. Norton JA, Fraker DL, Alexander HR, et al. Surgery to cure the Zollinger-Ellison Syndrome. N Engl J Med 1999; 341:635–644.

42. Lo CY, King-Yin L, Fan ST. Surgical strategy for insulinomas in multiple endocrine neoplasia type 1. Am J Surg 1998; 175:305–307.

43. Thompson NW. Management of pancreatic endocrine tumors in patients with multiple endocrine neoplasia type 1. Surg Oncol Clin North Am 1998; 7:881–891.

44. Moertel CG, Handley JA and Johnson LA. Streptozocin alone compared with streptozocin plus 5-fluorouracil in the treatment of advanced islet cell carcinoma. N Engl J Med 1980; 303:1189–1194.

45. Brentjens R, Saltz L. Islet cell tumors of the pancreas. Surgical clin North Am 2001; 81:527–542.

46. Jensen, RT, Fraker, DL. Zollinger-Ellison Syndrome: Advances in Treatment of Gastric Hypersecretion and the Gastrinoma. JAMA 1994;271:1429–1435.

47. Annibale B, Delle Fave G, Azzoni C, et al.. Three months of octreotide treatment decreases gastric acid secretion and argyrophil cell density in patients with Zollinger-Ellison syndrome and antral G-cell hyperfunction. Alimentary Pharmacol Therapeut 1994; 8:95–104.

28 Endoscopic Diagnosis and Management of Cholangiocarcinoma

VANESSA M. SHAMI, MD AND IRVING WAXMAN, MD

CONTENTS

1. BACKGROUND

Cholangiocarcinoma is rare with an increasing incidence with age. There are a variety of diagnostic studies available to evaluate the presence and extent of cholangiocarcinoma. Unfortunately, the majority of symptomatic patients present with advanced disease and are not candidates for curative resection. Palliation in the majority of cases consists of endoscopic decompression of the biliary tract to decrease the morbidity of jaundice, which includes pruritus, impaired hepatic and renal function, and associated coagulopathy. More recently, complementary palliative modalities such as photodynamic therapy (PDT) and brachytherapy have emerged.

2. INTRODUCTION

Cholangiocarcinoma is rare, representing less than 3% of all cancers with a reported incidence of 0.01–0.2% in large autopsy series (1,2). The incidence increases with age with two-thirds of all cases occurring in patients more than 65 yr old, with a peak incidence in the eighth decade of life (3). The distribution is slightly higher in males with a male to female ratio of 1.3:1 (4).

Predisposing factors for cholangiocarcinoma are listed in Table 1. Any condition that is associated with biliary stasis and chronic inflammation is a potential risk factor for the disease. The most common risk factor in the United States is primary sclerosing cholangitis (PSC) where occult cholangiocarcinoma has been reported in up to 40% of autopsy specimens and in up to 36% of liver explants after transplantation (5–8). The majority of cases of cholangiocarcinoma in America, however, are sporadic and have none of these risk factors identified.

Cholangiocarcinoma can develop anywhere along the biliary tree from the terminal ductules to the ampulla of Vater.

From: *Endoscopic Oncology: Gastrointestinal Endoscopy and Cancer Management.* Edited by: D. O. Faigel and M. L. Kochman © Humana Press, Totowa, NJ

Intrahepatic (peripheral) cholangiocarcinomas are rare and made up of 6–10% of all cholangiocarcinomas and typically present as solitary hepatic masses (9). Extrahepatic cholangiocarcinoma has been divided into three groups dependent on anatomic location. Proximal perihilar tumors are located in the common hepatic duct and/or the right and left hepatic ducts and are known as Klatskin tumors. They are the most common tumors accounting for up to two-thirds of all cholangiocarcinomas (9–11). The extent of duct involvement by Klatskin tumors may be classified according to Bismuth and Corlette (12) (Fig. 1). Middle extrahepatic tumors are bounded by the upper border of the duodenum and extend to the common hepatic bile duct. They comprise 17–20% of the cholangiocarcinomas. Lower or distal bile duct tumors arise between the ampulla of Vater and the upper border of the duodenum and comprise approx 18–27% of the tumors.

Painless jaundice is the most common clinical presentation in extrahepatic cholangiocarcinoma. In contrast, intrahepatic cholangiocarcinoma may present at a more advanced stage before causing symptoms of obstruction, because one unobstructed liver lobe often provides adequate biliary excretion to prevent jaundice. Therefore, patients with intrahepatic disease more often present with systemic manifestations such as fatigue and malaise. Other nonspecific complaints in patients presenting with extra- or intrahepatic cholangiocarcinoma include pruritus, abdominal pain, and weight loss, in part because of malabsorption caused by diminished bile excretion. Cholangitis is a rare clinical presentation in the noninstrumented patient. On physical examination, patients are usually jaundiced and rarely will have hepatomegaly, a palpable mass, or a palpable distended gallbladder (Courvoisier's sign).

There are no serum tests that are diagnostic for cholangiocarcinoma. Cholestasis with an elevated alkaline phosphatase, bilirubin, and γ-glutamyl transpeptidase is often noted. There may be prolongation of the prothrombin time secondary to a decrease in fat-soluble vitamin K. The value of carbohydrate

Table 1
Factors Predisposing to Cholangiocarcinoma

Acquired	Primary sclerosing cholangitis[a]
	Oriental hepatolithiasis
	Bile duct adenoma and biliary papillomatosis
Infectious	Liver flukes
	Opisthorcis viverrini
	Clonorchis sinensis
	Chronic typhoid
Congenital	Caroli's disease
	Choledochal cysts
	Congenital hepatic fibrosis
	Polycystic liver disease
	A long common channel
Exposures	Thorotrast

[a]The most common known predisposing factor of cholangiocarcinoma.

antigen 19-9 (CA 19-9) in cholangiocarcinoma is unclear but is elevated in up to 85% of patients *(13–15)*. CA 19-9 may also be elevated in benign etiologies of biliary obstruction as well as in the setting of pancreatic or gastric malignancies. Carcinoembryonic antigen and CA-125 may be elevated in 30% and 40–50% of patients with cholangiocarcinoma, respectively, but neither test is sensitive or specific.

Various histological types of cholangiocarcinoma are seen. The majority of intra- and extrahepatic cholangiocarcinomas are ductal adenocarcinomas. Rarely, papillary, mucinous, signet-ring cell, mucoepidermoid, adenosquamous, squamous, and cystadenocarcinoma types of cholangiocarcinoma present *(16,17)*.

3. DIAGNOSIS/STAGING

The diagnosis of cholangiocarcinoma is usually made on evaluation of obstructive jaundice or transaminase elevation. Goals of diagnostic and staging evaluation include: tissue confirmation, assessment of the extent and level of biliary tract and portal vein involvement, assessment of the liver for evidence of lobar atrophy or concomitant pathology, and evaluation of the extent or presence of nodal disease, and/or distant metastasis *(18)*. Tumor-node-metastasis (TNM) stage grouping for cholangiocarcinoma is as follows: stage 1 is tumor limited to the bile duct or extending just beyond the bile duct wall; stage 2 is local invasion and/or regional lymph node metastasis; stage 3 involves invasion of the main portal vein or its branches, common hepatic artery, or other adjacent structures such as the colon, stomach, duodenum, or abdominal wall; and stage 4 is metastatic disease *(19)*. Unfortunately, up to 50% of patients have stage 3 disease and 10–20% have stage 4 disease at presentation. The recommended algorithm for the diagnosis and staging of cholangiocarcinoma is summarized in Fig. 2.

3.1. RADIOLOGIC STUDIES
3.1.1. Ultrasound

Ultrasound (US) is an inexpensive, widely available, and noninvasive modality to evaluate patients presenting with obstructive jaundice. It can detect bile duct stones, differentiate obstructive from nonobstructive jaundice with a high accuracy, *(20)* and provide information about the level of obstruction *(21)*. One study *(22)* determined the sensitivity of US to correctly diagnose and establish the site and etiology of obstruction as 94% with a specificity of 96%.

In distal cholangiocarcinoma, a mass is often not visualized however in Klatskin tumors, US can visualize a mass in 83–89% of patients *(21,23)*. Additionally, duplex US can correctly diagnose vascular involvement such as the portal vein and hepatic artery in 85–91% of cases therefore assessing local unresectability. US, however, cannot reliably predict lymph node metastasis or show tumor infiltration into the hepatoduodenal ligament *(24)*. Additionally, US findings may not be able to differentiate peripheral cholangiocarcinoma from those cases of metastases from extrahepatic sites or hepatocellular carcinoma with a multinodular pattern *(25)*.

3.1.2. Computed Tomography

Computed tomography (CT) is widely available, and therefore, like US, is one of the most commonly performed tests for the initial evaluation of obstructive jaundice. Usually an abrupt termination of part of the biliary tree is noted with proximal dilation (Fig. 3). Recently, helical CT dual-phase imaging has been used. As opposed to conventional portal phase imaging, helical CT scans are acquired during both the arterial and portal phases of contrast enhancement. Peripheral cholangiocarcinoma is seen as a low attenuation irregular mass with minimal peripheral enhancement during both the arterial and portal venous phases *(26)*. Additionally, there is focal dilatation of the intrahepatic ducts around the tumor. The central part of the tumor does not enhance during these phases, whereas there may be prolonged enhancement at delayed-phase CT. Therefore, CT may reveal an intrahepatic mass lesion, dilated intrahepatic ducts, and localized lymphadenopathy. However, it does not usually define the extent of cholangiocarcinoma.

3.1.3. Magnetic Resonance Imaging/Magnetic Resonance Cholangiography

Magnetic resonance imaging (MRI)/magnetic resonance cholangiography (MRC) has the capacity to provide excellent noninvasive identification of the biliary system. This imaging modality has the advantage of being able to depict MRC, vascular anatomy (magnetic resonance angiography), and cross-sectional imaging of the liver to assess for nodal or distant metastases with a single technique *(27–29)* (Fig. 4). The MRI/MRC appearance of cholangiocarcinoma is that of a nonencapsulated tumor, hypointense on T1-weighted images and hyperintense on T2-weighted images *(30)*. Dilation of peripheral bile ducts distal to the lesion may be seen. MRI/MRC not only can determine the level of tumor involvement, but also can assess the extent of disease and visualize the biliary anatomy proximal to the obstruction often revealing isolated ducts not visualized at an endoscopic study *(31)*. Additionally, it avoids infection risk and other complications associated with endoscopic procedures and enables imaging of patients with altered surgical anatomy. However, MRI/MRC lacks the tissue sampling capability and therapeutic potential. Additionally, it has been criticized in delaying the appropriate care in patients who need therapeutic endoscopic or percutaneous intervention of obstructing bile duct lesions *(32)*.

MRI/MRC appears to be sensitive in detecting hilar cholangiocarcinomas *(33)*. In a retrospective study of 12

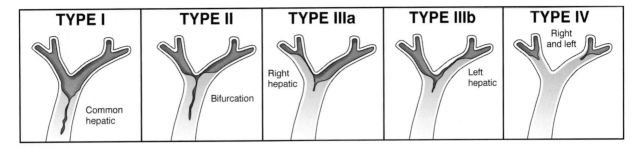

Fig. 1. The Bismuth and Corlette classification of Klatskin tumors.

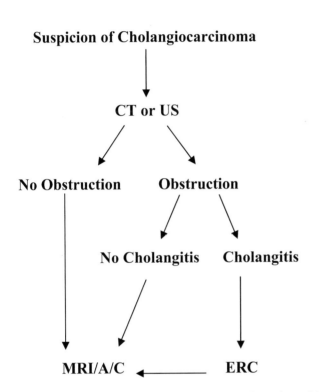

Fig. 2. The approach to the diagnosis and work-up of a patient with suspected cholangiocarcinoma.

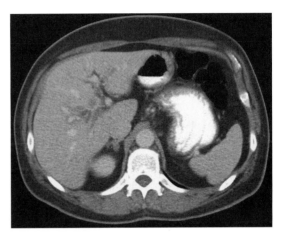

Fig. 3. A computed tomography scan of the abdomen in a patient presenting with obstructive jaundice reveals a mass in the porta hepatis with proximal intrahepatic biliary dilation suggestive of a Klatskin tumor.

patients with histologically confirmed hilar cholangiocarcinoma, MRI/MRC correctly diagnosed all cases. In other cases, MRI/MRC has been demonstrated to be as good as endoscopic retrograde cholangiography (ERC) in determining the level of bile duct obstruction and in differentiating benign strictures from malignant causes (29,34). Di Cesare et al. (35) reported the results of 21 patients with suspected malignant obstruction of the distal biliary tract that underwent MRC and ERC. MRC identified the presence and site of the distal biliary stenosis in all cases, although ERC detected the same in 20/21 cases. In another study (36), 88 patients with surgically proven cholangiocarcinoma were analyzed retrospectively. The accuracy of MRC in the location of hilar cholangiocarcinoma was 100% and extrahepatic cholangiocarcinoma was 52.2%, which increased to 91.3% when combined with enhanced MRI.

In summary, MRI/MRC is able to assess the extent of biliary involvement, as well as the presence of locally invasive and metastatic disease with a single technique. When available, it is the test of choice to assess for the presence and extent of cholangiocarcinoma.

3.1.4. Positron Emission Tomography

Fluorodeoxyglucose (FDG) is a glucose analog that accumulates in various malignant tumors because of their high glucose metabolic rates (Fig. 5). The role of FDG-PET in the diagnosis and staging of biliary tract cancers is still evolving.

In a recent study (37) FDG-PET was performed on 26 patients with adenocarcinoma of the biliary tract, 8 patients with benign lesions, and 20 control patients. The sensitivity and specificity for detecting malignancy was 92.3 and 92.9%, respectively. Although FDG-PET was good in detection of distant metastasis (7 of 10 cases), it only correctly detected regional or hepatoduodenal lymph node metastasis in 2 of 15 cases. In another study looking at hilar lesions (38), the sensitivity and specificity for detecting malignancy was 83 and 100%, respectively. Detection of distant metastasis had a significant influence on the treatment and strategy in as much as 20% of the patients. In another retrospective study of 21 patients with cholangiocarcinoma (39), PET was positive in all but one case of hilar cholangiocarcinoma. Unsuspected metastasis was detected in 4 of the 21 patients. In another study (40), 36 consecutive patients who underwent FDG-PET for suspected cholangiocarcinoma were reviewed. The sensitivity varied according to the morphology of the biliary cancer and was 85% for nodular and only 18% for infiltration morphology. Sensitivity for metastases was 65% but false-negative for carcinomatosis in three of three patients. There was one false-positive result in a patient with PSC and cholangitis. FDG-PET led to a change in surgical management in 30% owing to detection of unsuspected metastases.

In summary, the role of FDG-PET scanning in patients with suspected cholangiocarcinoma is evolving. Although helpful in detecting unsuspected metastatic disease, its role in local disease involvement is more controversial. One must caution its use in patients with cholangitis as this may result in a false-positive exam.

3.2. ENDOSCOPIC STUDIES

3.2.1. Endoscopic Retrograde Cholangiography

ERC is superior to MRC in the visualization of ampullary and duodenal cancers, affords the ability to obtain biopsy specimens or brushings, and may be more widely available. The ability to obtain a definite diagnosis is helpful especially in patients with unresectable disease where oftentimes oncologists want tissue confirmation to direct management. However, although the specificity of pathological diagnosis with endoscopic tissue sampling techniques approaches 100%, the sensitivity is low. Forceps biopsy has the highest yield with needle aspiration and fluid cytology having the lowest sensitivity *(41,42)*. Even the combination of brush cytology, FNA, and biopsy has a sensitivity of only 62% with a negative predictive value of 39% *(43)*.

ERC establishes the location of the tumor and the biliary extent of disease, both of which are critical in surgical planning *(44)*. However, more recent studies have demonstrated that MRC is at least as accurate as ERC in determining the location and extent of a pancreaticobiliary stricture *(45,46)*. When there is biliary obstruction, ERC should be followed by successful drainage to minimize the risk of infection *(47)*. ERC is particularly challenging in patients with complex hilar strictures because drainage of all obstructed branches in which contrast is injected is mandatory *(48,49)*. Therefore, ERC should be reserved for cases where a tissue diagnosis is needed, in patients presenting with cholangitis where therapeutic decompression is mandatory, or in cases where biliary decompression is desired before the initiation of systemic therapy in patients with unresectable disease.

3.2.2. Endoscopic Ultrasound

The definitive diagnosis of cholangiocarcinoma remains a challenge as the sensitivity for the detection of cholangiocarcinomas by brush cytology at ERC is 20–80% *(41,50–54)*. Consequently, other diagnostic modalities such as EUS-FNA have recently been investigated *(55–57)*. In one study, 28 patients with non-diagnostic sampling of biliary lesions underwent EUS-FNA *(56)*. The sensitivity, specificity, positive predictive value, negative predictive value, and accuracy were 86, 100, 100, 57, and 88% respectively. EUS-FNA had a positive impact on patient management in 84% of patients. In another study *(55)*, 44 patients with hilar strictures and inconclusive diagnosis underwent EUS-FNA. Accuracy, sensitivity, and specificity were 91, 89, and 100% respectively. EUS and EUS-FNA changed pre-planned surgical approach in 27 of 44 patients. These preliminary data suggest that EUS-FNA is a reasonable diagnostic alternative in cases where tissue confirmation is needed.

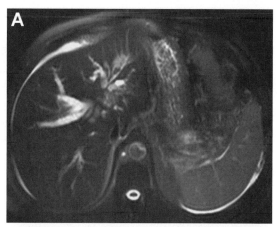

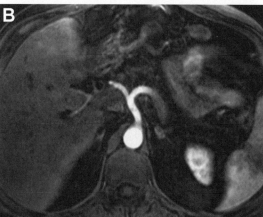

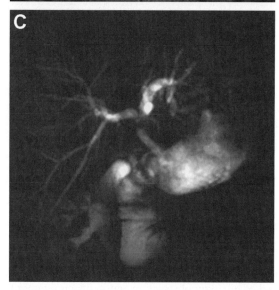

Fig. 4. **(A)** A magnetic resonance imaging T2-weighted image reveals focal thickening of the common hepatic duct at the level of the confluence with intrahepatic ductal dilatation. **(B)** A T1-weighted image reveals tumor involvement of the hepatic artery. **(C)** A magnetic resonance cholangiography reveals a filling defect of the proximal common hepatic duct extending to the confluence.

3.2.3. Intraductal Ultrasonography

Intraductal ultrasonography (IDUS) of the pancreaticobiliary system is currently under clinical evaluation. The small diameter of the current US probes (5–10 French [F]) and high frequencies (12.5–30 MHz), as well as the capacity to pass the

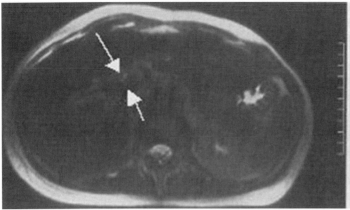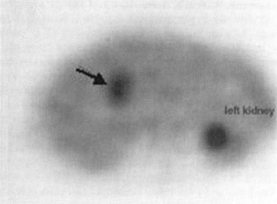

Fig. 5. A positron emission tomography scan in a patient with cholangiocarcinoma reveals increased uptake in the hilum and left kidney.

probes through the working channel of the duodenoscope has awoken interest in their application. The probes can be advanced in a transpapillary fashion under fluoroscopic control by free cannulation, or over a guide-wire.

By IDUS, using a 30-MHz probe, three layers can usually be identified. An outer echogenic layer representing an interface echo, middle hypoechoic layer representing the mucosa, muscularis propria, and fibrous layer of the subserosa, and inner echogenic layer which corresponds to the adipose layer of the subserosa and the serosa (58,59). Preliminary data on IDUS indicate that it is useful in assessing the extension of bile duct carcinoma into the portal vein and right hepatic artery, but does not sufficiently demonstrate the left and proper hepatic artery, i.e., vascular invasion outside the hepatoduodenal ligament, as well as distant metastasis (60–62). Menzel et al. (63) compared the accuracy of IDUS with conventional EUS in staging biliary carcinomas and assessing resectability in 56 patients. The study showed IDUS to be significantly superior to conventional EUS for T staging (77 vs 54%) with a reported accuracy and sensitivity of 89 vs 76% and 91 vs 76%, respectively. In addition, IDUS was better at predicting resectability (82 vs 76%) as compared with conventional EUS. IDUS has also been shown to be more accurate than cholangiography in assessing for intraductal spread (86 vs 43%) (64).

Recent reports of a newer technology three-dimensional (3D) IDUS, which reconstructs a 3D image from radial and linear intraductal scanning with the aid of computer software, suggest this technology might be better at assessing the extension of bile duct tumors and their relationship with surrounding organs (65,66). Tamada et al. (67) compared 3D IDUS to 2D imaging in assessing tumor extension of bile duct carcinoma. 3D reconstructions of the primary tumor and its relationship to surrounding structures allowed for better recognition of tumor involvement into the pancreas and portal vein as compared with 2D IDUS, suggesting that 3D technology may improve the accuracy for staging advanced disease (stage IV-A).

4. ENDOSCOPIC THERAPY

4.1. ENDOSCOPIC RETROGRADE CHOLANGIOGRAPHY

In patients with inoperable pancreaticobiliary malignancies, palliation by endoscopic decompression with biliary stent placement is the treatment of choice. Less commonly, pancreatic stents are placed to palliate the obstructive pain caused by main pancreatic duct stenosis.

4.1.1. Technique of Stent Placement

A cholangiogram is performed to identify the location and extent of the stricture (Fig. 6). A guidewire is then advanced across the stricture and into the more proximal biliary system. Dilation of the strictured area, either mechanical (with bougie or coaxial dilating catheters) or pneumatic dilation (using balloons) may be performed. Cytology, when indicated, may then be obtained with a cytology brush and/or biopsies. A plastic stent or metal stent is then advanced over the wire and across the stricture.

4.1.2. Endoscopic Decompression in Patients With Unresectable Cholangiocarcinoma

The goal in patients with unresectable cholangiocarcinoma is to palliate the morbidity of jaundice which includes pruritus, impaired hepatic and renal function, and associated coagulation problems. However, there are few studies examining the impact of endoscopic drainage on quality of life. Abraham et al. (68) performed a prospective cohort study on 50 patients to determine the clinical characteristics that have the greatest adverse impact on quality of life in patients with unresectable biliary obstruction and to quantify changes in quality of life after successful stent placement. Before endoscopic therapy, 70% were pruritic and 98% were icteric. Weight loss and elevated bilirubin level had the greatest impact on baseline quality of life domains in both univariate and multivariate analysis. After 1 mo of decompression, relief of jaundice was associated with significant improvements in social function and mental health; a bilirubin greater than 14 mg/dL was associated with a lack of improvement in social function. This study supports biliary decompression in jaundiced individuals with unresectable biliary tumors who have a reasonable life expectancy.

4.1.3. Surgical Bypass vs Endoscopic Stenting

Several studies have compared endoscopic stenting to surgical bypass for palliation in patients with unresectable malignant biliary obstruction. Although major complications were greater in the surgery group (69,70), all of the studies found no significant difference in patient survival between the two groups (69–74). Although initial hospitalization was reported to be

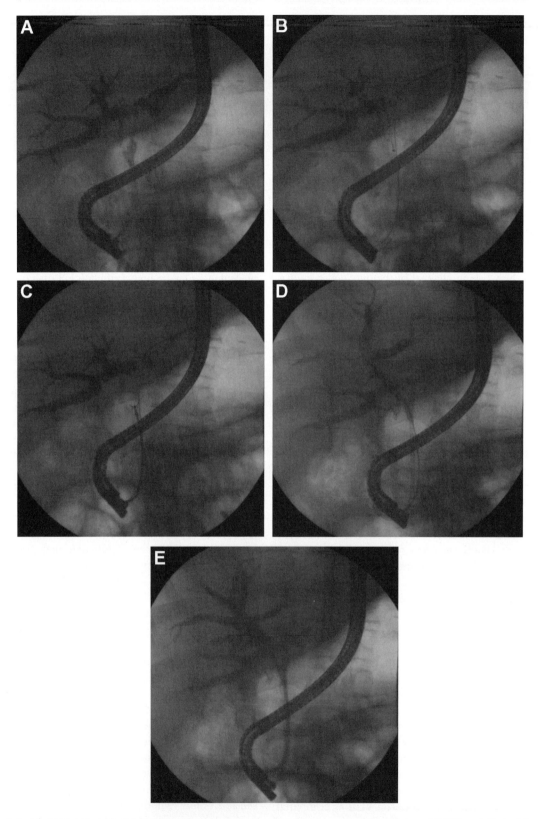

Fig. 6. **(A)** A cholangiogram in a patient who presents with obstructive jaundice reveals a Bismuth type IV filling defect of the hilum. **(B)** A guidewire is advanced into the left intrahepatic ductal system and brush cytology is being performed at the area of suspected tumor involvement. **(C)** Intraductal biopsies are being performed with a forceps for pathology. **(D)** A 10-French stent has been placed into the left intrahepatic system and balloon dilation is being performed of the right hepatic duct. **(E)** Another 10-French stent has been placed to drain the right intrahepatic system. Now both the left and right lobes of the liver are being decompressed.

shorter in the endoscopically treated group *(70,72,73)*, there was no significant difference in total days of hospitalization *(70,71)*. This is probably because of the more frequent readmissions noted in the endoscopically treated group secondary to stent occlusion *(70,72,73)*. Retrospective studies showed a lower cost for the endoscopic approach *(74,72)*. A recent meta-analysis is in favor of endoscopic biliary decompression in patients with a predicted survival of less than 6 mo and of surgery in patients with a longer life expectancy *(75)*. The above studies used plastic stents for biliary decompression and the outcome of surgical decompression vs endoscopic decompression with the longer patency metal biliary stents is still not known.

4.1.4. Endoscopic Decompression Pre-Operative in Patients With Resectable Disease

Although patients routinely undergo biliary decompression at major institutions prior to surgical resection, there is little data to support this. The rational for pre-operative decompression has been that hepatic reticuloendothelial cell function may return to normal and that biliary decompression may improve vitamin K absorption and consequently improve coagulopathy. Although some studies have found no effect on morbidity and mortality *(76–78)*, others have reported both increases and decreases in mortality and morbidity *(79–81)*. A meta-analysis on the effects of pre-operative biliary decompression on the outcome of surgery in patients with pancreatic reported no benefit to pre-operative endoscopic treatment.

In summary, the routine use of pre-operative biliary decompression is not recommended. Biliary drainage should be reserved for the minority of patients presenting with cholangitis, those who are severely malnourished, or those who may require neoadjuvant chemotherapy *(82)*.

4.1.5. Unilateral vs Bilateral Stenting in Hilar Malignancy

Palliation of jaundice usually requires drainage of 33–50% of the normal functioning liver. However, controversy exists as to whether unilateral or bilateral stenting should be performed. Cholangitis in the undrained segment of liver remains the major concern. Although some studies have shown that use of bilateral stents have resulted in fewer episodes of cholangitis and a reduction in the number of repeat procedures *(49)* or even survival *(83)*, other studies have refuted the necessity of draining both hepatic lobes *(84–86)*.

The literature suggests that ERC contrast filling of both lobes with subsequent decompression of only one lobe may increase the chance of cholangitis in the undrained segment. Therefore, more recently, MRC-guided endoscopic unilateral stent placement has been emphasized to reduce the incidence of post-procedure bacterial cholangitis in the undrained segment *(87)*. Large scale, prospective, randomized trials need to be performed to more definitively answer how much biliary decompression is needed in patients with unresectable hilar cancers.

4.1.6. Available Biliary Stents

There are both plastic and metal biliary stents available. Plastic stents are usually made of polyethylene and are available in 7, 8.5, 10, 11.5, and 12 F. Whenever feasible, 10-F stents are placed as there is evidence that stents have significantly longer patency rates compared with smaller diameter stents *(88,89)*,

whereas no advantage was found when 11.5-F stents were compared with 10-F stents *(90)*.

There are a variety of self-expandable metal stents available which can reach a diameter of 30-F. Different types include the Wallstent (braided stainless steel), the Diamond Ultraflex stent (braided Nitinol), the Zilver stent (laser cut Nitinol), and the Memotherm (braided Nitinol). These stents are assembled over a 7- to 8-F delivery catheter with radiopaque markers to ease their precise release within the bile ducts.

No significant differences have been reported in complications or overall survival between patients who have undergone metal vs plastic stent placement *(91,92)*. Although both types of stents work comparably well in biliary decompression, metal stents showed significantly longer patency rates vs plastic stents *(91–93)*. Metal stents were found to have a patency twice as long as plastic stents (9.1–10 vs 4–4.2 mo) *(91,93)*. Patients receiving metal stents required fewer ERC procedures as a result *(91–93)* with resultant lower overall cost.

In summary, there was no significant difference in relief of jaundice, peri-operative complications, and overall survival between patients receiving plastic vs metal stents. However, hospital stay and need for repeat ERC in patients with a longer life expectancy was lower with metal stents because of their longer patency. Therefore, insertion of a metal stent may be cost-effective in patients who will survive more than 6 mo. Kaassis et al. *(94)* showed that the presence or absence of liver metastasis to be a good indicator of stent strategy. They conduct that patients without hepatic involvement have a longer survival and are more apt to benefit from metal stent placement.

4.2. EUS-GUIDED CHOLANGIOGRAPHY

Although ERCP has become the procedure of choice for the management of obstructive jaundice *(95,96)*, the reported failure rate for biliary cannulation is 3–10% *(97,98)*. Common causes of failure include inexperience with the procedure, complex periampullary diverticuli, anatomic variation secondary to prior surgery (e.g., Billroth II anatomy), tumor involvement of the ampulla, stenosis of the biliary sphincter, and impacted stones *(99)*. The methods of selective biliary cannulation used in these instances include precut sphincterotomy *(100,101)*, second attempt at ERC, referral to a center of expertise, and percutaneous transhepatic cholangiography.

Access to the distal bile ducts can be obtained by EUS when the echoendoscope is placed in the antrum or duodenal bulb. A 24- or 19-gauge needle can then be used to access the bile duct and a guidewire can be advanced in an antegrade fashion through the ampulla. Conventional ERC can then be performed. In 1996 EUS-guided cholangiography was performed in 11 patients who failed ERC *(102)*. The biliary tree was successfully opacified in seven and this data was used to guide repeat ERC with precut sphincterotomy in five. In 2001, in a case of failed ERC a duodenocholedochal fistula was created and stented using EUS guidance *(103)*. In 2003, there were four additional similar cases reported *(104)*. Most recently two centers have reported success with EUS-guided cholangiography and subsequent biliary decompression in a total of seven patients with obstructive jaundice *(105,106)*. More experience in EUS-guided cholangiography with decompression is needed at experienced centers before the utility of this method is defined.

4.3. PHOTODYNAMIC THERAPY

In unresectable cholangiocarcinoma, palliative treatment has been limited to endoprosthesis placement, percutaneous drainage, or biliary surgical bypass. Adding chemotherapy to stenting has not appeared to improve prognosis (107). PDT is a new option for locoregional treatment of unresectable hilar cholangiocarcinoma (108–113).

PDT involves injection of a nontoxic photosensitizing drug with preferential retention by neoplastic tissue. This drug is then activated by illumination with light at an appropriate wavelength, which leads to photochemical destruction of tumor cells with apoptosis and/or necrosis (114–116). PDT has recently been shown to decrease cholestasis (30–33,111,112,117,118), improve quality of life (30,32, 33,111,112,118), and prolong survival in several studies. In the first prospective, randomized, multicenter study where PDT plus stenting was compared with stenting alone, the PDT group had significantly improved biliary drainage, quality of life, and survival (112). The advantage was felt to be so dramatic that the study was terminated prematurely. Additional large prospective randomized trials need to be performed before the exact role of PDT in this setting is defined.

4.4. BRACHYTHERAPY

There have been several, mostly retrospective series using intraluminal brachytherapy, usually in conjunction with external beam radiotherapy in patients with incompletely resected or unresectable cholangiocarcinoma (119–133). The majority of cases have been treated with percutaneous transhepatic drainage and brachytherapy delivered through the same route with iridium 192 wires. There have been a small number of cases reported of administration of brachytherapy by a nasobiliary route (128,130). Results have been conflicting and randomized prospective trials are needed to better determine whether brachytherapy has a survival advantage and should be offered to patients with incompletely resected or unresectable cholangiocarcinoma.

In summary, cholangiocarcinoma is a rare but deadly disease, which is usually asymptomatic until disease is wide spread. A definitive diagnosis is established by endoscopic brushings or biopsies, although the need for tissue in potentially resectable disease is questionable. MRI/MRC is the staging method of choice as it allows for assessment of lymph node involvement, vessel invasion, metastatic disease, in addition to providing a detailed cholangiogram. EUS has emerged as a powerful diagnostic and staging tool, although more studies are needed before its exact role in cholangiocarcinoma is defined. In patients with unresectable disease, endoscopic decompression appears to lower the morbidity of jaundice thereby improving quality of life. The role for preoperative decompression in potentially resectable patients, however, is still being defined. New endoscopic palliative therapies such as PDT and brachytherapy are now being investigated and larger, prospective trials are needed to determine the outcome of these patients.

REFERENCES

1. Kirschbaum JD, Kozoll DC. Carcinoma of the gallbladder and extrahepatic bile ducts. SGO 1941; 73:740–753.
2. Kuwayti K, Baggenstoss AH, Stauffer MH, Priestly JI. Carcinoma of the major intrahepatic and extrahepatic bile ducts exclusive of the papilla of Vater. Surg Gynecol Obstet 1957; 104:357–366.
3. Carriaga MT, Henson DE. Liver, gallbladder, extrahepatic bile ducts, and pancreas. Cancer 1995; 75:171–190.
4. Kemmer N, Waxman I. Biliary tract carcinoma. Curr Treat Options Gastroenterol 2000; 3:113–119.
5. Broome U, Olsson R, Loof L, et al. Natural history and prognostic factors in 305 Swedish patients with primary sclerosing cholangitis. Gut 1996; 38:610–615.
6. Pitt HA, Dooley WC, Yeo CJ, Cameron JL. Malignancies of the biliary tree. Curr Probl Surg 1995; 32:1–90.
7. Blumgart LH, Benjamin IS. Cancer of the bile ducts. In: Blumgart L, ed. Surgery of the Liver and Biliary Tract, 2nd ed. London: Churchill Livingstone; 1994:1051–1067.
8. Shaked A, Colonna JO, Goldstein L, Busuttil RW. The interrelation between sclerosing cholangitis and ulcerative colitis in patients undergoing liver transplantation. Ann Surg 1992; 215:598–605.
9. Nakeeb A, Pitt HA, Sohn TA, et al. Cholangiocarcinoma. Ann Surg 1996; 224:463–475.
10. Tompkins RK, Thomas D, Wile A, Longmire WPJ. Prognostic factors in bile duct carcinoma. Ann Surg 1981; 194:447–455.
11. Reding R, Buard JL, Lebeau G, Launois B. Surgical management of 552 carcinomas of the bile duct (gall bladder and periampullary excluded). Ann Surg 1991; 213:236–241.
12. Bismuth H, Corlette MB. Intrahepatic cholangio-enteric anastomosis in carcinoma of the hilus of the liver. Surg Gynecol Obstet 1975; 140:170–178.
13. Ramage JK, Donaghy A, Farrant JM, Iorns R, Williams R. Serum tumor markers for the diagnosis of cholangiocarcinoma in primary sclerosing cholangitis. Gastroenterology 1995; 108:865–869.
14. Patel AH, Harnois DM, Klee GG, LaRusso NF, Gores GJ. The utility of CA 19-9 in the diagnoses of cholangiocarcinoma in patients without primary sclerosing cholangitis. Am J Gastroenterol 2000; 95:204–207.
15. Hultcrantz R, Olsson R, Danielsson A, Jarnerot G, Loof L, Ryden BO. A 3-year prospective study on serum tumor markers used for detecting cholangiocarcinoma in patients with primary sclerosing cholangitis. J Hepatol 1999; 30:669–673.
16. Nakanuma Y, Minato H, Kida T, Terada T. Pathology of Cholangiocellular carcinoma. In: Tobe T, Kameda H, Okudaira M, Ohto M, eds. Primary liver cancer in Japan. Tokyo, Japan: Springer-Verlag; 1994:39–50.
17. Nakajima T, Kondo Y, Mayazaki M, Okui K. A histopathologic study of 102 cases of intrahepatic cholangiocarcinoma: histologic classification and modes of spreading. Hum Pathol 1988; 19:1228–1234.
18. Chamberlain RS, Blumgart LH. Hilar cholangiocarcinoma: A review and commentary. Ann Surg Oncol 2000; 7:55–66.
19. Greene FL, Page DL, Fleming ID, et al., In: F. Greene, et al., Extrahepatic Bile Ducts. American Journal of Cancer Staging Handbook, eds. 2002, Springer: New York; 163–169.
20. Gibson RN, Yeung E, Thompson JN, Carr DH, Hemingway AP, Bradpiece HA, et al. Biliary dilatation: defining level and cause by real-time US. Radiology 1986; 160:39–42.
21. Triller J, Losser C, Baer HU, et al. Radiological assessment of resectability. Eur J Radiol 1994; 4:9–17.
22. Sharma MP, Ahuja V. Aetiological spectrum of obstructive jaundice and diagnostic ability of ultrasonography: a clinician's perspective. Trop Gastroenterol 1999; 20:167–169.
23. Smits NJ, Reeders JWAJ. Current applicability of duplex Doppler ultrasonography in pancreatic head and biliary malignancies. In: Tytgat GNJ, Reeders JWAJ. eds. Ballieres Clinical Gastroenterology: Diagnostic Imaging of the Gastrointestinal Tract, Part II. London: Bailliere Tindall; 1995:153–172.
24. Smits NJ, Reeders JW. Imaging and staging of biliopancreatic malignancy: role of ultrasound. Ann of Oncol 1999; 10 Suppl 4:20–24.

25. Colli A, Cocciolo M, Mumoli N, et al. Peripheral intrahepatic cholangiocarcinoma: ultrasound findings and differential diagnosis from hepatocellular carcinoma. Eur J Ultrasound 1998; 7:93–99.
26. Han JK, Choi BI, Kim AY, et al. Cholangiocarcinoma: pictorial essay of CT and cholangiographic findings. Radiographics 2002; 22:173–187.
27. Schwartz LH, Coakley FV, Sun Y, Blumgart LH, Fong Y, Panicek DM. Neoplastic pancreaticobiliary duct obstruction: evaluation with breath-hold MR cholangiopancreatography. Am J Roentgenol 1998; 170:1491–1495.
28. Guthrie JA, Ward J, Robinson PJ. Hilar cholangiocarcinomas: T2-weighted spin-echo and gadolinium-enhanced FLASH MR imaging. Radiology 1996; 201:347–351.
29. Lee MG, Lee HJ, Kim MH, et al. Extrahepatic biliary disease: 3D MR cholangiopancreatography. Radiology 1997; 202:663–669.
30. Harisinghani MG, Hahn PF. Computed tomography and magnetic resonance imaging evaluation of liver cancer. Gastroenterol Clin North Am 2002; 31:759–776.
31. Sohn TA, Lillemoe KD. Tumors of the gallbladder, bile ducts, and ampulla. In Feldman M, Friedman L, Sleisenger M, eds. Sleisenger & Fortran's Gastrointestinal and Liver Disease: Pathophysiology, Diagnosis, Management, Philadelphia: Saunders; 2002:1153–1166.
32. Vitellas KM, Keogan MT, Freed KS, et al. Radiologic manifestations of sclerosing cholangitis with emphasis on MR cholangiopancreatography. Radiographics 2000; 20:959–975.
33. Altehoefer C, Ghanem N, Furtwangler A, Schneider B, Langer M. Breathhold unenhanced and gadolinium-enhanced magnetic resonance tomography and magnetic resonance cholangiography in hilar cholangiocarcinoma. Int J Colorectal Dis 2001; 16:188–192.
34. Reinhold C, Bret PM. Current status of MR cholangiopancreatography. Am J Roentgenol 1996; 166:1285–1295.
35. Di Cesare E, Puglielli E, Michelini O, et al. Malignant obstructive jaundice: comparison of MRCP and ERCP in the evaluation of distal lesions. Radiologia Medica 2003; 105:445–453.
36. Tian J, Wang J, Wang F, et al. Clinical value of MR cholangiopancreatography combining with dynamic enhanced MRI in the detection of cholangiocarcinoma. Chung Hua Kan Tsang Ping Tsa Chih 2003; 11:526–529.
37. Kluge R, Schmidt F, Caca K, et al. Positron emission tomography with [(18)F] fluoro-2-deoxy-D-glucose for diagnosis and staging of bile duct cancer. Hepatology 2001; 33:1029–1035.
38. Fritscher-Ravens A, Bohuslavizki KH, Broering DC, et al. FDG PET in the diagnosis of hilar cholangiocarcinoma. Nucl Med Commun 2001; 22:1277–1285.
39. Kim YJ, Yun M, Lee WJ, Kim KS, Lee JD. Usefulness of 18F-FDG PET in intrahepatic cholangiocarcinoma. Eur J Nuc Med Mol Imaging 2003; 30:1467–1472.
40. Anderson CD, Rice MH, Pinson CW, Chapman WC, Chari RS, Delbeke D. Fluorodeoxyglucose PET imaging in the evaluation of gallbladder carcinoma and cholangiocarcinoma. J Gastrointest Surg 2004; 8:90–97.
41. Howell DA, Beveridge RP, Bosco J, Jones M. Endoscopic needle aspiration biopsy at ERCP in the diagnosis of biliary strictures. Gastrointest Endosc 1992; 38:531–535.
42. Kubota V, Takaoka M, Tani K, et al. Endoscopic transpapillary biopsy for the diagnosis of patients with pancreaticobiliary ductal strictures. Am J Gastroenterol 1993; 88:1700–1704.
43. Jailwala J, Fogel EL, Sherman S, et al. Triple-tissue sampling at ERCP in malignant biliary obstruction. Gastrointest Endosc 2000; 51:383–390.
44. Jarnagin WR. Cholangiocarcinoma of the extrahepatic bile ducts. Semin in Surg Oncol 2000; 19:156–176.
45. Hall-Craggs MA, Allen CM, Owens CM, et al. MR cholangiography: clinical evaluation in 40 cases. Radiology 1993; 189:423–427.
46. Soto JA, Barish MA, Yucel ED, Seingenberg D, Ferrucci JT, Chuttani R. Magnetic resonance cholangiography: comparison with endoscopic retrograde cholangiopancreatography. Gastroenterology 1996; 110:589–597.
47. Hawes RH. Diagnostic and therapeutic uses of ERCP in pancreatic and biliary tract malignancies. Gastrointest Endosc 2002; 56:S201–205.
48. Sherman S. Endoscopic drainage of malignant hilar obstruction: Is one biliary stent enough or should we work to place two? Gastrointest Endosc 2001; 53:681–684.
49. Chang W, Kortan P, Haber GB. Outcome in patients with bifurcation tumors who undergo unilateral versus bilateral hepatic duct drainage. Gastrointest Endosc 1998; 47:354–362.
50. Ferrari AP, Lichtenstein DR, Slivka A, Chang C, Carr-Locke D. Brush cytology during ERCP for the diagnosis of biliary and pancreatic malignancies. Gastrointest Endosc 1994; 40:140–145.
51. Ryan ME. Cytologic brushings of ductal lesions during ERCP. Gastrointest Endosc 1991; 37:139–142.
52. Foutch PG, Kerr DM, Harlan JR, Manne RK, Kummet TD, Sanowki R. Endoscopic retrograde wire-guided brush cytology for diagnosis of patients with malignant obstruction of the bile duct. Am J Gastroenterol 1990; 85:791–795.
53. Glasbrenner B, Ardan M, Boeck W, Preclik G, Moeller P, Adler G. Prospective evaluation of brush cytology of biliary strictures during endoscopic retrograde cholangiopancreatography. Endoscopy 1999; 31:712–717.
54. Scudera PL, Kouzumi J, Jacobson IM. Brush cytology evaluation of lesions encountered during ERCP. Gastrointest Endosc 1990; 36:281–284.
55. Fritscher-Ravens A, Broering DC, Knoefel WT, et al. EUS-guided fine-needle aspiration of suspected hilar cholangiocarcinoma in potentially operable patients with negative brush cytology. Am J Gastroenterol 2004; 99:45–51.
56. Eloubeidi MA, Chen VK, Jhala NC, et al. Endoscopic ultrasound-guided fine needle aspiration biopsy of suspected cholangiocarcinoma. Clin Gastroenterol Hepatol 2004; 2:207–208.
57. Fritscher-Ravens A, Broering DC, Sriram PV, et al. EUS-guided fine-needle aspiration cytodiagnosis of hilar cholangiocarcinoma: a case series. Gastrointest Endosc 2000; 52:534–540.
58. Fujita N, Noda Y, Kobayashi G. Analysis of the layer structure of the gallbladder wall delineated by endoscopic ultrasound using the pinning method. Dig Endosc 1995; 7:353–356.
59. Noda Y, Fujita N, Kobayashi G, Kimura K, Yago A, Yuki T. Comparison of echograms by a microscanner and histological findings of the common bile duct, in vitro study. Jpn J Gastroenterol 1997; 94:172–179.
60. Tamada K, Ido K, Ueno N, Kimura K, Ichiyama M, Tomiyama T. Preoperative staging of extrahepatic bile duct cancer with intraductal ultrasonography. Am J Gastroenterol 1995; 90:239–246.
61. Kuroiwa M, Goto H, Hirooka Y, Furukawa T, Hayakawa T, Naitoh Y. Intraductal ultrasonography for the diagnosis of proximal invasion in extrahepatic bile duct cancer. J Gastroenterol Hepatol 1998; 13:715–719.
62. Fujita N, Noda Y, Kobayashi G, Kimura K, Yago A. Staging of bile duct carcinoma by EUS and IDUS. Endoscopy 1998; 30:A132–A134.
63. Menzel J, Poremba C, Dietl KH, Domschke W. Preoperative diagnosis of bile duct strictures—comparison of intraductal ultrasonography with conventional endosonography. Scand J Gastroenterol 2000; 35:77–82.
64. Tamada K, Nagai H, Yasuda Y, et al. Transpapillary intraductal US prior to biliary drainage in the assessment of longitudinal spread of extrahepatic bile duct carcinoma. Gastrointest Endosc 2001; 53:300–307.
65. Inui K, Nakazawa S, Yoshino J, et al. Ultrasound probes for biliary lesions. Endoscopy 1998; 30:A120–A123.
66. Kanemaki N, Nakazawa S, Inui K, Yoshino J, Yamao J, Okushima K. Three dimensional intraductal ultrasonography: preliminary results of a new technique for the diagnosis of diseases of the pancreaticobiliary system. Endoscopy 1997; 29:726–731.
67. Tamada K, Tomiyama T, Ohashi A, et al. Preoperative assessment of extrahepatic bile duct carcinoma using three-dimensional intraductal US. Gastrointest Endosc 1999; 50:548–554.
68. Abraham NS, Barkun JS, Barkun AN. Palliation of malignant biliary obstruction: a prospective trial examining impact on quality of life. Gastrointest Endosc 2002; 56:835–841.
69. Smith AC, Dowsett JF, Russell RC, Hatfield AR, Cotton PB. Randomised trial of endoscopic stenting versus surgical bypass in malignant low bile duct obstruction. Lancet 1994; 344:1655–1660.

70. Sherpard HA, Royle G, Ross AP, Diba A, Arthur M, Colins-Jones D. Endoscopic biliary endoprosthesis in the palliation of malignant obstruction of the distal common bile duct: a randomized trial. Br J Surg 1988; 75:1166–1168.

71. Anderson JR, Sorensen SM, Kruse A, Rokkjaer M, Matzen P. Randomised trial of endoscopic endoprosthesis versus operative bypass in malignant obstructive jaundice. Gut 1989; 30:1132–1135.

72. Raikar GV, Melin MM, Ress A, et al. Cost-effective analysis of surgical palliation versus endoscopic stenting in the management of unresectable pancreatic cancer. Ann Surg Oncol 1996; 3:470–475.

73. Leung JWC, Emergy R, Cotton PB, Russell RC, Vallon AG, Mason RR. Management of malignant obstructive jaundice at the Middlesex hospital. Br J Surg 1983; 70:584–586.

74. Brandabur JJ, Kozarek RA, Ball TJ, et al. Nonoperative versus operative treatment of obstructive jaundice in pancreatic cancer: cost and survival analysis. Am J Gastroenterol 1988; 83:1132–1139.

75. Taylor MC, Mcleod RS, Langer B. Biliary stenting versus bypass surgery for the palliation of malignant distal bile duct obstruction, a meta-analysis. Liver Transpl 2000; 6:302–308.

76. Lai ECS, Mok FPT, Fan ST, et al. Preoperative endoscopic drainage for malignant obstructive jaundice. Br J Surg 1994; 81:1195–1198.

77. Karsten TM, Allema JH, Reinders M, et al. Preoperative biliary drainage, colonisation of bile and postoperative complications in patients with tumours of the pancreatic head: a retrospective analysis of 241 consecutive patients. Eur J Surgery 1996; 162:881–888.

78. Lygidakis NJ, van der Heyde MN, Lubbers MJ. Evaluation of preoperative biliary drainage in the surgical management of pancreatic head carcinoma. Acta Chir Scand 1987; 153:665–668.

79. Marcus SG, Dobryansky M, Shamamian P, et al. Endoscopic biliary drainage before pancreaticoduodenectomy for periampullary malignancies. J Clin Gastroenterol 1998; 26:125–129.

80. Heslin MJ, Brooks AD, Hochwald SN, Harrison LE, Blumgart LH, Brennan MF. A preoperative biliary stent is associated with increased complications after pancreatoduodenectomy. Arch Surg 1998; 133:149–154.

81. Povoski SP, Karpeh MS, Conlon KC, Blumgart LH, Brennan MF. Preoperative biliary drainage: impact on intraoperative bile cultures and infectious morbidity and mortality after pancreaticoduodenectomy. J Gastrointest Surg 1999; 3:496–505.

82. Strasberg SM. ERCP and surgical intervention in pancreatic and biliary malignancies. Gastrointest Endosc 2002; 56:S213–S217.

83. Deviere J, Baize M, de Toeuf J, Cremer M. Long-term follow-up of patients with hilar malignant stricture treated by endoscopic internal biliary drainage. Gastrointest Endosc 1988; 34:95–101.

84. Polydorou AA, Chisholm EM, Romanos AA, et al. A comparison of right versus left hepatic duct endoprosthesis insertion in malignant hilar biliary obstruction. Endoscopy 1989; 21:266–271.

85. Polydorou AA, Cairns SR, Dowsett JF, et al. Palliation of proximal malignant biliary obstruction by endoscopic endoprosthesis insertion. Gut 1991; 32:685–689.

86. De Palma GD, Galloro G, Siciliano S, Iovino P, Catanzano C. Unilateral versus bilateral endoscopic hepatic duct drainage in patients with malignant hilar biliary obstruction: results of a prospective, randomized, and controlled study. Gastrointest Endosc 2001; 53:547–553.

87. Hintze RE, Abou-Rebyeh H, Adler A, Veltzke-Schlieker W, Felix R, Wiedenmann B. Magnetic resonance cholangiopancreatography-guided unilateral endoscopic stent placement for Klatskin tumors. Gastrointest Endosc 2001; 53:40–46.

88. Speer AG, Cotton PB, MacRae K. Endoscopic management of malignant biliary obstruction. Stents of 10 French gauge are preferable to stents of 8 French gauge. Gastrointest Endosc 1988; 34:412–417.

89. Pederson FM. Endoscopic management of malignant biliary obstruction. Is stent size of 10 French gauge better than 7 French gauge? Scand J Gastroenterol 1993; 28:185–189.

90. Pereira-Lima J, Jakobs R, Maier M, Benz C, Kohler B, Riemann JF. Endoscopic biliary stenting for the palliation of pancreatic cancer: results, survival predictive factors and comparison of 10 Fr with 11.5 Fr gauge stents. Am J Gastroenterol 1996; 91:2179–2184.

91. Davids PH, Groen AK, Rauws EA, Tytgat GN, Huigbregste K. Randomised trial of self-expanding metal stents versus polyethylene stents for distal malignant biliary obstruction. Lancet 1992; 340:1488–1492.

92. Prat F, Chapat O, Ducot B, Ponchon T, et al. A randomized trial of endoscopic drainage methods for inoperable malignant strictures of the common bile duct. Gastrointest Endosc 1998; 47:1–7.

93. Schamassmann A, Von Gunten E, Knuchel J, Scheurer U, Fehr HF, Halter F. Wallstents versus plastic stents in malignant biliary obstruction: effects of stent patency of the first and second stent on patient compliance and survival. Am J Gastroenterol 1996; 91:654–659.

94. Kaassis M, Boyer J, Dumas R, et al. Plastic or metal stents for malignant stricture of the common bile duct? Results of a randomized prospective study. Gastrointest Endosc 2003; 57:178–182.

95. Schofl R. Diagnostic endoscopic retrograde cholangiopancreatography. Endoscopy 2001; 33:147–157.

96. Fogel EL, Sherman S, Devereaux BM, Lehman GA. Therapeutic biliary endoscopy. Endoscopy 2001; 33:31–38.

97. Assouline Y, Liguory C, Ink O, et al. Endoscopic sphincterotomy for treatment of bile duct stones. New techniques and present results. Gastroenterol Clin Biol 1993; 17:251–258.

98. Lenriot JP, Le Neel JC, Hay JM, Jaeck D, Millat B, Fagniez PL. Endoscopic retrograde cholangiopancreatography and endoscopic sphincterotomy for biliary lithiasis. A prospective evaluation by surgeons. Gastroenterol Clin Biol 1993; 17:244–250.

99. Martin DF. Combined percutaneous and endoscopic procedures for bile duct obstruction. Gut 1994; 35:1011–1012.

100. Martin DF, Tweedle DE. Risks of precut papillotomy and the management of patients with duodenal perforation. Am J Surg 1992; 163:273–274 (comment).

101. Siegel JH. Precut papillotomy: a method to improve success of ERCP and papillotomy. Endoscopy 1980; 12:130–133.

102. Wiersema MJ, Sandusky D, Carr R, Wiersema LM, Erdel WC, Frederick PK. Endosonography-guided cholangiopancreatography. Gastrointest Endosc 1996; 43:102–106.

103. Giovannini M, Moutardier V, Pesenti C, Bories E, Lelong B, Delpero JR. Endoscopic ultrasound-guided bilioduodenal anastomosis: a new technique for biliary drainage. Endoscopy 2001; 33:898–900.

104. Burmester E, Niehaus J, Leineweber T, Huetteroth T. EUS-cholangiodrainage of the bile duct: report of 4 cases. Gastrointest Endosc 2003; 57:246–250.

105. Kahaleh M, Yoshida C, Kane L, Yeaton P. Interventional EUS cholangiography: A report of five cases. Gastrointest Endosc 2004; 60:138–142.

106. Mallery S, Matlock J, Freeman ML. EUS-guided rendezvous drainage of obstructed biliary and pancreatic ducts: report of 6 cases. Gastrointest Endosc 2004; 59:100–107.

107. Van Groeningen CJ. Intravenous and intra-arterial chemotherapeutic possibilities in biliopancreatic cancer. Ann Oncol 1999; 10:305–307.

108. Miura Y, Endo I, Togo S, et al. Adjuvant therapies using biliary stenting for malignant biliary obstruction. J Hepatobiliary Pancreat Surg 2001; 8:113–117.

109. Tsujino K, Landry JC, Smith RG, Keller JW, Williams WH, Davis LW. Definitive radiation therapy for extrahepatic bile duct carcinoma. Radiology 1995; 196:275–280.

110. McCaughan JS, Mertens BF, Cho C, Barabash RD, Payton HW. Photodynamic therapy to treat tumors of the extrahepatic biliary ducts. Arch Surg 1991; 126:111–113.

111. Ortner MA, Liebetruth J, Schreiber S, et al. Photodynamic therapy of nonresectable cholangiocarcinoma. Gastroenterology 1998; 114:536–542.

112. Ortner ME, Caca K, Berr F, et al. Successful photodynamic therapy for nonresectable cholangiocarcinoma: a randomized prospective study. Gastroenterology 2003; 125:1355–1363.

113. Wiedenmann M, Caca K, Frieder B, et al. Neoadjuvant photodynamic therapy as a new approach to treating hilar cholangiocarcinoma. Cancer 2003; 97:2783–2790.

114. Oleinick NL, Evans HH. The photobiology of photodynamic therapy: cellular targets and mechanisms. Radiat Res 1998; 150:S146–S156.

115. Hsi RA, Rosenthal DI, Glatstein E. Photodynamic therapy in the treatment of cancer: current state of the art. Drugs 1999; 57:725–734.

116. Webber J, Herman M, Kessel D, Fromm D. Current concepts in gastrointestinal photodynamic therapy. Ann Surg 1999; 230:12–23.

117. Dumoulin FL, Gerhardt T, Fuchs S, et al. Phase II study of photodynamic therapy and metal stent as palliative treatment for nonresectable hilar cholangiocarcinoma. Gastrointest Endosc 2003; 57:860–867.

118. Ortner MA. Photodynamic therapy for cholangiocarcinoma. J Hepatobiliary Pancreat Surg 2001; 8:137–139.

119. Gerhards MF, van Gulik TM, Gonzalez DG, Rauws EA, Gouma DJ. Results of postoperative radiotherapy for resectable hilar cholangiocarcinoma. World J Surg 2003; 27:173–179.

120. Dvorak J, Jandik P, Melichar B, et al. Intraluminal high dose rate brachytherapy in the treatment of bile duct and gallbladder cancers. Hepato-Gastroenterology 2002; 49:916–917.

121. Lu JJ, Bains YS, Abdel-Wahab M, et al. High-dose rate remote afterloading intracavitary brachytherapy for the treatment of extrahepatic biliary duct carcinoma. Cancer J 2002; 8:74–78.

122. Milella M, Salvetti M, Cerrotta A, et al. Interventional radiology and radiotherapy for inoperable cholangiocarcinoma of the extrahepatic bile ducts. Tumori 1998; 84:467–471.

123. Leung JT, Kuan R. Intraluminal brachytherapy in the treatment of bile duct carcinomas. Australas Radiol 1998; 41:151–154.

124. Leung J, Guiney M, Das R. Intraluminal brachytherapy in bile duct carcinomas. Aust NZ J Surg 1996; 66:74–77.

125. Bowling TE, Galbraith SM, Hatfield AR, Salono J, Spittle MF. A retrospective comparison of endoscopic stenting alone with stenting and radiotherapy in non-resectable cholangiocarcinoma. Gut 1996; 39:852–855.

126. Eschelman DJ, Shapiro MJ, Bonn J, et al. Malignant biliary duct obstruction: long-term experience with Gianturco stents and combined-modality radiation therapy. Radiology 1996; 200:717–724.

127. Kamada T, Saitou H, Takamura A, Nojima T, Okushiba SI. The role of radiotherapy in the management of extrahepatic bile duct cancer: an analysis of 145 consecutive patients treated with intraluminal and/or external beam radiotherapy. Int J Radiat Oncol Biol Phy 1996; 34:767–774.

128. Montemaggi P, Morganti AG, Dobelbower RR, et al. Role of intraluminal brachytherapy in extrahepatic bile duct and pancreatic cancers: is it just for palliation? Radiology 1996; 199:861–866.

129. Vallis KA, Benjamin IS, Munro AJ, et al. External beam and intraluminal radiotherapy for locally advanced bile duct cancer: role and tolerability. Radiother Oncol 1996; 41:61–66.

130. Montemaggi P, Costamagna G, Dobelbower RR, et al. Intraluminal brachytherapy in the treatment of pancreas and bile duct carcinoma. Int J Radiat Oncol Biol Phy 1995; 32:437–443.

131. Kuvshinoff BW, Armstrong JG, Fong Y, et al. Palliation of irresectable hilar cholangiocarcinoma with biliary drainage and radiotherapy. Br J Surg 1995; 82:1522–1525.

132. Alden ME, Mohiuddin M. The impact of radiation dose in combined external beam and intraluminal Ir-192 brachytherapy for bile duct cancer. Int J Radiat Oncol Biol Phy 1994; 28:945–951.

133. Minsky BD, Kemeny N, Armstrong JG, Reichman B, Botet J. Extrahepatic biliary system cancer: an update of a combined modality approach. Am J Clin Oncol 1991; 14:433–437.

29 Ampullary Neoplasia

Ian D. Norton, MBBS, PhD, FRACP

Contents

1. BACKGROUND

The optimal approach has yet to emerge for the management of sporadic periampullary adenomas and upper gastrointestinal (GI) neoplasia complicating familial adenomatous polyposis (FAP). There are no randomized trials comparing different surgical and/or endoscopic modalities. Such studies may not be feasible given the infrequency of these conditions and the long follow-up period required for such a study. In the meantime, selection of the optimal approach for an individual patient will rely on a careful evaluation of the disease severity and extent in that patient and the utilization of the best available endoscopic and surgical expertise.

2. INTRODUCTION

The ampulla of Vater is the most common site of neoplasia of the small intestine, related in part to the trophic effects of bile on the mucosa (1–4). This proliferation results in adenomatous transformation and, eventually in some cases, adenocarcinoma. Ampullary adenomas occur sporadically, but are particularly prevalent in FAP patients, occurring in 50–100% FAP subjects. Following proctocolectomy, the periampullary area is the most common site of malignancy in FAP subjects. The critical position of the ampulla and the lag time from adenoma to carcinoma makes this a potential site for surveillance and removal of significant ampullary adenomas. Endoscopic techniques play a central role in the management of these lesions. However, the optimal approach has yet to be determined.

Endoscopic approaches include surveillance, piecemeal resection, snare ampullectomy, and thermal ablation. Surgical

From: *Endoscopic Oncology: Gastrointestinal Endoscopy and Cancer Management.* Edited by: D. O. Faigel and M. L. Kochman © Humana Press, Totowa, NJ

options for advanced lesions include local transduodenal resection, pancreaticoduodenectomy, and pancreas-sparing duodenectomy. The appropriate management for each patient depends on many factors including the size of the lesion, degree of dysplasia, involvement of the pancreaticobiliary system, comorbidity, and local expertise.

3. PATHOLOGY

The vast majority of ampullary lesions are tubular or tubulovillous adenomas which arise from the intestinal-type epithelium of the ampulla (5). Foci of severe dysplasia or frank malignancy may be found within a lesion (6). Other forms of ampullary neoplasia are far less common. These include benign lesions (leiomyoma, lipoma, lymphangioma, hemangioma, and carcinoid) as well as malignancies, both primary and metastatic (lymphoma, melanoma, and metastatic small cell carcinoma) (7).

4. PATHOGENESIS

Regarding FAP syndrome, all nucleated cells in FAP patients contain one normal and one abnormal adenomatous polyposis coli (APC) gene (a germline mutation). In the colon, a somatic mutation in the previously normal (wild-type) APC allele is generally an early event in carcinogenesis. Accumulation of other somatic mutations (in genes such as p53 and K-ras) drives the progression toward malignancy (8). The situation with respect to periampullary malignancy appears to be similar except that somatic APC mutations may be relatively less frequent and K-ras mutations relatively more frequent (9). Another study has demonstrated p53 mutations associated with high-grade malignant change in periampullary tumors (10). A recent article has suggested that other familial factors, possibly unidentified modifier genes, may influence the development of periampullary

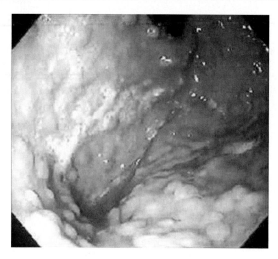

Fig. 1. Fundic cystic gland polyps. A common phenomenon seen in the proximal stomach of patients with FAP.

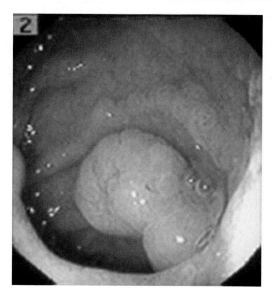

Fig. 3. Large, nonampullary duodenal adenoma.

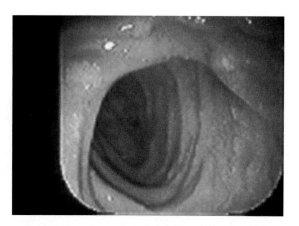

Fig. 2. Multiple tiny adenomata in the proximal duodenum ("military" appearance). Virtually pathognomonic of FAP syndrome.

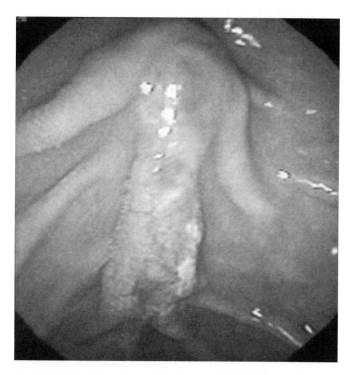

Fig. 4. Periampullary adenoma with typical inferior extension of the adenoma ("goatee" appearance).

adenomas in FAP kindreds explaining, at least in part, the familial segregation of periampullary disease observed in some FAP families *(11)*. This segregation was independent of the kindred's specific APC mutation. Spigelman and co-workers have reported a correlation between severity of duodenal polyposis and rectal polyposis following colectomy and ileorectal anastomosis *(12)*. They have suggested that other factor(s), possibly environmental, may be synergistic in some patients, resulting in more severe polyposis at both sites. The authors of this study caution, however, that paucity of rectal polyps does not obviate the need for ampullary surveillance.

The periampullary region is the site of the vast majority of significant small intestinal adenomas in both sporadic and FAP patients. These lesions seem to parallel mucosal exposure to bile, particularly concerning the characteristic inferior extension of early adenomas ("goatee" appearance). Bile has been shown to have proliferative *(1–3)* and mutagenic *(4)* effects of gut mucosa. Furthermore, the bile from patients with FAP has been shown to form more DNA adducts both in vitro and in vivo than bile from controls *(2,13)*, particularly at low pH (as found in the proximal duodenum) *(14)*. These DNA adducts have the potential to give rise to mutagenesis *(15)*.

In a situation analogous to that in the colon, these lesions appear to follow the adenoma–carcinoma sequence. In one study, adenomatous tissue was adjacent to or a component of 84% of periampullary cancers studied *(16)*. A retrospective study by Bleau supported the temporal progression of periampullary adenomas to carcinoma, with mean diagnosis of adenoma at age 39, high-grade dysplasia at age 47, and malignancy at age 54 *(17)*.

4.1. FAP SYNDROME

FAP is an autosomal-dominant condition with virtually complete penetration, affecting about 1 in 8000 in the United States *(18)*. Mutation of the *APC* gene on the long arm of chromosome 5 is responsible for most cases of FAP (19). The condition is classically characterized by the development of hundreds to thousands of adenomatous polyps in the colon with the inevitable progression of one or more of these adenomas to carcinoma (see Chapter 18). However, it is increasingly apparent that attenuated forms of FAP exist. These generally present with fewer colorectal polyps developing later in life than is typical of classic FAP and often distributed more proximally in the colon. Such patients do develop upper GI disease and in some the upper GI findings may be more marked than those in the colon (20,21). Thus, patients presenting with "sporadic" ampullary adenomas should undergo assessment of the colon.

Extracolonic disease is common in classic FAP but varies in severity from family to family and between individuals within families. At one extreme is Gardner's syndrome characterized by GI adenomatous polyps together with other benign neoplasms such as desmoid tumors, osteomas, and fibromas (22). Gardner's syndrome also results from germline APC mutations and is best regarded as part of the spectrum of FAP. Turcot's syndrome is characterized by central nervous system tumors, often glioblastomas or medulloblastomas (22), together with colonic polyposis. The inheritance of this disorder has been difficult to determine (22), because the association of central nervous system tumors and polyposis might arise through germline mutation of more than one gene (23). Germline APC mutations have been identified in some subjects with Turcot's syndrome, particularly those with cerebellar medulloblastomas and profuse colonic polyposis (23). For the purposes of this chapter, the term FAP incorporates Gardner's syndrome and those cases of Turcot's syndrome attributable to APC mutations.

The duodenum is the commonest site of malignancy in FAP patients following colectomy, occurring in 4.5–8.5% (24,25). Adenomas and carcinomas have also been encountered in the distal ileal segment and within ileoanal pouches 5–10 yr after proctocolectomy (26).

5. INCIDENCE

An understanding of the natural history of duodenal neoplasia in FAP patients is essential to the development of surveillance strategies and decisions regarding management in this condition. Periampullary tumors represent 5% of GI tumors and 36% of resectable pancreaticoduodenal tumors (10). The periampullary adenoma is an uncommon lesion in clinical practice, although not as rare as previously thought. An early review by Baggenstoss demonstrated 25 of these lesions in 4000 consecutive autopsies (0.62%), suggesting that the lesion may be subclinical (27). A review of the case notes in this study suggested that perhaps six of these lesions (24%) might have been symptomatic.

Asymptomatic adenomatous change of the ampulla is very common in FAP patients, occurring in up to 100% of subjects (17). The incidence of FAP-related duodenal and periampullary adenomas depends on the diligence of surveillance. A review of the Johns Hopkins FAP registry indicated that the relative risk of duodenal adenocarcinoma in FAP compared with the general population was 330 and the relative risk of

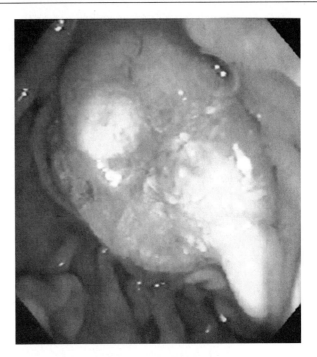

Fig. 5. Moderate-sized ampullary adenoma.

ampullary cancer was 123 (28). The combined absolute risk of duodenal cancer in FAP patients was, however, only 1/1698 years. Because follow-up was incomplete and most cancers occur later in life, this risk of malignancy may be an underestimate. A study from the United Kingdom reported development of malignancy in 3 of 70 patients followed over 40 mo (29). It is important to remember, therefore, that although adenomatous change in the duodenum may be almost universal in FAP only a small percentage of patients develop cancer. Several studies have indicated that the median age at onset of periampullary malignancy complicating FAP is in the sixth decade (11,25,28).

6. CLINICAL PRESENTATION

Lesions of the periampullary area may be asymptomatic but can also present relatively early with symptoms of pancreaticobiliary origin. Clinical presentation is usually a consequence of obstruction, resulting in abdominal pain, cholangitis or jaundice (7) or, less commonly, recurrent pancreatitis (30). Courvoisier's sign is occasionally present, suggesting advanced disease (31). Biochemical evidence of biliary obstruction is common in symptomatic patients (32). The diagnosis is usually unsuspected prior to visualization of the ampulla, with most patients thought to have pancreatic malignancy or choledocholithiasis.

7. ENDOSCOPIC MANAGEMENT OF PERIAMPULLARY ADENOMA

7.1. DIAGNOSIS

In patients with FAP, diagnosis of upper GI and particularly periampullary adenomas depends on the vigilance of the endoscopist. Examination with a side viewing duodenoscope is essential. Two recent studies have demonstrated that duodenoscopy with a forward-viewing endoscopy missed 50% of

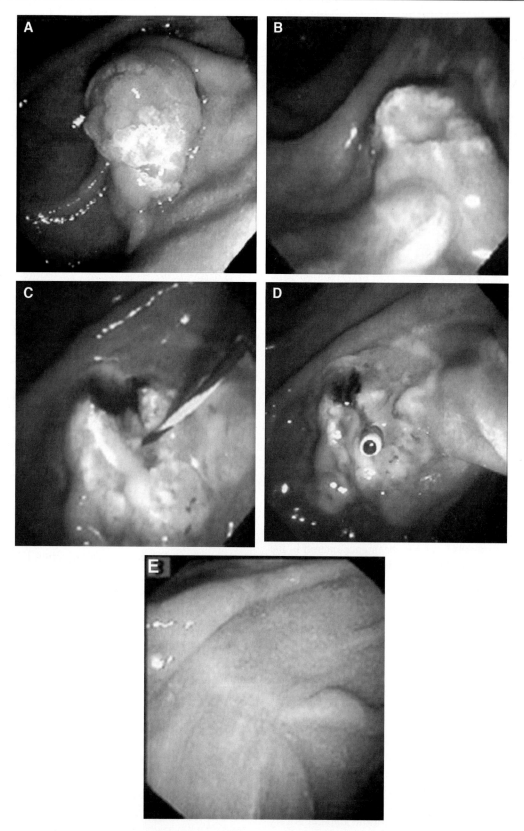

Fig. 6. Steps in snare ampullectomy: (**A**) ampullary adenoma; (**B**) appearance after snare removal using blended current; (**C**) pancreatic orifice accessed with a hydrophilic wire; (**D**) temporary (<1 wk) pancreatic stent placed following pancreatic sphincterotomy; (**E**) final result 3 mo later. (Color versions of A and E appear in the color insert following p. 84).

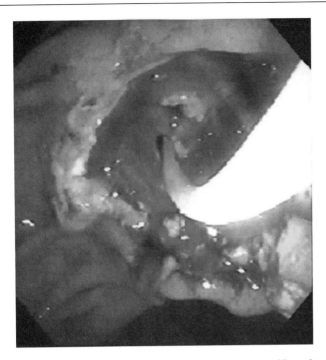

Fig. 7. Another example immediately postampullectomy. Note clear separation of pancreatic and biliary orifices. Most authors would advocate completion sphincterotomies to reduce the risk of subsequent orifice stenosis.

Table 1
Spigelman Scoring System for Staging of Ampullary Adenoma

Polyp number	Polyp size	Histology	Dysplasia	Points
1–4	1–4 mm	Tubular	Mild	1
5–20	5–10 mm	Tubulovillous	Moderate	2
>20	>10 mm	Villous	Severe	3
Stage 0	0			
Stage 1	1–4			
Stage 2	5–6			
Stage 3	7–8			
Stage 4	9–12			

gross lesions visible with the side-viewer (17,33). Careful biopsies of the ampulla may detect early adenomatous change in light of the somewhat "frond-like" appearance of many normal papillae. In one study six of eight normal-appearing ampullae demonstrated microscopic adenomatous change at biopsy (17). However, care should be taken to avoid the ampullary os, because even cold biopsies can result in pancreatitis. Most lesions demonstrate adenomatous-appearing proliferative tissues, but occasionally a mass will arise within the ampulla and present as a bulging ampulla covered with normal mucosa. Sphincterotomy to access the tissue is necessary in this situation. The differential diagnosis of a bulging ampulla includes choledocholithiasis, type III choledochal cyst, and perhaps duodenal wind-sock diverticulum (although this is not an ampullary lesion).

As a result of the poor sensitivity of endoscopic biopsies regarding malignant change, endoscopic retrograde cholangiography is an essential part of the management of a patient with an adenoma involving the ampulla. Sphincterotomy permits sampling of the intra-ampullary mucosa whereas extension along the pancreaticobiliary system will be revealed by cholangiopancreatography, a situation rendering the patient unsuitable for definitive endoscopic therapy.

Because management decisions will hinge on endoscopic biopsies, it is important to appreciate the limitations of endoscopic biopsy as an indication of dysplasia. Surface biopsies may underestimate the degree of dysplasia within the lesion. In one study, endoscopic biopsy failed to identify infiltrating malignancy in 7 of 23 cases (32%) (34). The accuracy of endoscopic biopsy was increased following biliary sphincterotomy and access to "deeper" tissue.

The role of endoscopic ultrasound (EUS) in this condition remains to be determined. There may be difficulty examining this area reliably owing to compression of the affected tissues. This difficulty is may be prevented by infusing water into the duodenum. In spite of this, EUS can afford excellent views of the region including the duct systems. Recent studies have indicated that EUS is useful in the tumor-node-metastasis staging of periampullary malignancy, with staging accuracy as high as 84% (34–38). In a recent study the T-stage accuracy was 82% and nodal accuracy was 71% (39). In another study, however, the diagnostic accuracy of EUS was only 44% in 23 patients with periampullary lesions (34). Intraductal ultrasound may provide useful information regarding intraductal extension. This approach requires further evaluation.

7.2. SURVEILLANCE

As early as 1950, Halsted advocated upper GI surveillance of FAP subjects (40). Given the risk of progression to malignancy, concerns regarding residual adenomatous tissue after ablation or resection and the ongoing proliferative nature of these lesions, surveillance appears justified, although no studies have demonstrated improved survival as a result. An ideal regimen for surveillance of these lesions has yet to be determined. As discussed earlier, virtually all patients with FAP will eventually have at least microscopic involvement of the ampulla and most will have multiple tiny adenomata spread over the proximal duodenum. It is impossible to remove all adenomatous tissue in FAP patients and the aim of surveillance in FAP patients is to sample tissue in order to detect advancement to high-grade dysplasia. Large lesions are more likely to contain foci of high-grade dysplasia or malignancy. Therefore it is our practice to remove or ablate lesions larger than 5 mm and grossly polypoid papillae. Sporadic adenomas, on the other hand, occur as isolated lesions, and the aim of surveillance is to detect recurrence at a previous site of therapy (either endoscopic or surgical).

The optimal time interval for surveillance in FAP patients remains to be determined. Two authors have suggested surveillance every 3–5 yr (41,42) Spigelman and co-workers have (retrospectively) developed a scoring system to determine which patients are most likely to progress to malignancy and therefore warrant more intense surveillance (see Table 1) (43). It is important to consider that patients with FAP may have adenomas beyond the ampulla and not seen with standard endoscopy. Therefore, an appropriate surveillance strategy in

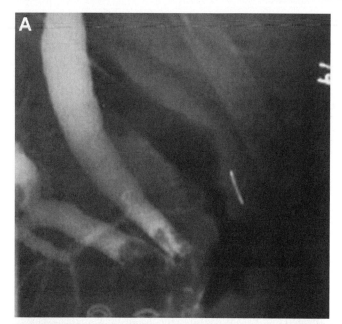

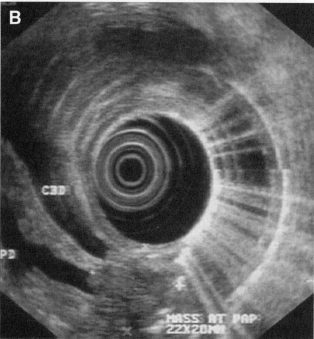

Fig. 8. Lesion not amenable to endoscopic removal owing to intra-ductal extension. (**A**) Endoscopic ultrasound image. (**B**) Endoscopic retrograde cholangiography image.

FAP patients might include extended duodenoscopy with either a colonoscope or push enteroscope.

7.3. THERAPY

The ideal endoscopic therapy for periampullary adenomas has not been established. Excision has the advantage of submitting ample tissue for histological examination. In practice, endoscopic therapy for these lesions usually involves excision of the bulk of the lesion followed by tissue ablation of residual adenoma at the conclusion of the initial endoscopic session and at follow-up examinations. Shemesh and co-workers *(44)* published their early experience with sphincterotomy and fulguration of adenomatous periampullary tissue in 1989. Four patients with recurrent disease

after local surgical resection were treated with fulguration. None had evidence of recurrence with a 12- to 24-mo follow-up.

The first step in endoscopic removal of the ampulla comprises assessment of intraductal extension of the adenoma. Any lesion extending beyond the wall of the duodenum is clearly beyond definitive endoscopic treatment. This is most easily determined by cholangiopancreatography or possibly EUS.

Endoscopic removal of the ampulla may be performed either in a single piece (snare ampullectomy), or using a piece-meal resection technique.

7.3.1. Snare Excision

This technique comprises removal of the tumor using a small snare in one piece. The procedure may be preceded by sub-mucosal saline injection. Advocates of this technique believe that it increased the distance between serosa and the snare, thus making the procedure safer. However, as the ampulla is teth-ered by the ductal complex, it does not rise in quite the same fashion as a colonic polyp and occasionally can become more difficult to effectively snare with a large cushion of saline.

A modification of the snare technique (not widely prac-ticed) is to inflate an occlusion balloon in the distal bile duct and retract the tissue toward the snare in an effort to better snare deep tissue *(45)*. Snare removal of the entire papilla was described in a large cohort by Binmoeller and co-workers in 1993 *(46)*. In a recent report of 28 ampullectomies from the Mayo Clinic immediate complications were minor bleeding ($n = 2$), mild pancreatitis ($n = 4$), and a duodenal perforation ($n = 1$). Papillary stenosis resulting in pancreatitis occurred in two patients (17%) at 4 and 24 mo. Follow-up endoscopy revealed recurrent/residual ampullary adenomatous tissue in two (10%) *(47)*. These recurrence rates following snare ampul-lectomy compare favorably with transduodenal ampullectomy *(34)*. Martin et al. *(48)* reported 14 consecutive patients treated with snare ampullectomy. One patient died from necrotizing pancreatitis and another required surgery for hemorrhage. The patient who died did not receive a prophylactic pancreatic stent. Recurrence has occurred in 4 out of 10 patients with a mean follow-up of 31 mo. Another study of eight patients *(49)* reported one episode of cholangitis following snare ampullec-tomy, but no other complications. Two patients had invasive malignancy in the snared specimen and went on to have pan-creaticoduodenectomy. The remaining six patients remain well with no recurrence at mean follow-up of 12 mo.

Clearly a major concern with snare ampullectomy is the potential for acute pancreatitis. This occurs in about 15–20% of cases *(46,47)* and can be fatal *(48)*. Identification of the pan-creatic orifice after snare ampullectomy may not be possible. In the Mayo series, about 50% of patients had a temporary stent placed (at the discretion of the endoscopist) but no differ-ence in pancreatitis rates was reported between those with and without stent insertion. Nonetheless it is possible that stenting the pancreatic duct may modify the severity of subsequent pancreatitis and it appears to be prudent.

7.3.2. Piecemeal Resection

Concerns regarding pancreatitis have led some authors to a piecemeal technique for adenoma resection performed after the insertion of a pancreatic stent. The patient initially undergoes a dual biliary and pancreatic sphincterotomy. The pancreatic orifice is then stented. Tissue is then raised on a cushion of submucosal saline and snared piecemeal. A potential concern with this technique is the adequacy of adenoma removal but small amounts of residual adenoma can usually be adequately removed after piecemeal excision with cautery techniques such as argon plasma coagulation or contact cautery techniques. In a recent report of this approach by Howell and co-workers, 13 patients with ampullary adenomas were treated. Ninety-two percent were disease-free after a mean of 2.7 procedures (mean follow-up 19 mo). One patient developed mild pancreatitis *(50)*.

Laser has been reported to be efficacious in ablation of periampullary adenomas. In a study by Lambert and co-workers, seven of eight lesions treated with Nd:YAG laser were completely ablated with follow-up of 14–53 mo *(51)*. However, complications such has pancreatitis, transmural burn, and perforation have generally led to the use of less aggressive ablative therapy *(17)* such as monopolar ablation following sphincterotomy. A fistulatome allows precise targeting of tissue for ablation. Argon plasma coagulation may be an attractive method for destroying residual tissue given its relatively shallow depth of injury.

8. SURGICAL THERAPY

The long-term results of endoscopic resection and ablative therapy are not known, whereas the limitations of endoscopic biopsy in excluding malignancy are well documented, with false-negative results of up to 56% *(34)*. The two surgical options for these lesions are pancreaticoduodenectomy (Whipple procedure) and transduodenal excision.

Gray has reported pancreaticoduodenectomy for five patients with benign adenomas and eight with adenomas containing foci of malignancy *(52)*. Two of the patients with benign lesions died in the peri-operative period, but the three survivors were free of disease at follow-up. Five of eight patients with invasive malignancy were also free of disease at follow-up. The cost of Whipple's procedure is higher potential morbidity and mortality *(34,53)*. Complications and hospital stay following this surgery are significantly longer than with local resection *(34)*.

Transduodenal excision is not a new technique, having been reported for ampullary lesions by Halsted in 1899 *(54)*. Transduodenal excision has been used as a less invasive surgical alternative to pancreaticoduodenectomy *(32,34,53,55,56)*. Unfortunately, transduodenal resection may be inadequate therapy in many patients. Recurrence of benign adenomas has been reported in 25–33% *(32,34,56)*. In one study, four of four subjects treated had recurrence of adenoma at 24-mo follow-up *(44)*. In a study of 12 patients, resection margins were inadequate in 50%, leading to conversion to pancreaticoduodenectomy in 3 patients *(34)*. In contrast to the above results, a more recent study by Posner and coworkers reported 89% total excision rate in 21 patients, 3 of whom had malignancy *(57)*. There was, however, one death.

FAP patients are a particularly difficult treatment group owing to the widespread nature of mucosal involvement. Recurrent duodenal adenomas following transduodenal resection (mean recurrence: 13 mo) has led one group to conclude that this is inadequate therapy for these patients *(58)*. Furthermore, the potential for desmoid formation following surgery is another factor favoring the use of nonsurgical (i.e., endoscopic) techniques.

9. PHARMACOLOGICAL TREATMENT

There is randomized controlled data that sulindac (Clinoril) slows the progression of polyps in the colon of patients with FAP syndrome *(59)*. Similar findings have been reported with the use of the COX-2 specific drug celecoxib (Celebrex); although recent data may temper this enthusiasm, as there is a long-term need for the medical therapy in this disease *(60)*. There is less compelling evidence for the use of non-steroidal anti-inflammatory drugs for progression of duodenal disease. The St Mark's group randomized 24 patients with advanced duodenal disease to 200 mg sulindac twice daily or placebo *(61)*. After 6 mo of treatment there was a reduction in epithelial proliferation in the sulindac group but no significant regression of large polyps. However, blinded review of videotapes demonstrated significant regression of small polyps (<2 mm) compared with the placebo group. This evidence supports the hypothesis that sulindac might also have an effect on polyp proliferation in the duodenum. However, it remains to be seen whether this will translate into a clinically significant benefit.

REFERENCES

1. Takano S, Matsushima M, Ertuk E, Bryan GT. Early induction of rat colonic orthithinedecarboxylase activity by n-methyl-n-nitro-n-nirtosoguaninidine or bile salts. Cancer Res 1981; 41:624–628.
2. Spigelman AD, Scates DK, Venitt S, Phillips RK. DNA adducts, detected by 32P-postlabelling, in the foregut of patients with familial adenomatous polyposis and in unaffected controls. Carcinogenesis 1991; 12:1727–1732.
3. Deschner EE, Raicht RF. Influence of bile on kinetic behavior of colonic epithelial cells of the rat. Digestion 1979; 19:322–327.
4. Spigelman AD, Crofton-Sleigh C, Venitt S, Phillips RK. Mutagenicity of bile and duodenal adenomas in familial adenomatous polyposis. Br J Surg 1990; 77:878–881.
5. Noda Y, Watanabe H, Iida M, et al. Histologic follow-up of ampullary adenomas in patients with familial *Adenomatous coli.* Cancer 1992; 70:1847–1856.
6. Yamaguchi K, Enjoji M. Adenoma of the ampulla of Vater: putative precancerous lesion. Gut 1991; 32:1558–1561.
7. Sobol S, Cooperman AM. Villous adenoma of the ampulla of Vater. An unusual cause of biliary colic and obstructive jaundice. Gastroenterology 1978; 75:107–109.
8. Polakis P. The adenomatous polyposis coli (APC) tumor suppressor. Biochim et Biophys Acta 1997; 1332:F127–F147.
9. Gallinger S, Vivona AA, Odze RD, et al. Somatic APC and K-ras codon 12 mutations in periampullary adenomas and carcinomas from familial adenomatous polyposis patients. Oncogene 1995; 10:1875–1878.
10. Scarpa A, Capelli P, Zamboni G, et al. Neoplasia of the ampulla of Vater. Ki-ras and p53 mutations. American Journal of Pathology 1993; 142:1163–1172.
11. Sanabria JR, Croxford R, Berk TC, Cohen Z, Bapat BV, Gallinger S. Familial segregation in the occurrence and severity of periampullary neoplasms in familial adenomatous polyposis. Am J Surg 1996; 171:136–140; discussion 140–141.
12. Spigelman AD, Williams CB, Phillips RK. Rectal polyposis as a guide to duodenal polyposis in familial adenomatous polyposis. J R Soc Med 1992; 85:77–89.
13. Scates DK, Spigelman AD, Phillips RK, Venitt S. DNA adducts detected by 32P-postlabelling, in the intestine of rats given bile from patients with familial adenomatous polyposis and from unaffected controls. Carcinogenesis 1992; 13:731–735.

14. Scates DK, Venitt S, Phillips RK, Spigelman AD. High pH reduces DNA damage caused by bile from patients with familial adenomatous polyposis: antacids may attenuate duodenal polyposis. Gut 1995; 36:918–921.

15. Venitt S. Biological Mechanisms. In: Raffle PAB, Adams PH, Baxter PJ, Lee WR, eds. Hunter's diseases of occupations. London: Edward Arnold, 1994:623–654.

16. Spigelman AD, Talbot IC, Penna C, et al. Evidence for adenoma-carcinoma sequence in the duodenum of patients with familial adenomatous polyposis. The Leeds Castle Polyposis Group (Upper Gastrointestinal Committee). J Clin Pathol 1994; 47:709–710.

17. Bleau BL, Gostout CJ. Endoscopic treatment of ampullary adenomas in familial adenomatous polyposis. J Clin Gastroenterol 1996; 22:237–241.

18. Powell SM, Petersen GM, Krush AJ, et al. Molecular diagnosis of familial adenomatous polyposis. N Engl J Med 1993; 328:1982–1987.

19. Groden J, Thliveris A, Samowitz W, Carlson M, Gelbert L, Albertsen H. Identification and characterization of the familial adenomatous polyposis gene. Cell 1991; 66:589–600.

20. Lynch HT, Smyrk T, McGinn T, et al. Attenuated familial adenomatous polyposis (AFAP). A Phenotypically and genotypically distinctive variant of FAP. Cancer 1995; 76:2427–2433 (see comments).

21. Leggett BA, Young JP, Biden K, Buttenshaw RL, Knight N, Cowen AE. Severe upper gastrointestinal polyposis associated with sparse colonic polyposis in a familial adenomatous polyposis family with an APC mutation at codon 1520. Gut; 41:518–521.

22. Boland CR, Kim YS. Gastrointestinal polyp syndromes. In: Sleisenger M, Fordtran J, eds., Gastrointestinal Disease. Vol. 2. Philadelphia: W. B. Saunders, 1993:1430–1448.

23. Paraf F, Jothy S, Van Meir EG. Brain tumor-polyposis syndromes: two genetic diseases? J Clin Oncol 1997; 15:2744–2758.

24. Arvantis ML, Jagelman DG, Fazio VW, Lavery IC, McGannon E. Mortality in patients with familial adenomatous polyposis. Diseases of the Colon and Rectum 1990; 33:639–642.

25. Jagelman DG, DeCosse JJ, Bussey HJ. Upper gastrointestinal cancer in familial adenomatous polyposis. Lancet 1988; 1:1149–1151.

26. Geller A, Wang KK, Batts KP, Gostout CJ. Ileostomy pouch polyposis in a patient with familial adenomatous polyposis. Gastrointest Endosc 1995; 41:377.

27. Baggenstoss AH. Major duodenal papilla: variations of pathologic interest and lesions of the mucosa. Arch Pathol 1938; 26:853–868.

28. Offerhaus GJ, Giardiello FM, Krush AJ, et al. The risk of upper gastrointestinal cancer in familial adenomatous polyposis. Gastroenterology 1992; 102:1980–1982 (see comments).

29. Nugent KP, Spigelman AD, Williams CB, Talbot IC, Phillips RK. Surveillance of duodenal polyps in familial adenomatous polyposis: progress report. J R Soc Med 1994; 87:704–706.

30. Guzzardo G, Kleinman MS, Krackov JH, Schwartz SI. Recurrent acute pancreatitis caused by ampullary villous adenoma. J Clin Gastroenterol 1990; 12:200–202.

31. Ponchon T, Berger F, Chavaillon A, Bory R, Lambert R. Contribution of endoscopy to diagnosis and treatment of tumors of the ampulla of Vater. Cancer 1989; 64:161–167.

32. Alstrup N, Burcharth F, Hauge C, Horn T. Transduodenal excision of tumours of the ampulla of Vater. Eur J Surg 1996; 162:961–967.

33. Church JM, McGannon E, Hull-Boiner S, et al. Gastroduodenal polyps in patients with familial adenomatous polyposis. DisColon Rectum 1992; 35:1170–1173.

34. Cahen DL, Fockens P, De Wit LT, Offerhaus GJA, Obertop H, Gouma DJ. Local resection or pancreaticoduodenectomy for villous adenoma of the ampulla of Vater diagnosed before operation. Br J Surg 1997; 84:948–951.

35. Tio TL, Tytgat GN, Cikot RJ, Houthoff HJ, Sars PR. Ampullo-pancreatic carcinoma: preoperative TNM classification with endosonography. Radiol 1990; 175:455–461.

36. Tio TL, Mulder CJ, Eggink WF. Endosonography in staging early carcinoma of the ampulla of Vater. Gastroenterology 1992; 102:1392–1395.

37. Tio TL, Sie LH, Kallimanis G, et al. Staging of ampullary and pancreatic carcinoma: comparison between endosonography and surgery. Gastrointest Endosc 1996; 44:706–713.

38. Rosch T, Braig C, Gain T, et al. Staging of pancreatic and ampullary carcinoma by endoscopic ultrasonography. Comparison with conventional sonography, computed tomography, and angiography. Gastroenterology 1992; 102:188–199.

39. Skordilis P, Mouzas IA, Dimoulios PD, Alexandrakis G, Moschandrea J, Kouroumalis E. Is endosonography an effective method for detection and local staging of the ampullary carcinoma? A prospective study. BMC Surg 2002; 2:25.

40. Halsted JA, Harris EJ, Bartlett MK. Involvement of the stomach in familial polyposis of the gastrointestinal tract. Gastroenterology 1950; 15:763–770.

41. Sarre RG, Frost AG, Jagelman DG, Petras RE, Sivak MV, McGannon E. Gastric and duodenal polyps in familial adenomatous polyposis: a prospective study of the nature and prevalence of upper gastrointestinal polyps. Gut 1987; 28:306–314.

42. Sawada T, Muto T. Familial adenomatous polyposis: should patients undergo surveillance of the upper gastrointestinal tract? Endoscopy 1995; 27:6–11.

43. Spigelman AD, Williams CB, Talbot IC, Domizio P, Phillips RK. Upper gastrointestinal cancer in patients with familial adenomatous polyposis. Lancet 1989; 2:783–785.

44. Shemesh E, Nass S, Czerniak A. Endoscopic sphincterotomy and endoscopic fulguration in the management of adenoma of the papilla of Vater. Surg Gynecol Obstet 1989; 169:445–448.

45. Aiura K, Imaeda H, Kitajima M, Kumai K. Balloon-catheter-assisted endoscopic snare papillectomy for benign tumors of the major duodenal papilla. Gastrointest Endosc 2003; 57:743–747.

46. Binmoeller KF, Boaventura S, Ramsperger K, Soehendra N. Endoscopic snare excision of benign adenomas of the papilla of Vater. Gastrointest Endosc 1993; 39:127–131 (see comments).

47. Norton ID, Gostout CJ, Baron TH, Geller A, Petersen BT, Wiersema MJ. Safety and outcome of endoscopic snare excision of the major duodenal papilla. Gastrointest Endosc 2002; 56:239–243.

48. Martin JA, Haber GB, Kortan PP, et al. Endoscopic snare ampullectomy for resection for resection of benign ampullary neoplasms. Gastrointest Endosc 1997; 45:AB139.

49. Greenspan AB, Waldon DT, Aliperti G. Endoscopic management of ampullary adenomas. Gastrointest Endosc 1997; 45:AB133.

50. Desilets DJ, Dy RM, Ku PM, et al. Endoscopic management of tumors of the major duodenal papilla: Refined techniques to improve outcome and avoid complications. Gastrointest Endosc 2001; 54:202–208. (see comment).

51. Lambert R, Ponchon T, Chavaillon A, Berger F. Laser treatment of tumors of the papilla of Vater. Endoscopy 1988; 20:227–231.

52. Gray G, Browder W. Villous tumors of the ampulla of Vater: local resection versus pancreatoduodenectomy. Southern Med J 1989; 82:917–920.

53. Knox RA, Kingston RD. Carcinoma of the ampulla of Vater. Br J Surg 1986; 73:72,73.

54. Halsted W. Contributions to the surgery of the bile passages, especially of the common bile duct. Boston Med Surg J 1899; 141:645–654.

55. Asbun HJ, Rossi RL, Munson JL. Local resection for ampullary tumors. Is there a place for it? Arch Surg 1993; 128:515–520.

56. Farouk M, Niotis M, Branum GD, Cotton PB, Meyers WC. Indications for and the technique of local resection of tumors of the papilla of Vater. Arch Surg 1991; 126:650–652.

57. Posner S, Colletti L, Knol J, Mulholland M, Eckhauser F. Safety and long-term efficacy of transduodenal excision for tumors of the ampulla of Vater. Surgery 2000; 128:694–701.

58. Penna C, Phillips RK, Tiret E, Spigelman AD. Surgical polypectomy of duodenal adenomas in familial adenomatous polyposis: experience of two European centres. Br J Surg 1993; 80:1027–1029.

59. Giardiello FM, Hamilton SR, Krush AJ. Treatment of colonic and rectal adenomas with sulindac in familial adenomatous polyposis. N Engl J Med 1993; 328:1313–1316.

60. Steinbach G, Lynch PM, Phillips RK. The effect of celecoxib, a cyclooxygenase-2 inhibitor, in familial adenomatous polyposis. N Engl J Med 2000; 342:1946–1952.

61. Debinski HS, Trojan J, Nugent KP, Spigelman AJ, Phillips RKS. Effect of sulindac on small polyps in familial adenomatous polyposis. Lancet 1995; 345:855–856.

30 Magnetic Resonance Imaging of Neoplasms of the Pancreatobiliary System

Evan S. Siegelman, MD and Wendy C. Hsu, MD

Contents

1. BACKGROUND

Magnetic resonance imaging (MRI) and magnetic resonance cholangiopancreatography (MRCP) are noninvasive imaging techniques that can detect, characterize, and stage neoplasms of the biliary system and pancreas. In patients with suspected pancreatic cancer, MRI/MRCP can help distinguish those patients who are unresectable from those who are potentially resectable. In patients with pancreatic cysts, MRI assists in the distinction among pseudocysts, benign cystic lesions, and cystic pancreatic malignancies. Limitations of current MRI techniques include the inability to detect subcentimeter peritoneal metastases and the lack of sensitivity for identifying microscopic metastases within normal-sized lymph nodes.

2. INTRODUCTION

MRI/MRCP is a noninvasive imaging modality that has been shown to be an accurate technique for diagnosing and staging neoplasms of the pancreatobiliary system. In some clinical circumstances, MRI/MRCP can replace endoscopic retrograde cholangiopancreatography (ERCP) as the study of choice for diagnostic evaluation of the pancreatobiliary tract. This chapter reviews the rationale, technique, and role of MRI/MRCP in the evaluation of neoplasms that involved the pancreas and bile ducts. Additional information concerning applications in nonneoplastic disease may be found in a concurrently published review *(1)*.

From: *Endoscopic Oncology: Gastrointestinal Endoscopy and Cancer Management.* Edited by: D. O. Faigel and M. L. Kochman © Humana Press, Totowa, NJ

3. RATIONALE FOR MRI/MRCP

MRI/MRCP has been advocated as a comprehensive diagnostic imaging modality of the pancreas and biliary system. MRI/MRCP is currently the single imaging modality that can most reliably provide information on the pancreatobiliary ducts, surrounding tissues, vasculature, and function in one session. Relative strengths and limitations of MRI/MRCP are presented in Table 1.

MRI is noninvasive, does not use ionizing radiation, and utilizes a safe intravenous contrast agent (Gadolinium chelate) that is not nephrotoxic and has a low rate of allergic reactions *(2)*. MRCP is less operator-dependent than modalities such as ERCP, sonography, and percutaneous transhepatic cholangiography (PTC). Menon et al. *(3)* found MRI/MRCP to be well tolerated and preferred by patients over ERCP, with patients reporting less pain and discomfort. MRI/MRCP has excellent soft tissue contrast, with especially high sensitivity for detection of fat, fluid, hemorrhage, and contrast enhancement. Images can be directly obtained in any specified plane, optimizing views, and thereby the information.

4. PANCREATOBILIARY MRI/MRCP TECHNIQUE

The abdomen from the diaphragm to the iliac crest is imaged when MRI is requested for evaluation of a potential neoplasm of the pancreatobiliary system. The specific sequences that are performed may vary by institution specific protocols. However, as a rule, both T1- and T2-weighted sequences are obtained in various planes, in addition to MRCP (heavily T2-weighted) sequences. Dynamic enhanced imaging with gadolinium is performed with breath-hold two or three dimensional T1-weighted gradient echo sequences. At some

Table 1
Strengths and Limitations of MRI/MRCP of the Pancreatobiliary System

Strengths	*Limitations*
• Comprehensive approach (ducts, surrounding tissue, vasculature, potentially function) • No ionizing radiation • Noninvasive • No sedation required • Non-nephrotoxic contrast agent: gadolinium • Excellent soft tissue contrast and sensitivity to contrast enhancement • Direct multiplanar sections • Shows ducts proximal to obstruction • Higher patient satisfaction over ERCP • Lower cost than ERCP	• Less sensitive for calcification and gas • Less sensitive for ampullary/periampullary lesions than ERCP • Lower spatial resolution than ERCP, CT • Longer scan times than CT • Artifacts • Less availability than CT, US

CT, computed tomography; ERCP, endoscopic retrograde cholangiopancreatography; US, ultrasound.

institutions, MRCP is performed exclusively without use of conventional MRI sequences or dynamic contrast-enhanced imaging. However, performing a complete abdominal MRI examination in addition to MRCP is often necessary for a complete patient evaluation.

MRCP is performed using heavily T2-weighted sequences that result in high signal from static or slow-moving fluid such as bile and pancreatic juice in the pancreatobiliary tract. Images are acquired or postprocessed to resemble the projection images obtained at ERCP. Currently, MRI techniques are used that can acquire an image in less than a second. These breath-hold techniques result in decreased artifacts from abdominal gas, respiratory motion, surgical clips, and biliary stents whereas increasing signal-to-noise ratio and spatial resolution.

Two complementary techniques are performed as part of MRCP. One technique acquires one or more thick (30–80 mm) slabs in the coronal and/or coronal oblique planes. The other technique obtains multiple thin (2–5 mm) sections in the axial and/or coronal planes. A maximal intensity projection can then be constructed from the thin-slice tomographic source images. On these heavily T2-weighted sequences, any fluid present within the imaging volume (e.g., fluid-filled stomach or bowel segment) will also be depicted as high signal intensity and in some cases may obscure visualization of the pancreatobiliary system.

5. MRI/MRCP EVALUATION OF SPECIFIC BILIARY OBSTRUCTION

A recent meta-analysis *(4)* reviewed 498 abstracts published from January 1987 to March 2003 and selected 67 studies (4711 patients) to assess the performance of MRCP in the evaluation of biliary obstruction. In the studies examined, findings on MRCP were compared with various gold standards including intraoperative cholangiography, ERCP, intravenous cholangiography, surgical exploration, or a combination of these procedures. MRCP was found to be highly accurate for diagnosing the presence of obstruction, with a sensitivity of 97% and specificity of 98%. MRCP identified the level of obstruction with a sensitivity of 98% and specificity of 98%. Accurate determination of the level and specific location of obstruction not only aids in the differential diagnosis, but also in choice of potential therapeutic intervention.

Patients with distal bile duct obstruction are better evaluated and treated via a retrograde endoscopic approach whereas those with proximal obstruction may be better treated by percutaneous transhepatic cholangiography or by selective intrahepatic duct cannulation at ERCP *(5)*.

With biliary obstruction, the increased ductal caliber increases the conspicuity of third and fourth order peripheral ducts on MRCP, which are not well depicted when normal in caliber. The biliary ducts both proximal and distal to an obstruction are well demonstrated on MRCP, whereas retrograde contrast injection at ERCP may not opacify ducts proximal to a high-grade obstruction, or do so at the risk of inducing sepsis if the ducts visualized are not subsequently successfully drained. The use of T1 and less-heavily-weighted T2 sequences provides information about surrounding tissues and assists in determining the nature of the obstruction. The ductal caliber seen on MRCP may more closely approximate the true caliber, which may be overestimated at ERCP owing to the distension effect of contrast injection.

Although MRCP is highly accurate for detecting and localizing biliary obstruction, it has variable accuracy ranging from 30 to 98% for differentiation between benign and malignant causes of obstruction. The sensitivity and specificity of MRCP in the evaluation of malignancy is 88 and 95%, respectively *(4)*. Some studies have only evaluated MRCP sequences in isolation, but the addition of T1, T2, and contrast-enhanced sequences can increase the sensitivity, specificity, and accuracy up to 20% *(6)*.

6. MRI/MRCP EVALUATION OF SPECIFIC NEOPLASTIC CONDITIONS OF THE PANCREATICOBILIARY SYSTEM

6.1. CHOLANGIOCARCINOMA

Cholangiocarcinoma (CCA) in or outside the setting of primary sclerosing cholangitis can be difficult to diagnose with available tests or imaging modalities, as findings may be nonspecific and subtle. The peripheral type of CCA typically presents at an advanced stage as a mass with peripheral duct dilation (Fig. 1). A suggestive MRI feature of peripheral CCA is central foci of low T2 signal, intensity that shows delayed

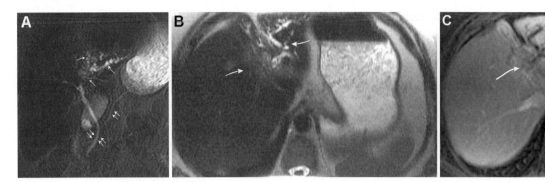

Fig. 1. Magnetic resonance imaging illustration of a peripheral cholangiocarcinoma (CCA). **(A)** Projection magnetic resonance cholangiopancre-atography image shows segmental biliary obstruction of the left hepatic ducts (curved arrows). The ducts occlude at the level of the tumor (arrow). Pancreatic divisum is revealed as the accessory pancreatic duct (double small arrows) drains into the minor papilla and does not communicate with the common bile duct B and C. **(B)** T2 and contrast enhanced **(C)** T1-weighted images shows the rim enhancing CCA (arrow) and dilated periph-eral ducts (curved arrows).

enhancement, a finding that correlates with intratumoral fibro-sis *(7,8)*. Rarely, liver metastases from colon carcinoma can result in peripheral duct dilation that can mimic peripheral CCA. Detection of the primary colon cancer can help establish a correct diagnosis (Fig. 2).

The hilar (Klatskin's) and extrahepatic types of CCA present earlier with obstructive signs and symptoms. These types cir-cumferentially infiltrate the duct walls, and might be depicted as an obstructing stricture with irregular contours and abrupt ter-mination, referred to as the "shoulder sign" that is suggestive of malignancy. Occasionally, a papillary growth projecting into the lumen may be revealed as a filling defect. MRI/MRCP has been advocated as the current optimal initial evaluation for suspected CCA, providing information on local extent, hepatic metastases, and vascular involvement (Fig. 3) *(9,10)*.

Enhancing bile duct walls that are more than 5 mm in width suggests a diagnosis of CCA, but is not a sensitive indicator of malignancy. Wall thickening and enhancement can be present in various infectious and inflammatory disorders of the biliary tract, including ascending cholangitis and primary sclerosing cholangitis. It is difficult to differentiate benign and malignant disease, but performance of MRCP can be improved by the use of T1- and T2-weighted and gadolinium-enhanced sequences to detect features such masses, abscesses, or cirrhosis that may help distinguish among the different entities. One should con-sider performing MRI/MRCP in the evaluation of suspected CCA prior to intervention, as inflammation related to stent placement can subsequently result in wall thickening and enhancement and lead to overestimation of the extent of dis-ease. In patients with inconclusive MRCP, ERCP or before bile duct brushing, positron emission tomography (PET) could be considered to potentially aid in the diagnosis and staging of a suspected CCA *(11)*.

7. EVALUATION OF THE PANCREAS AND PANCREATIC DUCT

The pancreatic duct is smaller in caliber than the common bile duct and is more difficult to evaluate in its entirety with MRI/MRCP unless it is dilated. Imaging sequences that are most effective for evaluating the pancreatic parenchyma often empha-size contrast differences between the high signal intensity on

T1-weighted images of the normal pancreatic tissue and the rela-tively lower signal intensity of many pathological processes. The pancreas demonstrates the highest signal intensity on T1-weighted imaging of all the parenchymal abdominal organs owing to its high-protein content. MRI is also highly sensitive for detection of presence of contrast enhancement. Patterns of enhancement depicted after gadolinium administration help differentiate vari-ous pathological conditions. The following reviews the various types of neoplastic conditions that involve the pancreas.

7.1. PANCREATIC DUCTAL ADENOCARCINOMA

A wide range of imaging modalities has been applied to detect and stage pancreatic adenocarcinoma including CT, percutaneous sonography, endoscopic sonography, MRI/MRCP, ERCP, and PET with variable success *(12)*. In a prospective study by Adamek et al. *(13)* MRI/MRCP was determined to be more accurate for detection of pancreatic adenocarcinoma than ERCP. MRI/MRCP was 84% sensitive and 97% specific compared with ERCP, which was 70% sensitive and 94% specific.

Studies have also shown that MRI is superior to nonhelical and single detector CT for the detection and staging of pancre-atic malignancy *(14)*, but in clinical practice, patients are often routinely referred for helical CT. The basis for better perform-ance of MRI over CT has been attributed to MRI's superior soft tissue contrast and sensitivity to contrast enhancement that renders small tumors more conspicuous. MRI/MRCP accu-rately evaluates for vascular involvement, regional invasion, and distant metastases—all factors that determine lesion resectability *(15,16)*. The accuracy of newer multidetector hel-ical CT scanning compared with MRI/MRCP has yet to be determined. One recent study suggests that the excellent spatial resolution of multidetector helical CT improves the detection of small (<2 cm) pancreatic tumors *(17)*.

Differentiating carcinoma from chronic pancreatitis based on imaging criteria can be difficult in some patients. The "double duct sign" at MRCP, as it is at ERCP, is highly suggestive of a pancreatic adenocarcinoma indicating mass effect in the head of the pancreas obstructing both the pancreatic and common bile ducts (Fig. 4A). However, this finding is not specific for pancreatic cancer and can also be present secondary to strictures from chronic pancreatitis, leading to false-positive diagnoses *(15)*. On conventional MRI sequences, presence of a focal

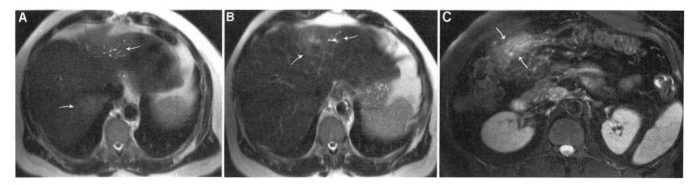

Fig. 2. Magnetic resonance findings of metastatic colon cancer that mimics intrahepatic cholangiocarcinoma (**A,B**). Two T2-weighted images show peripheral dilated left sided ducts (curved arrows in B) and a central heterogeneous left lobe mass (arrow). The presence of a second lesion (small arrow) in the liver dome is more suggestive of metastatic disease. (**C**) T2-weighted image obtained inferiorly shows the primary circumferential adenocarcinoma of the transverse colon (arrows).

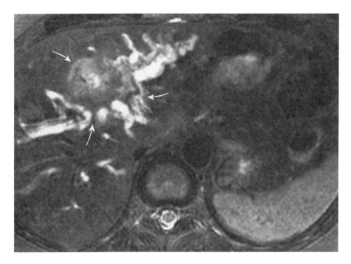

Fig. 3. MR illustration of a Klatskin tumor. Axial T2-weighted image shows a central heterogeneous mass (arrow at top of image) with associated dilation of both the left and right bile ducts (curved arrows).

mass that is lower in signal intensity on T1-weighted images relative to the normal surrounding higher signal intensity pancreatic parenchyma supports the diagnosis of adenocarcinoma. However, focal chronic pancreatitis may also appear well circumscribed and hypointense on T1-weighted imaging. Enhancement characteristics may also be similar, with delayed enhancement relative to the surrounding parenchyma reflecting the hypovascularity and fibrotic nature of both disease processes *(18)*. The presence of normal pancreatic tissue surrounding the mass favors malignancy. However, a nonborder deforming pancreatic head mass in a patient with chronic pancreatitis may represent either an adenocarcinoma that has resulted in secondary postobstructive chronic pancreatitis or benign inflammatory tissue.

Detection and characterization of lymph nodes and metastatic disease is also required in order to stage a patient with a potential pancreatic carcinoma. One of the limitations of current imaging techniques is that differentiating benign from malignant lymph nodes is often based on size criteria alone. Unfortunately, metastatic pancreatic carcinoma may be present in normal-sized nodes and both CT and MRI techniques are not accurate in predicting the presence or absence of tumor in nodes in patients with

pancreatic cancer *(19)*. More than half of resected lymph nodes in patient's with pancreatic adenocarcinoma that have a normal appearance at histology will reveal occult involvement by cancer with molecular biological techniques *(20–22)*. It is hoped that in the future novel contrast agents may help to characterize "micrometastases" to normal-sized nodes and exclude tumor in enlarged reactive nodes *(23,24)*.

Some centers use laparoscopy and laparoscopic ultrasonography in order to identify a subset of patients with occult unresectable disease (including malignant adenopathy and occult peritoneal metastases) who would not benefit from an attempt at curative resection *(25,26)*. However, others feel that laparoscopic staging does not detect enough patients with occult unresectable disease to warrant its routine use *(27)*. Because different surgeons have different opinions concerning what defines resectable or unresectable disease, one should engage in active discussion with ones surgical colleagues in order to understand the information desired to optimally stage a patient for treatment. Both MRI and multidetector CT can detected and characterize liver metastases from pancreatic cancer *(15,28)* (Fig. 4B,C). By establishing an accurate diagnosis of metastatic disease to the liver, the patient can avoid unnecessary attempt at curative laparotomy and can be referred for appropriate palliative care. Whereas endoscopic ultrasound produces high-resolution images of the primary tumor, often it is detection of disease outside of the field of view of the ultrasound probe that may ultimately determine an individual patient's treatment and prognosis.

7.2. ISLET CELL NEOPLASMS (NEUROENDOCRINE TUMORS)

Contrast-enhanced MRI/MRCP appears to be sensitive for detection of pancreatic islet cell tumors, although studies are often limited by small patient populations and different proportions of the various subtypes of tumors. Islet cell tumors are well demonstrated on multiple imaging sequences on MRI/MRCP *(29,30)*. Compared with CT, MRI demonstrates better soft tissue contrast and increased sensitivity for intravenous contrast enhancement that potentially makes smaller tumors more apparent.

The three most common types are insulinomas, gastrinomas, and nonfunctioning tumors. Most insulinomas are benign, whereas the majority of gastrinomas and nonfunctioning tumors

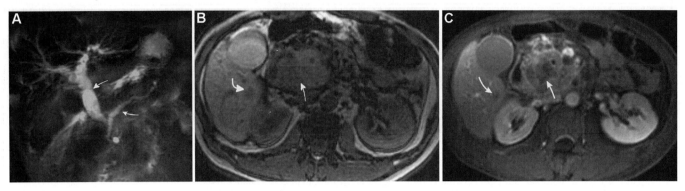

Fig. 4. Magnetic resonance cholangiopancreatography (MRCP) demonstration of the "double-duct" sign in a man with pancreatic cancer and liver metastases. (A) Coronal projection image from a MRCP shows a dilated common bile duct and pancreatic duct (arrows). The MRCP suggests of a diagnosis of a pancreatic head tumor. However, if interpreted in isolation, one can determine if a responsible tumor is resectable or unresectable. (B,C) Axial T1-weighted images obtained before (B) and after contrast show a T1 hypointense pancreatic cancer (arrows) in (B) that is hypoenhancing in (C). A hypovascular liver metastases establishes the presence of unresectable disease (curved arrow).

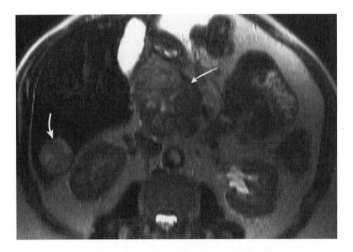

Fig. 5. Magnetic resonance demonstration of a primary nonfunctioning neuroendocrine tumor of the pancreas with metastatic disease to the liver. Axial T2-weighted image shows a heterogeneous low and high signal intensity mass (arrow) of the pancreatic neck with associated peripheral duct dilation. A similar appearing liver metastases is also revealed (curved arrow).

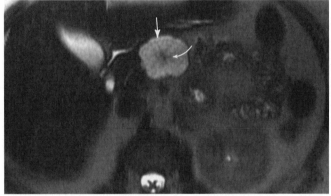

Fig. 6. Benign microcystic adenoma of the pancreas in an asymptomatic woman as revealed on magnetic resonance. Axial T2-weighted image shows a well-circumscribe high intensity lesion (arrow) made up of innumerable small cysts. Multiple internal septa coalesce in a central "scar" (curved arrow).

7.3. CYSTIC PANCREATIC NEOPLASMS

The pseudocyst accounts for about 90% of all cystic pancreatic lesions. The remaining 10% represent cystic neoplasms. The imaging findings of pancreatitis and pseudocysts are beyond the purview of this review. However, most pseudocysts have typical imaging features and are associated with other imaging findings of pancreatitis. However, in some lesions the differentiation between a pseudocyst and cystic pancreatic neoplasm can be difficult (31).

The appearances of the various cystic neoplasms can be nonspecific, but in some cases imaging with MRI/MRCP may be able to strongly suggest a specific diagnosis. Cystic structures are well depicted on MRI/MRCP, better than on CT, with fluid demonstrating very high signal intensity on T2- and heavily T2-weighted sequences. As a result, there is excellent contrast between the fluid and the solid components of pancreatic cystic lesions. This allows for a more confident assessment of the number and size of cysts as well as definition of cyst margins (32). Accurate assessment of these features is important for differentiation between serous and mucinous cystic neoplasms, with implications for patient management.

are malignant. Functional islet cell tumors are generally small (<2 cm) at the time of diagnosis because of clinical manifestations related to hormone elaboration. Functioning islet cell tumors typically show high signal intensity on T2-weighted images and appear lower in signal intensity than surrounding pancreas on T1-weighted images. They are hypervascular and demonstrate avid enhancement on arterial phase images, although exceptions occur when the tumor demonstrates scirrhous features.

Nonfunctioning tumors are often advanced at presentation with a diameter greater than 5 cm and carry a poorer prognosis. These are also hypervascular with enhancement characteristics similar to the functioning tumors. However, nonfunctioning tumors frequently demonstrate heterogeneous signal intensity with prominent areas of necrosis and cystic degeneration (Fig. 5). Symptoms are related to mass effect on the pancreatic duct and adjacent organs. Hypervascular liver metastases may be identified. In contrast to pancreatic ductal adenocarcinoma, islet cell tumors less often result in pancreatic ductal obstruction, vascular encasement, vascular thrombosis, or peritoneal metastases.

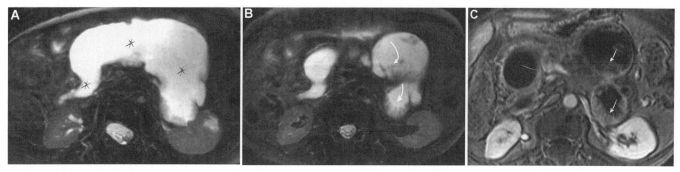

Fig. 7. Main branch intraductal papillary mucinous tumor as revealed on magnetic resonance. (A) Axial T2-weighted thick section image reveals a diffusely dilated pancreatic duct (*) that extends to the level of the ampulla. (B,C) T2-weighted (B) and contrast enhanced T1-weighted image reveals enhancing papillary projections—solid components within the duct (curved arrows).

Serous cystadenomas are benign and typically demonstrate multiple clustered cysts that measure less than 2 cm (Fig. 6). Larger tumors may have a characteristic fibrous central scar exhibiting delayed enhancement. Serous cystadenomas are managed conservatively. Mucinous cystic neoplasms are typically made up of uni- or multilocular macrocysts greater than 2 cm in diameter. Invasion of surrounding structures and presence of liver metastases indicate malignancy, but otherwise, imaging features are not specific for malignant transformation of mucinous tumors. Mucinous cystic neoplasms are all considered potentially malignant and thus are potentially surgical lesions.

Less common primary cystic lesions of the pancreas include intraductal papillary mucinous tumor (IPMT) and solid and papillary epithelial neoplasm. The gold standard for diagnosis of a main branch IPMT has been ERCP, which identifies the presence of intraductal mucin with direct inspection. However, some authors suggest that MRI/MRCP is not only complementary, but also superior to ERCP for evaluation of IPMT *(33)* (Fig. 7). Copious amounts of mucin may impede retrograde contrast injection resulting in incomplete examination at ERCP, whereas the mucin itself allows facilitates an excellent depiction of the pancreatic ducts on MRI/MRCP *(34)*. Features that are suggestive of malignancy of IPMT on MRCP include maximum main duct diameter of 15 mm, diffuse dilation of the main pancreatic duct, and mural nodules within the duct *(35)*. Regarding solid and papillary epithelial neoplasm, the appearance of a large well encapsulated, hemorrhagic mass in a young woman is virtually pathognomonic. The presence of hemorrhagic degeneration in these tumors is well characterized by MRI.

8. CONCLUSIONS

MRI/MRCP has been successfully used for diagnostic evaluation of a wide variety of pancreatobiliary neoplasms. In some circumstances, it has become the study of choice, replacing ERCP and other imaging modalities because of its safety and accuracy. In other scenarios, MRI/MRCP has proven reliable as a complementary or alternative imaging modality, providing additional information that determines need for treatment and directs choice of therapies. MRI/MRCP shows promise as a comprehensive "all-in-one" initial approach for diagnosis and staging of pancreatobiliary neoplasms.

REFERENCES

1. Hsu WC, Siegelman ES. Magnetic Resonance Imaging—Magnetic Resonance Cholangiogropancreatography of the Pancreatobiliary System. In: Ginsberg G, Amhad N, eds. The Clinician's Guide to Pancreatobiliary Disorders. 1st ed. Thorofare, NJ: Slack Incorporated, 2004.
2. Kirchin MA, Runge VM. Contrast agents for magnetic resonance imaging: safety update. Top Magn Reson Imaging 2003; 14:426–435.
3. Menon K, Barkun AN, Romagnuolo J, et al. Patient satisfaction after MRCP and ERCP. Am J Gastroenterol 2001; 96:2646–2650.
4. Romagnuolo J, Bardou M, Rahme E, Joseph L, Reinhold C, Barkun AN. Magnetic resonance cholangiopancreatography: a meta-analysis of test performance in suspected biliary disease. Ann Intern Med 2003; 139:547–557.
5. Schwartz LH, Lefkowitz RA, Panicek DM, et al. Breath-hold magnetic resonance cholangiopancreatography in the evaluation of malignant pancreaticobiliary obstruction. J Comput Assist Tomogr 2003; 27:307–314.
6. Kim MJ, Mitchell DG, Ito K, Outwater EK. Biliary dilatation: differentiation of benign from malignant causes—value of adding conventional MR imaging to MR cholangiopancreatography. Radiology 2000; 214:173–181.
7. Maetani Y, Itoh K, Watanabe C, et al. MR imaging of intrahepatic cholangiocarcinoma with pathologic correlation. AJR Am J Roentgenol 2001; 176:1499–1507.
8. Gabata T, Matsui O, Kadoya M, et al. Delayed MR imaging of the liver: correlation of delayed enhancement of hepatic tumors and pathologic appearance. Abdominal Imaging 1998; 23:309–313.
9. Yeh TS, Jan YY, Tseng JH, et al. Malignant perihilar biliary obstruction: magnetic resonance cholangiopancreatographic findings. Am J Gastroenterol 2000; 95:432–440.
10. Khan SA, Davidson BR, Goldin R, et al. Guidelines for the diagnosis and treatment of cholangiocarcinoma: consensus document. Gut 2002; 51 Suppl 6:VI1-9.
11. Kluge R, Schmidt F, Caca K, et al. Positron emission tomography with [(18)F]fluoro-2-deoxy-D-glucose for diagnosis and staging of bile duct cancer. Hepatology 2001; 33:1029–1035.
12. Tamm EP, Silverman PM, Charnsangavej C, Evans DB. Diagnosis, staging, and surveillance of pancreatic cancer. AJR Am J Roentgenol 2003; 180:1311–1323.
13. Adamek HE, Albert J, Breer H, Weitz M, Schilling D, Riemann JF. Pancreatic cancer detection with magnetic resonance cholangiopancreatography and endoscopic retrograde cholangiopancreatography: a prospective controlled study. Lancet 2000; 356:190–193.
14. Ichikawa T, Haradome H, Hachiya J, et al. Pancreatic ductal adenocarcinoma: preoperative assessment with helical CT versus dynamic MR imaging. Radiology 1997; 202:655–662.
15. Lopez Hanninen E, Amthauer H, Hosten N, et al. Prospective evaluation of pancreatic tumors: accuracy of MR imaging with MR cholangiopancreatography and MR angiography. Radiology 2002; 224:34–41.

16. Fischer U, Vosshenrich R, Horstmann O, et al. Preoperative local MRI-staging of patients with a suspected pancreatic mass. Eur Radiol 2002; 12:296–303.

17. Bronstein YL, Loyer EM, Kaur H, et al. Detection of small pancreatic tumors with multiphasic helical CT. AJR Am J Roentgenol 2004; 182:619–623.

18. Johnson PT, Outwater EK. Pancreatic carcinoma versus chronic pancreatitis: dynamic MR imaging. Radiology 1999; 212:213–218.

19. Roche CJ, Hughes ML, Garvey CJ, et al. CT and pathologic assessment of prospective nodal staging in patients with ductal adenocarcinoma of the head of the pancreas. AJR Am J Roentgenol 2003; 180:475–480.

20. Kanemitsu K, Hiraoka T, Tsuji T, Inoue K, Takamori H. Implication of micrometastases of lymph nodes in patients with extended operation for pancreatic cancer. Pancreas 2003; 26:315–321.

21. Beger HG, Gansauge F, Leder G. Pancreatic cancer: who benefits from curative resection? Can J Gastroenterol 2002; 16:117–120.

22. Demeure MJ, Doffek KM, Komorowski RA, Wilson SD. Adenocarcinoma of the pancreas: detection of occult metastases in regional lymph nodes by a polymerase chain reaction-based assay. Cancer 1998; 83:1328–1334.

23. Harisinghani MG, Saini S, Weissleder R, et al. MR lymphangiography using ultrasmall superparamagnetic iron oxide in patients with primary abdominal and pelvic malignancies: radiographic–pathologic correlation. AJR Am J Roentgenol 1999; 172:1347–1351.

24. Koh DM, Cook GJ, Husband JE. New horizons in oncologic imaging. N Engl J Med 2003; 348:2487–2488.

25. Zhao ZW, He JY, Tan G, Wang HJ, Li KJ. Laparoscopy and laparoscopic ultrasonography in judging the resectability of pancreatic head cancer. Hepatobiliary Pancreat Dis Int 2003; 2:609–611.

26. Hennig R, Tempia-Caliera AA, Hartel M, Buchler MW, Friess H. Staging laparoscopy and its indications in pancreatic cancer patients. Dig Surg 2002; 19:484–488.

27. Nieveen van Dijkum EJ, Romijn MG, Terwee CB, et al. Laparoscopic staging and subsequent palliation in patients with peripancreatic carcinoma. Ann Surg 2003; 237:66–73.

28. Catalano C, Laghi A, Fraioli F, et al. Pancreatic carcinoma: the role of high-resolution multislice spiral CT in the diagnosis and assessment of resectability. Eur Radiol 2003; 13:149–156.

29. Ly JN, Miller FH. MR imaging of the pancreas: a practical approach. Radiol Clin North Am 2002; 40:1289–1306.

30. Semelka RC, Custodio CM, Cem Balci N, Woosley JT. Neuroendocrine tumors of the pancreas: spectrum of appearances on MRI. Journal of Magnetic Resonance Imaging 2000; 11:141–148.

31. Scott J, Martin I, Redhead D, Hammond P, Garden OJ. Mucinous cystic neoplasms of the pancreas: imaging features and diagnostic difficulties. Clinical Radiology 2000; 55:187–192.

32. Minami M, Itai Y, Ohtomo K, Yoshida H, Yoshikawa K, Iio M. Cystic neoplasms of the pancreas: comparison of MR imaging with CT. Radiology 1989; 171:53–56.

33. Koito K, Namieno T, Ichimura T, et al. Mucin-producing pancreatic tumors: comparison of MR cholangiopancreatography with endoscopic retrograde cholangiopancreatography. Radiology 1998; 208:231–237.

34. Fukukura Y, Fujiyoshi F, Hamada H, et al. Intraductal papillary mucinous tumors of the pancreas. Comparison of helical CT and MR imaging. Acta Radiol 2003; 44:464–471.

35. Irie H, Honda H, Aibe H, et al. MR cholangiopancreatographic differentiation of benign and malignant intraductal mucin-producing tumors of the pancreas. AJR Am J Roentgenol 2000; 174:1403–1408.

31 Medical and Surgical Therapy of Pancreatic Cancer

Weijing Sun, md, Jon Morris, md, and Jeffrey Drebin, md, PhD, FACS

Contents

1. INTRODUCTION

Pancreatic adenocarcinoma is one of the most lethal malignancies, with an overall 5-yr disease-free survival rate of 1–2% for all patients. Most patients with pancreatic cancer are not diagnosed until they have developed locally advanced or regionally disseminated disease that is not amenable to attempted curative surgical resection. Chemotherapy and radiation therapy have only modest benefit in this stage of the disease and typical survival is 6 mo. Among those patients with apparently resectable disease who undergo surgical exploration, between 20 and 40% are found to be unresectable, dependent on the pre-operative evaluation. Even those pancreatic cancer patients who have a margin-negative resection have a 5-yr disease-free survival of less than 30%, and approximately half of patients surviving 5 yr will relapse between 6 and 10 yr. Thus, the treatment of pancreatic cancer remains a significant challenge to the surgical, radiation, and medical oncologist.

In recent years there have been a number of positive developments in the management of pancreatic cancer. Improvements in the pre-operative staging of pancreatic cancer have reduced the number of patients undergoing laparotomy for what proves to be unresectable disease. Advances in surgical

From: *Endoscopic Oncology: Gastrointestinal Endoscopy and Cancer Management.* Edited by: D. O. Faigel and M. L. Kochman © Humana Press, Totowa, NJ

technique and peri-operative management allow pancreatic cancer resections to be performed with very low mortality and tolerable morbidity. Resected patients, even when not cured, appear to have a substantially longer survival than patients managed with other modalities and, thus, at a minimum receive substantial palliation and extension of survival. Furthermore, evolving approaches to adjuvant chemoradiation therapy may substantially improve long-term survival following an attempted curative resection.

For patients who present with unresectable disease there has been an appropriate focus on optimizing quality of life. Nonoperative methods of relieving obstructive jaundice avoid the need for laparotomy in most patients. Appreciation of the importance of palliating pain is of great benefit to those patients who are not potentially curable. Furthermore, new approaches to chemotherapy offer the hope of extending both quality and quantity of life in many patients. This chapter will review current approaches to the management of patients with pancreatic cancer.

2. EPIDEMIOLOGY

Pancreatic carcinoma is a relatively uncommon malignancy but because of its high lethality it is a common cause of cancer death. There are approx 30,000 new cases diagnosed, and almost the same number of deaths recorded annually in the United States. Carcinoma of the pancreas ranks fifth behind carcinomas of the lung, colorectum, breast, and prostate as a cause of cancer death (1–3). Because of the relative rarity of breast cancer in men and the nonexistence of prostate cancer in women, pancreatic cancer is the fourth most common cause of cancer death in both men and in women, accounting for approx 6% of cancer deaths overall.

The incidence of pancreatic carcinoma has increased three- to fourfold in the 20th century, but appears to have leveled off in recent decades. This most likely reflects both improvements in the accuracy of diagnostic imaging techniques such as computed tomography (CT) and magnetic resonance (MR) scanning, as well as a genuine increase in incidence. The risk of developing pancreatic cancer increases with age (1,4); it has been estimated that this risk increases two- to threefold for each decade of life after age 40. Although patients typically present in their 60s and 70s, patients in their 40s and 50s are not uncommon. Pancreatic cancer is rarely seen in patients younger than 30 yr of age.

Adenocarcinoma of the pancreas has traditionally been viewed as occurring more commonly in men than women (relative risk 1.5:1), although recent data suggest that the relative risk in women is approaching that seen in men (1,3), perhaps resulting from increased tobacco use by women in the latter half of the 20th century. In the United States pancreatic cancer occurs more frequently in blacks than in whites (relative risk 2:1), and may be somewhat less common in Asians than whites (relative risk 0.7:1). Worldwide incidence rates are highest in industrialized countries and lowest in African and Asian countries (5), suggesting that environmental factors linked to a "Western lifestyle" substantially increases the risk of pancreatic cancer.

A number of environmental factors have been linked to the development of pancreatic carcinoma (6–25). Cigarette smoking significantly increases the risk of this form of cancer, as it does for a variety of other tumors. Dietary factors also appear to play a role. Dietary fat intake and obesity clearly increase the risk of developing pancreatic cancer, whereas vitamin C intake and consumption of fruits and vegetables may decrease the risk of pancreatic cancer. Although alcohol consumption by itself does not appear to be a risk factor for the development of pancreatic cancer, chronic pancreatitis, which may be related to alcohol consumption, substantially increases the risk of pancreatic cancer (8). Diabetes increases the risk of pancreatic cancer about twofold (9). Consumption of coffee and other caffeinated beverages, which had been suggested to be risk factors based on early studies, appear to be unrelated to the development of pancreatic cancer.

3. PATHOPHYSIOLOGY

Pancreatic malignancies arise in the head of the pancreas approx 75% of the time, with the remainder of lesions being distributed evenly in the body and tail of the gland (26). It is important to note that nonpancreatic tumors of the distal bile duct, duodenum, and ampulla of Vater, although much less common than pancreatic adenocarcinoma, compromise almost one-third of resectable tumors in the region of the pancreatic head. Furthermore, these tumors tend to be biologically less aggressive than pancreatic carcinomas, with 5-yr disease-free

Table 1
Staging for Pancreatic Cancer

Primary tumor (T)
TX	Primary tumor cannot be assessed
T0	No evidence of primary tumor
T1	Tumor <2 cm
T2	Tumor >2 cm, confined to the pancreas
T3	Tumor extends locally beyond the pancreas
T4	Tumor involves celiac or superior mesenteric arteries

Lymph nodes (N)
NX	Regional lymph nodes cannot be assessed
N0	No regional lymph node metastasis
N1	Regional lymph node metastasis

Distant metastases (M)
MX	Presence of distant metastasis cannot be assessed
M0	No distant metastasis
M1	Distant metastasis

Stage grouping
IA	T1, N0, M0
IB	T2, N0, M0
IIA	T3, N0, M0
IIB	T1–3, N1, M0
III	T4, N0–1, M0
IV	T1–4, N0–1, M1

survival following resection ranging from 30 to 50% (27–29). In some cases, it can be difficult to distinguish these tumor types from routine adenocarcinoma of the pancreas based on endoscopic, radiological, or needle cytology criteria. Only histological sectioning of a resected tumor mass can accurately classify the specific tumor type in some circumstances.

Pancreatic adenocarcinomas tend to be aggressive tumors, which disseminate early and tend to follow similar patterns of metastatic spread in most patients. Local invasion into adjacent structures is frequently seen, with encasement of the superior mesenteric, portal vein, and the superior mesenteric artery representing a common event that may preclude curative resection. Spread to regional lymphatics and perineural invasion is common, as is metastasis to the liver via the portal vein. Spread to peritoneal surfaces (carcinomatosis) is frequently seen in advanced disease, as are lung metastases.

The pathological staging of pancreatic cancer has recently been revised, and is based on the extent of tumor involvement of local and distant structures, as shown in Table 1. Stage I tumors are limited to the pancreas. Stage II tumors are regionally invasive, without involvement of the celiac or superior mesenteric arteries, but may involve regional lymph nodes. Stages I and II tumors are considered potentially amenable to resection with curative intent. Stage III lesions are defined by direct involvement of the celiac or superior mesenteric arteries and stage IV lesions are defined by the presence of distant metastases. Patients with stages III and IV disease are generally not considered resectable for cure, though palliative resections, along with resection of isolated liver metastases have been reported (30,31).

Although adenocarcinoma remains the most commonly identified pancreatic neoplasm, cystic lesions are identified with increasing frequency. Cystic neoplasms of the pancreas can be divided into benign tumors and malignant tumors (cystadenocarcinomas) *(26)*. Benign cystic tumors can be further divided on the basis of radiological factors and by analysis of cyst fluid into lesions with little predilection to become malignant, termed serous cystadenomas, and those with a significant risk of malignant degeneration, termed mucinous cystic neoplasms. Although previously classified as either benign mucinous cystadenomas or malignant cystadenocarcinomas, the term mucinous cystic neoplasm is preferred because of the malignant potential of all mucinous cystic tumors, as evidenced by the frequent identification of cystadenocarcinoma in patients suspected of harboring a mucinous cystadenoma. This nomenclature is further complicated by the relatively recent identification of a distinct lesion, the intraductal papillary mucinous neoplasm (IPMN).

Serous cystadenomas essentially never harbor areas of invasive carcinoma or metastasize, but can cause pancreatitis or obstructive symptoms related to local growth. In contrast, mucinous cystic neoplasms of the pancreas are less predictable in their biological behavior, with some malignant tumors remaining indolent for months to years. They may also be locally or regionally invasive without forming metastases. When mucinous tumors of the pancreas do disseminate they tend to form peritoneal implants but rarely develop liver or lung metastases. Because even serous cystadenomas can cause problems related to local extension *(3)*, an aggressive approach to the removal of most serous cystadenomas as well as all mucinous tumors of the pancreas is justified.

Although only formally identified in the past 20 yr, IPMNs have been retrospectively noted in pancreatectomy specimens obtained from prior decades *(32–34)*. This disorder is an abnormality of the pancreatic duct in which all or part of the pancreatic duct epithelium becomes dysplastic and may degenerate to overt malignancy. Segments or even the entire pancreatic duct may become ectatic and mucus-filled, giving a characteristic appearance when evaluated at endoscopic retrograde cholangiopancreatography (ERCP). Because of their predilection to harbor carcinoma *in situ* and even areas of invasive carcinoma, surgical resection of IPMNs is generally recommended, though a careful consideration of risks and benefits is necessary in patients with extensive disease that may require total pancreatectomy. There is at present no consensus on appropriate follow-up for patients who have undergone partial pancreatectomy for IPMNs, though MRI/MRCP and endoscopic ultrasound (EUS) are frequently employed in an effort to identify locally recurrent disease.

4. GENETICS

Research performed over the past several decades has demonstrated that the development of malignancy represents a multistep process in which distinct oncogenes are activated and tumor suppressor genes inactivated in a clonal population of cells. This process ultimately gives rise to a cell population that is resistant to molecular mechanisms that normally regulate cell proliferation and programmed cell death *(35)*. Molecular events underlying the development of pancreatic cancer have been studied extensively and a number of alterations in oncogenes and tumor suppressor genes that are thought to play a role in the development of this disease have been identified *(35–41)*. Common abnormalities include activating mutations in the *K-ras* oncogene (which occur in more than 90% of pancreatic cancers), overexpression of the *HER2-neu* oncogene (seen in 50–70% of pancreatic cancers) and loss of expression of the *CDKN2*, *p53*, and *DPC4* tumor suppressor genes (seen in 100, 70, and 50% of pancreatic cancers, respectively).

The identification and characterization of histologically distinct premalignant precursor lesions that give rise to pancreatic adenocarcinomas, termed pancreatic intraepithelial neoplasms (PanINs) suggest that the activation of oncogenes and loss of tumor suppressor genes occurs in a stepwise fashion. Activation of the *K-ras* oncogene is seen in very early preneoplastic lesions (PanIN1s) and even in secretions of patient with chronic pancreatitis and no known pancreatic cancer or mass *(26)*. Similarly, *HER2-neu* overexpression is frequently seen in early intraepithelial neoplasms. In contrast, loss of the *CDKN2*, *p53*, and *DPC4* tumor suppressor genes appear to be relatively late events in tumorigenesis and are seen in more advanced preneoplastic (PanIN2 and PanIN3) and frankly neoplastic lesions. Interestingly, a murine model in which activated *K-ras* genes are expressed in the pancreas along with *p53* tumor suppressor gene deletion results in the development of PanINs and pancreatic adenocarcinomas that pathologically and biologically appear to mimic human disease *(42)*.

Although the majority of pancreatic cancers appear to be sporadic, approx 5% of pancreatic malignancies are seen in patients with a familial history of pancreatic cancer *(43)*. Among patients with two first-degree relatives with pancreatic cancer the relative risk of developing pancreatic cancer is increased 18-fold. In patients with three or more affected relatives the increased risk is 57-fold. Such data strongly support the notion that familial pancreatic cancer is a real entity *(43)*.

An additional unknown percentage of pancreatic cancers may reflect the presence of an overall cancer family syndrome that is less strikingly specific for the pancreas. For example, it has been shown that among a subset of kindreds with the familial atypical mole malignant melanoma syndrome there an approx 20-fold increased risk for the development of pancreatic cancer *(41)*, although the relative risks for other forms of cancer is not substantially increased. Molecular analysis has demonstrated that this subset of FAMM patients has a germline alteration in the *CDKN2* tumor suppressor gene *(41)*. Similarly, patients at risk for breast cancer as a result of inherited *BRCA2* gene abnormalities also have a risk of pancreatic cancer at least 10-fold higher than that of the general population *(35,44)*. Other familial syndromes associated with an increased risk of pancreatic cancer include the hereditary nonpolyposis colon cancer syndrome, familial adenomatous polyposis, and ataxia telangiectasia. Furthermore, the hereditary pancreatitis syndrome, caused by a mutation in the trypsinogen gene, carries a 40–70% risk of pancreatic cancer. Thus genetic factors, while of variable penetrance, clearly plays a role in the predisposition to pancreatic cancer development in many patients.

5. DIAGNOSIS AND STAGING

Patients with pancreatic cancer often are vaguely unwell for a number of months prior to the development of overt symptoms. Though the development of "painless jaundice" is often thought of as a typical presenting feature of patients with pancreatic cancer, most patients in fact have mild to moderate abdominal pain. The presence of back pain is a particularly ominous symptom, which may reflect retroperitoneal nerve invasion by tumor. The development of obstructive jaundice is related to the anatomic location of the primary tumor. It is almost universal in tumors of the pancreatic head but is quite rare in patients with primary tumors of the pancreatic tail.

The presence of weight loss is relatively common. This may reflect duodenal obstruction by tumor, an as yet poorly understood inhibitory effect of pancreatic cancer on gastric motility and/or effects of tumor-related cytokines on host metabolism. Findings on physical examination are often nonspecific. Jaundice is common, as noted above, but not specific for the presence of a malignancy. The presence of a palpable pancreatic mass or gallbladder (Courvoisier's sign) is uncommon and usually observed only in thin patients. Hepatomegaly owing to liver congestion or the presence of metastatic disease is similarly seen in the minority of patients at the time of initial diagnosis. Accurate diagnosis and staging of pancreatic cancer is largely dependent on radiological and endoscopic imaging.

Patients suspected of having a pancreatic malignancy are generally evaluated by thin-cut contrast-enhanced CT scanning. This is of use in identifying the tumor mass as well as assessing the liver for metastasis. Vascular involvement of superior mesenteric vein, portal vein, and celiac and superior mesenteric arteries can often be determined by dedicated CT scanning with fine cuts and intravenous and mouth contrast. Transabdominal ultrasonography is useful in identifying the primary tumor mass, particularly in the pancreatic head, but is less sensitive than CT and provides less information regarding local and regional dissemination. MR imaging has not proven superior to CT scanning for assessment of the primary tumor, metastatic disease or vascular encasement. Occasional patients with CT findings suggestive but not diagnostic of vascular encasement may benefit from preoperative visceral angiography, though improvements in CT methodology, particularly the use of dynamic contrast infusion and spiral techniques, have largely supplanted angiography.

Positron emission tomography (PET) using 18-fluorodeoxyglucose (FDG) has not proved useful in the diagnosis or staging of pancreatic cancer. Initial hopes that FDG-PET would distinguish chronic pancreatitis from pancreatic neoplasia have not been supported in clinical studies (45,46). Furthermore, FDG-PET misses a substantial number of lymph node metastases and peritoneal metastases. Most importantly, the addition of FDG-PET to CT-based diagnostic algorithms appears to rarely alter subsequent diagnostic or therapeutic maneuvers. Whether PET technology using agents that detect cell proliferation rather than cell metabolism will improve these results is currently under evaluation.

Patients with a pancreatic mass on CT and no evidence of metastatic disease or vascular encasement require no further

testing and can be taken to the operating room for surgical resection. At the time of definitive surgery a laparoscopic evaluation of resectability may be performed, as discussed later. It is not necessary to obtain a tissue diagnosis pre-operatively. Indeed, because of the frequent presence of a dense reactive stroma surrounding small islands of cancer cells, cytological assessment of pancreatic malignancies is notoriously inaccurate, rendering absence of malignant cells on percutaneous or endoscopic biopsy of little value in patient management. An additional concern with percutaneous techniques is the possibility of tumor dissemination as a result of the biopsy process, as has been suggested in some studies (47).

Patients with jaundice but no mass on CT are generally evaluated by EUS and/or ERCP. This evaluation may reveal a mass, or an irregular or tapering biliary stricture characteristic of an obstructing periampullary tumor. Sometimes the biliary stricture is seen in conjunction with a pancreatic duct stricture—the "double-duct" sign—which is highly suspicious for the presence of a malignancy. Irregular strictures of the pancreatic duct may also be seen in patients with pancreatic carcinoma. Such endoscopic findings, even in the absence of a pancreatic mass on CT scanning, justify proceeding to surgical resection. Endoscopic brushings and biopsies may confirm the presence of a pancreatic neoplasm, but have a relatively high false-negative rate, as discussed earlier. An aggressive surgical approach to patients with suspicious biliary strictures, particularly in those patients without a history of previous gallstone disease, will often result in removal of tumors at a relatively early stage.

The risks and benefits of decompressing the biliary tree before resecting a pancreatic cancer remain controversial (48–51). Although the rationale for relieving obstructive jaundice and normalizing liver function pre-operatively is logical, several randomized prospective trials have failed to show a benefit of preoperative biliary stenting by ERCP or percutaneous techniques. There are procedure-related complications in patients who undergo ERCP and stenting prior to resection, and the presence of an endoscopically placed stent appears to increase the risk of postoperative morbidity, particularly the development of infectious complications, in patients undergoing pancreaticoduodenectomy (51).

Probably the critical factor in deciding whether to preoperatively decompress a jaundiced patient who will definitely be taken for surgical exploration is the interval to surgery. If the patient can be operated on in a few days and is not symptomatic from jaundice it may be best to proceed directly to surgery; if there will be a delay in scheduling surgery or if the patient is extremely symptomatic from jaundice, it may be best to stent the patient—both for comfort and to possibly help improve the nutritional status.

Another important endoscopic technique that plays a major role in the diagnosis and staging of patients with pancreatic malignancies is EUS (52). EUS can assess tumor size, portal and mesenteric vascular involvement and regional nodal involvement. EUS can also obtain tissue samples for histological analysis from virtually all pancreatic lesions, and from suspicious lymph nodes located close to the stomach and duodenum. It has the advantage of not requiring a general anesthetic and can be performed outside an operating suite with conscious sedation. Like all sonographic procedures, the quality of clinical information achieved with EUS is highly operator-dependent. Furthermore, EUS may have more difficulty evaluating lesions, such as peritoneal or liver metastases, which are located at sites distant from the lumen of the gastrointestinal tract and are best evaluated with cross-sectional imaging or laparoscopy.

A number of tumor-associated antigens detectable in the serum of patients with pancreatic carcinoma have been described, the most useful being CA19-9 (53). CA19-9 is a mucin-associated carbohydrate antigen produced by normal pancreatic cells, as well as pancreatic carcinoma cells. CA19-9 can be detected in serum and pancreatic juice. As with other tumor markers, the use of CA19-9 in the management of patients with pancreatic cancer is plagued by problems related to sensitivity and specificity. Small tumors often fail to produce enough CA19-9 to be detectable above the accepted serum threshold of 35 units/mL. Non-neoplastic disorders of the pancreas and biliary tract, particularly pancreatitis, are associated with elevations of CA19-9, which may reach several hundred units per milliliter. Patients with CA19-9 levels in the thousands almost definitely have pancreatic cancer, but are generally quite symptomatic from their tumors and often unresectable. Thus there is little use for CA19-9 in screening asymptomatic populations. There may be a role for monitoring CA19-9 in patients postoperatively following tumor resection, but in the absence of effective therapy for recurrent disease this is also of questionable value except in research protocols.

Analysis of tumor markers in pancreatic cyst aspirates may be of use in distinguishing pseudocysts from cystic neoplasms and in separating serous cystadenomas from mucinous tumors if radiologic criteria alone are inadequate. Interestingly, CA19-9 levels in cyst aspirates are of little use in separating these different lesions. However, it has been shown that analyzing the combination of amylase, carcinoembryonic antigen, and CA-125 allows fairly accurate separation among the different cystic lesions of the pancreas (54,55). These studies are particularly useful in the elderly or medically frail patient in whom resection of a cystic lesion of the pancreas poses an unusually high risk. When cyst fluid analysis suggests a low likelihood of malignancy, such high-risk patients can be managed nonoperatively.

The development of laparoscopic staging procedures represents a significant advance in the management of patients with pancreatic cancer and other periampullary tumors (47,56–59). Among patients that appear to have a resectable pancreatic cancer based on spiral CT scanning techniques, there is a 20–30% incidence of either locally advanced disease or of small hepatic or peritoneal implants, undetected by radiological imaging, which preclude curative resection. With advances in nonoperative palliation of advanced disease, particularly improvements in biliary stenting as discussed below, there may be no need for formal laparotomy in patients with disease not amenable to curative resection. Avoiding unnecessary laparotomy is an important goal of palliating patients with advanced disease, which may be facilitated by laparoscopic evaluation.

Simple laparoscopy and biopsy allows the evaluation of visceral and peritoneal surfaces and may reveal disease undetectable by other techniques. Patients may then avoid unnecessary open surgical procedures if adequate palliation of jaundice can be achieved with percutaneous or transhepatic biliary stent placement. Staging laparoscopy, with frozen section evaluation of biopsy specimens if necessary, can be carried out in 15–20 min and can be followed by formal laparotomy and tumor resection under the same anesthetic. Available data suggests that this technique alone can reduce the incidence of unresectable disease at laparotomy by more than 50% (57,59). The addition of other techniques, including laparoscopic peritoneal washings and intraoperative ultrasound, may further improve the ability to discriminate patients who will benefit from laparotomy, although with a further increase in time and expense.

6. TREATMENT

6.1. SURGICAL RESECTION

For patients with potentially resectable pancreatic malignancies, defined as those that have not yet metastasized to distant sites, encased the portal or superior mesenteric veins, or invaded the roots of the celiac or superior mesenteric arteries, surgical resection remains the best hope for achieving prolonged disease-free survival. Most resectable tumors occur in the head of the pancreas and are resected by pancreaticoduodenectomy (Whipple procedure) (60,61). Although there are variations in technical approach among different surgeons, in all cases the head of the pancreas, distal bile duct, and most of the duodenum and proximal jejunum are resected en bloc. In many cases, the entire duodenum, as well as the gastric antrum, are included with the resection specimen. Reconstruction involves the performance of pancreatic, biliary and gastric, or duodenal anastomoses to the remaining jejunum.

Pancreaticoduodenectomy is a demanding technical operation, requiring meticulous dissection around portal and mesenteric blood vessels and three distinct anastomoses; the morbidity and mortality associated with the Whipple procedure can be significant. Indeed, in the mid-1970s it was seriously questioned whether patients with resectable pancreatic malignancies might be better managed with palliative bypass procedures (62). Over the past several decades, however, there has been a steady improvement in the results reported following pancreaticoduodenectomy with regard to morbidity and mortality, with a corresponding improvement in long-term survival of resected patients.

During the past 30 yr, peri-operative mortality rates have declined from 20% to less than 5% in many institutions around the world. Near-zero mortality rates, which we define as 2% or lower, are being reported with increasing frequency (61). These mortality rates are so low that many hundreds of cases would be required to determine precise mortality rates. Nonetheless, it is safe to make the general statement that extremely low mortality rates are now the norm for pancreaticoduodenectomies performed in specialized centers.

The reason(s) for the precipitous decline in perioperative mortality rates is not completely understood. It appears, in part, to reflect concentration of pancreaticoduodenectomy procedures at high volume centers (63); low volume centers still have peri-operative mortality rates of 15–20% in national surveys. A substantial degree of this improvement is related to surgeon experience (64). As with other complex procedures, surgeons that do pancreatic surgery more often in general do it better. Other contributing factors are improvements in intensive care, diagnostic and interventional radiology, and nutritional support. Prophylaxis and management of infection, venous thromboembolism, and gastrointestinal hemorrhage have also improved greatly during this period. As a result, postoperative cardiopulmonary complications and gastrointestinal hemorrhage, which used to be fairly common, have been sharply reduced.

Although mortality rates have improved significantly, pancreaticoduodenectomy remains a procedure in which major morbidity is common. Improvements in surgical technique have reduced the incidence of leakage at biliary-enteric anastomoses (biliary fistula) and gastric- or duodenal-enteric anastomoses to less than 3% in most series (61). In contrast, leakage at the pancreaticoenteric anastomosis (pancreatic fistula) is still a major complication of pancreaticoduodenectomy, occurring in 10–20% of patients in most series (61). In reported case series there does not appear to have been much improvement in the incidence of this complication over the years. However, in the current era, leakage at the pancreaticojejunostomy is less morbid, generally leading to an increased length of hospital stay but rarely to reoperation or death (65). Furthermore, a number of recent reports suggest that modifications of technique for performing the pancreaticoenteric anastomosis are associated with reduction in leak rates to less than 5% (66).

Probably the most common postoperative complication seen in patients undergoing pancreaticoduodenectomy is delayed gastric emptying. Although not well understood, it is thought that disruption of enterogastric signaling following duodenectomy is responsible for the gastric motility problems so frequently seen. Although once thought to be more common in patients undergoing pyloric preservation, randomized studies have demonstrated that delayed emptying is equally common in patients undergoing classic Whipple resection with hemigastrectomy (67). Delayed gastric emptying is seen in 10–20% of patients and may range in severity from mild nausea and inability to eat, to persistent vomiting requiring nasogastric suction for days to weeks postoperatively. Problems with gastric emptying are rarely life threatening but can significantly prolong postoperative hospitalization. A randomized prospective trial of erythromycin demonstrated modest but statistically significant benefits in improving gastric emptying after pancreaticoduodenectomy, presumably through the effects of erythromycin on motilin receptors (68).

With improvements in peri-operative morbidity and mortality, there has also been some improvement in 5-yr survival rates for patients undergoing pancreaticoduodenectomy for pancreatic cancer. Five-year survival rates following Whipple resection for ampullary, bile duct, and duodenal malignancies have always been reasonable, ranging from 30 to 50% in most

series, although resection of a mucinous tumor of the pancreas results in 5-yr survival rates of more than 75%. In contrast, the long-term survival of patients with pancreatic adenocarcinoma has generally been extremely poor. A recent review of the world literature dating back over the past 50 yr suggests that the overall 5-yr survival of patients following attempted curative resection for adenocarcinoma of the pancreas is on the order of 4% (69). Furthermore, some of these patients recurred beyond 5 yr, suggesting that they in fact had not been cured by resection of their tumors.

Several large case series from high-volume centers suggest that better long-term results are now being obtained, with 20–30% of resected patients with documented pancreatic adenocarcinoma surviving 5 yr (70–72). In patients with negative resection margins, small tumors, and no evidence of lymph node metastases the results may be even better, with more than 40% of such patients expected to survive 5 yr. It is important to note, however, that these survival curves are based on actuarial rather than actual survival and not all recent series have noted such results. Those who believe that results have improved point to improvements in diagnosis, surgical technique, and the use of adjuvant chemotherapy and radiation therapy as possible contributing factors.

Patients with adenocarcinoma of the pancreas involving the body or tail of the pancreas are generally not symptomatic until their tumors have reached an advanced stage and thus are rarely resectable at the time of diagnosis. Furthermore, the long-term outcome following attempted surgical resection of more distal pancreatic adenocarcinomas is poor (73,74). Probably the one subset of patients most likely to benefit from distal pancreatectomy are those with mucinous tumors of the pancreas. These tumors have a high cure rate following surgical resection and thus warrant aggressive surgical measures regardless of their size or anatomic location.

7. ADJUVANT THERAPY OF PANCREATIC CANCER

Although operative results have improved dramatically over the past 20 yr owing to better staging, improved surgical techniques, and advances in peri-operative care, the overall outcome for pancreatic cancer is still very disappointing. The number of patients amenable to therapeutic resection is less than 20%. Even for those patients with complete resection, the median survival is only around 20 mo with high recurrence rates both locally and distantly. For the past 20 yr, numerous studies have been performed in an effort to identify effective adjuvant (postoperative) therapy that could improve the long-term survival of resected patients.

The modest success of surgical resection in producing long-term survival of patients with pancreatic tumors has led to a number of studies using chemotherapy and radiation therapy in an effort to diminish local and systemic recurrence following surgery. The classic study of adjuvant therapy for pancreatic carcinoma was performed by the Gastrointestinal Tumor Study Group (GITSG). This study prospectively randomized patients undergoing resection with curative intent to either no additional therapy or to combined bolus 5-fluorouracil (5-FU) and external beam radiation therapy. Despite small numbers of patients in each arm of the study, a significant difference in outcome was observed between the two groups, with treated patients surviving 20 mo, vs 11 mo for untreated controls *(75)*. Two-year survival was also markedly improved by chemoradiation (46 vs 18%). The GITSG subsequently completed a confirmatory trial in a larger patient population *(76)*.

Case series from several institutions, although nonrandomized, also support a beneficial role for adjuvant 5-FU chemotherapy and radiation therapy in patients undergoing resection of pancreatic carcinoma *(77,78)*. In contrast, a multi-institutional study conducted in Europe (ESPAC-1) suggested that chemoradiation was of no benefit following resection of pancreatic or other periampullary tumors, although chemotherapy alone might have had some modest benefit *(79)*. However, this study used a dose of radiation substantially lower than that used by most United States institutions and had other substantial methodological flaws that bring its findings into question. Additional multi-institutional studies, in both the United States and Europe, are currently evaluating the benefit of postoperative chemoradiation following pancreatic cancer resection. Given the limited benefit of standard adjuvant treatments, enrollment in clinical trials should be encouraged.

8. PATIENTS WITH LOCALLY ADVANCED DISEASE

8.1. DOWNSTAGING

A substantial fraction of pancreatic cancer patients present with locally advanced disease, either encasement of the superior mesenteric or portal veins or involvement of the celiac or superior mesenteric arteries, which precludes curative resection. This has led to a number of studies attempting to use chemoradiation to "downstage" the tumor and permit a margin-negative surgical resection *(80–82)*. Unfortunately the results of these studies have generally been poor, with 0–10% of patients achieving sufficient tumor shrinkage to permit surgical resection; survival after resection may also be more limited than that usually seen following pancreaticoduodenectomy.

9. PRIMARY RADIATION THERAPY

Pancreatic cancer is a relatively radioresistant malignancy, with doses in excess of 7000 cGy required to eradicate all viable tumor cells *(83–87)*. Unfortunately the tolerances of surrounding tissues, including liver, stomach, kidney, and small bowel do not permit this dose to be achieved clinically. Efforts to boost the tumor radiation dose using brachytherapy or intra-operative radiation therapy in combination with external beam radiation have succeeded in decreasing local recurrence but have not substantially impacted survival because of the development of metastatic disease outside the radiation field *(84–87)*. Radiation therapy does play a role in the adjuvant treatment of resected patients, as described earlier, and can modestly extend survival in patients with advanced disease *(88)*. Furthermore, radiation therapy can substantially ameliorate pain in patients with disseminated disease *(89)*.

10. CHEMOTHERAPY FOR ADVANCED DISEASE

Chemotherapy for pancreatic cancer has had a minimal impact on the survival of patients with advanced disease *(89)*.

For many years, 5-FU-based therapy, either as a single agent or in combination with other drugs, was the principal treatment strategy employed in patients with advanced pancreatic cancer. Studies suggested that such therapy resulted in at best a modest survival advantage compared with patients receiving supportive care alone.

The development and approval of gemcitabine as a first-line agent for the treatment of advanced pancreatic cancer represents an advance in both therapeutic armamentarium and in the approach to identifying agents of benefit to patients with this disease. Because of the problems with dense tumor stroma, it was considered probable that some patients who did, in fact, benefit from therapy might not show classic criteria for partial response—a 50% decrease in the perpendicular diameters of a radiologically detectable tumor mass. Therefore, a new set of "clinical benefit response" criteria were developed.

Using these clinical benefit response criteria, it was demonstrated in a prospective randomized study that gemcitabine resulted in substantial clinical benefit in about 25% of patients as compared with less than 5% of patients who received 5-FU *(90)*. This study also demonstrated a modest, but statistically significant extension of median survival in patients receiving gemcitabine (5.4 vs 4.3 mo, $p < 0.05$). Furthermore, the fraction of patients surviving more than 1 yr was approximately ninefold higher in the gemcitabine group (18 vs 2%). It is worth noting that the fraction of patients achieving a partial radiological response in this study was less than 5% and was not significantly different in the two treatment groups. Thus this study has not only identified an agent that improves the quality and the quantity of life for patients with advanced pancreatic cancer, it has also demonstrated the limitations of traditional radiological measures of tumor response and the importance of alternative criteria in testing novel agents for the treatment of patients with pancreatic cancer.

The identification of gemcitabine as an active agent in pancreatic cancer has led to the study of additional regimens employing single-agent gemcitabine on different dosing schedules *(91)*, or gemcitabine-based combinations *(92,97)* (*see* Table 2). Although additional studies are ongoing, it appears that gemcitabine-based combination therapies may be modestly more active in terms of median survival than single-agent gemcitabine but at the cost of increased toxicity. Even with the application of more potent gemcitabine-based combination therapies, survival of more than 1 yr is uncommon in patients with advanced disease.

The emerging development of molecularly targeted therapeutics offers the hope of more potent and less toxic approaches to treatment of pancreatic cancer. A number of novel agents are currently in phase 2 trials in pancreatic cancer, either alone or in combination with gemcitabine. These include agents that block ras function (such as farnesyl-transferase inhibitors), monoclonal antibodies, and drugs that inhibit tumor angiogenesis, and a number of distinct signal-transduction inhibitors including monoclonal antibodies to the EGF receptor and HER2/neu protein as well as chemical inhibitors of signaling kinase cascades. Preliminary reports suggest that adding an angiogenesis inhibitor (bevacizumab)

Table 2
Combination of Gemcitabine with Different Chemotherapy Agents vs Gemcitabine Alone

Regimen	No. of pts.	RR (%)	p	PFS (mo)	p	MS (mo)	p	Reference
Gemcitabine + 5-FU vs gemcitabine alone	327	6.9 vs 5.6	—	3.4 vs 2.2	0.022	6.7 vs 5.4	0.09	92
Gemcitabine + irinotecan vs gemcitabine alone	360	16.1 vs 4.4	<0.001	(TTP) 3.4 vs 3.0	NS	6.3 vs 6.6	NS	93
Gemcitabine + cisplatin vs gemcitabine alone	195	10.2 vs 8	NS	4.6 vs 2.5	0.016	7.6 vs 6.0	0.12	94
Gemcitabine + exatecan vs gemcitabine alone	349	8.2 vs 7.1	NS	(TTP) 4.1 vs 3.8		6.7 vs 6.2	0.52	95
Gemcitabine + pemetrexed vs gemcitabine alone	565	14.8 vs 7.1	0.004	3.9 vs 3.3	0.110	6.2 vs 6.3	0.848	96

RR, relative risk; PFS, progression-free survival; MS, median survival; TTP, time to progression.

or an EGF-receptor kinase inhibitor (erlotinib) to gemcitabine modestly potentiates the effects of single-agent gemcitabine. It is hoped that other novel agents, or the use of these agents in combination, will have substantially greater activity in pancreatic cancer patients and may, thus, represent a real advance in the management of patients with this disease.

11. PALLIATIVE MANAGEMENT OF PATIENTS WITH ADVANCED DISEASE

Modern approaches to surgical management of pancreatic carcinoma and the use of adjuvant therapy have made pancreatic resection safer and more effective. Such therapy has resulted in significant extension of survival for many patients. However, long-term eradication of disease is still the exception among patients with pancreatic carcinoma undergoing attempted curative resection. Furthermore, only 10–20% of patients with pancreatic carcinoma present at an early enough stage to be eligible for resection. Thus, the vast majority of patients with pancreatic cancer either present with advanced disease or develop it in the setting of tumor recurrence. For physicians involved in the palliative management of patients with advanced pancreatic cancer there are a number of important issues to be addressed.

11.1. PAIN

Advanced pancreatic cancer can be extremely painful and most patients experience moderate or severe pain in the course of their illness. Pancreatic malignancies commonly invade neural and perineural tissues. Invasion of neural structures in the retroperitoneum by the growing pancreatic tumor mass is associated with a steady unrelenting pain that can be psychologically devastating. There are a number of important aspects to the management of such patients, including the use of long-acting analgesics in appropriate doses, and consideration for celiac plexus ablation. Although the use of long-acting oral or topical narcotic preparations should be well understood by all physicians that care for patients with advanced cancer, the use of celiac plexus blockade is less often appreciated.

Probably the best study of celiac plexus ablation was performed by Lillemoe and colleagues (98). They randomized patients with unresectable disease, who were undergoing laparotomy for palliative biliary and gastric bypass, to receive injections of either 50% alcohol or saline into the celiac ganglia bilaterally. The study was carried out in a double-blind, prospective fashion, and outcomes of interest included pain,

narcotic usage and survival among treated patients. This study convincingly demonstrated that patients undergoing chemical splanchnicectomy had significant relief of pain and required less narcotic usage than patients receiving saline. The benefit of such therapy appeared to last for 4–6 mo. Interestingly, in the subset of patients with moderate to severe pain at the time of treatment there was a statistically significant survival advantage among those treated with alcohol injection. Although celiac plexus block can be easily and safely performed at the time of a palliative surgical bypass procedure, it can also be performed percutaneously, with or without CT guidance, in patients who have no other indication for laparotomy.

11.2. JAUNDICE

Most patients with tumors of the periampullary region present with jaundice. Although pancreaticoduodenectomy is an effective method of relieving jaundice, most patients present with disease too extensive for attempted curative surgical resection. There are multiple approaches to the management of jaundice in such patients, including endoscopic and percutaneous biliary stent placement, and surgical biliary bypass. There have been several trials comparing surgical with nonsurgical approaches to biliary tract obstruction (99). In general these trials have demonstrated a lower initial morbidity among those undergoing nonoperative stenting. However, the stent occlusion rates were significantly higher than the failure rates of surgical biliary bypass, resulting in more frequent bouts of cholangitis and the need for multiple procedures over time in patients managed nonoperatively.

The greater long-term morbidity among stented patients was felt to be approximately equivalent to the greater short-term morbidity among patients undergoing surgical bypass, leading to the conclusion that the treatments were approximately equivalent (99). It has been suggested that patients with a relatively short life expectancy owing to extensive disease (i.e., stage IV), and those with increased operative risk because of other medical problems, might be best managed with biliary stenting. In contrast, patients thought to have less extensive but still unresectable disease (stage III) and who are felt to be reasonable operative candidates might benefit more from surgical biliary bypass.

The development of expandable wall stents has changed this treatment algorithm. Wall stents can be placed endoscopically or percutaneously, but unlike older stent technology, wall stents have a significantly longer time to stent failure. In one recent study it was demonstrated that the stent occlusion rate among patients receiving wall stents was less than 30% at 10 mo *(100)*. As the median survival of patients with advanced pancreatic cancer ranges from 4 to 8 mo and rarely exceeds 1 yr, most patients receiving a metal endoprosthetic will be typically palliated for life. The rare patients who outlive the functional life of a metal endoprosthetic can generally be salvaged by endoscopic or percutaneous techniques. It is, therefore, our practice to spare patients with unresectable pancreatic tumors the morbidity and mortality of surgical biliary bypass in favor of metal endoprosthetic placement.

It is worth noting, however, there are still times when surgical biliary bypass is preferred. The most common is when a patient undergoing laparotomy for attempted curative resection is found to have unresectable disease. In such cases it is our practice to perform surgical gastric and biliary bypass as well as an intra-operative chemical splanchnicectomy. Another group of patients who benefit from surgical biliary bypass are those with duodenal obstruction at the time of diagnosis. Such patients generally require laparotomy for creation of a gastrojejunostomy, and should have a surgical biliary bypass under the same anesthetic. The precise type of biliary bypass created is largely a choice of the operating surgeon. Although choledochojejunostomy to a defunctionalized jejunal loop is the preferred approach to surgical biliary bypass, cholecystojejunostomy may be an acceptable alternative except in cases in which the tumor is encroaching on the cystic duct *(101)*.

11.3. GASTRIC OUTLET / DUODENAL OBSTRUCTION

Approximately 15% of patients with periampullary tumors have symptoms of gastric outlet obstruction at the time of diagnosis, and another 20–30% of patients will develop symptomatic duodenal obstruction in the course of their disease. Surgical gastrojejunostomy is the preferred approach to palliating such patients. When carcinomatosis involving the small bowel is also present, it is our practice to place a gastrostomy tube along with performing surgical bypass of the gastric and/or intestinal obstruction. Patients with carcinomatosis almost invariably reobstruct in a matter of weeks and the presence of a gastrostomy tube can greatly facilitate terminal care by avoiding the need for nasogastric suction in most patients.

12. CONCLUSION

Pancreatic cancer remains one of the most lethal malignancies. Most patients present with disease that is too advanced to permit an attempt at curative resection and most patients who undergo resection will eventually recur. Radiation and chemotherapy are of only modest benefit in extending survival in unresectable patients. However, there have been a number of promising advances including enhanced understanding of the molecular mechanisms leading to pancreatic carcinogenesis, improvements in staging, optimization of surgical techniques, and improvements in adjuvant therapy for patients with resectable disease and a focus on effective palliation for patients with more advanced disease. It is hoped that our understanding of molecular mechanisms will lead to the development of more effective diagnostic approaches and targeted therapeutics for the management of patients with this disease.

REFERENCES

1. Howe GR. Epidemiology of cancer of the pancreas. In: Pancreatic Cancer, (Cameron, JL, ed.), B.C. Decker, London, 2001, pp. 1–12.
2. Bell RH Jr. Neoplasms of the exocrine pancreas. In: Bell, RH, Rikkers LF Mulholland MW, eds. Digestive Tract Surgery: A Text and Atlas, Lippincott-Raven Publishers; Philadelphia, PA, 1996: 849–878.
3. Drebin JA and Strasberg SM. Carcinoma of the pancreas and tumors of the periampullary region. In: Winchester DP, Jones RS and Murphy GP, eds. Cancer Surgery for the General Surgeon, Lippincott, Williams & Wilkens; Philadelphia, PA, 1999:195–211.
4. Parkin DM, Muir CS, Whelan SL, et al. Cancer Incidence in Five Continents, Vol VI, Lyon, International Agency for Research on Cancer. 1992, p. 301.
5. Akoi K, Ogawa H. Cancer of the pancreas: international mortality trends. World Health Stat Rep 1978; 31:2–27.
6. Fuchs CS, Colditz GA, Stampfer MJ, Giovannucci EL, Hunter DJ, Rimm EB, Willett WC, Speizer FE. A prospective study of cigarette smoking and the risk of pancreatic cancer. Archives of Int Med 1996; 56(19):2255–2260.
7. Ahlgren JD. Epidemiology and risk factors in pancreatic cancer. Seminars in Oncology 1996; 3(2):241–250.
8. Lowenfels AB, Maisonneuve P, Cavallini G, et al. Pancreatitis and the risk of pancreatic cancer. International Pancreatitis Study Group. NEJM 1993; 328(20):1433–1437.
9. Gullo L, Pezzilli R, Morselli-Labate AM for the Italian Pancreatic Cancer Study Group. Diabetes and the risk of pancreatic cancer. NEJM 1994; 331(2):81–84.
10. Zheng W, McLaughlin JK, Gridley G, et al. A cohort study of smoking, alcohol consumption and dietary factors for pancreatic cancer. Cancer Causes Control 1993; 4:477–482.
11. Kalopothaki V, Tzonou A, Hseih CC, et al. Tobacco, ethanol, coffee, pancreatitis, diabetes mellitus, and cholelithiasis as risk factors for pancreatic carcinoma. Cancer Causes Control 1993; 4:375–382.
12. Friedman GC, Van den Eeden SK. Risk factors for pancreatic cancer: an exploratory study. Int J Epidemiol 1993; 22:30–37.
13. Kahn H. The Dorn study of smoking and mortality among U.S. veterans: report on eight and one-half years of observation. NCI Monogr 1966; 19:11–25.
14. Chyou PH, Nomura AM, Stemmermann GN. A prospective study on the attributable risk of cancer due to cigarette smoking. Am J Public Health 1992; 82:37–40.
15. Lyon JL, Mahoney AW, French TK, Moser R Jr. Coffee consumption and the risk of cancer of the exocrine pancreas: a case control study in a low-risk population. Epidemiology 1992; 3:164–170.
16. Adami HO, McLaughlin JK, Hsing AW, et al. Alcoholism and cancer risk: a population-based cohort study. Cancer Causes Control 1992; 3:419–425.
17. Kato I, Nomura AM, Stemmermann GN, Chyou PH. Prospective study of the association of alcohol with cancer of the upper aerodigestive tract and other sites. Cancer Causes Control 1992; 3:145–151.
18. Bueno de Mesquita HG, Maisonneuve P, Moerman CJ, et al. Lifetime consumption of alcoholic beverages, tea and coffee and exocrine carcinoma of the pancreas: a population-based case-control study in the Netherlands. Int J Cancer 1992; 50:514–522.
19. Gold EB, Goldin SB: Epidemiology of and risk factors for pancreatic cancer. Surg Oncol Clin North Am 1998; 7:67–91.
20. Mack TM, Peters JM, Yu MC, et al. Pancreas cancer is unrelated to the workplace in Los Angeles. Am J Ind Med 1985; 7:253–266.
21. Gold EB, Gordis L, Diener MD, et al. Diet and other risk factors for cancer of the pancreas. Cancer 1985; 55:460–467.
22. Kalapthaki V, Tzonou A, Hseih CC, et al. Nutrient intake and cancer of the pancreas: a case-control study in Athens, Greece. Cancer Causes Control 1993; 4:383–389.

23. Olsen GW, Mandel JS, Gibson RW, et al. Nutrients and pancreatic cancer: a population-based case-control study. Cancer Causes Control 1991; 2:291–297.

24. Mack TM, Yu MC, Hanisch R, et al. Pancreas cancer and smoking, beverage consumption and past medical history. J Natl Cancer Inst 1986; 76:49–60.

25. Hsing AW, Hansson LE, McLaughlin JK, et al. Pernicious anemia and subsequent cancer: a population-based cohort study. Cancer 1993; 71:745–750.

26. Wilenitz RE, Hruban RH. Pathology of Pancreatic Cancer. In: Pancreatic Cancer, Cameron, JL, ed. B.C. Decker; London, 2001:37–66.

27. Fong Y, Blumgart LH, Lin E, Fortner JG, Brennan MF. Outcome of treatment for distal bile duct cancer. Br J Surg 1996; 83(12): 1712–1715.

28. Rose DM, Hochwald SN, Klimstra DS, Brennan MF. Primary duodenal adenocarcinoma: a ten-year experience with 79 patients. J Am Coll Surg 1996; 183(2):89–96.

29. Talamini MA, Moesinger RC, Pitt HA, Sohn TA, Hruban RH, Lillemoe KD, Yeo CJ, Cameron JL. Adenocarcinoma of the ampulla of Vater. A 28-year experience. Ann Surg 1997; 225:590–599.

30. Lillemoe KD, Cameron JL, Yeo CJ, Taylor AS, Nakeeb A, et al. Pancreaticoduodenectomy; does it have a role in the palliation of pancreatic cancer? Ann Surg 1996; 223:718–728.

31. Howard JM. Pancreaticoduodenectomy (Whipple resection) with resection of hepatic metastases for carcinoma of the exocrine pancreas. Arch Surg 1997; 132:1049–1055.

32. D'Angelica M, Brennan MF, Suriawinata AA, Klimstra D, Conclon KC. Intraductal papillary mucinous neoplasms of the pancreas: an analysis of clinicopathologic features and outcome. Ann Surg 2004; 239:400–408.

33. Salvia R, Fernandez-del Castillo C, Bassi C, et al. Main-duct intraductal papillary mucinous neoplasms of the pancreas: clinical predictors of malignancy and long-term survival following resection. Ann Surg 2004; 239:678–687.

34. Sohn TA, Yeo CJ, Cameron JL, et al. Intraductal papillary mucinous neoplasms of the pancreas: an updated experience. Ann Surg 2004; 239:788–799.

35. Kern SE, Hruban RH. Molecular Genetics of Adenocarcinoma of the Pancreas. In: Pancreatic Cancer, Cameron JL, ed. B.C. Decker; London, 2001:13–24.

36. Almoguera C, Shibata D, Forrester K, Martin J, Arnheim N, Perucho M. Most human carcinomas of the exocrine pancreas contain mutant c-K-ras genes. Cell 1988; 53:549–554.

37. Day JD, Digiuseppe JA, Yeo C, et al. Immunohistochemical evaluation of HER-2/neu expression in pancreatic adenocarcinoma and pancreatic intraepithelial neoplasms. Human Pathology 1996; 27(2):119–124.

38. Abbruzzese JL, Evans DB, Raijman I, et al. Detection of mutated c-Ki-ras in the bile of patients with pancreatic cancer. Anticancer Research 1997; 17(2A):795–801.

39. Caldas C, Hahn SA, da Costa LT, et al. Frequent somatic mutations and homozygous deletions of the p16 (MTS1) gene in pancreatic adenocarcinoma. Nature Genetics 1994; 8:27–32.

40. Redston MS, Caldas C, Seymour AB, et al. p53 mutations in pancreatic carcinoma and evidence of common involvement of homocopolymer tracts in DNA microdeletions. Cancer Res 1994; 54(11):3025–3033.

41. Goldstein AM, Fraser MC, Struewing JP, et al. Increased risk of pancreatic cancer in melanoma-prone kindreds with p16INK4 mutations. NEJM 1995; 333(15):970–974.

42. Hingorani SR, Wang L, Multani AS, et al. Trp53R172H and KrasG12D cooperate to promote chromosomal instability and widely metastatic pancreatic ductal adenocarcinoma in mice. Cancer Cell 2005; 7:469–483.

43. Hruban RH, Offerhaus GJA, Kern SE. Familial pancreatic cancer. In: Pancreatic Cancer, (Cameron, JL, ed.), B.C. Decker, London, 2001, pp.25–36.

44. Kern SE. Advances from genetic clues in pancreatic cancer. Curr Opin Oncol 1998; 10:74–78.

45. Kasperk RK, Riesener KP, Wilms K, Schumpelick V. Limited value of positron emission tomography in treatment of pancreatic cancer: surgeon's view. World J Surg 2001; 25(9):1134–1139.

46. Kalady MF, Clary BM, Clark LA, et al. Clinical utility of positron emission tomography in the diagnosis and management of periampullary neoplasms. Ann Surg Onc 2002; 9(8):799–806.

47. Warshaw AL. Implications of peritoneal cytology for staging of early pancreatic cancer. Am J Surg 1991; 161:26–30.

48. Pitt HA, Gomes AS, Lois JF, et al. Does preoperative percutaneous biliary drainage reduce operative risk or increase hospital cost? Ann Surg, 1985; 201:545–553.

49. Lygridakis NJ, van der Heyde MN, Lubbers NJ. An evaluation of preoperative biliary drainage in the surgical management of pancreatic head carcinoma. Acta Chir. Scand. 1987; 153:665–668.

50. Lai ECS, Mok, FPT, Fan ST, et al. Preoperative endoscopic drainage for malignant obstructive jaundice. Br J Surg 1994; 81:1195–1198.

51. Povoski SP, Karpeh MS Jr, Conlon KC, et al. Association of preoperative biliary drainage with postoperative outcome following pancreaticoduodenectomy. Ann Surg 1999; 23(2):131–142.

52. Ahmad NA, Shah JN, Kochman ML. Endoscopic ultrasonography and endoscopic retrograde cholangiopancreatography imaging for pancreaticobiliary pathology: the gastroenterologist's perspective. Radiologic Clinics of North America 2002; 40(6):1377–1395.

53. Safi F, Roscher R, Beger HG. The clinical relevance of the tumor marker CA 19-9 in the diagnosing and monitoring of pancreatic carcinoma. Bulletin du Cancer 1990; 77:83–91.

54. Lewandrowski KB, Southern JF, Pins MR, Compton CC, Warshaw AL. Cyst fluid analysis in the differential diagnosis of pancreatic cysts: a comparison of pseudocysts, serous cystadenomas, mucinous cystic neoplasms and mucinous cystadenocarcinoma. Ann Surg 1993; 217(1):41–47.

55. Yang JM, Southern JF, Warshaw AL, Lewandrowski KG. Proliferation tissue polypeptide antigen distinguishes malignant mucinous cystadenocarcinomas from benign cystic tumors and pseudocysts. Am J Surg 1996; 171(1):126–129.

56. John TG, Greig JD, Carter DC, and Garden OJ. Carcinoma of the pancreatic head and periampullary region: tumor staging with laparoscopy and laparoscopic ultrasound. Ann Surg 1995; 221:165–170.

57. Callery MP, Strasberg SM, Doherty GM, Soper NJ, Norton JA. Staging laparoscopy with laparoscopic ultrasonography: optimizing resectability in hepatobiliary and pancreatic malignancy. J Am Coll Surg 1997; 185(1):33–39.

58. Conlon KC. Dougherty E. Klimstra DS. Coit DG. Turnbull AD. Brennan MF. The value of minimal access surgery in the staging of patients with potentially resectable peripancreatic malignancy. Ann Surg 1996; 223:134–140.

59. Vollmer C, Drebin JA, Middleton WD, et al. Utility of staging laparoscopy in subsets of peripancreatic and biliary malignancies. Ann Surg 2002; 235:1–7.

60. Whipple AO, Parsons WB, Mullins CR. Treatment of carcinoma of the ampulla of Vater. Ann Surg 1935; 102:763–776.

61. Strasberg SM, Drebin JA, Soper NJ. Evolution and current status of the Whipple procedure: an update for gastroenterologist. Gastroenterology 1997; 113:983–994.

62. Crile G. The advantages of bypass operations over radical pancreatoduodenectomy in the treatment of pancreatic carcinoma. Surg Gynecol Obstet 1970; 130:1049–1053.

63. Birkmeyer JD, Siewers AE, Finlayson EV, et al. Hospital volume and surgical mortality in the United States. NEJM 2002; 346(15): 1128–1137.

64. Birkmeyer JD, Stukel TA, Siewers AE, et al. Surgeon volume and operative mortality in the United States. NEJM 2003; 349(22): 2117–2127.

65. Cullen, JJ, Sarr, MG, and Ilstrup, DM. Pancreatic Anastomotic Leak After Pancreaticoduodenectomy: Incidence, Significance and Management. Am J Surg 1994; 168:295–298.

66. Strasberg SM, Drebin JA, Mokadam NA, et al. Prospective trial of a blood supply based technique of pancreaticojejunostomy: effect

on anastomotic failure in the Whipple procedure. J Am College Surgeons 2002; 194:746–758.

67. Stojadinovic A, Hoos A, Brennan MF, Conlon KC. Randomized clinical trials in pancreatic cancer. Surg Onc Clinics of North Am 2002; 11(1):207–229.

68. Yeo, CJ, Barry, MK, Sauter, PK, et al. Erythromycin Accelerates Gastric Emptying After Pancreaticoduodenectomy. Ann Surg 1993; 218:229–238.

69. Gudjonsson G. Carcinoma of the pancreas: critical analysis of costs, results of resections, and the need for standardized reporting. J Am Coll Surg 1995; 181:483–503.

70. Yeo CJ, Cameron JL, Lillemoe KD, et al. Pancreaticoduodenectomy for cancer of the head of the pancreas: 201 patients. Ann Surg 1995; 221(6):721–733.

71. Trede M. Schwall G, Saeger HD. Survival after pancreatoduodenectomy. 118 consecutive resections without an operative mortality. Ann Surg 1990; 21(4):447–458.

72. Janes RH, Niederhuber JE, Chmiel JS, et al. National patterns of care for pancreatic cancer. Results of a survey by the Commission on Cancer. Ann Surg 1996; 223:261–272.

73. Brennan MF, Moccia RD, Klimstra D. Management of adenocarcinoma of the body and tail of the pancreas. Ann Surg 1996; 223(5): 506–511.

74. Nordback IH, Hruban RH, Boitnott JK, Pitt HA, Cameron JL. Carcinoma of the body and tail of the pancreas. Am J Surg 1992; 164:26–31.

75. Kalser, MH and Ellenberg, SS. Pancreatic cancer: adjuvant combined radiation and chemotherapy following curative resection. Arch Surg 1985; 120:899–903.

76. Gastrointestinal Tumor Study Group. Further evidence of effective adjuvant combined radiation and chemotherapy following curative resection of pancreatic cancer. Cancer 1987; 59:2006–2010.

77. Yeo CJ, Cameron JL, Sohn TA, et al. Six hundred fifty consecutive pancreaticoduodenectomies in the 1990's: pathology, complications, outcomes. Ann Surg 1997; 226: 248–260.

78. Neoptolemos JP, Stocken DD, Friess H, et al. A randomized trial of chemoradiotherapy and chemotherapy after resection of pancreatic cancer. N Engl J Med 2004; 350:1200–1210.

79. Picozzi VJ, Kozarek RA, Traverso LW. Interferon-based adjuvant chemoradiation therapy after pancreaticoduodenectomy for pancreatic adenocarcinoma. Am J Surg 2003; 185(5):476–480.

80. Spitz FR, Abbruzzese JL, Lee JE, et al. Preoperative and postoperative chemoradiation strategies in patients treated with pancreaticoduodenectomy for adenocarcinoma of the pancreas. J Clin Oncol;1997; 15(3):928–937.

81. Hoffman JP, Lipsitz S, Pisansky T, Weese JL, Solin L, Benson AB. Phase II trial of preoperative radiation therapy and chemotherapy for patients with localized, resectable adenocarcinoma of the pancreas: an eastern cooperative oncology group study. J Clin Oncol 1997; 16:317–323.

82. White RR, Hurwitz HI, Morse MA, et al. Neoadjuvant chemoradiation for localized adenocarcinoma of the pancreas. An Surg Onc 2001; 8(10):758–765.

83. Bastidas JA, Poen JC, Niederhuber JE. Pancreas. In: Abeloff MD, Armitage JA, Lichter AS, Niederhuber JE, eds. Clinical Oncology 2nd Edition Churchill Livingstone; Philadelphia, 2000:1749–1783.

84. Gotoh M, Monden M, Sakon M, et al: Intraoperative irradiation in resected carcinoma of the pancreas and portal vein. Arch Surg 1992; 127:1213–1215.

85. Staley CA, Lee JE, Cleary KR, et al. Preoperative chemoradiation, pancreaticoduodenectomy, and intraoperative radiation therapy for adenocarcinoma of the pancreatic head. Am J Surg 1996; 171: 118–125.

86. Hiraoka T, Uchino R, Kanemitsu K, et al. Combination of intraoperative radiation with resection of the cancer of the pancreas. Int J Pancreatol 1990; 7:201–207.

87. Zerbi, A, Fossati V, Parolini D, et al. Intraoperative radiation therapy adjuvant to resection in the treatment of pancreatic cancer. Cancer 1994; 73:2930–2935.

88. Blackstock, AW, Cox, AD, and Tepper, JE. Treatment of pancreatic cancer: current limitations, future possibilities. Oncology 1996; 10:301–307.

89. El Kamar FG, Grossbard ML, Kozuch PS. Metastatic pancreatic cancer: emerging strategies in chemotherapy and palliative care. The Oncologist 2003; 8:18–34.

90. Burris HA, Moore MI, Anderson J, et al. Improvement in survival and clinical benefit with gemcitabine as first-line therapy for patients with advanced pancreatic cancer: a randomized trial. J Clin Oncol 1997; 15:2403–2413.

91. Tempero MJ, Plunkett J, van Haperen VR, et al. Randomized phase II comparison of dose-intense gemcitabine: thirty-minute infusion and fixed dose rate infusion in patients with pancreatic adenocarcinoma J Clin Oncol 2003; 21(18):3402–3408.

92. Berlin JD,Catalano P, Thomas JP, et al. Phase III study of gemcitabine in combination with fluorouracil versus gemcitabine alone in patients with advanced pancreatic carcinoma: Eastern Cooperative Oncology Group Trial E2297. J Clin Oncol 2002; 20: 3270–3275.

93. Rocha Lima CMS, Rotche R, Jeffery M, et al. A randomized phase 3 study comparing efficacy and safety of gemcitabine (GEM) and irinotecan (I), to GEM alone in patients (pts) with locally advanced or metastatic pancreatic cancer who have not received prior systemic therapy. Pro Am Soc Clin Oncol 2003; 22:a251 (A1005).

94. Heinemann V, Quietzsch D, Gieseler F, et al. A phase III trial comparing gemcitabine plus cisplatin vs. gemcitabine alone in advanced pancreatic carcinoma. Pro Am Soc Clin Oncol 2003; 22:a250 (A1003).

95. O'Reilly EM, Abou-Alfa GK, Letourneau R, et al. A randomized phase III trial of DX-8951f (exatecan mesylate; DX) and gemcitabine (GEM) vs. gemcitabine alone in advanced pancreatic cancer (APC). Pro Am Soc lin Oncol 2004; 23:A4006.

96. Richards DA, Kindler HL, Oettle H, et al. A randomized phase III study comparing gemcitabine + pemetrexed versus gemcitabine in patients with locally advanced and metastatic pancreas cancer. Pro Am Soc Clin Oncol 2004; 23:A4007.

97. Louvet C, Labianca R, Hammel P, et al. GemOx (gemcitabine + oxaliplatin) versus Gem (gemcitabine) in non resectable pancreatic adenocarcinoma: Final results of the GERCOR/GISCAD Intergroup Phase III. Pro Am Soc Clin Oncol 2004; 23:A4008.

98. Lillemoe KD, Cameron JL, Kaufman HS, Yeo CIJ, Pitt HA, Sauter PK. Chemical splanchnicectomy in patients with unresectable pancreatic cancer: a prospective randomized trial. Ann Surg 1993; 217:447–457.

99. Lillemoe KD, Pitt HA. Palliation: surgical and otherwise. Cancer Supplement 1996; 78(3):605–614.

100. Neuhaus H, Hagenmuller F, Griebel M, Classen M. Percutaneous cholangioscopic or transpapillary insertion of self-expanding biliary metal stents. Gastrointest Endosc 1991; 37(1):31–37.

101. Urbach DR, Bell CM, Swanstrom LL, Hansen PD. Cohort study of surgical bypass to the gallbladder or bile duct for the palliation of jaundice due to pancreatic cancer. Ann Surg 2003; 237(1):86–93.

32 Endoscopic Ultrasound for Thoracic Disease

Timothy Woodward, md, Massimo Raimondo, md, and Michael B. Wallace, md, mph

Contents

1. OBJECTIVES

The focus of this chapter is to examine the role of endoscopic ultrasound (EUS) in the management of mediastinal lesions. EUS, owing to its diagnostic accuracy, tissue sampling capability, low morbidity, and time and cost savings has become an integral part of the multidisciplinary approach to the imaging and management of thoracic diseases. It is the intent of this chapter to outline the benefit of EUS as an adjunct to modalities such as bronchoscopy, positron emission tomography (PET), and computed tomography (CT) imaging in the evaluation of mediastinal diseases.

2. ENDOSONOGRAPHIC EQUIPMENT

Cross-sectional endosonographic imaging is obtained from within the esophagus using a radial EUS endoscope. The image provided is that of a 270–360° circular plane centered on the endoscope (Fig. 1). When the endoscope is parallel to the spine, the axial EUS image obtained closely resembles a CT scan of the mediastinum (Fig. 2). Conventional nomenclature places the abdominal aorta at 5 o'clock with the spine at 6 o'clock. Current devices allow for switching between 7.5 and 12.5 or 20 MHz. Higher frequencies allow for either more detailed study of the esophageal wall (e.g., differentiating the submucosal and muscularis propria layers), and lower frequencies allow deeper evaluation of surrounding parenchymal structures.

Electronic linear array or curved array transducers obtain images in a sector configuration. In order to examine the entire 360° of the gastrointestinal tract, the endoscope must be rotated along the longitudinal axis. There are two major advantages of the linear array echoendoscope when compared to the radial echoendoscope. First, a linear system may incorporate pulse wave Doppler allowing detection and characterization of

From: *Endoscopic Oncology: Gastrointestinal Endoscopy and Cancer Management.* Edited by: D. O. Faigel and M. L. Kochman © Humana Press, Totowa, NJ

blood flow. Secondly, alignment of the imaging plane parallel to the endoscope shaft allows for fine needle aspiration to be performed under direct EUS guidance.

3. ENDOSONOGRAPHIC ANATOMY OF THE MEDIASTINUM

The esophagus presents an excellent window for visualization of surrounding structures in the mediastinum. Present nomenclature divides the mediastinum into three parts: the upper section (upper esophageal sphincter to aortic arch), middle (aortic arch to subcarinal region, just distal to the azygos vein), and lower (subcarinal region to cardia). Figure 3 demonstrates paraesophageal structures and organs. The trachea is seen only as an air column; thus its wall cannot be delineated. Lymph nodes may be visible along the length of the esophagus, even in normal individuals. They may be especially pronounced in the subcarinal region. Peri-aortic tissue is seen alongside the distal esophagus.

Lymph nodes can be identified in the posterior mediastinum, retroperitoneum, and celiac regions. Posterior mediastinal lymph nodes are predominantly left-sided and communicate with the para-aortic lymph nodes of the abdomen; hence thorough evaluation of the celiac region is important. Additionally, metastases may be seen in the left adrenal gland and left lobe of the liver. Corresponding to the American Thoracic Society's mediastinal map for lymphadenopathy (Fig. 4), stations visible to EUS include the following: subcarinal (station 7); subaortic (station 5); paraesophageal (station 8); inferior pulmonary ligament region (station 9); and main bronchial (station 10). Lymph nodes in the left paratracheal (station 2) and left lower paratracheal (station 4) stations can be imaged and sampled, whereas the right paratracheal stations are inaccessible owing to air interference from the trachea. Stations removed from the esophagus, i.e., lobar (station 12), interlobar (station 11), and those anterior and lateral to the trachea (stations 3 and 6)

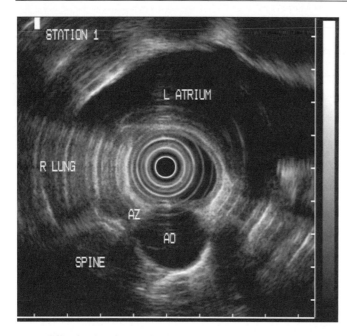

Fig. 1. 360° circular plane endosonographic image of the mediastinum.

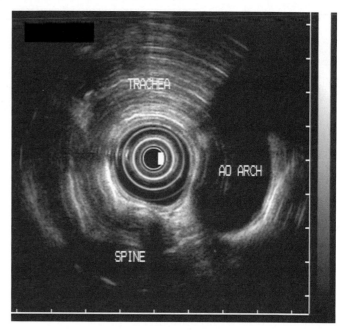

Fig. 3. Paraesophageal structures as seen by endosonographic evaluation.

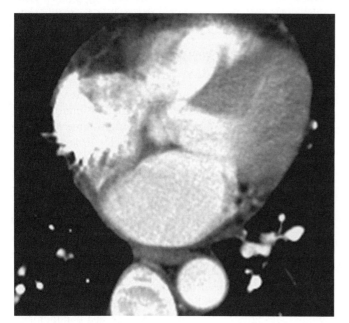

Fig. 2. Representative computed tomography image of the mediastinum.

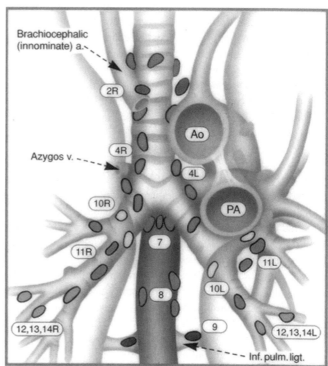

Fig. 4. American Thoracic Society mediastinal map of lymph node stations.

cannot be imaged with EUS, but may be accessible to new endobronchial ultrasound technologies.

4. CURRENT APPLICATIONS FOR THE MEDIASTINUM

4.1. ESOPHAGEAL CANCER

Adenocarcinoma of the esophagus and esophagogastric junction has increased markedly in incidence over the past several decades. The survival rate in esophageal carcinoma is closely related to the disease stage at initial diagnosis. Accurate pretreatment staging is essential for optimal management. The primary role of EUS in esophageal cancer is in staging. Diagnosis is usually established by endoscopy with subsequent endoscopic biopsy for histology. Esophageal carcinoma usually presents as a circumscribed, hypoechoic wall thickening by EUS (Fig. 5). As a result of tumor penetration, the endosonographic wall layers are destroyed. This endosonographic disruption corresponds well with surgical tumor-node-metastasis (TNM) staging, in which the extent of local tumor invasion into the esophageal wall (T classification) (see Table 1) and the presence or absence of local lymph nodes (N classification) suitably

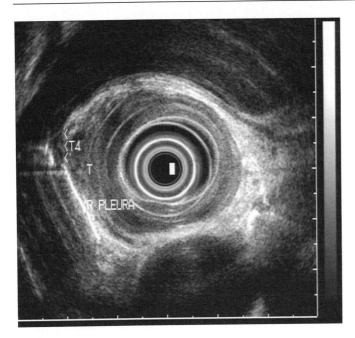

Fig. 5. Esophageal carcinoma presenting as circumscribed, hypoechoic wall thickening by endosonography.

Table 1
Endosonographic T Classification System
for Esophageal Carcinoma

T1: Tumor through the mucosa and submucosa but leaving the muscularis propria intact
T2: Tumor infiltrating the muscularis propria
T3: Tumor extending through the muscularis layer
T4: Tumor involving surrounding paraesophageal structures (e.g., the aorta, left atrium)

mirrors the surgical specimen. EUS is thus the only imaging modality currently clinically available able to visualize tumor infiltration through the individual layers of the esophageal wall.

Almost one-third of esophageal cancers obstruct the passage of an EUS scope and force the decision to either dilate or stage from the top of the lesion only. Although early studies suggested dilation carried significant risk *(1)*, more recent studies with smaller caliber (and thus less dilation required) echoendoscopes suggest that dilation is safe, and identifies up to 20% more patients with advanced disease *(2,3)*.

In experienced hands, EUS T classification accuracy rates have been reported to range between 80 and 90%. Lymph node staging is somewhat problematic. To distinguish malignant from benign nodes, sonographic criteria have been developed. Malignancy is suggested by the following: lymph node size 1 cm or larger, hypoechogenicity, and spherical shape (Fig. 6). When matched with surgical specimens from studies, the combination of these criteria achieves an accuracy ranging between 70 and 80%. Problems may ensue, however, when the findings are equivocal (e.g., a hypoechoic lymph node less than a centimeter in size).

Fine-needle aspiration (FNA) of lymph nodes is useful in lymph nodes distant from the primary (e.g., celiac adenopathy; Fig. 6) but should not be done in lymph nodes adjacent to the tumor owing to the issue of potential tissue contamination via passage of the needle through the primary lesion. A recent study in which 125 patients with esophageal carcinoma revealed that EUS-FNA was superior to CT in nodal staging, both in sensitivity (83 vs 29%) and accuracy (87 vs 51%) *(4)*. EUS staging had direct impact on therapy primarily by detecting locally advanced and nodal disease which in this study led to multimodality chemoradiotherapy.

Several studies have suggested that patients with T4 tumors do not benefit from surgical resection. Although modern helical

CT has improved the detection of T4 disease, recent studies suggest that up to 25% of T4 cases are missed by helical CT but are detected by EUS *(5)*. Detected T1 lesions would direct therapy to either surgery alone or potentially, albeit controversial, endoscopic mucosal resection or photodynamic therapy. T1 lesions, however, are rarely seen in the United States and Europe. The primary clinical impact of EUS in the management of esophageal cancer appears to be within the context of neoadjuvant therapy. In centers that incorporate pre-operative chemotherapy and radiotherapy in the treatment of esophageal cancers, EUS T and N staging significantly affect candidate selection. It should be noted, however, that standard criteria for T and N staging do not appear to hold following radiation therapy, thus making EUS less useful in the restaging exams prior to surgery. Patients with EUS-FNA-proven celiac adenopathy prior to surgery have demonstrated a higher incidence of recurrent cancer and overall worse survival *(6)*.

A recent prospective study of 42 patients compared the role of EUS, CT, and PET in the staging of esophageal adenocarcinoma. EUS was found to be the only effective method for detecting invasion depth of a tumor, although overstaging was demonstrated in this study. CT was insufficiently sensitive in detecting distant metastases and locoregional nodal disease. PET was able to identify organ metastases, but lacked overall accuracy in primary and locoregional disease. Accuracy for lymph node metastasis was 63% for PET, 66% for CT, and 75% for EUS *(7)*. A cost-effectiveness analysis comparing EUS, CT, PET, and laparoscopy/thoracoscopy staging indicated that the combinations of CT plus EUS or PET plus EUS were the most cost-effective approaches. Using all three staging procedures in an individual was not cost-effective *(8)*. This was likely owing to the fact that when PET and EUS were both used, CT scan added very little because PET is more accurate than CT for distant metastases and EUS is more accurate that CT for locoregional disease.

4.2. LUNG CANCER

Lung cancer is the most common neoplasm in the Western world. Management depends on histological type and stage of the disease at diagnosis. Although the tumor is usually diagnosed by bronchoscopy, staging is dependent on various imaging procedures. The prognosis for non-small cell lung cancer (NSCLC) correlates closely with the presence of mediastinal adenopathy. Mediastinal lymph node involvement is reported in 28–38% of patients at the time of diagnosis. Patients with large subcarinal nodes or contralateral adenopathy are considered unresectable. The 5-yr survival for unresectable disease is less than 5%. The current staging system for lung cancer uses

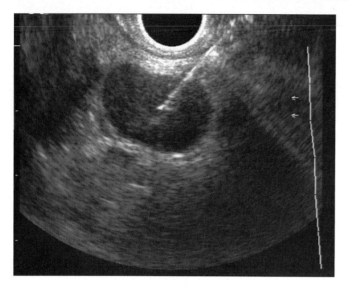

Fig. 6. Endosonographic directed fine-needle aspiration of celiac lymph node.

The American Joint Committee on Cancer TNM system that incorporates pathological evaluation of the primary tumor along with anatomic data (*see* Table 2).

Therapies for patients with NSCLC include surgery, chemotherapy, and radiation therapy. These therapies are dependent on the histology of the cancer, mediastinal lymph node involvement, and distant metastases. The pre-operative identification of these patients can prevent unnecessary surgery. Surgery is most appropriate for patients in whom disease is confined to the lung and hilar lymph nodes (stages I and II). Surgery is of benefit and offers the best chance of cure in stage I disease. There is no lymph node involvement in stage I disease, whereas in stage II disease ipsilateral hilar and/or peribronchial nodes are present (N1). Neoadjuvant therapy with chemo/radiation before surgery may improve survival in stage II disease. Metastases to the mediastinal lymph node confer a worse prognosis. Surgery combined with chemoradiotherapy may be of benefit in patients with limited ipsilateral mediastinal lymph node metastases, but patients with contralateral (N3) nodal disease or distant metastases do poorly with surgery.

EUS is suitable to evaluate common sites of spread of lung cancer such as the mediastinal lymph nodes, left adrenal gland, liver, and direct invasion of the mediastinal structures (esophagus, trachea, great vessels, or heart) by the primary tumor. Over the past decade, EUS has emerged as a valuable adjunct in the evaluation of lymph nodes and masses in the posterior mediastinum. In a prospective, triple blinded trial, EUS-FNA has been shown to be superior to CT and PET scanning in the mediastinal evaluation of lung cancer patients verified by surgical pathology. In this study, CT and PET were compared with EUS. The sensitivity, specificity, and accuracy of all three modalities were comparable when either CT or PET scanning correctly predicted the nodal stage. The tissue diagnosis obtained from the EUS-guided FNA was extremely helpful. EUS with FNA was the most useful modality even with small mediastinal lymph nodes (<1 cm) (9). An important limitation

to EUS-FNA is the inability to see structures anterior to the trachea because of the poor ultrasound penetration through air. In this regard, CT and PET are complementary to EUS in targeting patients that may benefit most from EUS-FNA (e.g., those with posterior mediastinal lymph nodes) (9).

Several prospective studies of patients with lung cancer demonstrate a sensitivity and specificity of EUS-guided FNA in detecting metastases to the posterior mediastinal lymph nodes of 88–96% and 80–100%, respectively (10–13). In patients with enlarged mediastinal lymph nodes on CT who would otherwise be candidates for mediastinoscopy or thoracoscopy, EUS-FNA was able to pathologically confirm advanced (stages III or IV) disease, thus avoiding surgical staging, in 70%. EUS-guided FNA is very safe, and there have been no reports of complications or mediastinitis in EUS-FNA of lymph nodes even in the absence of prophylactic antibiotics (10–13).

The choice of which lymph nodes to sample with EUS-FNA (or any other sampling method) remains difficult. There are frequently 15–20 lymph nodes visualized at the time of EUS, and most are less than 1 cm. Traditional imaging features which are suggestive of metastases (round shape, sharp distinct borders, homogeneous hypoechoic node, and nodes greater than 10 mm in short axis diameter) are useful, but imperfect (14). The location of the primary tumor may also predict the site of metastases. It has been demonstrated that right and left lower lobe tumors, as well as right middle lobe and left lingular tumors tend to spread to subcarinal lymph nodes. Left upper lobe tumors tend to spread to the aortopulmonary window (Fig. 7). Unfortunately, none of these characteristics is highly reliable at diagnosing or excluding malignancy in lymph nodes. In a large multivariate analysis, the predictive accuracy of image characteristics and tumor location (relative to lymph node location) was poor. It was suggested from the study that FNA or other biopsy methods be used whenever feasible and in which the pathological diagnosis would alter management of the patient (15).

The evaluation of patients without enlarged or PET-positive lymph nodes is more controversial. Even grossly negative lymph nodes may harbor "micrometastases." Recurrence of disease is common after completely resected early stage NSCLC suggesting a subclinical burden of disease. Although these patients frequently undergo direct thoracotomy for resection, up to 30% will have metastatic lymph nodes identified at surgery. A recent publication suggests that EUS may identify advanced disease in up to 25% of patients with a "normal" mediastinum on CT scan (16). This data, combined with the previous studies on patients with enlarged or PET-positive lymph nodes, suggests that EUS may be useful in all potentially operable patients.

We have recently investigated whether EUS-FNA combined with highly sensitive reverse transcriptase polymerase chain reaction techniques, can detect gene abnormalities that may be indicate the presence of cancer cells. In a prospective study, we performed EUS-FNA on 98 patients with NSCLC without CT or PET evidence of mediastinal involvement. Samples were sent for cytology and real-time reverse transcriptase polymerase chain reaction. In the cytology positive group, gene expression was above the respective clinical threshold in 93%

Table 2
Current Staging System for Lung Cancer (American Joint Committee on Cancer)

- Tis: Carcinoma *in situ*
- T1: Tumor that is 3 cm or less, does not invade visceral pleura, without bronchoscopic evidence of invasion more proximal than a lobar bronchus
- T2: Tumor that has any of the following features: size more than 3 cm; involvement of the mainstem bronchus with a proximal extent at least 2 cm from the carina; invasion of the visceral pleura; obstructive pneumonitis that extends to the hilar region
- T3: Tumor of any size with any of the following features: invasion of the chest wall, diaphragm, mediastinal pleura or parietal pericardium; involvement of a mainstem bronchus within 2 cm of the carina but without invasion of the carina; association with obstructive pneumonitis of the entire lung
- T4: Invasion of the mediastinum, heart, great vessels, trachea, esophagus, vertebral body, or carina; association with a malignant pleural or pericardial effusion; presence of satellite tumor nodule(s) within lobe of lung containing the primary tumor

Nodes
- N0: No regional lymph node involvement
- N1: Involvement of ipsilateral peribronchial, intrapulmonary, and/or ipsilateral hilar lymph nodes
- N2: Involvement of ipsilateral mediastinal and/or subcarinal lymph nodes
- N3: Contralateral mediastinal or contralateral hilar lymph nodes, or either ipsilateral or contralateral involvement of scalene or supraclavicular lymph nodes

of samples. Remarkably, in the cytology negative lymph nodes, 30% overexpressed at least one of the gene markers. It is postulated that this group will have the highest rate of recurrence *(17–19)*. Further studies need to be conducted; however, results suggest that EUS-FNA will provide a means of detecting micrometastases in normal appearing lymph nodes.

EUS can also be used to evaluate whether the primary lung tumor invades the mediastinum. Tumors within the lung parenchyma are not seen or poorly seen at EUS owing to the air-filled structures surrounding the tumor. However, when the tumor abuts or invades the mediastinum, it can be directly visualized from the esophagus. Our group recently reported the accuracy of EUS for the T staging of lung cancer and found the sensitivity to be 87% and specificity 98% *(20)*. We observed a tendency to overstage when the only evidence of invasion was loss of interface between the tumor and the mediastinal soft tissue (Fig. 8). In 10 such cases, 3 were incorrectly staged (all overstaged). A more reliable, although less sensitive, indicator of invasion is visualization of tumor within a mediastinal organ (aorta, heart, esophagus, or FNA of a malignant pleural effusion [*see* Fig. 9]). Given the significant implications of misstaging T4 disease (avoiding potentially curative surgery), it is preferable to base T staging on the more stringent criteria.

4.3. THYROID AND CANCERS OF THE HEAD AND NECK

Thyroid cancer is generally associated with a favorable prognosis. However, advanced local involvement and distant metastases incur significant mortality. Curative resection improves the prognosis in advanced thyroid cancer *(21)*. Thyroid cancers that have invaded the esophageal wall as far as the muscular layer require a full thickness resection, although cancers that invade only the adventitia can be managed with a simple shaving *(22)*. Although CT and MRI are able to detect esophageal invasion, these modalities are insufficient for a precise determination of depth.

Because the thyroid is near the esophagus, the gland can be detected by EUS through the esophageal wall. EUS has been used successfully for diagnosing depth and extension of thyroid cancer (*see* Fig. 10). A study published recently compared

EUS with esophagography and MRI in 59 patients in whom esophagopharyngeal invasion by thyroid cancer was suspected (large tumors with poor mobility). The diagnostic specificity and accuracy of EUS (82.9 and 82.7%) in assessing invasion into the muscularis propria were greater than MRI (60 and 65.4%) and esophagography (58.8 and 60%) *(23)*. Interestingly, if the tumor is located in the upper lobe of the thyroid, EUS determination of invasion becomes difficult owing to an increased swallowing reflex at that location, contributing to imaging difficulty. In addition, changes occur in the muscularis propria toward the inferior constrictor muscle of the pharynx in which the layer definition becomes unclear. Thus, EUS is the best modality for assessing esophagopharyngeal invasion into the muscularis propria, however, if the lesion is located in the upper portion of the thyroid lobe, accurate diagnosis becomes limited for physiological and anatomical reasons.

ENT malignancies can also metastasize to the mediastinum. Risk factors for mediastinal disease include hypopharyngeal cancers, cancers with high-grade histology, and those with bulky or bilateral cervical lymph node involvement. EUS has recently been evaluated as a staging tool for detecting mediastinal lymph node metastases and local invasion of the esophagus. In a study by Wildi et al., among 17 cases with suspected local invasion on CT scan, EUS demonstrated invasion of the esophagus ($n = 4$) and pleura ($n = 1$). Twelve tumors showed no visible invasion of adjacent structures. Another 17 examinations were performed for suspected mediastinal metastatic disease. In eight cases EUS-FNA confirmed metastatic disease, whereas only benign changes were shown in the other nine cases *(24)*.

4.4. MISCELLANEOUS MEDIASTINAL PROCESSES AND MEDIASTINAL MASSES OF UNKNOWN ORIGIN

Sarcoidosis is a systemic disease that is often diagnosed following evaluation of hilar or mediastinal adenopathy on chest radiograph. In the past, diagnostic studies included blind transbronchial biopsy or more invasive surgical procedures, such as mediastinoscopy. Several studies have recently demonstrated the utility of EUS-FNA in establishing the diagnosis of sarcoid. In a retrospective, descriptive review, of 108 consecutive patients who underwent EUS-FNA of mediastinal nodes for various clinical

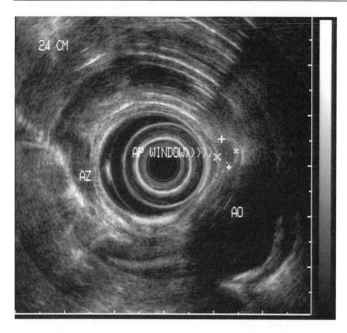

Fig. 7. Left upper lobe lung tumor with aortopulmonary window involvement.

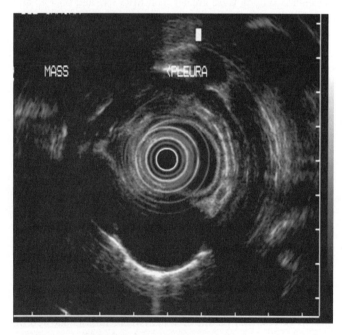

Fig. 8. Endosonographic representation of loss of interface between lung tumor and the mediastinal soft tissue.

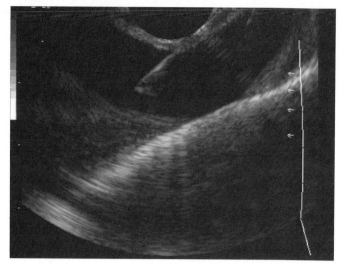

Fig. 9. Malignant pleural effusion as visualized by endosonographic examination.

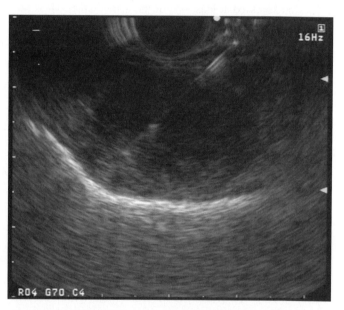

Fig. 10. Thyroid cancer as visualized by endosonographic examination.

indications, 6 were found to have cytological evidence of sarcoidosis, with a central hyperechoic strand evident in 4 *(25)*. These preliminary studies suggest that mediastinal lymph nodes in patients with sarcoidosis have specific echocharacteristics, and EUS-FNA can be used for confirmatory tissue diagnosis.

Benign mediastinal cysts, which account for about 20% of mediastinal masses, represent diagnostic challenges. In one series, 20 patients were identified who underwent 23 EUS examinations for suspected mediastinal cysts, follow-up of a known cyst, or for a mediastinal mass of unknown origin *(26)*. In 19 patients, the definitive diagnosis of a mediastinal cyst was established. CT or MRI was performed in 18 patients; only 4 were diagnostic of a cyst. The cyst contents were aspirated by EUS-FNA in three patients. A fourth case, a solid-appearing duplication cyst, misdiagnosed by EUS, was sampled by EUS with FNA and core biopsy. The patient developed mediastinitis 4 d later. Thoracotomy revealed an infected bronchogenic cyst. Thus, EUS provides a minimally invasive approach to the diagnosis of mediastinal cysts. However, caution must be used when undertaking tissue sampling in this setting.

EUS-FNA in the evaluation of unexplained mediastinal masses has recently been studied from the standpoint of its impact on patient management. A recent multicenter study examined the diagnostic accuracy of EUS-FNA on a heterogeneous group of patients presenting with idiopathic mediastinal lesions *(27)*. In order to evaluate the clinical impact of EUS-FNA, the history of each patient up to referral for EUS-FNA was reviewed. A board of thoracic specialists was asked to decide the course of evaluation if EUS-FNA had not been available and this diagnostic strategy was compared to the actual clinical course of events after EUS-FNA. For patients known to have lung cancer before EUS-FNA, 18 out of 34 patients (53%) demonstrated mediastinal involvement as N2/N3 disease. All of the 18 malignant EUS-FNA diagnoses were recorded as true positive. In 16 patients with known lung cancer EUS-FNA of the suspected mediastinal lesion demonstrated the mass to be benign. Fourteen patients went to either thoracotomy and/or mediastinoscopy. Two patients had a positive lymph node, one adjacent to the esophagus, and the other in the aortopulmonary window. The two remaining patients had documented invasive or metastatic disease by other studies. Of 50 patients with unknown disease, EUS-FNA demonstrated mediastinal malignancy in 36 of these patients (72%.) In three patients, benign diseases (sarcoidosis, mediastinal abscess, and leiomyoma of the esophagus) were diagnosed. Regarding the overall clinical impact of EUS-FNA in this series for 93% of patients mediastinoscopy or thoracotomy/thoracoscopy were avoided.

5. SUMMARY

EUS with needle aspiration is a safe, accurate, and minimally invasive method for evaluating masses in the mediastinum. Lung cancer, as a result of the large number of potential cases, will likely be the most important application of mediastinal EUS. Although CT and PET scanning are helpful for targeting lymph node FNA, EUS still detects a significant number of metastases even in the setting of negative CT and PET of the mediastinum. EUS should be considered in all potentially operative candidates with lung cancer. Future potential applications include EUS assistance in the staging evaluation and management decisions for head and neck cancer.

REFERENCES

1. Van Dam J, Rice TW, Catalano MF, Kirby T, Sivak MV, Jr. High-grade malignant stricture is predictive of esophageal tumor stage. Risks of endosonographic evaluation. Cancer 1993; 71:2910–2917.
2. Wallace MB, Hawes RH, Sahai AV, Van Velse A, Hoffman BJ. Dilation of malignant esophageal stenosis to allow EUS guided fine-needle aspiration: safety and effect on patient management. Gastrointest Endosc 2000; 51:309–313.
3. Pfau PR, Ginsberg GG, Lew RJ, Faigel DO, Smith DB, Kochman ML. Esophageal dilation for endosonographic evaluation of malignant esophageal strictures is safe and effective. Am J Gastroenterol 2000; 95:2813–2815.
4. Vazquez-Sequeiros E, Wiersema MJ, Clain JE, et al. Impact of lymph node staging on therapy of esophageal carcinoma. Gastroenterology 2003; 125:1626–1635.
5. Romagnuolo J, Scott J, Hawes RH, et al. Helical CT versus EUS with fine needle aspiration for celiac nodal assessment in patients with esophageal cancer. Gastrointest Endosc 2002; 55:648–654.
6. Eloubeidi MA, Wallace MB, Hoffman BJ, et al. Predictors of survival for esophageal cancer patients with and without celiac axis lymphadenopathy: impact of staging endosonography. Ann Thorac Surg 2001; 72:212–219; discussion 219,220.
7. Rasanen JV, Sihvo EI, Knuuti MJ, et al. Prospective analysis of accuracy of positron emission tomography, computed tomography, and endoscopic ultrasonography in staging of adenocarcinoma of the esophagus and the esophagogastric junction. Ann Surg Oncol 2003; 10:954–960.
8. Wallace MB, Nietert PJ, Earle C, et al. An analysis of multiple staging management strategies for carcinoma of the esophagus: computed tomography, endoscopic ultrasound, positron emission tomography, and thoracoscopy/laparoscopy. Ann Thorac Surg 2002; 74:1026–1032.
9. Fritscher-Ravens A, Bohuslavizki KH, Brandt L, et al. Mediastinal Lymph Node Involvement in Potentially Resectable Lung Cancer: Comparison of CT, Positron Emission Tomography, and Endoscopic Ultrasonography With and Without Fine-Needle Aspiration. Chest 2003; 123:442–451.
10. Gress FG, Savides TJ, Sandler A, et al. Endoscopic ultrasonography, fine-needle aspiration biopsy guided by endoscopic ultrasonography, and computed tomography in the preoperative staging of non-small-cell lung cancer: a comparison study. Ann Intern Med 1997; 127:604–612.
11. Wallace MB, Silvestri GA, Sahai AV, et al. Endoscopic ultrasound-guided fine needle aspiration for staging patients with carcinoma of the lung. Ann Thorac Surg 2001; 72:1861–1867.
12. Fritscher-Ravens A, Soehendra N, Schirrow L, et al. Role of trans-esophageal endosonography-guided fine-needle aspiration in the diagnosis of lung cancer. Chest 2000; 117:339–345.
13. Laudanski J, Kozlowski M, Niklinski J, Chyczewski L. The preoperative study of mediastinal lymph nodes metastasis in lung cancer by endoscopic ultrasonography (EUS) and helical computed tomography (CT). Lung Cancer 2001; 34 Suppl 2:S123—S126.
14. Bhutani MS, Hawes RH, Hoffman BJ. A comparison of the accuracy of echo features during endoscopic ultrasound (EUS) and EUS-guided fine-needle aspiration for diagnosis of malignant lymph node invasion. Gastrointest Endosc 1997; 45:474–479.
15. Schmulewitz N, Wildi SM, Varadarajulu S, et al. Accuracy of EUS criteria and primary tumor site for identification of mediastinal lymph node metastasis from non-small-cell lung cancer. Gastrointest Endosc 2004; 59:205–212.
16. Wallace MB, Ravenel J, Block MI, et al. Endoscopic ultrasound in lung cancer patients with a normal mediastinum on computed tomography. The Annals of Thoracic Surgery 2004; 77:1763–1768.
17. Wallace M, Block M, Gillanders W, et al. Detection of micrometastases in mediastinal lymph nodes in non-small cell lung cancer patients by EUS-FNA and real-time rtPCR. Chest 2003:in press.
18. Mitas M, Cole DJ, Hoover L, et al. Real-time reverse transcription-PCR detects KS1/4 mRNA in mediastinal lymph nodes from patients with non-small cell lung cancer. Clin Chem 2003; 49:312–315.
19. Wallace MB, Block M, Hoffman BJ, et al. Detection of telomerase expression in mediastinal lymph nodes of patients with lung cancer. Am J Respir Crit Care Med 2003; 167:1670–1675.
20. Varadarajulu S, Schmulewitz N, Wildi SF, et al. Accuracy of EUS in staging of T4 lung cancer. Gastrointest Endosc 2004; 59:345–348.
21. McConahey WM, Hay ID, Woolner LB, van Heerden JA, Taylor WF. Papillary thyroid cancer treated at the Mayo Clinic, 1946 through 1970: initial manifestations, pathologic findings, therapy, and outcome. Mayo Clin Proc 1986; 61:978–996.
22. Gillenwater AM, Goepfert H. Surgical management of laryngotracheal and esophageal involvement by locally advanced thyroid cancer. Semin Surg Oncol 1999; 16:19–29.
23. Koike E, Yamashita H, Noguchi S, et al. Endoscopic ultrasonography in patients with thyroid cancer: its usefulness and limitations for evaluating esophagopharyngeal invasion. Endoscopy 2002; 34:457–460.
24. Wildi SM, Fickling W, Day T, et al. Endoscopic ultrasound in the diagnosis and staging of neoplasms of the head and neck. Endoscopy 2004; 36:624–630.
25. Mishra G, Sahai AV, Penman ID, et al. Endoscopic ultrasonography with fine-needle aspiration: an accurate and simple diagnostic modality for sarcoidosis. Endoscopy 1999; 31:377–382.
26. Wildi SM, Hoda RS, Fickling W, et al. Diagnosis of benign cysts of the mediastinum: the role and risks of EUS and FNA. Gastrointest Endosc 2003; 58:362–368.
27. Larsen SS, Krasnik M, Vilmann P, et al. Endoscopic ultrasound guided biopsy of mediastinal lesions has a major impact on patient management. Thorax 2002; 57:98–103.

Index